Clinics in Developmental Medicine

NEUROENDOCRINE DISORDERS IN CHILDREN

Clinics in Developmental Medicine

Neuroendocrine Disorders in Children

Edited by

MEHUL T DATTANI
UCL Institute of Child Health
London, UK

PETER C HINDMARSH
Institute of Child Health
London, UK

LUCINDA CARR
Great Ormond Street Hospital for Children
London, UK

IAIN CAF ROBINSON
National Institute of Medical Research
London, UK

2016
Mac Keith Press

© 2016 Mac Keith Press
6 Market Road, London, N7 9PW

Managing Director: Ann-Marie Halligan
Production Manager and Commissioning Editor: Udoka Ohuonu
Project Management: Lumina Datamatics

First published in this edition in 2016

British Library Cataloguing-in-Publication data
A catalogue record for this book is available from the British Library

Cover design: David Hibberd

ISBN: 978-1-909962-50-7

Typeset by Lumina Datamatics, Chennai, India

Manufacturing managed by Jellyfish Solutions Ltd

Mac Keith Press is supported by Scope

CONTENTS

Contents

AUTHORS' APPOINTMENTS

Kyriaki S Alatzoglou Consultant Paediatrician, Chelsea and Westminster Hospital, London, UK

Patrick Aubourg Professor of Paediatrics, Genetics and Neurology, Paris-Sud University; Chief of Paediatric Neurology Department, Bicêtre Hospital, France

Elizabeth Baranowski Springboard Fellow, Department of Paediatric Endocrinology and Diabetes, Birmingham Children's Hospital; Clinical Research Fellow, Institute of Metabolism and Systems Research, University of Birmingham, UK

Pierre-Marc G Bouloux Consultant Endocrinologist, Centre for Neuroendocrinology, Royal Free Hospital, London, UK

Mary-Jane Brassill Research Fellow, Molecular Endocrinology and Diabetes, Department of Medicine, Imperial College London, UK

Erika Brolin Doctoral Student, Department of Pharmaceutical Biosciences, Uppsala University, Sweden

Fergus J Cameron Head of Diabetes Research Group, Murdoch Childrens Research Institute; Consultant Endocrinologist, Royal Children's Hospital, Department of Paediatrics, University of Melbourne, Victoria, Australia

Jean-Claude Carel Professor, Head of the Department of Paediatric Endocrinology and Diabetes; Head of Diabetes, Robert Debré University Hospital and Paris Diderot University, Paris, France

Lucinda Carr Consultant Paediatric Neurologist, Great Ormond Street Hospital, London, UK

Benjamin G Challis Clinical Lecturer, The University of Cambridge Metabolic Research Laboratories, Institute of Metabolic Science, Cambridge, UK

Evangelia Charmandari	Professor of Paediatric and Adolescent Endocrinology, Division of Endocrinology, Metabolism and Diabetes, First Department of Pediatrics, National and Kapodistrian University of Athens Medical School, 'Aghia Sophia' Children's Hospital, Athens, Greece
Tim Cheetham	University Reader, Institute of Genetic Medicine, Newcastle University; Honorary Consultant Paediatrician, Department of Paediatric Endocrinology, Royal Victoria Infirmary, Newcastle Upon Tyne, UK
Wassim Chemaitilly	Director, Division of Endocrinology, St Jude Children's Research Hospital, Memphis TN, USA
George P Chrousos	Division of Endocrinology and Metabolism and Diabetes, First Department of Pediatrics, National and Kapodistrian University of Athens Medical School 'Aghia Sophia' Children's Hospital, Athens, Greece, Clinical Research Center, Biomedical Research Foundation of the Academy of Athens, Greece
Mehul T Dattani	Professor and Head of Clinical Service in Endocrinology; Head of Section of Genetics and Epigenetics in Health and Disease; Genetics and Genomic Medicine Programme; UCL Institute of Child Health/Great Ormond Street Hospital for Children, London, UK
Nicolas de Roux	Head of the Molecular Genetics Laboratory in Endocrine Disorders, Robert Debré Hospital and Paris Diderot University, France
I Sadaf Farooqi	Professor of Metabolism and Medicine, Wellcome Trust - MRC Institute of Metabolic Science, Addenbrooke's Hospital, Cambridge, UK
Hoong-Wei Gan	Clinical Research Fellow, Section for Genetics and Epigenetics in Health and Disease, Genetics and Genomic Medicine Programme, UCL Institute of Child Health, London, UK
Apostolos I Gogakos	Molecular Endocrinology Group, Department of Medicine, Imperial College London, UK
Alfhild Grönbladh	Researcher, Department of Pharmaceutical Biosciences, Uppsala University, Sweden

Tulay Guran   Centre for Endocrinology, Diabetes and Metabolism, School of Clinical and Experimental Medicine, University of Birmingham, UK

Mathias Hallberg   Professor, The Beijer Laboratory, Department of Pharmaceutical Biosciences, Uppsala University, Sweden

Peter C Hindmarsh   Professor of Paediatric Endocrinology, Developmental Endocrinology Research Group, Institute of Child Health, University College London, UK

Melissa Hines   Professor of Psychology and Director, Gender Development Research Centre, University of Cambridge, UK

Terrie Inder   Brigham and Women's Hospital, Harvard Medical School, Boston, MA, USA

Jenny Johansson   Researcher, Department of Pharmaceutical Biosciences, Uppsala University, Sweden

Anna Jonsson   Department of Pharmaceutical Biosciences, Uppsala University, Sweden

Nils Krone   Academic Unit of Child Health, Department of Oncology and Metabolism, University of Sheffield, UK

Juliane Léger   Professor of Paediatrics, Paediatric Endocrinology and Diabetology Department, Robert Debré Hospital, Paris, France

John G Logan   Research Associate, Molecular Endocrinology Group, Department of Medicine, Imperial College London, UK

Simon M Luckman   Brackenbury Chair of Physiology, Faculty of Biology, Medicine and Health, University of Manchester, UK

Joseph Majzoub   Chief, Division of Endocrinology, Boston Children's Hospital; Thomas Morgan Rotch Professor of Pediatrics, Professor of Medicine, Harvard Medical School, MA, USA

Laetitia Martinerie   Consultant, Pediatric Endocrinology Department, Robert Debré Hospital, Paris, France

Juan-Pedro Martinez-Barbera	Professor in Developmental Biology and Cancer, Birth Defects Research Centre, Developmental Biology and Cancer Research Programme, Institute of Child Health, University College London, UK
Elisabeth A Northam	Senior Neuropsychologist, Department of Psychology, The Royal Children's Hospital, Melbourne; Senior Research Fellow, Cell Biology/Clinical Sciences, Murdoch Childrens Research Institute; Associate Professor, School of Psychological Sciences, The University of Melbourne, Australia
Fred Nyberg	Senior Professor, Department of Pharmaceutical Biosciences, Uppsala University, Sweden
Iain CAF Robinson	National Institute for Medical Research, London, UK
Joanne F Rovet	Senior Scientist, Neuroscience and Mental Health Program, Research Institute, The Hospital for Sick Children; Professor of Paediatrics, University of Toronto, Canada
Martin O Savage	Emeritus Professor of Paediatric Endocrinology, Barts and the London School of Medicine and Dentistry, London, UK
Terry Segal	Consultant in General Paediatrics and Adolescent Medicine, University College Hospital, London, UK
Robert K Semple	Reader in Endocrinology and Metabolism, Wellcome Trust-MRC Institute of Metabolic Science, University of Cambridge, UK
Bhavni Shah	Paediatric and Adolescent Registrar, University College London Hospital, UK
Dominique Simon	MD, Pediatric Endocrinology Department, Robert Debré Hospital, Paris, France
Charles A Sklar	Attending Pediatrician, Full Member, Department of Pediatrics, Memorial Sloan Kettering Cancer Center, NY, USA

Helen A Spoudeas   Consultant/ Honorary Senior Lecturer Paediatric Endocrinology, London Centre for Paediatric Endocrinology and Diabetes, Neuroendocrine Division, Great Ormond Street and University College Hospitals, London, UK

Ramesh Srinivasan   Consultant Paediatrician, Department of Paediatrics, University Hospital of North Tees, Stockton on Tees, UK

Helen L Storr   Reader and Honorary Consultant in Paediatric Endocrinology, Centre for Endocrinology, William Harvey Research Institute, Barts and the London School of Medicine, Queen Mary University London, UK

Julian A Waung   Clinical Research Fellow, Molecular Endocrinology Group, Department of Medicine, Imperial College London, UK

Emma A Webb   NIHR Academic Clinical Lecturer, Institute of Metabolism and Systems Research, College of Medical and Dental Sciences, University of Birmingham, UK

Graham R Williams   Professor of Endocrinology, Molecular Endocrinology Group, Department of Medicine, Imperial College London, UK

Delphine Zenaty   Department of Paediatric Endocrinology, Robert Debré Hospital, Paris, France

FOREWORD

Neuroendocrine Disorders in Children, is a modern-day *tour de force* with contributions from a group of true international experts. The importance of this topic has been recognized by many academic institutions that have now created pediatric centers for pituitary and neuroendocrine disorders that provide age-specific specialized interdisciplinary care for the diagnosis, evaluation, and treatment of tumors and other disorders involving the pituitary gland and hypothalamus. The book begins with an excellent review chapter of the regulation of growth hormone secretion and physiology starting in fetal life. Chapter 2 is a comprehensive review of disorders of the hypothalamic-pituitary-somatotroph axis leading to growth failure, including, but not limited to, a comprehensive review of genetic abnormalities. Chapters 3 and 4 provide current thinking with regard to the effects of growth hormone (and IGF-I) on brain structure and neurological/cognitive/behavioral function. Subsequent chapters (often in pairs) cover in great detail the relevant embryology and physiology in the first, followed by clinical disorders and the genetic basis of disease (as appropriate), diagnostic modalities and treatment of essentially all relevant neuroendocrine issues in the second. Areas covered include disorders of salt and water balance and thyroid and weight regulation. Genetic disorders involving brain and adipose peptides associated with morbid obesity are well delineated in Chapter 10, with comorbidities and treatment of obesity eloquently presented in Chapter 11 (including some excellent summary tables). Chapter 12 discusses the late endocrine and metabolic effects of cancer and its treatments as they relate to the neuroendocrine system. A comprehensive review of all aspects of craniopharyngioma, including new genetic information, is provided in Chapter 13. The current physiology and pathophysiology of the hypothalamic-pituitary-adrenal (HPA) axis is nicely summarized in Chapter 14, while the bi-directional interplay of the HPA axis and stress/stress disorders is eruditely discussed in Chapter 15. Chapter 16 presents a modern review of adrenoleukodystrophy. Everything one needs to know about pediatric Cushing disease follows in Chapter 17. Chapter 18 provides detailed physiology and pathophysiology of the hypothalamic-pituitary-ovarian and -testicular axes. Chapter 19 provides a superb review of hypogonadotropic hypogonadism in both males and females, including detailed reviews of the many genetic causes (in an easy-to-read table) and treatment approaches to fertility recovery. Chapter 20 provides an excellent review of central precocious puberty, including etiology, diagnosis, and management. Chapter 21 is a welcome inclusion that examines the psychological and behavioral consequences of sex steroid exposure on the brain, with an emphasis on androgens in various naturally occurring human conditions. Chapters 22 and 23 nicely delve into the metabolic and physiological effects of hyper- and hypoglycemia, including the actions of glucose, on the brain.

In summary, *Neuroendocrine Disorders in Children* is a comprehensive, state-of-the-art text that replaces older books from the 1980's (Gupta) and 1990's (Savage), integrating molecular biology and genetics into our thinking about the pathophysiology and treatment of pediatric hypothalamic-pituitary disease, offering a one-stop shop for brain-hypothalamic-pituitary hormonal physiology and pathophysiology, and serving as an extremely useful reference for physicians young and old.

Mitchell E. Geffner MD

Professor of Pediatrics

Keck School of Medicine, University of Southern California;

Chief, Center for Endocrinology, Diabetes and Metabolism

Children's Hospital Los Angeles,

CA, USA

PREFACE

The effects of hormones on brain function have been studied for many years, but many questions have remained unanswered. Recent advances in our understanding of the molecular basis of a number of endocrine and neurological disorders as well as advances in neuroimaging with more sophisticated techniques have led to major novel insights in neuroendocrinology. The availability of new tools, such as optogenetics, will in the future pave the way to major discoveries in the mechanisms of hormone action that impact on brain function.

This book tackles the subject of neuroendocrine disorders in childhood. The editors represent basic neuroendocrinology, clinical paediatric endocrinology and neurology. Each editor has tried to bring in their unique expertise to the book. We have tried to encompass a broad range of topics and we are fortunate that many clinicians and scientists who are renowned experts in their respective areas have agreed to participate in this project and contributed state-of the-art chapters. We are very grateful to them for their input in spite of their demanding schedules. This has allowed us to put together a book that is highly translational; insights from basic science have been incorporated into the description of a number of clinical problems.

We hope that the book will be of value to undergraduates as well as post-graduates, and will aid those clinicians who look after children with complex neuroendocrine disorders, many of whom have significant neurodisability. We believe that the book will also be of benefit to other members of the multi-disciplinary team looking after children with neuroendocrine disorders. We hope that the book will go some way towards improving the understanding of these disorders, with the ultimate aim of improving the clinical management of these children and benefitting them and their families. Finally, we hope that the book will help basic scientists and clinical researchers to identify gaps in our knowledge of the pathogenesis and management of these disorders and stimulate further basic, clinical and translational research in neuroendocrinology.

We are grateful to the team at Mac Keith Press, particularly Udoka Ohuonu, Alessy Beaver and Ann-Marie Halligan, for helping us to bring the project to a satisfactory conclusion and hope that you enjoy reading the final product.

Mehul Dattani, Peter, Hindmarsh, Lucinda Carr, Iain Robinson
May 2016

1
NEUROENDOCRINE REGULATION OF GROWTH HORMONE SECRETION

Peter C Hindmarsh and Iain CAF Robinson

Introduction

The entire process of human growth represents a continuum to which birth is largely incidental. Postnatal growth can be considered to consist of at least three distinct phases: infancy, childhood and puberty. The infancy component is largely a continuation of the longitudinal growth process observed *in utero*. This displays a peak length velocity around 27 to 28 weeks of gestation, with a decline in growth rate during the last trimester of pregnancy. This declining growth rate continues during the first 3 years of life, reaching a plateau at or around the fourth year of life and continues at this rate until the commencement of the pubertal growth spurt (Karlberg 1987).

The factors influencing these distinct growth periods are different. We know relatively little directly about the factors influencing fetal and early infant growth. However, we know from animal experiments that nutrition plays a key role partly through regulation of insulin-like growth factor (IGF) secretion, and there is good evidence that these factors are likely to play similar roles in human fetal growth. With the appearance of the growth hormone receptor (GHR) in both liver and growth plate at around 6 months of postnatal life, growth hormone–dependent IGF production and action assume a greater importance, and, during the childhood years, growth is largely dependent on the growth hormone secretory status of the individual. The final step in the growth process, the pubertal growth spurt, comprises a 50% contribution from sex steroids and 50% contribution from growth hormone. Growth hormone secretion (GHS) from the anterior pituitary represents the final common pathway by which a series of inputs that regulate growth are processed. This regulation takes place predominantly at the level of the hypothalamus with further integration between the hypothalamic factors taking place at the level of the pituitary somatotrophs.

Growth hormone regulation

Our understanding of the regulation of GHS stemmed from the pioneering work of Geoffrey Harris and his group in Oxford who suggested that release of growth hormone from the pituitary, like other pituitary hormones, was under the control of a releasing factor secreted from the hypothalamus into the pituitary portal circulation to activate hormone release. Before this was identified, however, Brazeau et al. (1973) identified a growth hormone release–inhibiting factor (somatostatin), which led to a radical change in the thinking

1

around the control of GHS, as prior to this it was assumed that the original concept of one releasing hormone for one pituitary hormone prevailed. The final demonstration of a growth hormone–stimulating factor came in 1982 when growth hormone–releasing hormone (GHRH) was isolated and characterised from two pancreatic tumours (Guillemin et al. 1982; Rivier et al. 1982).

During the search for the growth hormone–releasing factor, little was made of a further stimulating molecule earlier described by Bowers et al. (1980), which, although synthetic in nature, formed the basis for the identification of an endogenous receptor capable of activating growth hormone release (Howard et al. 1996), used in turn to identify its naturally occurring ligand, ghrelin, an acylated peptide mostly produced in the stomach (Kojima et al. 1999). Interestingly, despite their powerful effects to inhibit or stimulate GHS pharmaco-logically, deletion of either somatostatin (Low et al. 2001) or ghrelin or its receptors (Sun et al. 2008) has surprisingly little effects on growth in experimental animals. In contrast, GHRH and its receptor are both essential for normal GHS. Deletion or mutations of GHRH receptors in animals and humans cause profound growth hormone deficiency (GHD) and dwarfism/short stature (Lin et al. 1993; Maheshwari et al. 1998), as does deletion of GHRH in mice (Alba and Salvatori 2004). Curiously, to date, GHRH deletion has not yet been reported as a cause of human GHD.

ONTOGENY OF GROWTH HORMONE SECRETION

The human fetal pituitary gland synthesises and secretes growth hormone from 8 to 10 weeks of gestation, and pituitary growth hormone content increases from about 20ng at 10 weeks to 1000ng at 16 weeks of gestation. Fetal plasma growth hormone concentrations in cord blood samples are in the range 1–4nmol/l during the first trimester and increase to a mean peak of approximately 6nmol/l at mid-gestation. Plasma growth hormone concentra-tions fall progressively during the second half of gestation to a mean value of 1.5nmol/l at term. Pituitary growth hormone mRNA and growth hormone content generally parallel the increase in plasma growth hormone concentration between 16 and 24 weeks of gestation. This pattern of ontogenesis of plasma growth hormone reflects a progressive maturation of hypothalamic-pituitary and forebrain function. The responses of plasma growth hormone to somatostatin, GHRH and to insulin and arginine are mature at term in human infants (Suganuma et al. 1989).

The high plasma growth hormone concentrations at mid-gestation after the development of the pituitary portal vascular system may reflect unrestrained secretion. Studies of 9- to 16-week-old human fetal pituitary cells in culture have shown a predominant response to GHRH and a limited effect of somatostatin, which suggests that the inhibitory action of somatostatin develops later in gestation (Goodyear et al. 1987). This interpretation has been substantiated by *in vivo* studies in the sheep fetus, which have shown a failure of soma-tostatin to inhibit GHRH-stimulated growth hormone release early in the third trimester and maturation of the inhibitory effect of somatostatin near term. Thus, a predominant GHRH enhancement and limited somatostatin inhibition of GHS at mid-gestation presum-ably relate to a limited capacity for inhibition of growth hormone release by somatomedin feedback. In addition, there may be unrestrained GHS at the pituitary cell level or

2

immaturity of limbic and forebrain inhibitory circuitry that modulates hypothalamic function, or both. Whatever the mechanisms, control of GHS matures progressively during the last half of gestation and the early weeks of postnatal life so that mature responses to sleep, glucose and L-dopa are present by 3 months of age.

POSTNATAL PERIOD

GHS in the immediate postnatal period is characterised by high circulating concentrations and a lack of a defined pulsatility (Miller et al. 1993). The relationship between growth hormone and IGF-1 is inverse as opposed to the positive relationship seen in childhood. These findings probably reflect more the relatively growth hormone insensitive state of the fetus/newborn infant than a major perturbation in the hypothalamo-pituitary-growth hormone axis *per se*, and the move to the child/adult growth hormone–IGF-1 relationship is probably a reflection of gradually increased postnatal expression of the GHR in the liver.

PATTERN IN CHILDHOOD AND ADULTHOOD

During childhood and adolescence, this picture changes dramatically. In a state of adequate nutrition, GHS becomes the predominant determinant of height velocity. Strikingly, the growth hormone secretory pattern is highly pulsatile, with discrete pulses of growth hormone separated by low troughs of growth hormone in the bloodstream. Because of this, multiple frequent sampling is essential in order to define clearly the true heights of the growth hormone peaks. If sampling were too infrequent, the true peak heights would be underestimated or small peaks missed altogether. Figure 1.1 shows a typical growth hormone profile in a 9-year-old boy, generated by taking blood samples for growth hormone measurement every 20 minutes. The upper panel shows the actual plasma growth hormone concentration measured whereas the lower panel is a mathematical derivative of the actual secretion of growth hormone that the pituitary would have to make to generate the concentration profile in the peripheral blood. The profile is characterised by episodes of growth hormone release generating peak growth hormone concentrations interspersed with periods of time when GHS is effectively switched off and growth hormone concentrations are undetectable. This appears to be the predominant pattern in males, whereas in females in many species, although the peak concentrations tend to be similar, the most striking difference is that there is an elevation in the trough concentrations so that at all times growth hormone concentrations are detectable. One further point to note is that the pulses occur at fairly regular intervals of one every 3 hours so that, for normal individuals, most of the growth hormone concentration signal is contained in the amplitude of the pulses, rather than in the basal secretion between the pulses.

The reason for a fixed periodicity is unclear. This may relate to the cycling of GHRH and somatostatin release into the hypophyseal portal circulation for which there are experimental data in different animal species. The pituitary appears refractory to repeated stimulation with GHRH given on an hourly basis and maximum responsivity is only re-established once a 3-hourly stimulatory regimen is approximated. This has been modelled experimentally in animals, where varying concentrations of somatostatin can give rise to pulsatile growth hormone release, even in the presence of continuous GHRH exposure and where

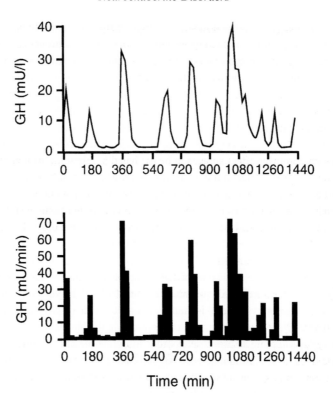

Figure 1.1. Upper panel shows 24-hour serum growth hormone concentration profile with a deconvoluted estimate of the pituitary secretion of growth hormone needed to generate the serum concentrations shown in the lower panel.

rapid withdrawal of somatostatin generates a 'rebound' peak of growth hormone release (Clark et al. 1988). An additional important effect of GHRH is to stimulate *de novo* growth hormone synthesis so that more growth hormone is available for release in large amplitude pulses.

The reason why there is a relatively long time interval between growth hormone pulses with respect to peripheral tissue responses is also unclear. Circulatory time from the pituitary to the target tissues is quick. Generation of IGF-1 by growth hormone is relatively slow and certainly slower in terms of maximum production than that expected from a feedback effect on a 3-hourly basis. Insulin secretion has a periodicity of 13 minutes and execution of the metabolic action (plasma glucose lowering) is completed before the next insulin pulse, but this is not obviously the case for growth hormone. It may relate to the importance of the growth hormone–signalling kinetics at the receptor and post-receptor pathways in different tissues (see below).

In humans the pulse amplitude of the growth hormone bursts is directly related to the height velocity in childhood (Hindmarsh et al. 1987). During puberty, GHS doubles under the influence of the sex steroids in order to generate the pubertal growth spurt. This increase comes about as a result of an increase in growth hormone pulse amplitude with growth hormone pulse frequency remaining unchanged. During early adulthood there is a gradual decline in the amount of growth hormone secreted, and in later decades the amount secreted declines significantly, and is similar to that observed in children with GHD. This is not because of a lack of growth hormone secretory reserve, as much larger amounts of growth hormone can be released in elderly patients if they are treated with growth hormone secretagogues (Bowers et al. 2004).

Sex steroids increase the amount of growth hormone that can be synthesised and secreted. The predominant effect appears to be mediated by estradiol, as non-aromatisable androgens do not increase GHS and the increase in secretion can be blocked by prior treatment with an estrogen receptor blocker, tamoxifen. Thyroxine is required for transcription of the growth hormone gene, so a reversible impairment of growth hormone release is often observed in hypothyroid states which can be restored with appropriate thyroid hormone replacement. The glucocorticoid cortisol acutely increases growth hormone release in response to GHRH administration. Likewise adrenocorticotropic hormone (ACTH) will increase the growth hormone response to GHRH compared to GHRH administration alone but corticotrophin-releasing hormone suppresses the GHS despite generating similar ACTH and cortisol concentrations. This suggests a complex series of integrative actions at the level of the hypothalamus and pituitary.

At both levels, other interactions take place with glucose, amino acids and free fatty acids, modulating growth hormone release. There is also a rich literature on the effect of a variety of neurotransmitters such as acetylcholine and dopamine. Many of these studies are essentially pharmacological in nature. In experimental animals, it has proved possible to identify living GHRH neurons and study the effects of neurotransmitters and peptides such as ghrelin directly on GHRH neuronal activity (Osterstock et al. 2010), but disentangling the physiological roles of these transmitters in human growth hormone regulation remains challenging.

GHS is entrained to the sleep–wake cycle but not to the same extent as cortisol, body temperature or blood pressure. The majority of growth hormone release takes place in association with stage IV sleep, irrespective of whether sleep takes place at night or during the day. Certainly, the strong association between sleep and nocturnal GHS would be a useful event to prevent nocturnal hypoglycaemia during this period of fast. Technically the growth hormone secretory pattern is not circadian. That said, a considerable number of circadian clock–driven systems impinge on the growth hormone axis. The close approximation of the growth hormone secretory pattern to those pathways that are clock driven might allow for better integration and avoid poor synchronisation with these critical pathways (Bass and Takahashi 2012).

Generation of growth hormone pulses

As mentioned above, in both rodents and humans there is evidence to support the concept of an inverse relationship between the secretion of the two hypothalamic peptides: somatostatin and GHRH. GHRH is involved in both the release and synthesis of growth hormone whilst somatostatin inhibits growth hormone release. Normal growth hormone pulsatility requires endogenous GHRH though growth hormone responses to exogenous GHRH are variable and reveal varying periods of responsiveness and refractoriness. There are several possible explanations for this. First, the phenomenon may be intrinsic to the growth hormone–secreting cells. This would require an internal sexually dimorphic somatotroph clock, which at this stage appears unlikely. Second, acute down-regulation of the GHRH receptors or their intracellular signalling systems may take place. In some children with GHD, GHRH administration leads to some attenuation of the growth hormone response with time. However, GHRH receptor down-regulation appears to be an unlikely explanation as down-regulation only takes place at very high GHRH concentrations, certainly well above those usually encountered physiologically, and does not occur with chronic GHRH exposure from ectopic GHRH-producing tumours, which maintain very high levels of pulsatile growth hormone over a raised baseline (Thorner et al. 1982), and cause acromegaly. This would also seem to rule out the possibility that it is simply an acute depletion of a small readily releasable pool of growth hormone, since blockade of endogenous somatostatin immediately allows growth hormone release in response to GHRH during a refractory period (Tannenbaum and Ling 1984).

A more likely explanation is that the pattern reflects variation in endogenous soma- tostatin tone, imposing an ultradian rhythm in GHRH responses. Evidence for this comes from the observation that continuous GHRH administration leads to pulsatile growth hormone release, implying modulation by another factor, somatostatin (Vance et al. 1985). Although somatostatin readily suppresses pulsatile GHS in rats and humans, its effects are short-lived and rapid release of growth hormone takes place on its removal. This rebound secretion can be detected *in vitro* but is even more pronounced *in vivo* (Clark et al. 1988). Somatostatin withdrawal can produce growth hormone rebound secretion in humans but for regular repeatable growth hormone release to take place, it is the combination of soma- tostatin withdrawal coupled with GHRH administration that is the most efficacious (Fig 1.2; Hindmarsh et al. 1991). Of course, it should be recalled that, in clinical practice, somatostatin analogues with much longer half-lives and/or depot formulations are used, so that growth hormone oversecretion can usually be effectively inhibited over long periods.

The interplay between GHRH and somatostatin operates with an additional degree of complexity, in that the release of a pulse of growth hormone comes about by coordinated activity at both GHRH and growth hormone cell levels. The classic description of the GHRH neuronal distribution in the hypothalamus comes from immunohistochemical sec- tions. This presents a concept of a grouping or nucleus of cells. In fact this static histological approach belies a complex interaction that takes place between GHRH cells, possibly aided by interneurons, to allow a more coordinated release of GHRH to occur (perhaps analogous to what is being revealed for kisspeptin and the GnRH neuronal pulses; see Chapter 19).

This close relationship between GHRH and somatostatin acting as integrators of other signals, for example, sleep, is complicated by the discovery of ghrelin, which differs sub- stantially from GHRH in both its structure and its receptor (GHSR type 1a). The receptor is strongly expressed in the hypothalamus, and present in the pituitary, but has also been identified in many other regions of the central nervous system and peripheral endocrine and non-endocrine tissues in humans (Gnanapavan et al. 2002). As mentioned above,

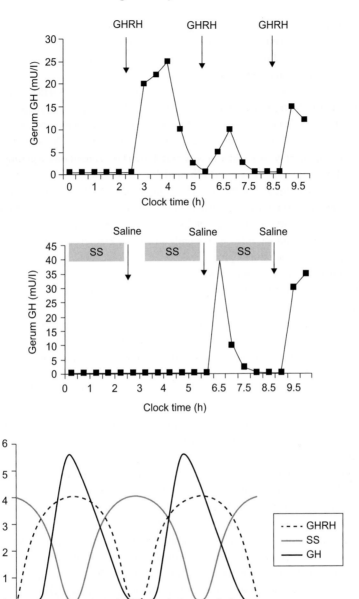

Figure 1.2. Generation of a growth hormone pulse. Upper panel shows the effect of three similar intravenous bolus injections of growth hormone–releasing hormone (GHRH) generating different growth hormone pulse amplitudes. The middle panel shows the effect of a somatostatin infusion followed by abrupt withdrawal leading to increasing growth hormone pulse amplitudes. The lower panel integrates these observations to show the most likely interaction of GHRH (dotted line) and somatostatin (gray line) in the generation of a growth hormone pulse (black line).

ghrelin was isolated from the stomach and is an octanoylated peptide of 28 amino acids (Kojima et al. 1999). Though it is expressed predominantly in the stomach, lower amounts are present within the bowel, pancreas, kidney, the immune system, placenta, pituitary, testis, ovary and hypothalamus.

Ghrelin stimulates GHS directly, and also via a direct effect on GHRH neurons (Osterstock et al. 2010). It also can stimulate prolactin and ACTH secretion at higher doses. Additionally, it influences endocrine pancreatic function and glucose metabolism, gonadal function, appetite and behaviour. It is important to measure acylated ghrelin (Nass et al. 2008) as its desacylated form (which is present in significant amounts in the circulation) is inactive on the GHSR1a and does not release growth hormone. When specific assays are used, there is a good correlation between acylghrelin and amplification of GHS in adults (Nass et al. 2011). However, the role of endogenous ghrelin in normal growth during childhood remains unclear.

An important observation is that ghrelin acts synergistically with GHRH to generate increased growth hormone release. A number of other endogenous agents effect growth hormone pulsatility including opioids, calcitonin and glucagon, but these have not been used to manipulate growth hormone secretory patterns to alter growth and their physiological relevance to the control of endogenous growth hormone pulsatility remains unclear.

There is good evidence that growth hormone feeds back to inhibit its own release and this may have a bearing on the temporal control of growth hormone pulsatility. Experiments indicate that exogenous growth hormone acts directly on the hypothalamus rather than on the pituitary (where endogenous concentrations would be very high). The most likely acute mode of feedback of growth hormone to regulate its own secretion is through increased secretion of somatostatin into the portal blood as well as inhibition of GHRH production. The blood–brain barrier is relatively permeable in the ventral part of the hypothalamus, and both somatostatin and GHRH neurons express GHRs, so a short-loop direct feedback can readily operate. Of more importance for chronic feedback, growth hormone exerts negative feedback by the generation of increased levels of peripheral IGF-1, which in turn inhibits growth hormone synthesis and release chiefly at the pituitary level.

The entry rate of endogenous growth hormone into the circulation is governed by the kinetics of growth hormone release from the somatotropes. Its availability to the tissues from the bloodstream is also affected by the amount of growth hormone bound to its circulating binding protein (derived from the extracellular growth hormone-binding domain of the GHR). With regard to coordinated release of growth hormone pulses from the pituitary, Lafont et al. (2010) have used novel imaging techniques in transgenic mice to demonstrate that pituitary somatotrophs form networks in the pituitary gland and that GHRH can alter local blood flow around these networks, which may facilitate the coordinated delivery of GHRH to the secretory cells and the acute release of growth hormone necessary to generate a pulse of growth hormone leaving the gland.

Given the pulsatile nature of growth hormone, the precise role of the growth hormone–binding protein in human is far from clear. There is a correlation with growth hormone status but only at the very extremes and the effect of growth hormone treatment is highly variable. The presence of a growth hormone–binding protein retains more growth hormone in the circulation than in its absence, so it could act to modify the presentation of growth hormone to the receptors, allowing large peaks to stimulate cellular GHRs acutely, but 'mopping up' trough levels of growth hormone, providing competition for the cellular GHRs in target tissues.

WHY REGULATE GROWTH HORMONE SECRETION IN PULSES?
Given the pulsatile nature of GHS in all species tested to date, it is suggested that this could have evolved as the most efficient method of stimulating GHRs and growth. It has been recently suggested that signalling through the GHR probably does not involve simply dimerisation of GHR monomers, but rather binding and changing the conformation of pre-formed inactive GHR dimers to an activated state (Brooks et al. 2014). How the presentation of high concentrations of growth hormone in pulses followed by rapid disappearance compares with a more continuous lower level of growth hormone for this receptor transactivation remains to be clarified. However, it is clear that the pattern of growth hormone is important in determining a number of different target organ effects, yet with essentially the same GHR type present (Gebert et al. 1997).

There is sexual dimorphism in the pulsatile patterns of growth hormone in both rodents and humans (Jaffe et al. 1998). For example, in the rodent, the pattern of hormone secretion, either pulsatile (male mode) or continuous (female mode), has an impact on the growth of the animal, expression of a number of liver enzymes and the determination of the level of growth hormone–binding protein in the circulation as well as GHR expression (Gevers et al. 1996; Gebert et al. 1997). The tissue response is also variable in that the liver will generate significant amounts of IGF-1 in response to growth hormone irrespective of its mode of administration whereas adequate expression of IGF-1 in the muscle in animals is highly dependent on the pulsatile mode of administration.

There is a wealth of earlier data showing that growth hormone replacement by daily injections in children is highly effective for their growth (Smith et al. 1988), and in experimental studies, it has been clearly demonstrated that giving growth hormone replacement in a pulsatile pattern that mimics the endogenous profile reproduces the normal growth pattern in GHD animal models (Clark et al. 1995; Gevers et al. 1996; Fig 1.3) This is not to say that continuous growth hormone exposure is ineffective – indeed in rodents it elicits a completely different pattern of responses from some growth hormone–dependent genes, and probably does so in humans, given the same post-receptor mechanisms. For example, the pattern of fat distribution around the abdomen is more influenced by the trough concentrations than peak concentrations of growth hormone in humans (Hindmarsh et al. 1999).

There is good evidence that this pattern dependence is somehow mediated via the signalling pathways of the GHR, primarily the kinetics of GHR activation of the JAK/STAT and MAPkinase pathways and their downstream targets (Waxman and O'Connor 2006), which may require differing periods of receptor 'on/off' to elicit optimal responses (Gebert et al. 1997). In this context, the growth hormone–binding proteins could play a role in modifying the pharmacodynamics of receptor activation, and hence the pattern of growth hormone signalling in different tissues.

It is important to bear in mind that the pulsatile pattern of growth hormone can be dramatically altered in some physiological (pregnancy secretion of placental growth

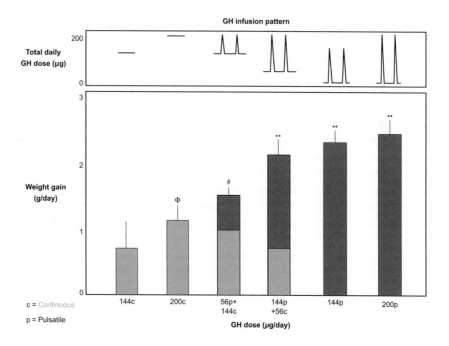

Figure 1.3a. Pulsatile growth hormone is better than continuous growth hormone for growth stimulation in rats with growth hormone deficiency (GHD). Dwarf GHD rats were given IV infusions of two daily amounts of growth hormone either continuously (first two bars), in mixed continuous and pulsatile patterns (middle two bars), or in a pulsatile pattern of eight pulses per day (last two bars). The larger the pulsatile component of the infusion, the greater the growth response. From Gevers et al. (1996).

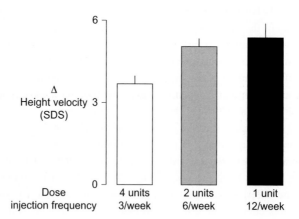

Figure 1.3b. The growth response in children depends on the frequency of growth hormone injections. Increasing the frequency of growth hormone injections in children with growth hormone deficiency from 3 times per week to 6 or 12 injections per week produced greater growth responses for the same weekly amount of growth hormone. From Smith et al. (1988).

10

hormone) or pathological (acromegaly) conditions. Whilst there is evidence that in humans IGF-1 generation occurs best when growth hormone is presented in an intermittent rather than continuous mode at least in the physiological situation (Achermann et al. 1999), it is clearly raised by increased continuous baseline growth hormone exposure (even at relatively low levels), for example, in poorly controlled acromegaly. This remains a controversial area, as there are efforts in the pipeline by the pharmaceutical industry to develop growth hormone preparations or analogues that are intrinsically, or by formulation, more long-acting in nature, and provide continuous growth hormone exposure. These could have advantages in avoiding the inconvenience of daily injections of growth hormone, and will clearly generate some growth, but seem to aim away from a more physiological pattern of intermittent growth hormone exposure in normal childhood growth. The long-term conse-quences of using more continuous growth hormone exposure to stimulate growth in children with GHD remain to be established. On the other hand, since current growth hormone injections are given via the subcutaneous route, the pharmacokinetics of subcutaneous growth hormone delivery will clearly spread out the pulses, and so the pattern achieved cannot be described as completely physiological either. It may be that, in the future, a more complex replacement therapy pattern of growth hormone may be developed, just as is cur-rently under way with insulin pump therapy for insulin replacement.

REFERENCES

Achermann JC, Brook CGD, Robinson ICAF et al. (1999) Peak and trough growth hormone (GH) concentra-tions influence growth and serum insulin-like growth factor-1 (IGF-1) concentrations in short children. *Clin Endocrinol* 50: 301–308.

Alba M and Salvatori R (2004) A mouse with targeted ablation of the growth hormone-releasing hormone gene: A new model of isolated growth hormone deficiency. *Endocrinology* 145(9): 4134–4143.

Bass J and Takahashi JS (2012) Circadian integration of metabolism and energetics. *Science* 330: 1349–1354.

Bowers CY, Granda R, Mohan S, Kuipers J, Baylink D, Veldhuis JD (2004) Sustained elevation of pulsatile growth hormone (GH) secretion and insulin-like growth factor I (IGF-I), IGF-binding protein-3 (IGFBP-3), and IGFBP-5 concentrations during 30-day continuous subcutaneous infusion of GH-releasing peptide-2 in older men and women. *J Clin Endocr Metab* 89: 2290–2300.

Bowers CY, Momany F, Reynolds GA et al. (1980) Structure-activity relationships of a synthetic pentapeptide that specifically releases growth hormone in vitro. *Endocrinology* 106: 663–667.

Brazeau P, Vale W, Burgus R et al. (1973) Hypothalamic polypeptide that inhibits the secretion of immuno-reactive pituitary growth hormone. *Science* 178: 77–79.

Brooks AJ, Dai W, O'Mara ML et al. (2014) Mechanism of activation of protein kinase JAK2 by the growth hormone receptor. *Science* 344(6185): 1249783.

Clark RG, Carlsson LM, Rafferty B and Robinson IC (1988) The rebound release of growth hormone (GH) following somatostatin infusion in rats involves hypothalamic GH-releasing factor release. *J Endocrinol* 119: 397–404.

Clark RG, Jansson JO, Isaksson O and Robinson IC (1985) Intravenous growth hormone: Growth responses to patterned infusions in hypophysectomized rats. *J Endocrinol* 104: 53–61.

Gebert CA, Park SH and Waxman DJ (1997) Regulation of signal transducer and activator of transcription (STAT) 5b activation by the temporal pattern of growth hormone stimulation. *Mol Endocrinol* 11: 400–414.

Gevers EF, Wit JM and Robinson ICAF (1996) Growth, growth hormone (GH) – binding protein and GH receptors are differentially regulated by peak and trough components of the GH secretory pattern in the rat. *Endocrinology* 137: 1013–1018.

Gnanapavan S, Kola B, Bustin SA et al. (2002) The tissue distribution of the mRNA of ghrelin and subtypes of its receptor, GHS-R, in humans. *J Clin Endocrinol Metab* 87: 2988.

Goodyear CG, Sellen JM, Fuks M et al. (1987) Regulation of growth hormone secretion from human fetal pituitaries, interactions between growth hormone releasing factor and somatostatin. *Reprod Nutr Dev* 27: 461–470.

Guillemin R, Brazeau P, Bohien P, Escu F, Ling N and Wehrenburg WB (1982) Growth hormone releasing factor from a human pancreatic tumour that caused acromegaly. *Science* 218: 585–587.

Hindmarsh PC, Brain CE, Robinson ICAF, Matthews DR and Brook CGD (1991) The interaction of growth hormone releasing hormone and somatostatin in the generation of GH pulse in man. *Clin Endocrinol* 35: 353–360.

Hindmarsh PC, Dennison E, Pincus SM et al. (1999) A sexually dimorphic pattern of growth hormone secretion in the elderly. *J Clin Endocrnol Metab* 84: 2679–2685.

Hindmarsh PC, Smith PJ, Brook CGD and Matthews DR (1987) The relationship between growth velocity and growth hormone secretion in short prepubertal children. *Clin Endocrinol* 27: 581–591.

Howard AD, Feighner SD, Cully DF et al. (1996) A receptor in pituitary and hypothalamus that functions in growth hormone release. *Science* 273(5277): 974–977.

Jaffe CA, Ocampo-Lim B, Guo W et al. (1998) Regulatory mechanisms of growth hormone secretion are sexually dimorphic. *J Clin Invest* 102: 153–164.

Karlberg J. (1987) On the modelling of human growth. *Stat Med* 6: 185–192.

Kojima M, Hosoda H, Date Y et al. (1999) Ghrelin is a growth-hormone-releasing acylated peptide from stomach. *Nature* 402: 656–660.

Lafont C, Desarménien MG, Cassou M et al. (2010) Cellular in vivo imaging reveals coordinated regulation of pituitary microcirculation and GH cell network function. *P Natl Acad Sci USA* 107: 4465–4470.

Lin SC, Lin CR, Gukovsky I, Lusis AJ, Sawchenko PE and Rosenfeld MG (1993) Molecular basis of the little mouse phenotype and implications for cell type-specific growth. *Nature* 364: 208–213.

Low MJ, Otero-Corchon V, Parlow AF et al. (2001) Somatostatin is required for masculinization of growth hormone-regulated hepatic gene expression but not of somatic growth. *J Clin Invest* 107: 1571–1580.

Maheshwari HG, Silverman BL, Dupuis J and Baumann G (1998) Phenotype and genetic analysis of a syndrome caused by an inactivating mutation in the growth hormone-releasing hormone receptor: Dwarfism of Sindh. *J Clin Endocrnol Metab* 83: 4065–4074.

Miller JD, Esparza A, Wright NM et al. (1993) Spontaneous growth hormone release in term infants: Changes during the first four days of life. *J Clin Endocrnol Metab* 76: 1058–1062.

Nass R, Farhy LS, Liu J et al. (2008) Evidence for acyl-ghrelin modulation of growth hormone release in the fed state. *J Clin Endocrinol Metab* 93: 1988–1994.

Nass R, Gaylinn BD and Thorner MO (2011) The role of ghrelin in GH secretion and GH disorders. *Mol Cell Endocrinol* 340(1): 10–14.

Osterstock G, Escobar P, Mitutsova V et al. (2010) Ghrelin stimulation of growth hormone-releasing hormone neurons is direct in the arcuate nucleus. *PLoS One* 5(2): e9159.

Rivier J, Spiess J, Thorner MO and Vale W (1982) Characterisation of a growth hormone-releasing factor from a human pancreatic islet tumour. *Nature* 300: 276–278.

Smith PJ, Hindmarsh PC and Brook CG (1988) Contribution of dose and frequency of administration to the therapeutic effect of growth hormone. *Arch Dis Child* 63: 491–494.

Suganuma N, Seo H, Yamamoto N et al. (1989) The ontogeny of growth hormone in the human fetal pituitary. *Am J Obstet Gynecol* 160: 729–733.

Sun Y, Butte NF, Garcia JM and Smith RG (2008) Characterization of adult ghrelin and ghrelin receptor knockout mice under positive and negative energy balance. *Endocrinology* 149: 843–850.

Tannenbaum GS and Ling N (1984) The interrelationship of growth hormone (GH)-releasing factor and somatostatin in generation of the ultradian rhythm of GH secretion. *Endocrinology* 115: 1952–1957.

Thorner MO, Perryman RL, Cronin MJ et al. (1982) Somatotroph hyperplasia. Successful treatment of acromegaly by removal of a pancreatic islet tumor secreting a growth hormone-releasing factor. *J Clin Invest* 70: 965–977.

Vance ML, Kaiser DL, Evans WS et al. (1985) Pulsatile growth hormone secretion in normal man during a continuous 24-hour infusion of human growth hormone releasing factor (1–40). Evidence for intermittent somatostatin secretion. *J Clin Invest* 75: 1584–1590.

Waxman DJ and O'Connor C (2006) Growth hormone regulation of sex-dependent liver gene expression. *Mol Endocrinol* 20: 2613–2629.

2

DISORDERS OF THE HYPOTHALAMO-PITUITARY-SOMATOTROPH AXIS LEADING TO GROWTH FAILURE

Kyriaki S Alatzoglou and Mehul T Dattani

Introduction

Short stature is the commonest reason for referral to the paediatric endocrine clinic; the diagnostic approach to an abnormal growth pattern requires evaluation for underlying illness, skeletal defects or syndromes, central nervous system abnormalities and genetic defects (Wit et al. 2011). Growth hormone, secreted by the somatotroph cells of the anterior pituitary gland, is a major regulator of growth and metabolism. Congenital or acquired disorders affecting the growth hormone–insulin-like growth factor-1 (IGF-1) axis manifest primarily as growth failure. Genetic defects may affect any part of this axis including the development of somatotrophs; the control, production and secretion of growth hormone (manifesting as growth hormone deficiency [GHD]) or its action on peripheral tissues; and the synthesis of IGF-1 and its downstream signalling (manifesting as growth hormone insensitivity or resistance).

The commonest genes implicated in the aetiology of GHD are those encoding growth hormone (*GH1*) and the growth hormone–releasing hormone receptor (*GHRHR*). However, isolated GHD may also result from heterozygous mutations in early developmental transcription factors that affect directly or indirectly the early stages of the development of the anterior pituitary and somatotrophs, such as *HESX1*, *SOX3*, *SOX2* or *OTX2*. As these transcription factors are implicated in the development of the eyes, forebrain and midline structures or even extrapituitary organs, the resulting GHD may be part of a wider syndrome (syndromic GHD). In addition, GHD may be the first presentation before the development of multiple pituitary hormone deficiencies as in the case with mutations in transcription factors involved in the later stages of pituitary cell differentiation such as *PROP1* or *POU1F1*. More rarely isolated GHD may result from recessive and dominant mutations in the growth hormone secretagogue receptor (*GHSR*) (Pantel et al. 2006), or biallelic mutations in components of the minor spliceosome (*RNPC3*) (Argente et al. 2014). These recent studies in pedigrees with isolated GHD have furthered our understanding of the genetic aetiology of GHD.

For the purposes of this review we will first summarise key aspects of the development of pituitary somatotrophs, the growth hormone–producing cells, before focusing on the genetic aetiology of GHD; we will then outline some of the acquired disorders that may affect the hypothalamo-pituitary axis.

Development of the hypothalamo-pituitary-somatotroph axis

The pituitary gland has a dual embryonic origin: the anterior and intermediate lobes are derived from the oral ectoderm, whilst the posterior pituitary is derived from the neural ectoderm. The development of the pituitary and the specification of the hormone-producing cells is a complex process that requires the coordinated spatial and temporal expression of a number of transcription factors and signalling molecules (Kelberman et al. 2009); this process has been extensively studied in rodents and reflects that in humans.

Outline of pituitary development

During murine development the first sign of pituitary development appears by embryonic day (E) 7.5 as a thickening of the ectoderm in the middle of the anterior neural ridge, forming the pituitary or hypophyseal placode, which is in continuity with the future hypothalamo-infundibular region located posteriorly. By E8.5, which corresponds to 4–6 weeks of gestation in human embryos, the placode appears as a thickening of the roof of the oral ectoderm and it invaginates dorsally to form the rudimentary Rathke's pouch (E9.0). At these early stages, inductive signals from the diencephalon (Bmp4, Fgf8) are required for the induction and formation of the pouch, and the maintenance of the apposition between the oral and neural ectoderm is critical for normal pituitary development. The definitive Rathke's pouch, which will give rise to the anterior and intermediate lobes, is developed by E10.5 and is separated from the underlying oral ectoderm at E12.5. Between E12.5 and E15.5, the progenitors of the hormone-secreting cells proliferate ventrally from the pouch to populate the forming anterior lobe.

During the early stages of the morphogenesis of the pituitary, signalling molecules from the ventral diencephalon (Bmp4, Fgf8, Fgf4, Nkx2.1, Wnt5α), the oral ectoderm (sonic hedgehog), the surrounding mesenchyme (Bmp2, Chordin) and the pouch itself (Bmp2, Wnt4) contribute to establish signalling gradients and the expression of transcription factors, which will determine the positional identity of ventral pituitary cells. The sequential activation and silencing of different families of transcription factors will result in the normal development of the gland and the maturation of hormone-producing cells. Insults to this developmental process can result in congenital hypopituitarism; mutations in genes implicated in the early stages of pituitary development tend to result in syndromic forms of hypopituitarism such as septo-optic dysplasia (SOD), in association with extra-pituitary defects and midline abnormalities, whilst mutations in genes required for the specification of particular cell types or encoding specific hormone subunits give rise to isolated pituitary hormone deficiencies, the most common of which is isolated GHD (Fig 2.1; Kelberman et al. 2009; McCabe et al. 2011).

These signalling molecules and transcription factors contribute to the development of the hypothalamo-pituitary axis at multiple levels, directly or indirectly. In addition there is increasing evidence of overlap in the aetiology of conditions that were previously considered to be discrete, such as Kallmann syndrome, SOD and combined pituitary hormone deficiencies, as mutations in the same array of genes (*KAL-1, PROKR2, FGF8, FGFR1*) have now been implicated in their aetiology (Raivio et al. 2012; McCabe et al. 2013). For

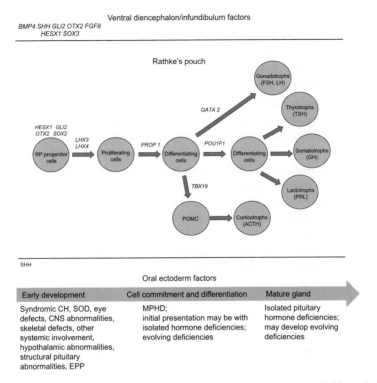

Figure 2.1. Outline of pituitary development and possible phenotypes of congenital hypopituitarism. SOD, septo-optic dysplasia; CNS, central nervous system; EPP, ectopic posterior pituitary; MPHD, multiple pituitary hormone deficiency; FSH, follicle stimulating hormone; LH, luteinizing hormone; TSH, thyroid-stimulating hormone; GH, growth harmone; PRL, prolactin; ACTH, adrenocorticotropic hormone; POMC, pro-opiomelanocortin; RP, rathke's Pouch.

example *FGF8* is expressed in the infundibulum by E9.5 and mediates the expansion of Rathke's pouch by inducing the expression of *LHX3* and *LHX4*. *FGF8* hypomorphic mice have variable phenotypes and may present with a markedly hypoplastic anterior pituitary gland, defects in the maturation of luteinizing hormone–producing cells, absent posterior pituitary, midline defects and a marked reduction of the arginine vasopressin and oxytocin neurons in hypothalamic nuclei. In humans heterozygous *FGF8* mutations have previously been reported in association with Kallmann syndrome; we recently reported the first auto-somal recessive case of holoprosencephaly attributed to *FGF8*, as well as heterozygous *FGF8* mutations in association with SOD. This suggests that the observed hypopituitary phenotypes may be the result of reduced functional *FGF8* in the diencephalon, leading to deficiencies in the neuroendocrine hypothalamus (McCabe et al. 2011).

Specification of somatotrophs

With respect to the development of somatotroph cells, they appear by E15.5 in the antero-lateral wings of the developing gland, following the appearance of corticotrophs and thy-rotrophs. In this process the onset of expression of the activator *PROP1* by E12.5 and its maintenance until E15.5 are critical steps as they are required for the emergence of the *POU1F1* lineage (somatotrophs, lactotrophs, thyrotrophs). In turn *POU1F1* is detected by E13.5 and reaches its peak level of expression in the differentiated somatotrophs by E16, and its expression is maintained in adulthood. Activation of *POU1F1* is required for the production of growth hormone, the expression of *GHRHR* and the postnatal expansion of growth hormone–producing cells. In fact, the appearance of differentiated somatotrophs is marked by the expression of the growth hormone gene and is followed by a dramatic increase in the number of somatotrophs and their migration by E18.5 throughout the central and lateral parts of the anterior lobe (Nogami and Hisano 2008; Kelberman et al. 2009).

There is increasing evidence that in addition to the role of the cell-type-specific factors (*PROP1*, *POU1F1*), other extracellular factors (hormones, neuropeptides, signalling molecules), diverse molecular pathways and the developing capillary pituitary network are also required for the establishment, proliferation and maintenance of somatotrophs (Alatzoglou et al. 2014). Hypothalamic growth hormone–releasing hormone (GHRH) is secreted by neurons of the arcuate nucleus of the hypothalamus and stimulates proliferation of somatotrophs and transcription and release of pituitary growth hormone. However, the timing of GHRH expression during pituitary development still remains unclear. In rats, GHRH neurons first appear at E11.5 and during the functional maturation of fetal somatotrophs, *GHRHR* mRNA is detected at the same stage as the onset of growth hormone gene expression. Other factors involved in the development and maturation of somatotrophs include glucocorticoids, components of the adenosine monophosphate activated protein kinase pathway, hypothalamic acetylcholine signalling via neuronal M3 receptors, thyroid hormones and retinoic acid (Nogami and Hisano 2008). The mechanisms and extent of the contribution of these various factors in vivo remains to be established.

In addition, during pituitary development, there is close relationship and interplay between the development of the capillary network and the emergence of hormone-producing cells. In fact, studies of the pituitary of the *PROP1$^{-/-}$* murine model have shown that the failure of normal cell differentiation occurs in parallel with a reduction in the normal vascularisation of the pituitary and an abnormal pattern of expression of vascular endothelial factors (Ward et al. 2006). On the other hand, somatotrophs in the normal adult pituitary are in close proximity to the vascular network with clusters and strands of cells being surrounded by capillaries. Recent elegant imaging studies reveal that the organisation of somatotrophs, as well as the other hormone-producing cells, within the anterior pituitary is far from random. Somatotrophs are organised into a functional and structural network that facilitates their coordinated physiological response to different stimuli. This organisation into a cellular continuum is maintained postnatally, thus ensuring the plasticity of the system and its adaptation throughout life (Le Tissier et al. 2012).

Isolated growth hormone deficiency

The reported incidence of congenital isolated GHD is in the range of 1:4 000–10 000 live births, with the majority of cases being sporadic whilst familial cases account for anything between 3% and 30% in various studies. Depending on the pattern of inheritance, isolated GHD has been classified in four genetic types: autosomal recessive (types IA and IB),

TABLE 2.1
Genetic forms of isolated growth hormone deficiency

Type	Inheritance	Phenotype	Gene	Mutations
IA	AR	Undetectable GH; anti-GH antibodies on treatment	*GH1*	Deletions (6.7kb–7.0kb–7.6kb–45kb); frameshift, nonsense
IB	AR	Low, detectable GH; no antibodies on rhGH treatment	*GH1/GHRHR* ? other	Splice site, missense, nonsense, frameshift
II	AD	Variable short stature (severe to normal height); may have evolving endocrine deficits	*GH1*	Splice site, splice site enhancers, missense
III	X-linked	+/− intellectual disability; IGHD or in combination with other hormone deficiencies; EPP	*SOX3*	PA tract deletions, expansions; gene deletions or duplications
		Agamma/ hypogammaglobulinaemia	*BTK,* not known	

IGHD, isolated growth hormone deficiency; GH, growth hormone; AR, autosomal recessive; AD, autosomal dominant; rhGH, recombinant human GH; EPP, ectopic posterior pituitary; PA, polyalanine tract.

autosomal dominant (type II) and X-linked recessive (type III; Table 2.1; Mullis 2011). The prevalence of mutation detection depends on the cohort studied and the criteria used for defining GHD. In our cohort, we identified mutations in up to 11% of patients screened, with a higher prevalence in familial cases (34%) compared to those with sporadic isolated GHD. The commonest genes implicated in its aetiology are *GH1* and *GHRHR* (Alatzoglou and Dattani 2010).

GH1 and *GHRHR* genes

The gene encoding growth hormone (*GH1*) is located on the long arm of chromosome 17 (17q22-24) within a cluster of five homologous genes (chorionic somatomammotropin pseudogene [*CSHP*], chorionic somatomammotropin gene [*CSH-1*], *GH-2* and *CSH-2*). *GH1* consists of five exons and its full-length product is a 191 amino acid (22kDa) peptide representing about 75% of the circulating growth hormone. Alternative splicing may result in complete skipping of exon 3 and the generation of a 17.5kDa variant which lacks amino acids 32–71 and represents 1%–5% of the circulating growth hormone. Another product of aberrant splicing is the 20kDa molecule that represents 5%–10% of circulating growth hormone (Mullis 2011).

The gene encoding the receptor for GHRH (*GHRHR*) maps to chromosome 7p15 and consists of 13 exons spanning approximately 15kb. It encodes a 423 amino acid G-protein coupled receptor comprising seven trans-membrane domains. The expression of *GHRHR* is up-regulated by *POU1F1* and is required for the proliferation of somatotropes. The role

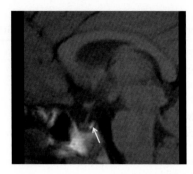

Figure 2.2. MRI of patient with isolated growth hormone deficiency Type IB because of a homozygous mutation in *GH1* (p.C182X). There is severe anterior pituitary hypoplasia with only a rim of pituitary tissue seen. The posterior pituitary is located within the sella (arrow indicates the bright spot of the posterior pituitary). (Adapted from Alatzoglou KS et al. *JCEM* 2009; 94(9): 3191–3199. Copyright 2009, The Endocrine Society, with permission.)

of *GHRHR* in the proliferation of somatotropes has been first demonstrated in a spontaneous occurring dwarf mouse model (*little* mouse) that harbours a single nucleotide substitution in codon 60 (D60G) that eliminated binding of *GHRH* to the receptor, resulting in severe anterior pituitary hypoplasia with a decrease in the number of somatotrophs.

GH1 mutations associated with growth hormone deficiency

AUTOSOMAL RECESSIVE *GH1* MUTATIONS

Homozygous *GH1* deletions of various sizes (6.5–45kb) were first described in families with severely affected members with a phenotype characterised by early severe growth failure (height standard deviation score [SDS] <−4.5), undetectable growth hormone concentrations and poor response to treatment with the development of antibodies. Similar phenotypes can result from homozygous or compound heterozygous mutations that result in a severely truncated or absent growth hormone molecule. Newer recombinant forms of human growth harmone are however more effective in promoting growth.

On the other hand, patients with type IB GHD due to *GH1* mutations also have marked short stature with low but detectable growth hormone concentrations and a good response to recombinant human growth hormone (rhGH) treatment. A number of homozygous or compound heterozygous *GH1* and *GHRHR* mutations result in this phenotype and have been reported in patients from consanguineous pedigrees or specific ethnic backgrounds (Fig 2.2).

ABNORMAL SPLICING AND DEFECTS IN GROWTH HORMONE RELEASE

The commonest genetic form of isolated GHD is autosomal-dominant (type II) isolated GHD with patients exhibiting significant variability with regard to the time of presentation and degree of growth failure that may range from severe short stature to even normal height. They have low but detectable growth hormone with or without anterior pituitary hypoplasia

18

on MRI; there is now increasing recognition that they may develop additional pituitary hormone deficiencies including adrenocorticotropic hormone (ACTH), thyroid-stimulating hormone (TSH) prolactin and gonadotrophin deficiency and require life-long follow-up. In order to explain this greatly variable and evolving phenotype, we should consider the mechanism by which heterozygous *GH1* mutations cause isolated GHD. These genetic changes result in the production of the 17.5kDa isoform at various concentrations, which in turn exerts a dominant negative effect on the production of the 22kDa molecule. In vitro and in vivo studies have demonstrated the dose-dependent deleterious effect of the 17.5kDa molecule. It is retained in the endoplasmic reticulum, triggers a mis-folded protein response and the accumulation of macrophages and results in the disruption of the Golgi apparatus and therefore impairs the trafficking and secretory pathway of growth hormone and other hormones such as ACTH, TSH and luteinizing hormone (McGuinness et al. 2003).

In addition heterozygous missense *GH1* mutations (p.P89L, p.R183H, p.V110F) have been shown to impair growth hormone release at the cellular level, affect the correct folding of the molecule or, as in the case of the p.R178H, disrupt the zinc-dependent dimerisation and packaging of growth hormone resulting in reduced secretion (Alatzoglou and Dattani 2010).

EFFECTS ON GROWTH HORMONE ACTION AND BIOACTIVITY

Heterozygous missense *GH1* mutations may also impair growth by a complex mechanism that affects not only the secretion of growth hormone but also its bioactivity. For instance, the recently reported p.R178H mutation seems to have a dual mechanism of action so that, in addition to the dimerisation of the growth hormone molecule, it also affects its binding affinity for the growth hormone receptor (GHR), resulting in reduced activation of the downstream signalling pathway (Mullis 2011).

Another heterozygous *GH1* mutation (p.R77C) has been reported in a patient with growth retardation and delayed pubertal development, who showed normal catch-up growth with rhGH replacement therapy. However, there is no clear phenotype–genotype correlation as the same mutation has also been identified in family members of normal height. Patients do not always have short stature; they may have normal or slightly increased growth hormone secretion (GHS) and low IGF-1 and growth hormone–binding protein (GHBP) concentrations. Functional studies did not show any difference between the mutant and wild-type growth hormone molecule in terms of binding to the GHR and activation of the downstream JAK2/STAT5 pathway. However, it is possible that the mutation results in reduced capability to induce the *GHR/GHBP* gene transcription, compared to the wild-type molecule (Petkovic et al. 2007). Other heterozygous missense mutations (p.P59L) may result in reduced binding affinity for the GHR and decreased activation of the downstream signalling pathway (Mullis 2011).

GHRHR mutations associated with isolated growth hormone deficiency
Wajnrajch et al. first reported two patients of a consanguineous pedigree who had severe isolated GHD resulting from a homozygous *GHRHR* mutation (p.E72X) causing premature termination and a truncated protein missing all trans-membrane domains of the receptor.

Since then a number of homozygous or compound heterozygous mutations have been reported in *GHRHR* (missense, nonsense, splice site, deletions or regulatory mutations), leading to autosomal recessive, type IB isolated GHD. Patients are usually of consanguine-ous pedigrees and of ethnic backgrounds including the Indian subcontinent, Pakistan, Sri Lanka, Somalia and Brazil. Children usually have severe growth failure with height SDS reported up to −7.4, undetectable growth hormone concentrations, a blunted growth hormone response to various stimuli with low IGF-1 and IGFBP3, and a good response to treatment with rhGH. Compared to patients with recessive *GH1* mutations, mid-facial hypoplasia, neonatal hypoglycaemia and microphallus are not common. The mean adult height for untreated patients is in the range of 130cm and 113.5cm for males and females, respectively (Alatzoglou and Dattani 2010; Mullis 2011).

Because of the role of GHRH on the proliferation of somatotroph cells, the finding of anterior pituitary hypoplasia on MRI has been considered to be almost invariable in these patients. However, recent reports suggest a variability in the size of the anterior pituitary even among family members having the same *GHRHR* mutation. This finding may be explained by the fact that patients were of different age and by the lack of well-defined age-matched reference standards. With regard to their mechanism of action, mutations in *GHRHR* may impair ligand binding and signal transduction, or affect the trafficking and localisation of the receptor to the cell membrane. Interestingly a heterozygous change in *GHRH* has been recently reported in patients with sporadic isolated GHD. Although a digenic effect cannot be excluded in these patients, it has been proposed that this may represent a novel form of isolated GHD caused by dominant mutations in *GHRHR* with variable penetrance (Godi et al. 2009).

Control of growth hormone secretion and isolated growth hormone deficiency
As mutations in known genes are identified in a relatively small percentage of patients with isolated GHD, it is conceivable that other, yet unidentified, factors are implicated in its aetiology. Among the possible candidates are factors associated with the regulation and/or secretion of growth hormone. In this respect, *GHRH* is an obvious candidate; however, a multicentre study did not identify any functionally significant changes in *GHRH* in patients with isolated GHD (Franca et al. 2011).

The GHSR is expressed in the hypothalamic-pituitary area, and its endogenous ligand, ghrelin, has a role in the regulation of the release of growth hormone. Recessive and domi-nant mutations in *GHSR* (p.W2X, p.R237W, p.A204E) have been reported to result in phenotypes that range from normal to partial GHD or isolated GHD, with a mechanism of action that is not fully elucidated but may be associated with loss of the constitutive activity of the receptor (Pantel et al. 2009). Functionally significant changes in *GHSR* are rare and the effect of its polymorphisms on the determination of height is unclear.

The muscarinic cholinergic receptor (mAchR) is another candidate as the cholinergic pathway plays a role in the regulation of GHS, with central cholinergic stimulation resulting in an increase in growth hormone release. Although no functional changes in mAchR were identified in a study of families with autosomal recessive GHD, its contribution to other types of isolated GHD cannot be excluded (Mohamadi et al. 2009).

Syndromic growth hormone deficiency

Syndromic GHD may result from mutations in early transcription factors in association with other developmental abnormalities (including variants of SOD and ocular defects), skeletal defects and intellectual impairment, with or without other pituitary hormone deficiencies.

SOX3 and X-linked growth hormone deficiency

X-linked recessive GHD has been initially reported in males in association with agammaglobulinaemia. Although the *BTK* gene has been associated with this condition, its genetic aetiology remains unknown.

SOX3, a member of the SOX (SRY-related high mobility group box) family of transcription factors, has been implicated in the aetiology of X-linked hypopituitarism with a highly variable phenotype (Table 2.2). This single exon gene maps on chromosome Xq27 and encodes a transcript that consists of a short N-terminal domain of unknown function, a 79 amino acid DNA binding high mobility group domain, and a longer C-terminal domain, containing four polyalanine stretches involved in transcriptional activation.

Patients with over- or under-dosage of *SOX3* present with isolated GHD or combined pituitary hormone deficiencies, with or without intellectual disability or learning difficulties and an ectopic/undescended posterior pituitary on MRI (Woods et al. 2005). In different pedigrees large (3.9–13Mb) or sub-microscopic (685.6kb) duplications at the Xq26-27 locus encompassing *SOX3* have been associated with the phenotype. In addition, expansion of the first polyalanine tract of *SOX3* by 7 or 11 residues or an in-frame deletion resulting in the loss of six alanine residues have been reported in association with variable phenotypes (isolated GHD or combined pituitary hormone deficiencies). In vitro experiments have shown a variable mechanism of action that could account for the phenotype. For example, polyalanine tract expansions result in reduced transcriptional activation of target genes because of retention of the mutant protein in the cytoplasm with failure of the protein to translocate to the nucleus (Woods et al. 2005). Conversely, polyalanine tract deletions result in increased transcriptional activation in vitro, and this may be comparable to increased dosage of the gene as observed with genetic duplications (Alatzoglou et al. 2011). The variability in the size of the polyalanine tract in *SOX3* is an uncommon cause of hypopituitarism or isolated GHD, and even within the same family, patients may have diverse phenotypes with or without associated intellectual disability (Burkitt Wright et al. 2009; Alatzoglou et al. 2011). To date there have been no reported point mutations in *SOX3* leading to functional compromise.

Growth hormone deficiency with ocular defects

Homozygous and heterozygous mutations in *HESX1*, a member of the paired-like family of homeodomain transcription factors, are associated with SOD. In humans, the first homozygous *HESX1* mutation was described in two siblings from a consanguineous pedigree who presented with hypopituitarism in association with SOD (optic nerve hypoplasia, absent corpus callosum and septum pellucidum) and an ectopic/undescended posterior pituitary. Homozygous and heterozygous *HESX1* mutations are an uncommon cause of

TABLE 2.2
Variable phenotypes in patients with changes in *SOX3* dosage

Mutation	Size	Endocrine phenotype	MRI	Other	References
Duplication	3.9–13Mb	GHD; panhypopituitarism	NA	Developmental delay, learning difficulties; spina bifida	Solomon et al. 2002; Hol et al. 2000
Duplication	685.6kb	GHD, evolving TSHD; panhypopituitarism	APH, EPP	No intellectual disability	Woods et al. 2005
	33bp, +11PA	IGHD	NA	Intellectual disability	Laumonnier et al. 2002
Duplication, in-frame		Panhypopituitarism	APH, EPP	No intellectual disability	Woods et al. 2005
	+7PA	IGHD	APH, EPP	Intellectual disability or normal intelligence	Burkitt Wright et al. 2009; Alatzoglou et al. 2011
Deletion, in frame	del9PA	Not reported	Not available	Intellectual disability	Laumonnier et al. 2002
	18bp, del6PA	GHD, TSHD, GnD	Enlarged AP with cystic lesion, small corpus callosum; normal stalk and PP	Female patient, normal intelligence	Alatzoglou et al. 2011
SOX3 gene deletion	2.3Mb	GHD, TSHD, GnD	APH, normal PP; persistent craniopharyngeal canal	Haemophilia B, developmental delay	Alatzoglou et al. 2014

PA, polyalanine tract; del denotes deletion; + denotes expansion; GHD, growth hormone deficiency; IGHD, isolated growth hormone deficiency; TSHD, thyroid-stimulating hormone (thyrotrophin) deficiency; GnD, gonadotrophin deficiency; AP, anterior pituitary; APH, anterior pituitary hypoplasia; EPP, ectopic posterior pituitary; NA, not available.

hypopituitarism and SOD (less than 1% of cases) and have since been described in patients with highly variable phenotypes without obvious genotype–phenotype correlation. On rare occasions heterozygous *HESX1* mutations (p.E149K, p.S170L or p.T181A) may be associated with isolated GHD. These patients exhibit a relatively milder phenotype compared with the severe manifestations of SOD, and they may or may not have optic nerve hypoplasia. They have an ectopic/undescended posterior pituitary on MRI, and anterior pituitary hypoplasia is common but not always present (as in the cases of the p.S170L mutation; Thomas et al. 2001; McCabe et al. 2011).

OTX2 (orthodentic homeobox 2) is another early transcription factor, important for the formation of anterior structures and the forebrain that has been implicated in the aetiology of 2%–3% of anophthalmia/microphthalmia syndromes in humans. To date more than 20 heterozygous mutations have been reported in patients with variable ocular malformations. The reported pituitary phenotype of patients with heterozygous *OTX2* mutations ranges from partial to complete GHD or hypopituitarism with or without an ectopic posterior pituitary on MRI. In rare cases, patients may not even exhibit an ocular phenotype (p.N233S). Even among patients with the same mutation (p.S188X), there is no clear genotype–phenotype correlation, as they may present with hypopituitarism or even normal pituitary function (Dateki et al. 2010). Ashkenazi et al. reported a heterozygous *OTX2* mutation (p.R90S) in a patient with unilateral anophthalmia and learning difficulties in association with isolated GHD, a hypoplastic anterior pituitary and an ectopic posterior pituitary on MRI. A similar phenotype has been reported in a patient with a 15 base pair deletion leading to frameshift (c.221_236del15). On the other hand, a heterozygous whole gene deletion has been described in a patient with isolated GHD, bilateral ocular defects and anterior pituitary hypoplasia but with a normally positioned posterior pituitary on MRI. Because of lack of follow-up data, it is not clear if in these cases the manifested GHD will remain as the only endocrine deficit or if additional pituitary hormone deficiencies will develop over time (Ashkenazi-Hoffnung et al. 2010; Dateki et al. 2010).

GHD may also be part of the endocrine phenotype in patients with heterozygous *SOX2* mutations. *SOX2*, as the previously described *SOX3*, is a single exon gene and member of the SOX family of transcription factors. Heterozygous de novo mutations have been initially reported in patients with bilateral anophthalmia or severe microphthalmia in association with other developmental defects (oesophageal atresia, genitourinary tract abnormalities, spastic diplegia, developmental delay). Subsequently we showed that *SOX2* haploinsufficiency was associated with hypogonadotrophic hypogonadism, sensorineural hearing loss, anterior pituitary hypoplasia and variable structural defects on MRI (hippocampal abnormalities, defects of the corpus callosum, hypothalamic hamartomas or slow-progressing hypothalamo-pituitary tumours); GHD may rarely be part of the endocrine spectrum (Kelberman et al. 2009).

Recently, Jayakody et al. generated a transgenic murine model with selective absence of *SOX2* in the developing Rathke's pouch. These embryos survived to birth but had significant anterior pituitary hypoplasia detectable from E12.5 to E14.5, with normal intermediate and posterior lobes, and had a marked reduction in the expression of *POU1F1* with severe disruption of the differentiation of somatotrophs and thyrotrophs. In this model the reduced proliferation of perilumenal progenitors probably results in a reduced pool of undif-ferentiated precursors, which is insufficient to allow the subsequent differentiation of enough numbers of hormone-producing cells at late gestation, leading to reduced numbers of somatotrophs and severe pituitary hypoplasia (Jayakody et al. 2012). The observation that at least some patients with *SOX2* mutations manifest GHD in addition to hypogonado-trophic hypogonadism supports this notion.

In humans, mutations in *PITX2* are associated with Axenfeld–Rieger syndrome, a het-erogeneous disorder characterised by malformation of the anterior segment of the eye (hypoplasia of the iris, corneal abnormalities), dental hypoplasia, craniofacial and brain abnormalities and a protuberant umbilicus. Some of the reported patients to date have reduced growth hormone concentration and anterior pituitary hypoplasia, whilst others may have an abnormal sella turcica but without endocrine deficit. Although these observations suggest a role for *PITX2* in pituitary development, its importance and contribution remain to be identified (Kelberman et al. 2009).

Growth hormone deficiency caused by mutations in other early transcription factors and novel genes

In case of mutations affecting other transcription factors implicated in the early stages of pituitary development, GHD, resulting in growth failure, is one of the commonest, if not the first, manifestation. For example, a defect in the development of somatotrophs and GHD, in association with other deficits (TSH, gonadotrophin or prolactin deficiency with/without ACTH deficiency), are constant findings in patients with recessive mutations in *LHX3*. The pituitary MRI may reveal a normal, hypoplastic or enlarged anterior pituitary. Other associated features may include a short neck with limited rotation, spinal abnormali-ties and variable sensorineural hearing loss (Pfaffle and Klammt 2011).

All reported patients with heterozygous *LHX4* mutations had GHD and short stature on presentation, in association with variable endocrine deficits (ACTH, TSH, gonadotro-phin deficiency) or panhypopituitarism. However, there is remarkable variability in the phenotype even within the same family, ranging from panhypopituitarism to GHD with partial TSH deficiency or even partial GHD and short stature, diagnosed later in life, with no additional hormone deficiencies in a parent (Pfaffle and Klammt 2011). Neuroradiologic findings include a hypoplastic, normal or enlarged anterior pituitary, a hypoplastic corpus callosum and Chiari malformation, with almost a third of cases having an ectopic posterior pituitary. Neck rotation and hearing are normal. More recently, the first homozygous mis-sense *LHX4* variant (c.377C>T, p.T126M) was reported in siblings from a consanguineous pedigree who were born small for gestational age and had severe panhypopituitarism with anterior pituitary aplasia and an ectopic/undescended posterior pituitary, and all died within the first week of life (Gregory et al. 2015b).

GHD may be one of the clinical manifestations in patients with mutations in compo-nents of the sonic hedgehog signalling pathway. For instance a heterozygous *GLI2* variant (c1552G>A; p.E518K) was reported in a patient with GHD and a low normal free T4 who had anterior pituitary hypoplasia and an absent posterior pituitary on MRI (Gregory et al. 2015a). In addition, a 26.6Mb deletion encompassing *GLI2* and other genes was reported in a patient with developmental delay, short stature and impaired growth who had a small anterior pituitary and a cavum septum pellucidum but a normal posterior pituitary (Gregory et al. 2015a). Heterozygous *GLI2* variants have been reported in a number of patients with variable phenotypes ranging from panhypopituitarism to isolated GHD, with/without an ectopic posterior pituitary on MRI or other clinical features such as midline clefts or poly-dactyly (Flemming et al. 2013; Franca et al. 2013; Arnhold et al. 2015). Mutations in known genes account for only a small percentage of congenital GHD. The detailed phenotypic study of families with GHD and the application of novel techniques, such as whole exome sequencing (WES), will result in the identification of novel genes involved in various steps of the development of the anterior pituitary gland or the control and secretion of growth hormone, resulting in the clinical manifestation of GHD. A recent example is the identifica-tion of biallelic *RNPC3* mutations in three sisters with severe isolated GHD who presented with postnatal growth failure (height SDS between −5 and −6.6) and mild microcephaly (Argente et al. 2014). The patients had undetectable stimulated growth hormone and basal IGF-1 and IGFBP-3 concentrations, with a low-normal prolactin and anterior pituitary hypoplasia on MRI, whilst the other pituitary hormones were not affected at the time of diagnosis. The probands were compound heterozygous for a missense (c.1320C>A, p.P474T) and nonsense (c.1504C>T, p.R502X) mutation in *RNPC3* and their unaffected parents were heterozygous carriers (Argente et al. 2014). *RNPC3* codes for a 65-kDa protein of the minor spliceosome (U11/U12-65K protein) that is essential for the intron-recognition complex. These mutations that were shown to have a deleterious effect on the stability of the complex were the first reported in patients with GHD, thus representing a novel genetic aetiology for congenital GHD.

Growth hormone deficiency and mutations in late transcription factors
Apart from mutations in the above-mentioned early transcription factors, GHD may be the first or only manifestation of genetic defects in factors involved in later stages of the dif-ferentiation of the cells of the somatotroph lineage.

As already mentioned, the activation of *PROP1* is required for the emergence of the gonadotroph lineage, as well as for cells of the *POU1F1* lineage, that include somatotrophs, lactotrophs and thyrotrophs. The Ames dwarf mouse (*df*) has a naturally occurring mutation in the homeodomain of *PROP1* that lowers its binding activity to DNA; targeted deletion of *PROP1* in transgenic murine models (*df/df*) results in animals deficient in growth hormone, prolactin, TSH and gonadotrophins. In humans, mutations in *PROP1* are the most common genetic cause of combined pituitary hormone deficiencies, with mutations being identified in up to 60% of familial cases, with a lower incidence in sporadic cases. Homo-zygous *PROP1* mutations are typically associated with growth hormone, TSH, prolactin and gonadotrophin deficiency, although the timing and extent of the hormone deficits vary considerably and the full phenotype may not be evident from the outset. For instance, patients with a homozygous *PROP1* mutation (p.R120C) may first present in childhood with GHD before the development of TSH, prolactin and gonadotrophin deficiency later in life. In rare cases, somatotroph function may be retained, as in the report of a patient who attained normal final height without growth hormone replacement (Prince et al. 2011).

With regard to *POU1F1*, studies of two naturally occurring murine mutants have shed light on the function and phenotypes associated with mutations in this gene. In humans, autosomal recessive and dominant *POU1F1* mutations are associated with GHD, manifesting as a severe growth deficit in the first years of life, prolactin and variable TSH deficiency with a hypoplastic anterior pituitary. However, we have reported on an adult patient with isolated GHD and a hypoplastic anterior pituitary who, although was homozygous for a *POU1F1* mutation (p.E230K), did not develop other pituitary hormone deficiencies (Turton et al. 2005).

Acquired disorders of the hypothalamo-pituitary axis

Growth failure may be the first manifestation of a number of pathological conditions affecting the hypothalamo-pituitary axis, ranging from tumours to infection, vascular causes or damage secondary to trauma, surgery or irradiation (Table 2.3).

Tumours of the hypothalamo-pituitary area may cause endocrine deficits and growth failure either directly (mass effect, direct pressure, reduced synthesis and transport of hypothalamic-releasing hormones) or secondary to treatment (surgery, radiotherapy). Growth failure and endocrine disorders are the first presenting symptoms in about one-third of patients with tumours of the hypothalamo-pituitary area, before the development of neuro-ophthalmic signs; however, the endocrine manifestations are easily missed resulting in delayed diagnosis (Taylor et al. 2012).

In children, craniopharyngiomas are the most common neoplasm of the hypothalamo-pituitary area, accounting for up to 80% of tumours in this location and 5%–15% of

TABLE 2.3
Acquired causes of growth hormone deficiency

Tumours in/around pituitary area	Craniopharyngioma, pituitary adenoma, germinoma, optic glioma, dysgerminoma, ependymoma, meningioma, metastatic tumours (childhood Hodgkin disease, nasopharyngeal carcinoma)
Cystic lesions	Rathke's cleft cyst, arachnoid, dermoid
Cranial irradiation	Radiotherapy for CNS tumours, haematologic malignancies or bone marrow transplant
Traumatic brain injury	Post-accident, neurosurgery, child abuse
Vascular insults	Subarachnoid hemorrhage, pituitary apoplexy, other vascular causes
Inflammation/infection	Meningitis, encephalitis, pituitary abscess, sarcoidosis, tuberculosis, autoimmune processes (lymphocytic hypophysitis)
Infiltration	Langerhans cell histiocytosis, iron overload (haemochromatosis, thalasaemia)
Psychosocial deprivation	

GHD, growth hormone deficiency; CNS, central nervous system.

intracranial tumours. Craniopharyngiomas are rare, sporadic, epithelial tumours of embryonal origin derived from remnants of Rathke's pouch; the most commonly encountered type in children is adamantinomatous craniopharyngioma (ACP). Although ACPs are histologically benign, they have the tendency to infiltrate vital surrounding tissues, including the hypothalamus and optic chiasm, making their complete excision difficult, if not impossible, with increased incidence of tumour recurrence (Karavitaki et al. 2006; Muller 2014).

Activating mutations in the gene encoding β-catenin (*CTNNB1*), a component of the Wnt-signalling pathway, have long been identified in ACPs. However, a recent breakthrough in the understanding of the molecular pathogenesis of ACPs is the generation of a murine model that expresses a degradation-resistant mutant form of β-catenin in early progenitors of Rathke's pouch. Most mutant mice die perinatally by 4 weeks age and those that survive exhibit pituitary hyperplasia and marked hypopituitarism with severe disruption of the differentiation of the POU1F1-lineage, resulting in extreme growth retardation. Ultimately all animals develop lethal pituitary tumours which closely resemble human ACPs. The tumorigenic effect of the activated mutant β-catenin is observed only when it is expressed in undifferentiated progenitors and not when committed or differentiated cells are targeted to express the protein. This demonstrates that mutated β-catenin in pituitary progenitor/stem cells has a causative role in the aetiology of murine tumours resembling human ACPs (Gaston-Massuet et al. 2011). The development of a murine model for human ACPs will have implications for further studies on the pathogenesis and treatment of ACPs.

With regard to the other tumours affecting the hypothalamo-pituitary area, pituitary adenomas represent less than 3% of supratentorial tumours in childhood and about 3.5%–6% of all surgically treated paediatric pituitary tumours. In most cases, they are hormonally active, arising from any of the five cell types of the anterior pituitary, with corticotrophinomas being the commonest in pre-pubertal children, whilst non-functioning pituitary adenomas are rare (2.7%). Pituitary adenomas occur in isolation or may be part of a genetic syndrome, such as multiple endocrine neoplasia type 1, McCune–Albright syndrome or Carney complex. Their clinical presentation results from pituitary hormone hypersecretion or deficiencies, disruption of growth and sexual maturation and pressure effects. For example, in the case of Cushing disease caused by an ACTH-secreting pituitary adenoma, there is a characteristic growth pattern of short stature (height SDS less than −2 in 40%) with a discrepancy between height and BMI SDS (Savage and Storr 2014; Nieman et al. 2015). The pathogenesis of pituitary adenomas is not clear but there is evidence that dysregulation in hormone receptor signalling and changes in molecules that regulate cell cycle or are important for adhesion to the extracellular matrix, as well as changes in growth factors, may be implicated. GHD is the second commonest endocrinopathy in patients with Langerhans cell histiocytosis, occurring in almost 40% of patients who have pituitary involvement. In these cases, GHD is commonly associated with diabetes insipidus, with a median interval of 3–3.5 years between the diagnosis of diabetes insipidus and the development of GHD (Taylor et al. 2012).

Insult to the hypothalamo-pituitary-somatotroph axis may also occur after serious traumatic brain injury. GHD and hypopituitarism may manifest months or even years after a serious traumatic brain injury, but the extent and characteristics of this potential complication in the paediatric population are still unknown. In the reported cases, somatotroph cells are the most vulnerable (85%), followed by gonadotrophs (80%), thyrotrophs (75%) and corticotrophs (50%). The majority of patients have multiple anterior pituitary hormone deficiencies, with rare cases having isolated GHD. At least in some cases, there is evidence that the presenting hypopituitarism is of hypothalamic origin, but irrespective of the mechanism, growth failure is the presenting symptom in more than half of patients, followed by delayed or arrested puberty. However, in the majority of cases the diagnosis of hypopituitarism is considered with extreme delay, with the potential serious implications of the undiagnosed pituitary deficiency (Einaudi and Bondone 2007).

Conclusion

Congenital and acquired disorders can affect the hypothalamo-pituitary-somatotroph axis and manifest as growth failure. There is increasing understanding that genetic factors may affect the axis at multiple levels and have a digenic/oligogenic effect. The development of transgenic animal models not only helps to elucidate the mechanisms implicated in normal pituitary development and the genetic causes of GHD, but may also provide a tool for the understanding and even treatment of other disorders affecting the hypothalamo-pituitary axis such as ACPs. The identification of novel genes implicated in the genetic aetiology of GHD and their diverse mechanisms of action will challenge the 'traditional' classification of congenital isolated GHD.

REFERENCES

Alatzoglou KS, Azriyanti A, Rogers N et al. (2014) SOX3 deletion in mouse and human is associated with persistence of the craniopharyngeal canal. *J Clin Endocrinol Metab* 99: E2702–E2708.

Alatzoglou KS and Dattani MT (2010) Genetic causes and treatment of isolated growth hormone deficiency- an update. *Nat Rev Endocrinol* 6: 562–576.

Alatzoglou KS, Kelberman D, Cowell CT et al. (2011) Increased transactivation associated with SOX3 polyalanine tract deletion in a patient with hypopituitarism. *J Clin Endocrinol Metab* 96: E685–E690.

Argente J, Flores R, Gutierrez-Arumi A et al. (2014) Defective minor spliceosome mRNA processing results in isolated familial growth hormone deficiency. *EMBO Mol Med* 6: 299–306.

Arnhold IJ, Franca MM, Carvalho LR, Mendonca BB and Jorge AA (2015) Role of GLI2 in hypopituitarism phenotype. *J Mol Endocrinol* 54: R141–R150.

Ashkenazi-Hoffnung L, Lebenthal Y, Wyatt AW et al. (2010) A novel loss-of-function mutation in OTX2 in a patient with anophthalmia and isolated growth hormone deficiency. *Hum Genet* 127: 721–729.

Burkitt Wright EM, Perveen R, Clayton PE et al. (2009) X-linked isolated growth hormone deficiency: Expanding the phenotypic spectrum of SOX3 polyalanine tract expansions. *Clin Dysmorphol* 18: 218–221.

Dateki S, Kosaka K, Hasegawa K et al. (2010) Heterozygous orthodenticle homeobox 2 mutations are associated with variable pituitary phenotype. *J Clin Endocrinol Metab* 95: 756–764.

Einaudi S and Bondone C (2007) The effects of head trauma on hypothalamic-pituitary function in children and adolescents. *Curr Opin Pediatr* 19: 465–470.

Flemming GM, Klammt J, Ambler G et al. (2013) Functional characterization of a heterozygous GLI2 missense mutation in patients with multiple pituitary hormone deficiency. *J Clin Endocrinol Metab* 98: E567–E575.

Franca MM, Jorge AA, Alatzoglou KS et al. (2011) Absence of GH-releasing hormone (GHRH) mutations in selected patients with isolated GH deficiency. *J Clin Endocrinol Metab* 96: E1457–E1460.

Franca MM, Jorge AA, Carvalho LR et al. (2013) Relatively high frequency of non-synonymous GLI2 variants in patients with congenital hypopituitarism without holoprosencephaly. *Clin Endocrinol (Oxford)* 78: 551–557.

Gaston-Massuet C, Andoniadou CL, Signore M et al. (2011) Increased Wingless (Wnt) signaling in pituitary progenitor/stem cells gives rise to pituitary tumors in mice and humans. *Proc Natl Acad Sci U.S.A* 108: 11482–11487.

Godi M, Mellone S, Petri A et al. (2009) A recurrent signal peptide mutation in the growth hormone releasing hormone receptor with defective translocation to the cell surface and isolated growth hormone deficiency. *J Clin Endocrinol Metab* 94: 3939–3947.

Gregory LC, Gaston-Massuet C, Andoniadou CL et al. (2015a) The role of the sonic hedgehog signalling pathway in patients with midline defects and congenital hypopituitarism. *Clin Endocrinol (Oxford)* 82: 728–738.

Gregory LC, Humayun KN, Turton JP, McCabe MJ, Rhodes SJ and Dattani MT (2015b) Novel lethal form of congenital hypopituitarism associated with the rirst recessive LHX4 mutation. *J Clin Endocrinol Metab* 100: 2158–2164.

Hol FA, Schepens MT, van Beersum SE et al. (2000) Identification and characterization of an Xq26-q27 duplication in a family with spina bifida and panhypopituitarism suggests the involvement of two distinct genes. *Genomics* 69: 174–181.

Jayakody SA, Andoniadou CL, Gaston-Massuet C et al. (2012) SOX2 regulates the hypothalamic-pituitary axis at multiple levels. *J Clin Invest* 122: 3635–3646.

Karavitaki N, Cudlip S, Adams CB and Wass JA (2006) Craniopharyngiomas. *Endocr Rev* 27: 371–397.

Kelberman D, Rizzoti K, Lovell-Badge R, Robinson IC and Dattani MT (2009) Genetic regulation of pituitary gland development in human and mouse. *Endocr Rev* 30: 790–829.

Laumonnier F, Ronce N, Hamel BC et al. (2002) Transcription factor SOX3 is involved in X-linked mental retardation with growth hormone deficiency. *Am J Hum Genet* 71: 1450–1455.

Le Tissier PR, Hodson DJ, Lafont C, Fontanaud P, Schaeffer M and Mollard P (2012) Anterior pituitary cell networks. *Front Neuroendocrinol* 33: 252–266.

McCabe MJ, Alatzoglou KS and Dattani MT (2011) Septo-optic dysplasia and other midline defects: The role of transcription factors: HESX1 and beyond. *Best Pract Res Clin Endocrinol Metab* 25: 115–124.

Mohamadi A, Martari M, Holladay CD, Phillips JA III, Mullis PE and Salvatori R (2009) Mutation analysis of the muscarinic cholinergic receptor genes in isolated growth hormone deficiency type IB. *J Clin Endocrinol Metab* 94: 2565–2570.

Muller HL (2014) Craniopharyngioma. *Endocr Rev* 35: 513–543.

Mullis PE (2011) Genetics of GHRH, GHRH-receptor, GH and GH-receptor: Its impact on pharmacogenetics. *Best Pract Res Clin Endocrinol Metab* 25: 25–41.

Nieman LK, Biller BM, Findling JW et al. (2015) Treatment of Cushing's syndrome: An endocrine society clinical practice guideline. *J Clin Endocrinol Metab* 100: 2807–2831.

Nogami H and Hisano S (2008) Functional maturation of growth hormone cells in the anterior pituitary gland of the fetus. *Growth Horm IGF Res* 18: 379–388.

Pantel J, Legendre M, Nivot S et al. (2009) Recessive isolated growth hormone deficiency and mutations in the ghrelin receptor. *J Clin Endocrinol Metab* 94: 4334–4341.

Pfaffle R and Klammt J (2011) Pituitary transcription factors in the aetiology of combined pituitary hormone deficiency. *Best Pract Res Clin Endocrinol Metab* 25: 43–60.

Prince KL, Walvoord EC and Rhodes SJ (2011) The role of homeodomain transcription factors in heritable pituitary disease. *Nat Rev Endocrinol* 7: 727–737.

Savage MO and Storr HL (2014) Fundamental principles of clinical and biochemical evaluation underlie the diagnosis and therapy of Cushing's syndrome. *J Pediatr Endocrinol Metab* 27: 1029–1031.

Solomon NM, Nouri S, Warne GL, Lagerstrom-Fermer M, Forrest SM and Thomas PQ (2002) Increased gene dosage at Xq26-q27 is associated with X-linked hypopituitarism. *Genomics* 79: 553–559.

Taylor M, Couto-Silva AC, Adan L et al. (2012) Hypothalamic-pituitary lesions in pediatric patients: endocrine symptoms often precede neuro-ophthalmic presenting symptoms. *J Pediatr* 161: 855–863.

Thomas PQ, Dattani MT, Brickman JM et al. (2001) Heterozygous HESX1 mutations associated with isolated congenital pituitary hypoplasia and septo-optic dysplasia. *Hum Mol Genet* 10: 39–45.

Turton JP, Reynaud R, Mehta A et al. (2005) Novel mutations within the POU1F1 gene associated with variable combined pituitary hormone deficiency. *J Clin Endocrinol Metab* 90: 4762–4770.

Woods KS, Cundall M, Turton J et al. (2005) Over- and underdosage of SOX3 is associated with infundibular hypoplasia and hypopituitarism. *Am J Hum Genet* 76: 833–849.

3

THE EFFECT OF GROWTH HORMONE ON THE BRAIN

Fred Nyberg, Alfhild Grönbladh, Erika Brolin, Anna Jonsson, Jenny Johansson and Mathias Hallberg

Introduction

Growth hormone is recognised as one of the major hormonal compounds produced by somatotrophs in the anterior pituitary. The human variant of growth hormone consists of a single polypeptide chain of 191 amino acids. Its secretion is controlled by the hypothalamic hormones, growth hormone–releasing hormone (GHRH) and somatostatin. Whereas GHRH stimulates its release, somatostatin acts an inhibitor of growth hormone secretion (GHS). Several other peptides known to elicit stimulatory effects on growth hormone release, for example, ghrelin, have also been described. Growth hormone regulates its own secretion through interactions with catecholamines in the median eminence of the hypothalamus (Andersson et al. 1983).

The three-dimensional structure of growth hormone is stabilised by two disulfide bonds and includes four helices that are required for functional interaction with its receptor (de Vos et al. 1992). The growth hormone receptor (GHR) is a single membrane-spanning cell surface protein member of the class 1 cytokine receptor superfamily. Like other members of the family, GHR lacks intrinsic kinase activity, and signal transduction is mediated by phosphorylation of Janus kinase (JAK)2, a cytoplasmic tyrosine kinase that associates to the so-called box 1 in the membrane proximal region of the GHR cytoplasmic domain (Carter-Su et al. 1994). Binding of growth hormone to GHR induces receptor dimerisation and the activation of the intracellular signal transduction pathway leading to Stat5b phosphorylation, and thereby the effects of growth hormone (Carter-Su et al. 2015).

It is widely agreed that the major effect of growth hormone is to promote growth and metabolism. Thus, the hormone is known to stimulate muscle and bone growth. It also promotes lipolysis and reduces liver uptake of glucose. It is known to exert many of its effects through its two mediators insulin-like growth factor-1 (IGF-1) and IGF-2. Growth hormone exerts some of its effects by binding to receptors on target cells, where it activates the MAPK/ERK or the JAK/STAT pathways. The production of IGF-1 is stimulated through the JAK/STAT pathway (Carter-Su et al. 2015).

During the past decades the effects that growth hormone may exert on the central nervous system (CNS) have received attention among many investigators. A variety of

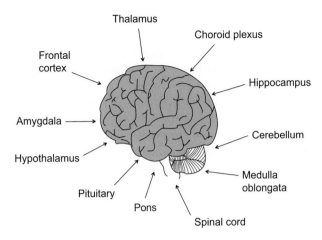

Figure 3.1. Brain regions expressing growth hormone receptor gene transcripts.

clinical studies have reported beneficial effects of the hormone on cognitive functions. Growth hormone replacement therapy in children as well as in adult patients with growth hormone deficiency (GHD) has been shown to induce significant improvements in alertness, cognitive capabilities and psychological well-being (Arwert et al. 2006; Geisler et al. 2012; Chaplin et al. 2015). Experimental animal studies have shown that growth hormone treatment may restore behavioural abnormalities induced by various drugs and impaired pituitary function (Le Greves et al. 2006; Gronbladh et al. 2012; Nyberg and Hallberg 2013).

An important contribution to the understanding of all effects seen for growth hormone on brain function comes from the discovery and characterisation of GHR in the CNS (for review, see [Nyberg 2000]). Thus, specific binding sites for the hormone have been identified in brain areas related to various behaviours influenced by growth hormone treatment (Fig 3.1). Studies on CNS circuits that are affected by stimulation of these receptor sites have contributed new knowledge about the mechanisms involved in growth hormone actions on the brain (Nyberg and Hallberg 2013).

Another issue to which attention should be paid is the route by which growth hormone may reach its responsive sites in the brain. In this respect, it is necessary to discuss the relevance of local production of growth hormone within certain areas of the CNS as well as the ability of the hormone to penetrate the blood–brain barrier (BBB).

This chapter aims to give a brief review about current knowledge of growth hormone effects on brain function. It will highlight characteristics of growth hormone–responsive targets in the CNS and discuss mechanisms behind interactions of the hormone with various signal systems of importance for the CNS behaviours attributed to the hormone. A particular focus will be on the ability of growth hormone to promote neuroprotection and to restore drug-induced brain damage. In particular, growth hormone replacement has been demonstrated to promote cognitive capabilities.

Evidence for growth hormone to cross biological barriers to reach its targets in the brain

An important aspect related to the actions of growth hormone on its brain targets concerns its ability to penetrate the BBB or the blood–cerebrospinal fluid (CSF) barrier (BCB). Over the past decades, clinical observations have suggested that the hormone may induce profound effects on the CNS. This is indicated by studies confirming that growth hormone replacement in children with GHD induces several psychological improvements, such as increased attention and visual-spatial memory (Huisman et al. 2008). Indeed, IQ score and educational level are suggested to correlate positively to the serum concentrations of IGF-1, considered as a serum marker for the growth hormone status (Rosen et al. 1994; Deijen et al. 1996). Also, in adult patients with GHD, treatment with the hormone has been demonstrated to affect brain function.

Further evidence favouring an ability of the hormone to cross the BBB or the BCB comes from studies of the CSF concentrations of growth hormone and IGF-1. Growth hormone replacement in adults has confirmed increased concentrations of both growth hormone and IGF-1 in CSF (Johansson et al. 1995). Moreover, following growth hormone therapy, a positive correlation between the exogenous dose of growth hormone and the detected concentration of the hormone in the CSF has been reported (Burman et al. 1996).

Furthermore, the presence of specific binding sites for growth hormone in many areas within the CNS (Nyberg 2000) provides logical evidence for the ability of the hormone to penetrate the BBB or BCB. To successfully reach its responsive sites in the brain, the pituitary-secreted hormone should be able to leave the circulatory system and cross the BBB or the BCB. In this context it should be mentioned that it has also been speculated that the hormone may be locally produced in the brain. For instance, evidence for a local production of growth hormone has been demonstrated in the adult hippocampal formation since its gene transcript was identified in this brain area (Donahue et al. 2006). Earlier, the hormone was identified in brain tissues using immunological techniques (Hojvat et al. 1982).

The mechanism underlying the penetrance of growth hormone through the BBB has been discussed. It is generally believed that the high density of growth hormone binding in the choroid plexus is compatible with a receptor-mediated mechanism for the hormone to cross the BBB (Coculescu 1999). Further evidence that growth hormone may cross the BBB has emerged from studies using cell systems, where it was indicated that the hormone may passively diffuse into the brain (Pan et al. 2005). The growth hormone mediator IGF-1 was shown to cross the BBB via a saturable transport system, and was detected in the brain 20 minutes following intravenous injection (Pan and Kastin 2000). Another route for growth hormone to reach the brain is related to its regulatory function of its own release. Thus, the hormone may reach the brain and directly interact with neurons in the median eminence.

An alternative pathway for growth hormone to produce effects on the CNS, which has also been considered, is that the hormone may release mediators from peripheral tissues or organs, which in turn may cross the BBB. One example of this is, as mentioned above, the growth factor, IGF-1, which easily penetrates the BBB to find its receptors in the brain. Indeed, high densities of IGF-1 receptors have been identified in the CNS (Werther et al. 1989).

Growth hormone receptors in the brain

The presence of specific receptor sites for growth hormone in the brain (Fig 3.1) has been documented by a number of studies performed over the past decades (for review, see Nyberg [2000]). Specific binding sites have been characterised both in human (Lai et al. 1991, 1993) and the rat (Zhai et al. 1994) brain. The expression of the GHR gene transcript in various brain areas of both humans and rodents has been confirmed (Thornwall-Le Greves et al. 2001; Le Greves et al. 2006). The cDNA sequence of GHR in the rat hippocampus, hypothalamus and spinal cord has been elucidated (Le Greves et al. 2006).

By sodium dodecyl-sulfate gel electrophoresis of the cross-linked growth hormone–GHR complex, the molecular weight of the GHR protein in various brain regions was estimated in both human (Lai et al. 1991, 1993) and rat (Zhai et al. 1994). It was found that the brain protein differed in size compared to that predicted from the liver variant of GHR (Lai et al. 1993). However, cloning experiments indicated that the DNA sequence of *GHR* in the brain did not differ from that determined for the gene in the peripheral liver (Le Greves et al. 2006). From these observations it was suggested that the brain entity represented a truncated form of the hormone.

Regarding the distribution of GHR within the CNS it is obvious that GHR is expressed in several brain areas as well as in the spinal cord (Lai et al. 1993; Zhai et al. 1994; Nyberg 2000). High density of growth hormone binding is present in choroid plexus, hippocampus, hypothalamus and the pituitary. Of note, a particularly high density of growth hormone binding is found in choroid plexus, both in human and in rat (Zhai et al. 1994; Nyberg 2000).

The somatotrophic axis interacts with brain circuits involved in various behaviours

In addition to its involvement in the hypothalamic regulation of its own release, growth hormone seems to have targets related to various behaviours in many other regions of the brain. The specific binding sites and the messages of the receptor proteins identified in the above-mentioned brain structures reveal that the hormone may be implicated in several important brain functions. They may also be essential for many aspects related to the modifiable brain. These aspects have been recognised in several processes that occur in the brain during degeneration as well as protection. One important aspect is ageing.

GROWTH HORMONE AND IGF-1 AND THEIR ROLE IN THE AGEING PROCESS

Of the changes in human that are related to ageing, hypofunction in the growth hormone/IGF-1 axis provides a most pronounced example. The decline in the somatotrophic axis may account for several of the alterations in brain function that are observed during ageing and that concern physiological capabilities. There is a spectrum of potential alterations linked to GHD that can be attributed to many of these inabilities, both in elderly and in adolescents and young adults. The impaired cognitive functions observed in humans – decreased mood and well-being, sleep deprivation, decreased motor abilities, decreased energy and decreased motivation – are conditions associated with a waning release of growth hormone that subsequently leads to a decrease in circulating IGF-1. These disabilities all contribute to an impaired quality of life (Giordano et al. 2005). The decline in the secretion of growth hormone with increasing age is generally mirrored by a concomitant decrease in the concentration of IGF-1 in plasma. IGF-1 is the best marker of growth hormone status. Furthermore, the decline in the pituitary secretion of growth hormone in humans is accompanied by a corresponding decline in the expression levels of the *GHR* gene transcript (Nyberg 2000) as well as in the density of the GHR protein in the brain (Lai et al. 1991, 1993).

GROWTH HORMONE AND ITS MEDIATOR IGF-1 ARE SHOWN TO INDUCE NEUROPROTECTIVE EFFECTS
The neuroprotective effects of both growth hormone and IGF-1 are well documented. It seems that a growing body of evidence suggests that the somatotrophic axis is integrally involved not only in the growth and development of the normal CNS but also in the repair of trauma to the brain and spinal cord (Torres Aleman 2005; Harvey et al. 2009; Nyberg 2009). Several of the neuroprotective effects reported for growth hormone and IGF-1 emerged from effects of these substances on adult cell genesis (Anderson et al. 2002; Aberg et al. 2006; Aberg 2010). For instance, in the hippocampus, IGF-1 was shown to promote oligodendrocyte recruitment and increase newborn cells with the endothelial phenotype. These effects on the endothelial cell phenotype induced by IGF-1 may provide an explanation of the observed enhancement in the cerebral arteriole density that follows the administration of growth hormone (Anderson et al. 2002). These observations emphasise that IGF-1 has the capacity to act as a regenerative agent in the CNS. On the other hand, growth hormone, which is less studied in this context, is also suggested to exert similar effects, probably through its ability to release IGF-1 (Le Greves et al. 2005).

Brain injury in experimental rats may induce the IGF-1 gene transcript within reactive microglia. The translation product, the IGF-1 protein, may have a dual role (Scheepens et al. 2000). First, the growth factor may act directly on the stressed cells as an agent that is neurotrophic and anti-apoptotic. In a second phase, IGF-1 may act as a prohormone for the generation of two active peptides, the tripeptide Gly-Pro-Glu, released from the N-terminal of IGF-1, and the remaining sequence of IGF-1, the des-N-(1–3) IGF-1. Notably, both these IGF-1 fragments were found to possess specific neuroprotective properties (Scheepens et al. 2000). The same study also revealed that injections of growth hormone into the CNS 2 hours subsequent to a hypoxic-ischemic brain injury in juvenile rats indeed gave rise to significant neuroprotection, in areas distinct from the neuroprotective effect induced by IGF-1. It was also reported that some of the neuroprotective effects of growth hormone are mediated directly through the GHR without any involvement of IGF-1 (Scheepens et al. 2000). It was suggested in a latter study that smaller peptide fragments, derived from IGF-1, could have advantages over growth factors in the treatment of brain injury (Guan and Gluckman 2009). It is possible that these peptide fragments could be modified and designed with suitable properties to overcome many of the limitations associated with tentative endogenous peptides with respect to their potential role as pharmaceutical agents (Guan and Gluckman 2009; Guan et al. 2000).

Both growth hormone and IGF-1 may reduce the outcome of spinal cord trauma in the rat. As an example, topical application of both hormones was shown to reduce trauma-induced oedema formation and cell damage (Sharma et al. 1998; Nyberg and Sharma 2002). Additional studies that indicated that growth hormone may improve spinal cord conduction and attenuate oedema formation and cell injury in the spinal cord provided further support for a beneficial role of the hormone in injuries to the cord (Winkler et al. 2000). Growth hormone injection in rats exposed to chronic sustained hypoxia increased the hippocampal expression of the IGF-1 gene transcript, reduced the hypoxia-induced hippocampal injury and attenuated hypoxia-induced cognitive deficits (Li et al. 2011). It was concluded that exogenous growth hormone may provide a viable therapeutic intervention to protect hypoxia-vulnerable brain regions from neuronal damage and subsequent deficits in neuro-cognitive function (Li et al. 2011).

Furthermore, in humans, injury to the brain and to spinal cord are associated with a decline in the circulatory levels and the responsivity of both growth hormone and IGF-1 (for a review, see Nyberg [2000]). As both growth hormone and IGF-1 exhibit a wide array of neuroprotective activities, as evidenced in both in vitro studies using various cell systems and in vivo studies with experimental animal models, it is tempting to speculate upon a possible potential therapeutic utility of both hormones in this context. A study using murine hippocampal cells demonstrated that growth hormone may counteract opioid-induced cell damage and apoptosis (Svensson et al. 2008), and in a very recent study, it has been indicated that the hormone may reverse opioid-induced cognitive impairments, also in humans (Rhodin et al. 2014), emphasising the importance of the somatotrophic axis in therapeutic strategies for the treatment of various types of drug-induced damage to the brain.

GROWTH HORMONE HAS A ROLE IN FOOD INTAKE AND APPETITE

The ability of growth hormone to stimulate appetite is well known. Thus, patients with GHD increase their food intake during growth hormone replacement therapy. It is also known from experiments with transgenic mice that overexpress growth hormone in the CNS that a differentiation of the effect of the hormone on body fat mass from that on appetite is possible (Giordano et al. 2005). Hence, in parallel with a central stimulatory effect on appetite and lipolysis, growth hormone overexpression in the CNS causes hyperphagia-induced obesity. Moreover, ghrelin stimulates release of growth hormone and increases food intake (Lim et al. 2010). However, it is worth noting that the acute effect of ghrelin in this respect is dependent on GHR signalling that is functionally intact (Egecioglu et al. 2010).

The role of the 36 amino acid residue neuropeptide Y (NPY) in the regulation of appetite is well known. There are now several studies on food intake that have verified a link between NPY and growth hormone (Konturek et al. 2004; Dimaraki and Jaffe 2006). Furthermore, it was previously reported that a growth hormone secretagogue receptor and NPY are co-localised in the rat hypothalamic arcuate nucleus (Willesen et al. 1999). In addition, studies that show expression of the GHR gene transcript in visceral sensory and motor structures in the rat brain suggest a role of growth hormone in the regulation of food intake and energy homeostasis (Kastrup et al. 2005).

GROWTH HORMONE IN COGNITION AND MEMORY FUNCTION

It is now well established, as deduced from reports from many laboratories, that growth hormone and IGF-1 have potential roles in memory acquisition and cognitive function (Nyberg and Hallberg 2013). Data from replacement therapy with growth hormone in adult patients with GHD suggest that both growth hormone and IGF-1 may enhance both long-term and working memory (Deijen et al. 1996; Popovic 2005; Arwert et al. 2006; Wass and Reddy 2010). For example, growth hormone replacement during a 6-month period in patients with GHD improved both long-term memory and working memory (Arwert et al. 2006). This memory improvement was concomitant with a decreased activation in the ventrolateral prefrontal cortex (PFC) in the brain as visualised by functional magnetic resonance imaging. However, it is worth noting, and somewhat discouraging, that in spite of all reports that indicate beneficial effects of growth hormone on the impaired cognitive functions seen in patients with GHD, there are no convincing studies that imply that the hormone would improve cognitive disabilities in elderly non-GHD individuals who are healthy (Arwert et al. 2005).

With respect to the underlying mechanisms that account for the observed beneficial effects of growth hormone on cognitive function, it is postulated that growth hormone induces these effects, at least partly, through its mediator IGF-1, which is able to penetrate the BBB and reach its responsive sites in the CNS (Pan et al. 2005). Thus, both of the large peptides, growth hormone and IGF-1, may cross the BBB and interact with specific receptors in the CNS (Pan et al. 2005). Several brain areas, including the hippocampus, contain high concentrations of GHR, as previously mentioned (Nyberg 2000, 2007). Moreover, after peripheral administration of growth hormone in rats, the expression of the GHR mRNA is up-regulated in the hippocampus of young, but not elderly, rats (Le Greves et al. 2002). Furthermore, chronic treatment with growth hormone and IGF-1 significantly improves learning and memory in aged rats with impaired growth hormone production (Le Greves et al. 2006). It is suggested that growth hormone may exert its beneficial effects on neuro-cognition by increasing neurogenesis, vascular density and glucose utilisation (Aberg et al. 2006). At the molecular level it is believed that growth hormone may alter the composition of the subunits of the *N*-methyl-D-aspartate (NMDA) receptor in brain areas implicated in learning and memory (Sonntag et al. 2000, 2005; Le Greves et al. 2002, 2006). Data from animal experiments with rats demonstrated that growth hormone may influence the NMDA receptor subunits in a mode that is in consonance with improved memory and cognitive capabilities. A similar outcome was shown with IGF-1 (Sonntag et al. 2000). It has been demonstrated in both in vivo and in vitro experiments that growth hormone is able to increase regeneration and prevent apoptosis in hippocampal cells (Aberg et al. 2006; Svensson et al. 2008).

Reversal of drug-induced impairments by growth hormone replacement

During the past few years, we have directed studies on the ability of growth hormone to reverse behavioural symptoms induced by various drugs. It is established that the hormone may improve a number of psychological deficits seen in individuals with insufficient production of growth hormone. As mentioned above, these impairments include attention,

36

energy, motivation, cognitive capabilities and well-being. The beneficial effects of growth hormone in this regard have been confirmed in both humans and experimental animals (for reviews, see Nyberg and Burman [1996]; Nyberg [2000]; Aberg et al. [2006]; Geisler et al. [2012]).

However, in addition to various forms of brain trauma and impaired pituitary function, a deficient somatotrophic axis leading to impaired neurocognition may result from other conditions, for example, diabetes and drug addiction. We have recently observed that streptozotocin-induced diabetes in mice affected the expression of GHR in the PFC and induced learning impairment (Enhamre et al. 2012). Thus, our study indicated that the *GHR* gene transcript is up-regulated in the PFC of diabetic mice compared to controls. Moreover, a significant correlation between the expression of GHR mRNA and performance in the Barnes maze during the acquisition phase was confirmed in diabetic, but not control, mice. These findings suggest that diabetes induces an imbalance in the growth hormone/IGF-1 system, leading to altered activity in the PFC and associated cognitive deficiencies (Enhamre et al. 2012). In a subsequent study, diabetic and control mice were subjected to treatment with recombinant human growth hormone for 10 consecutive days (Enhamre-Brolin et al. 2013). In the latter phase of this treatment regimen, we tested the cognitive abilities of the mice using the Barnes maze behavioural assay. In this test, we observed a profound effect of the hormone when analysing the search patterns used by the animals in the maze. The hormonal treatment significantly counteracted the cognitive disabilities expressed as lack of direct search strategies on the last day in this cognitive test system.

As mentioned above, a decline in the function of the growth hormone/IGF-1 axis is seen during ageing. This decline is known to occur concomitant to decreased cognitive capability. Among the harmful long-term effects recognised in individuals abusing addictive drugs is accelerated obsolescence expressed as impaired cognition (for review, see Nyberg [2012]). As mentioned above, there is clear evidence that growth hormone therapy may improve cognitive function in both human and experimental animals (Nyberg and Burman 1996; Falleti et al. 2005; Nyberg and Hallberg 2013). It is also reported that the hormone may counteract and reverse opioid-induced damage of hippocampal cells, as observed in primary cultures of cells from mouse fetus (Svensson et al. 2008). In addition, we have observed that rats exposed to anabolic androgenic steroids (AAS) will undergo a decline in their cognitive capacity (Magnusson et al. 2009). The ability of steroids to induce damage in brain areas like the hippocampus has recently been confirmed in other laboratories (Tugyan et al. 2013). Thus, the study demonstrated that abuse of these steroids caused a decline in the number of neurons in several brain areas, including hippocampus, parietal cortex and PFC, and increased oxidative damage. We recently examined the ability of growth hormone to impact on cognitive disabilities induced by AAS (Gronbladh et al. 2012). Male rats were subjected to treatment with the steroid nandrolone decanoate every third day for 3 weeks and thereafter treated with recombinant human growth hormone for 10 consecutive days. During the hormone replacement the spatial performance was tested in the Morris water maze (MWM). Our results indicated a significant positive effect of growth hormone on memory functions. Although, in this study, the AAS treatment did not exhibit any pronounced alteration in memory of the experimental animals compared to controls, as recorded in the MWM, growth hormone replacement was shown to improve spatial memory in intact rats and it was also demonstrated to reverse certain effects induced by the steroid (Gronbladh et al. 2012).

In a progressive clinical study we have noted impairments in the somatotrophic axis in patients with chronic pain who have been subjected to long-term opioid treatment. In a case study focused on one of these patients, we observed a clear decline in cognitive ability. Interestingly, following 6 months' replacement therapy with growth hormone, a notable improvement in certain cognitive domains, such as visuospatial performance, was observed. In parallel to this, we noted increased hippocampal activity as documented by MRI (Rhodin et al. 2014). This observation raises the possibility to use growth hormone replacement therapy to repair cognitive deficiencies induced by addictive drugs.

Conclusion

In this chapter, we have highlighted some essential aspects pertaining to the relevance of specific receptors for growth hormone identified in the brain. Current knowledge about the regional distribution of these receptors as well as their biochemical characteristics has been described. We have also discussed possible pathways for the hormone to leave the circulatory system and find its targets in the brain. The chapter also includes text on the interaction of growth hormone with brain circuits related to certain behaviours that could be influenced by this hormone, and extrapolating from this, the potential role of growth hormone as a therapeutic agent has been discussed. In particular, we have focused on the role of growth hormone as a neuroprotective agent with strong emphasis on its ability to improve cognitive disabilities, as shown in both humans and experimental animals. It seems that the hormone may be of clinical use, not only for its growth promoting effect, but also with respect to its ability to stimulate regeneration of nerve cells. Thus, current research suggests that growth hormone may be useful for the treatment of a variety of disorders associated with cognitive impairment, for example, that resulting from CNS trauma or from brain damage induced by addictive drugs.

REFERENCES

Aberg ND (2010) Role of the growth hormone/insulin-like growth factor 1 axis in neurogenesis. *Endocr Dev* 17: 63–76.

Aberg ND, Brywe KG and Isgaard J (2006) Aspects of growth hormone and insulin-like growth factor-I related to neuroprotection, regeneration, and functional plasticity in the adult brain. *Scientific World Journal* 6: 53–80.

Anderson MF, Aberg MA, Nilsson M and Eriksson PS (2002) Insulin-like growth factor-I and neurogenesis in the adult mammalian brain. *Dev Brain Res* 134: 115–122.

Andersson K, Fuxe K, Eneroth P, Isaksson O, Nyberg F and Roos P (1983) Rat growth hormone and hypothalamic catecholamine nerve terminal systems. Evidence for rapid and discrete reductions in dopamine and noradrenaline levels and turnover in the median eminence of the hypophysectomized male rat. *Eur J Pharmacol* 95: 271–275.

Arwert LI, Veltman DJ, Deijen JB, van Dam PS, Delemarre-van deWaal HA and Drent ML (2005) Growth hormone deficiency and memory functioning in adults visualized by functional magnetic resonance imaging. *Neuroendocrinology* 82: 32–40.

Arwert LI, Veltman DJ, Deijen JB, van Dam PS and Drent ML (2006) Effects of growth hormone substitution therapy on cognitive functioning in growth hormone deficient patients: a functional MRI study. *Neuroendocrinology* 83: 12–19.

Burman P, Hetta J, Wide L, Mansson JE, Ekman R and Karlsson FA (1996) Growth hormone treatment affects brain neurotransmitters and thyroxine [see comment]. *Clin Endocrinol (Oxford)* 44: 319–324.

Carter-Su C, Argetsinger LS, Campbell GS, Wang X, Ihle J and Witthuhn B (1994) The identification of JAK2 tyrosine kinase as a signaling molecule for growth hormone. *Proc Soc Exp Biol Med* 206: 210–215.

Carter-Su C, Schwartz J and Argetsinger LS (2015) Growth hormone signaling pathways. *Growth Horm IGF Res* 28: 11–15.

Chaplin JE, Kristrom B, Jonsson B, Tuvemo T and Albertsson-Wikland K (2015) Growth hormone treatment improves cognitive function in short children with growth hormone deficiency. *Horm Res Paediatr* 83: 930–399.

Coculescu M (1999) Blood-brain barrier for human growth hormone and insulin-like growth factor-I. *J Pediatr Endocrinol Metab* 12: 113–124.

de Vos AM, Ultsch M and Kossiakoff AA (1992) Human growth hormone and extracellular domain of its receptor: crystal structure of the complex. *Science* 255: 306–312.

Deijen JB, de Boer H, Blok GJ and van der Veen EA (1996) Cognitive impairments and mood disturbances in growth hormone deficient men. *Psychoneuroendocrinology* 21: 313–322.

Dimaraki EV and Jaffe CA (2006) Role of endogenous ghrelin in growth hormone secretion, appetite regulation and metabolism. *Rev Endocr Metab Disord* 7: 237–249.

Donahue CP, Kosik KS and Shors TJ (2006) Growth hormone is produced within the hippocampus where it responds to age, sex, and stress. *Proc Natl Acad Sci USA* 103: 6031–6036.

Egecioglu E, Jerlhag E, Salome N et al. (2010) Ghrelin increases intake of rewarding food in rodents. *Addict Biol* 15: 304–311.

Enhamre E, Carlsson A, Gronbladh A, Watanabe H, Hallberg M and Nyberg F (2012) The expression of growth hormone receptor gene transcript in the prefrontal cortex is affected in male mice with diabetes-induced learning impairments. *Neurosci Lett* 523: 82–86.

Enhamre-Brolin E, Carlsson A, Hallberg M and Nyberg F (2013) Growth hormone reverses streptozotocin-induced cognitive impairments in male mice. *Behav Brain Res* 238: 273–278.

Falleti MG, Sanfilippo A, Maruff P, Weih L and Phillips KA (2005) The nature and severity of cognitive impairment associated with adjuvant chemotherapy in women with breast cancer: A meta-analysis of the current literature. *Brain Cogn* 59: 60–70.

Geisler A, Lass N, Reinsch N et al. (2012) Quality of life in children and adolescents with growth hormone deficiency: Association with growth hormone treatment. *Horm Res Paediatr* 78: 94–99.

Giordano R, Lanfranco F, Bo M et al. (2005) Somatopause reflects age-related changes in the neural control of GH/IGF-I axis. *J Endocrinol Invest* 28: 94–98.

Gronbladh A, Johansson J, Nostl A, Nyberg FJ and Hallberg M (2012) Growth hormone improves spatial memory and reverses certain anabolic androgenic steroid-induced effects in intact rats. *J Endocrinol* 216: 31–41.

Guan J and Gluckman PD (2009) IGF-1 derived small neuropeptides and analogues: A novel strategy for the development of pharmaceuticals for neurological conditions. *Br J Pharmacol* 157: 881–891.

Guan J, Krishnamurthi R, Waldvogel HJ, Faull RL, Clark R and Gluckman P (2000) N-terminal tripeptide of IGF-1 (GPE) prevents the loss of TH positive neurons after 6-OHDA induced nigral lesion in rats. *Brain Res* 859: 286–292.

Harvey S, Baudet ML and Sanders EJ (2009) Growth hormone-induced neuroprotection in the neural retina during chick embryogenesis. *Ann NY Acad Sci* 1163: 414–416.

Hojvat S, Baker G, Kirsteins L and Lawrence AM (1982) Growth hormone (GH) immunoreactivity in the rodent and primate CNS: distribution, characterization and presence posthypophysectomy. *Brain Res* 239: 543–557.

Huisman J, Aukema EJ, Deijen JB et al. (2008) The usefulness of growth hormone treatment for psychological status in young adult survivors of childhood leukaemia: an open-label study. *BMC Pediatr* 8: 25.

Johansson JO, Larson G, Andersson M et al. (1995) Treatment of growth hormone-deficient adults with recombinant human growth hormone increases the concentration of growth hormone in the cerebrospinal fluid and affects neurotransmitters. *Neuroendocrinology* 61: 57–66.

Kastrup Y, Le Greves M, Nyberg F and Blomqvist A (2005) Distribution of growth hormone receptor mRNA in the brain stem and spinal cord of the rat. *Neuroscience* 130: 419–425.

Konturek SJ, Konturek JW, Pawlik T and Brzozowski T (2004) Brain-gut axis and its role in the control of food intake. *J Physiol Pharmacol* 55: 137–154.

Lai Z, Roos P, Zhai O et al. (1993) Age-related reduction of human growth hormone-binding sites in the human brain. *Brain Res* 621: 260–266.

Lai ZN, Emtner M, Roos P and Nyberg F (1991) Characterization of putative growth hormone receptors in human choroid plexus. *Brain Res* 546: 222–226.

Le Greves M, Le Greves P and Nyberg F (2005) Age-related effects of IGF-1 on the NMDA-, GH- and IGF-1-receptor mRNA transcripts in the rat hippocampus. *Brain Res Bull* 65: 369–374.

Le Greves M, Steensland P, Le Greves P and Nyberg F (2002) Growth hormone induces age-dependent alteration in the expression of hippocampal growth hormone receptor and N-methyl-D-aspartate receptor subunits gene transcripts in male rats. *Proc Natl Acad Sci USA* 99: 7119–7123.

Le Greves M, Zhou Q, Berg M et al. (2006) Growth hormone replacement in hypophysectomized rats affects spatial performance and hippocampal levels of NMDA receptor subunit and PSD-95 gene transcript levels. *Exp Brain Res* 173: 267–273.

Li RC, Guo SZ, Raccurt M et al. (2011) Exogenous growth hormone attenuates cognitive deficits induced by intermittent hypoxia in rats. *Neuroscience* 196: 237–250.

Lim CT, Kola B, Korbonits M and Grossman AB (2010) Ghrelin's role as a major regulator of appetite and its other functions in neuroendocrinology. *Prog Brain Res* 182: 189–205.

Magnusson K, Birgner C, Bergstrom L, Nyberg F and Hallberg M (2009) Nandrolone decanoate administration dose-dependently affects the density of kappa opioid peptide receptors in the rat brain determined by autoradiography. *Neuropeptides* 43: 105–111.

Nyberg F (2000) Growth hormone in the brain: Characteristics of specific brain targets for the hormone and their functional significance. *Front Neuroendocrinol* 21: 330–348.

Nyberg F (2007) Growth hormone and brain function. In: Ranke MM, Price DA, and Reiter EO (eds) *Growth hormone therapy in pediatrics 20 years of KIGS*. Basel: Karger, 450–460.

Nyberg F (2009) The role of the somatotrophic axis in neuroprotection and neuroregeneration of the addictive brain. *Int Rev Neurobiol* 88: 399–427.

Nyberg F (2012) Cognitive impairments in drug addicts. In: González-Quevedo A (ed) *Brain damage – Bridging between basic research and clinics*. In Tech, Rijeka, Croatia, pp. 221–243.

Nyberg F and Burman P (1996) Growth hormone and its receptors in the central nervous system–location and functional significance. *Horm Res* 45: 18–22.

Nyberg F and Hallberg M (2013) Growth hormone and cognitive function. *Nat Rev Endocrinol* 9: 357–365.

Nyberg F and Sharma HS (2002) Repeated topical application of growth hormone attenuates blood-spinal cord barrier permeability and edema formation following spinal cord injury: an experimental study in the rat using Evans blue, ([125])I-sodium and lanthanum tracers. *Amino Acids* 23: 231–239.

Pan W and Kastin AJ (2000) Interactions of IGF-1 with the blood-brain barrier in vivo and in situ. *Neuroendocrinology* 72: 171–178.

Pan W, Yu Y, Cain CM, Nyberg F, Couraud PO and Kastin AJ (2005) Permeation of growth hormone across the blood-brain barrier. *Endocrinology* 146: 4898–4904.

Popovic V (2005) GH deficiency as the most common pituitary defect after TBI: clinical implications. *Pituitary* 8: 239–243.

Rhodin A, von Ehren M, Skottheim B et al. (2014) Recombinant human growth hormone improves cognitive capacity in a patient exposed to chronic opioids *Acta Anaesthesiol Scand* 58: 759–765.

Rosen T, Wiren L, Wilhelmsen L, Wiklund I and Bengtsson BA (1994) Decreased psychological well-being in adult patients with growth hormone deficiency. *Clin Endocrinol (Oxford)* 40: 111–116.

Scheepens A, Williams CE, Breier BH, Guan J and Gluckman PD (2000) A role for the somatotropic axis in neural development, injury and disease. *J Pediatr Endocrinol Metab* 13(Suppl 6): 1483–1491.

Sharma HS, Nyberg F, Westman J, Alm P, Gordh T and Lindholm D (1998) Brain derived neurotrophic factor and insulin like growth factor-1 attenuate upregulation of nitric oxide synthase and cell injury following trauma to the spinal cord. An immunohistochemical study in the rat. *Amino Acids* 14: 121–129.

Sonntag WE, Bennett SA, Khan AS et al. (2000) Age and insulin-like growth factor-1 modulate N-methyl-D-aspartate receptor subtype expression in rats. *Brain Res Bull* 51: 331–338.

Sonntag WE, Ramsey M and Carter CS (2005) Growth hormone and insulin-like growth factor-1 (IGF-1) and their influence on cognitive aging. *Ageing Res Rev* 4: 195–212.

Svensson AL, Bucht N, Hallberg M and Nyberg F (2008) Reversal of opiate-induced apoptosis by human recombinant growth hormone in murine foetus primary hippocampal neuronal cell cultures. *Proc Natl Acad Sci USA* 105: 7304–7308.

Thornwall-Le Greves M, Zhou Q, Lagerholm S, Huang W, Le Greves P and Nyberg F (2001) Morphine decreases the levels of the gene transcripts of growth hormone receptor and growth hormone binding protein in the male rat hippocampus and spinal cord. *Neurosci Lett* 304: 69–72.

Torres Aleman I (2005) Role of insulin-like growth factors in neuronal plasticity and neuroprotection. *Adv Exp Med Biol* 567: 243–258.

Tugyan K, Ozbal S, Cilaker S et al. (2013) Neuroprotective effect of erythropoietin on nandrolone decanoate-induced brain injury in rats. *Neurosci Lett* 533: 28–33.

Wass JA and Reddy R (2010) Growth hormone and memory. *J Endocrinol* 207: 125–126.

Werther GA, Hogg A, Oldfield BJ, McKinley MJ, Figdor R and Mendelsohn FA (1989) Localization and characterization of insulin-like growth factor-I receptors in rat brain and pituitary gland using in vitro autoradiography and computerized densitometry*. A distinct distribution from insulin receptors. *J Neuroendocrinol* 1: 369–377.

Willesen MG, Kristensen P and Romer J (1999) Co-localization of growth hormone secretagogue receptor and NPY mRNA in the arcuate nucleus of the rat. *Neuroendocrinology* 70: 306–316.

Winkler T, Sharma HS, Stalberg E, Badgaiyan RD, Westman J and Nyberg F (2000) Growth hormone attenuates alterations in spinal cord evoked potentials and cell injury following trauma to the rat spinal cord. An experimental study using topical application of rat growth hormone. *Amino Acids* 19: 363–371.

Zhai Q, Lai Z, Roos P and Nyberg F (1994) Characterization of growth hormone binding sites in rat brain. *Acta Paediatr Suppl* 406: 92–95.

4
IMPACT OF DISORDERS OF THE GROWTH HORMONE–IGF-1 AXIS ON NEUROLOGICAL FUNCTION

Emma A Webb and Mehul T Dattani

Even among human beings, children when compared with adults, and dwarf adults, when compared with others, may have some characteristics in which they are superior, but in intelligence at any rate, they are inferior. And the reason is that in many of them the principle of the soul is sluggish and corporeal.

(Aristotle, Parts of animals, IV.x.)

Introduction

Aristotle first suggested that there may be an association between 'dwarfism' and impaired cognition. Evidence is accumulating that the growth hormone axis plays an important role in normal brain growth and development (Russo et al. 2005), with an ongoing role in determining childhood and adult cognitive function (Gluckman et al. 1992; Woods et al. 1996; Werther et al. 1998). There is also evidence to suggest that insulin-like growth factor-1 (IGF-1) and IGF-binding protein-3 (IGFBP-3) deficiency, such as that found in children and adults with growth hormone deficiency (GHD), are associated with cognitive deficits and changes in brain structure (Hansen-Pupp et al. 2011; Webb et al. 2012), with cognitive improvements seen following growth hormone treatment (Chaplin et al. 2015).

Evidence to suggest a role for the growth hormone–IGF-1 axis in brain development

The growth hormone–IGF-1 axis is summarised in Chapter 3 (Nyberg). A large body of evidence suggests that IGF and IGF receptors and growth hormone and growth hormone receptors (GHRs) are expressed in the parts of the brain responsible for learning and memory. Growth hormone is produced both in the pituitary and, to a lesser degree, by other tissues in the central nervous system (CNS), for example, the hippocampus (Baumann 1991; Donahue et al. 2006). There is also evidence to support the transport of growth hormone into the CNS across the blood–brain barrier. There is a high density of GHRs in the choroid plexus (Lobie et al. 1993; Johansson et al. 1995), and several studies report an increase in cerebrospinal fluid (CSF) IGF-1 and growth hormone after peripheral recombinant human growth hormone (rhGH) administration (Hynes et al. 1987; Burman et al. 1996). Peripheral rhGH administration also increases levels of CSF neurotransmitters including vasoactive intestinal peptide, noradrenaline, homovanillic acid (dopamine metabolite) and glutamate (an excitatory amino acid that acts as a ligand for the N-methyl-D-aspartate (NMDA) receptor, which in turn is involved in memory formation in the hippocampus; Burman et al. 1993).

Growth hormone–binding sites are found on various cell types in the brain including neurons, astrocytes, oligodendrocytes and microglia. In the rodent, growth hormone has been identified in the amygdala, cortex, hippocampus and thalamus (Hojvat et al. 1982), and the GHR in the choroid plexus, cortex, hippocampus, hypothalamus, striatum and spinal cord, with levels being higher in females than in males (Mustafa et al. 1994). The human brain has a similar pattern of GHR expression with concentrations being highest in the choroid plexus, thalamus, hypothalamus, pituitary, putamen and hippocampus (Lai et al. 1991; Lai et al. 1993). The putamen plays an important role in the processing of social perceptions, with the hippocampal and perihippocampal regions playing roles in learning and memory (Milner and Penfield 1955; Penfield and Milner 1958; McClelland and Goddard 1996). Interestingly GHR expression is two- to four-fold higher in the hippocampus than elsewhere in the brain, suggesting that growth hormone may play an important role in memory formation. GHR concentration is highest in the fetal and infant brain when GHRs located specifically in areas known to be actively involved in neurogenesis within the juvenile brain, including the hippocampal dentate gyrus, the olfactory bulb and the subventricular zone (Turnley et al. 2002; Lobie et al. 1993). Subsequently GHR concentrations decline with increasing age (Lobie et al. 1993; Harvey et al. 2002).

There is accumulating evidence that in addition to growth hormone, IGF-1 also plays an important role in brain growth, development and myelination, and that it has an ongoing role in determining childhood and adult cognitive function (Woods et al. 1996; Camacho-Hubner et al. 2002). IGF-1 is actively transported across the blood–brain barrier (Reinhardt and Bondy 1994), acting to stimulate the viability and function of a variety of different neuronal cell types through the IGF receptor family (Caroni and Grandes 1990). It promotes neuronal DNA synthesis in addition to myelination, stabilises tubulin mRNA, enhances oligodendrocyte proliferation and increases neuron and glia survival and neuromuscular synaptogenesis (Sonntag et al. 2000; Lynch et al. 2001). IGF-1 stimulates neuronal acetylcholine release (Araujo et al. 1989) and activates the NMDA receptor. In addition to its neurotrophic effects it also has several neuroprotective effects, limiting neuronal loss after ischaemic injury (Pulford et al. 1999) and improving neurological functioning in rats when administered after spinal cord injury (Scheepens et al. 1999; Winkler et al. 2000). *IGF-1* gene expression has been found in humans in the hypothalamus, hippocampus, olfactory bulb, cerebellum, neocortex and striatum (Sonntag et al. 2000) with IGF-1 receptors being most dense in the hippocampus, amygdala, caudate nucleus, cortex, cerebellum, prefrontal and parahippocampal cortex (Adem et al. 1989). Together these regions make up the neural circuit known as the social brain (Baron-Cohen et al. 1999).

In humans, fetal cord IGF-1 and IGFBP-3 concentrations have been reported to be related to head circumference at birth (Geary et al. 2003), and in children, one study found that serum IGF-1 concentrations correlated positively with verbal intelligence (Gunnell et al. 2005). Amongst elderly patients, those with higher concentrations of IGF-I perform better on tests of cognitive function and have lower rates of cognitive decline (Aleman et al. 1999).

Human disease models also exist where either the *IGF-I* gene is deleted or there is impairment in the functioning of the GHR, leading to reduced production of *IGF-1*. Deletion of the *IGF-1* gene is universally associated with significant intrauterine growth retardation, microcephaly, significant cognitive impairment and postnatal growth failure (Woods et al. 1996). Although all reported patients with *IGF-1* gene mutation presented with microcephaly, brain magnetic resonance imaging (MRI) revealed apparently normal patterns of myelination (Woods et al. 1996; Camacho-Hubner et al. 2002; Netchine et al. 2009). It has been hypothesised that the increase in serum IGF-II found in these patients may also be present in the brain of individuals with *IGF-1* gene mutations, and this may in some way compensate for their IGF-1 deficiency. In IGF-1 knockout mice it has been shown that IGF-II can compensate in part for IGF-I actions on myelination (Ye et al. 2002). Individuals with an *IGF-1* receptor gene mutation also exhibit prenatal and postnatal growth retardation, microcephaly, mild intellectual disability, learning disorders and/or altered behavioural characteristics (Abuzzahab et al. 2003; Walenkamp et al. 2006). On the other hand, individuals with *GHR* mutations have varying cognitive phenotypes. Guevara-Aguirre et al. have reported on an Ecuadorian population with a single-point mutation (E180 splice mutation) in the GHR, preventing dimerisation and normal functioning. In this population, which has elevated concentrations of growth hormone but undetectable IGF-1, intelligence has been found to be normal or slightly higher than in the general population (Guevara-Aguirre et al. 1991; Kranzler et al. 1998). This contrasts with the initial reports of growth hormone insensitivity or Laron syndrome in an Israeli cohort with a different pathogenic mutation, in which affected individuals were found to have significantly reduced cognitive performance (Laron 1984; Laron and Klinger 1994). Individuals with *STAT5B* mutations also appear to have normal brain development and cognitive functions, although detailed neurocognitive and imaging studies have not been performed in these patients (David et al. 2011). The normal functioning of the GHR does not therefore appear to be a prerequisite for normal cognitive development. Scheepens et al. (2005) have suggested that this may indicate 'some central role for high levels of growth hormone acting via a receptor that does not require homodimerization'. The evidence that IGF-1 is not important in brain development is not however conclusive with antenatal reductions in IGF-1 concentrations such as those found in children with intra-utereine growth retardation (IUGR) (Lassarre et al. 1991) also being associated with significant impairments in cognitive performance (Morsing et al. 2011).

IGF-binding proteins (IGFBPs) are also expressed during brain development with IGFBP-2, IGFBP-3, IGFBP-4 and IGFBP-5 being the most abundant IGFBPs in the brain. Overexpression of IGFBP-1, IGFBP-2 and IGFBP-3 in transgenic murine models is associated with reductions in brain growth and myelination, thought to be secondary to decreased bioavailability of IGF-1 (Ni et al. 1997; Hoeflich et al. 1999; Silha et al. 2005). However, the exact roles of the IGFBPs in neural development remain to be fully elucidated.

Several neuropsychological studies have documented impairments in cognitive functioning in adults with childhood-onset GHD (Deijen et al. 1996, 1998) and adult-onset GHD (Burman et al. 1995; Deijen et al. 1996; Lijffijt et al. 2003; Scheepens, Moderscheim and Gluckman 2005; van Dam 2005). When compared to individuals without GHD, adults with GHD have consistently been found to have impairments in attention, memory and executive function with some evidence for improvements in certain areas of cognitive functioning (memory and atten- tion tasks) in adults receiving growth hormone replacement (Falleti et al. 2006).

Cognitive impact of growth hormone deficiency in childhood

There are only a small number of studies in the literature pertaining to the cognitive impact of isolated GHD on children (Table 4.1). In a majority of these studies, children with idio- pathic isolated GHD have been reported to have a normal IQ. However, despite having IQs within the normal range, a high percentage of patients with GHD have to repeat a class (Holmes et al. 1984, 1985; Frisch et al. 1990) and have difficulties with problem solving (Drotar et al. 1980). Steinhausen et al. reported that children with GHD scored lower in two subtests of the Leistungsprtif system intelligence test measuring spatial orientation and speed of closure when compared to controls despite there being no difference in full-scale IQ between the two groups (Steinhausen and Stahnke 1976, 1977). Subsequently Stabler et al. (1998) investigated the benefit of growth hormone treatment in 72 individuals with isolated GHD and 59 with idiopathic short stature (ISS), and reported a reduction in IQ prior to the start of growth hormone treatment between short study individuals (GHD and short-stature patients) and healthy controls. However, there was no difference in IQ scores between chil- dren with short stature and children with GHD at baseline. Importantly children with GHD were defined as having a peak growth hormone to stimulation as less than 10μg/L (*n*=109) and as having ISS when >10μg/L (*n*=86). Some centres only recognise a growth hormone peak of <10μg/L as being diagnostic for GHD and some children may therefore have been wrongly diagnosed with GHD in this study. More recently Webb et al. studied 15 children with isolated GHD (peak growth hormone <6.7ng/ml) and 14 with ISS (peak growth hormone >10ng/ml) (Webb et al. 2012). When compared to controls, children with isolated GHD had significantly lower full scale IQ (FSIQ), Verbal Comprehension Index and Process- ing Speed Index scores, although the mean FSIQ and Verbal Comprehension Index of both groups lay within the average Wechsler Intelligence Scales for Children (4th edition) range (as in previous studies). In children with isolated GHD, Verbal Comprehension Index scores also correlated significantly with IGF-1 and IGFBP-3 standard deviation score (SDS) and FSIQ correlated significantly with IGFBP-3 SDS, but not IGF-1 SDS. Concentrations of IGF-1 and IGFBP-3 explained 49% of the variance in Verbal Comprehension Index in the isolated GHD group. When compared to controls, children with isolated GHD also had significant reductions in motor skills scores, with significantly lower scores on the manual dexterity, balance and total scores of the Movement Assessment Battery for Children 2 test (Webb et al. 2012). The conclusions of all of these studies suggest that GHD impacts on cognitive development (Steinhausen and Stahnke 1977; Stabler et al. 1998; Webb et al. 2012).

TABLE 4.1

Studies to assess the impact of growth hormone deficiency and growth hormone replacement on cognition in the paediatric population

Author(s) (age of recruits)	Number of participants and diagnosis	Assessment tools used	Study conclusions
Webb et al., 2012 (5–11 years, mean 8.6 years)	15 isolated growth hormone deficiency (GHD) 14 ISS Assessed before growth hormone treatment	–WISC-IV –MABC, 2nd edition –CBCL –MRI brain	–FSIQ, VIQ, Processing Speed Index and motor skills scores significantly lower in children with isolated GHD in association with reductions in white matter integrity in the corticospinal tract and corpus callosum and selective reductions in neural volumes –No difference in CBCL scores between isolated GHD and ISS groups
Stabler et al., 1998 (5–16 years, mean 11.2 years)	72 isolated GHD 59 ISS Assessed before and after 3 years growth hormone therapy Normal stature children assessed at baseline	–IQ –CBCL	–CBCL scores for total behaviour problems were higher ($p<0.001$) in children with short stature at baseline than in children with normal stature –IQ and achievement scores did not change with growth hormone therapy –After growth hormone treatment, CBCL scores for total behaviours were improved (effect larger in those with isolated GHD ($p<0.001$) than in those with ISS ($p<0.003$)) –Growth hormone improved scores on internalizing subscales (withdrawn: $p<0.007$, somatic complications $p<0.001$, anxious/depressed $p<0.001$) and on attention, social problems and thought problems ($p=0.001$)
Steinhausen and Stahnke, 1977 (9–19 years, mean 14.9 years)	16 GHD (6 isolated GHD/10 MPHD) 16 children with short stature Assessed before growth hormone treatment	–Thurstone's test of primary mental abilities –Wechsler scales –Personality test –Children's personality questionnaire of Cattell	–Impaired social and coping behaviour in all short children –Reduced spatial orientation and speed of closure in children with GHD –No difference in IQ –Children with GHD less aggressive, excitable, dominant and tense, but more conscientious than the children with short stature

WISC-IV, Wechsler Intelligence Scales for Children, 4th edition; MABC, Movement Assessment Battery for Children; CBCL, Child Behavior Checklist; ISS, idiopathic short stature

Effect of growth hormone deficiency on brain structure

Since its introduction, MRI has proved valuable in defining the gross structural abnormalities present in individuals with pathological conditions. For example, in individuals with idiopathic GHD, the anterior pituitary gland is frequently small, the posterior pituitary ectopic and the infundibulum thin or absent (Tillmann et al. 2000). Recent advances in MRI have enabled more detailed examination of brain structure (Basser et al. 1994; Fischl et al. 2002), with techniques including volumetric and diffusion tensor imaging (DTI) being used to investigate the phenotype of individuals with pathological conditions, including isolated GHD, in more depth. Automated software analysis of volumetric imaging generates neural volumes, which can then be entered into statistical analyses to assess whether significant associations are present, for example, between neural volumes, IGF-1 and IGFBP-3 SDS in children with isolated GHD. DTI provides quantitative indices of brain development, enabling the visualisation of white matter microstructure and characterisation of white matter anatomy including the degree of connectivity between different regions of the brain (Basser, Mattiello and LeBihan 1994; Basser and Pierpaoli 1996). The diffusion of water molecules within the brain is affected by the underlying tissue microstructure; this enables the study of the orientation and integrity of neural fibres, a useful tool when assessing the impact of physiological and pathological processes on neurological development (Beaulieu 2002). Fractional anisotropy, which describes the degree of diffusion directionality and correlates with axonal density and degree of myelination, ranging from 0 for isotropic diffusion to 1 for anisotropic diffusion, is calculated by relating the amount of diffusion along the major axis to that along the minor axes (Beaulieu 2002). Fractional anisotropy can be affected by a range of microstructural differences in neural tissue including axonal membranes, myelin sheaths, percentage brain water, compactness of fibre tracts and amount of axonal space (Beaulieu 2002), with studies conducted in the paediatric population having found that fractional anisotropy correlates with neurocognitive function (Schmithorst et al. 2005).

Calculation of neural volumes has been performed in children born extremely preterm (<31 weeks at birth), in whom there is a relative IGF-1 and IGFBP-3 deficiency postnatally. In these children, Hansen-Pupp et al. (2011) identified significant associations between IGF-1 and IGFBP-3, verbal IQ, total brain volume, unmyelinated white matter and cerebellar volumes. Volumetric imaging has also been carried out in children with isolated GHD. The splenium of the corpus callosum, left and right pallidum, left thalamus and left accumbens volumes were found to be significantly smaller in children with isolated GHD than in children with ISS.

Interestingly, the pattern of neural volume changes identified in this study was not limited to areas with a high density of growth hormone and IGF-1 receptor expression (prefrontal cortex, cerebellum, thalamus, putamen, hippocampus, caudate) (Araujo et al. 1989; Lai et al. 1991, 1993; Bondy and Lee 1993), but was restricted to certain structures (the right hippocampus, globus pallidum, thalamus and cerebellum), suggesting that these structures may be more vulnerable to variations in the growth hormone–IGF-1 axis. As not all structures with a high concentration of growth hormone and IGF-1 receptors were affected, it may also be that the effects of variations in the growth hormone–IGF-1 axis are being mediated via the activation of other biochemical processes. For example, IGF-1 has also been found to stimulate acetylcholine release from hippocampal neurons (Araujo et al. 1989), and to impact on NMDA-R2a and NMDA-R2b receptor density. Normal CNS functioning is dependent, in part, on glutamate signalling through the NMDA receptor (Kadotani et al. 1996). Another possibility is that these findings are secondary to the selective neuronal vulnerability of these brain regions to the underlying disease process (Wang and Michaelis 2010). In animal models of GHD, a significant reduction in glucose metabolism throughout the brain has been identified, with levels of glucose utilisation being significantly reduced in the thalamus and hippocampus (Kodl et al. 2008). The thalamus and globus pallidum form an integral part of the motor system and therefore require high concentrations of energy in the form of adenosine triphosphate (ATP) to function normally. Growth hormone and IGF-1 act centrally to modulate neural ATP concentrations (Sonntag et al. 2006). ATP controls neurotransmitter synthesis, release and reuptake, and is also required to maintain the transmembrane ion gradients necessary for signal conduction (Fahn 1976). Regions of high energy demand such as the thalamus and globus pallidum are more susceptible to injury than other brain regions with lower energy requirements (selective neuronal vulnerability). The increased sensitivity of these neural regions to reduced ATP availability may lead to increased cell injury or cell death, which may in turn be visualised on brain MRI as reduced neural volumes in these areas.

DTI has also been performed in children with isolated GHD who were naïve to growth hormone therapy. Corpus callosum and bilateral corticospinal tract fractional anisotropy were shown to be significantly lower in children with isolated GHD than in children with ISS (Fig 4.1) (Webb et al. 2012).

In children with isolated GHD, corpus callosum volume and fractional anisotropy correlated significantly with reductions in cognitive and motor skills scores (Webb et al. 2012). Corpus callosum size also correlated significantly with IGF-1 and IGFBP-3 SDS, suggesting that the differences in the size of the corpus callosum identified were not secondary to midline brain abnormalities which have not been identified by conventional MRI acquisition, but may be related to the severity of the underlying GHD.

In children with isolated GHD, bilateral corticospinal tract fractional anisotropy correlated significantly with performance on the Movement Assessment Battery for Children 2 test and with Processing Speed Index (which has many motor components), and corpus callosum fractional anisotropy correlated significantly with FSIQ (Webb et al. 2012). There is evidence from murine studies to suggest that IGF-1 may play a specific role in corticospinal tract development with murine in vivo and in vitro studies having previously shown that IGF-1 acts specifically to significantly enhance corticospinal motor neuron outgrowth, development and maturation (Ozdinler and Macklis 2006). The study reported above (Webb et al. 2012) provides further evidence to suggest that abnormalities in the growth hormone–IGF-1 axis also affect corticospinal tract development in humans, leading to reduced fractional anisotropy in individuals with GHD; and that these changes have functional consequences, namely impairments in motor skills performance.

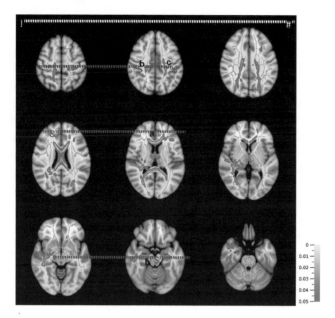

Figure 4.1. Functional MRI and tract-based spatial statistics analysis comparing fractional anisotropy in children with isolated growth hormone deficiency (GHD) and children with short stature. Areas of the mean fractional anisotropy skeleton in green represent regions where there were no significant differences in fractional anisotropy values; areas in red/yellow are regions where the fractional anisotropy was significantly lower in the isolated GHD group, as observed in the corpus callosum (a), right and left corticospinal tract (b and c). Colour map indicates the degree of significance for red and yellow regions. Adapted from Webb et al., *Brain* 2012; 135:216–227, Oxford University Press, with permission. (A colour version of this figure can be seen in the plate section at the end of the book.)

Effect of growth hormone replacement on cognition

Chaplin et al. recently published evidence to support a beneficial effect of growth hormone replacement on FSIQ, performance IQ and processing speed in children with GHD (Chaplin et al. 2015). This study included children with a mean age of 7.3 years (range 3–11 years at the start of treatment). Children with GHD had an improvement in FSIQ of >5 IQ points and in performance IQ of >8 IQ points over the 24-month study period. The one previous large study by Stabler et al. which only assessed verbal intelligence, academic achievement, social competence and behaviour yearly for 3 years after the onset of growth hormone treatment, reported no significant changes in verbal IQ and achievement scores following growth hormone therapy. Importantly Stabler et al. performed an abbreviated assessment of IQ, not measuring FSIQ, performance IQ and processing speed. However, after growth hormone treatment, child behaviour checklist scores for total behaviour were improved. This effect was found to be larger in those with isolated GHD ($p<0.001$) than in those with ISS ($p<0.003$) (Stabler et al. 1998). Growth hormone treatment in individuals with GHD also improved scores on internalising subscales (withdrawn: $p<0.007$, somatic complications $p<0.001$, anxious/depressed $p<0.001$) and on attention, social problems and thought problems (*p*=0.001). Other studies looking at the effect of growth hormone on cognition have studied this question in groups of children who have an abnormal growth hormone axis (Prader–Willi syndrome) and children born small for gestational age (SGA), but not classic GHD. The study in children with Prader–Willi syndrome, who have low circulating concentrations of IGF-1, suggests that growth hormone replacement is associated with cognitive benefits (improved motor skills and performance IQ) in this group (Siemensma et al. 2012). However, it is difficult to extrapolate these findings to children with GHD as children with Prader–Willi syndrome have significant hypotonia, which also improves with GHD treatment. It is therefore not surprising that performance on tests of motor skills and the performance component of the IQ test improve with improved muscle strength.

In a proportion of children born SGA, the growth hormone axis is abnormal. Whilst they do not fulfill the criterion standard for the diagnosis of GHD, up to 60% of children born SGA have been reported to have low serum growth hormone concentrations during a 24h growth hormone profile, and the majority have low IGF-I concentrations (de Waal et al. 1994). When growth hormone therapy was administered to children born SGA, significant improvements in overall intellectual performance and behavioral scores were identified compared to untreated matched children born SGA (van Pareren et al. 2004).

Conclusion

There is now good evidence that the growth hormone–IGF-1 axis plays an important role in brain and cognitive development in children and that growth hormone therapy impacts positively on cognitive performance and behaviour (Stabler et al. 1998; Chaplin et al. 2015). At present the main aims of growth hormone treatment remain the optimisation of final height, bone mass and body composition. Treatment is therefore often not started in infancy when growth hormone is not the main driver of growth. The published evidence from Chaplin et al. which documents significant improvements in cognitive performance after initiation of growth hormone treatment in children aged 3–11 years challenges current clinical practice. Further early intervention studies are therefore now required to determine whether growth hormone treatment should be started in infancy to prevent the development of brain and cognitive functioning abnormalities, as this would have major implications for clinical practice.

REFERENCES

Abuzzahab MJ, Schneider A, Goddard A et al. (2003) IGF-I receptor mutations resulting in intrauterine and postnatal growth retardation. *N Engl J Med* 349(23): 2211–2222 available from: PM:14657428

Adem A, Jossan SS, d'Argy R et al. (1989) Insulin-like growth factor 1 (IGF-1) receptors in the human brain: quantitative autoradiographic localization. *Brain Res* 503(2): 299–303 available from: PM:2557967

Aleman A, Verhaar HJ, de Haan EH et al. (1999) Insulin-like growth factor-I and cognitive function in healthy older men. *J Clin Endocrinol Metab* 84(2): 471–475 available from: PM:10022403

Araujo DM, Lapchak PA, Collier B, Chabot JG and Quirion R (1989) Insulin-like growth factor-1 (somatomedin-C) receptors in the rat brain: Distribution and interaction with the hippocampal cholinergic system. *Brain Res* 484(1–2): 130–138 available from: PM:2540883

Baron-Cohen S, Ring HA, Wheelwright S et al. (1999) Social intelligence in the normal and autistic brain: An fMRI study. *Eur J Neurosci* 11(6): 1891–1898 available from: PM:10336657

Basser PJ, Mattiello J and LeBihan D (1994) Estimation of the effective self-diffusion tensor from the NMR spin echo. *J Magn Reson B* 103(3): 247–254 available from: PM:8019776

Basser PJ and Pierpaoli C (1996) Microstructural and physiological features of tissues elucidated by quantitative-diffusion-tensor MRI. *J Magn Reson B* 111(3): 209–219 available from: PM:8661285

Baumann G (1991) Growth hormone heterogeneity: genes, isohormones, variants, and binding proteins. *Endocr Rev* 12(4): 424–449 available from: PM:0001760996

Beaulieu C (2002) The basis of anisotropic water diffusion in the nervous system – A technical review. *NMR Biomed* 15(7–8): 435–455 available from: PM:12489094

Bondy CA and Lee WH (1993) Patterns of insulin-like growth factor and IGF receptor gene expression in the brain. Functional implications. *Ann NY Acad Sci* 692: 33–43 available from: PM:8215043

Burman P, Broman JE, Hetta J et al. (1995) Quality of life in adults with growth hormone (GH) deficiency: Response to treatment with recombinant human GH in a placebo-controlled 21-month trial. *J Clin Endocrinol Metab* 80(12): 3585–3590 available from: PM:8530603

Burman P, Hetta J and Karlsson A (1993) Effect of growth hormone on brain neurotransmitters. *Lancet* 342(8885): 1492–1493 available from: PM:7504154

Burman P, Hetta J, Wide L, Mansson JE, Ekman R and Karlsson FA (1996) Growth hormone treatment affects brain neurotransmitters and thyroxine [see comment]. *Clin Endocrinol (Oxford)* 44(3): 319–324 available from: PM:8729530

Camacho-Hubner C, Woods KA, Clark AJ and Savage MO (2002) Insulin-like growth factor (IGF)-I gene deletion. *Rev Endocr Metab Disord* 3(4): 357–361 available from: PM:12424437

Caroni P and Grandes P (1990) Nerve sprouting in innervated adult skeletal muscle induced by exposure to elevated levels of insulin-like growth factors. *J Cell Biol* 110(4): 1307–1317 available from: PM:2157718

Chaplin J, Kristrom B, Jonsson B, Tuvemo T and Albertsson-Wikland K (2015) Growth hormone treatment improves cognitive function in short children with growth hormone deficiency. *Horm Res Paediatr* 83: 390–399 available from: PM:375529

David A, Hwa V, Metherell LA et al. (2011) Evidence for a continuum of genetic, phenotypic, and biochemical abnormalities in children with growth hormone insensitivity. *Endocr Rev* 32(4): 472–497 available from: PM:21525302

Deijen JB, de Boer H, Blok GJ and van der Veen EA (1996) Cognitive impairments and mood disturbances in growth hormone deficient men. *Psychoneuroendocrinology* 21(3): 313–322 available from: PM:8817729

Deijen JB, de Boer H and van der Veen EA (1998) Cognitive changes during growth hormone replacement in adult men. *Psychoneuroendocrinology* 23(1): 45–55 available from: PM:9618751

De Waal WJ, Hokken-Koelega AC, Stijnen T, de Muinck Keizer-Schrama SM and Drop SL (1994) Endogenous and stimulated GH secretion, urinary GH excretion, and plasma IGF-I and IGF-II levels in prepubertal children with short stature after intrauterine growth retardation. The Dutch Working Group on Growth Hormone. *Clin Endocrinol (Oxford)* 41: 621–630.

Donahue CP, Kosik KS and Shors TJ (2006) Growth hormone is produced within the hippocampus where it responds to age, sex, and stress. *Proc Natl Acad Sci USA* 103(15): 6031–6036 available from: PM:16574776

Drotar D, Owens R and Gotthold J (1980) Personality adjustment of children and adolescents with hypopituitarism. *Child Psychiatry Hum Dev* 11(1): 59–66 available from: PM:7398444

Fahn S (1976) Biochemistry of the basal ganglia. *Adv Neurol* 14: 59–89 available from: PM:7932

Falleti MG, Maruff P, Burman P and Harris A (2006) The effects of growth hormone (GH) deficiency and GH replacement on cognitive performance in adults: A meta-analysis of the current literature. *Psychoneuroendocrinology* 31(6): 681–691 available from: PM:16621325

Fischl B, Salat DH, Busa E et al. (2002) Whole brain segmentation: Automated labeling of neuroanatomical structures in the human brain. *Neuron* 33(3): 341–355 available from: PM:11832223

Frisch H, Hausler G, Lindenbauer S and Singer S (1990) Psychological aspects in children and adolescents with hypopituitarism. *Acta Paediatr Scand* 79(6–7): 644–651 available from: PM:2386056

Geary MP, Pringle PJ, Rodeck CH, Kingdom JC and Hindmarsh PC (2003) Sexual dimorphism in the growth hormone and insulin-like growth factor axis at birth. *J Clin Endocrinol Metab* 88(8): 3708–3714 available from: PM:12915659

Gluckman P, Klempt N, Guan J et al. (1992) A role for IGF-1 in the rescue of CNS neurons following hypoxic-ischemic injury. *Biochem Biophys Res Commun* 182(2): 593–599 available from: PM:1370886

Guevara-Aguirre J, Rosenbloom AL, Vaccarello MA et al. (1991) Growth hormone receptor deficiency (Laron syndrome): Clinical and genetic characteristics. *Acta Paediatr Scand Suppl* 377: 96–103 available from: PM:1785320

Gunnell D, Miller LL, Rogers I and Holly JM (2005) Association of insulin-like growth factor I and insulin-like growth factor-binding protein-3 with intelligence quotient among 8- to 9-year-old children in the Avon Longitudinal Study of Parents and Children. *Pediatrics* 116(5): e681–e686 available from: PM:16263982

Hansen-Pupp I, Hovel H, Hellstrom A et al. (2011) Postnatal decrease in circulating insulin-like growth factor-I and low brain volumes in very preterm infants. *J Clin Endocrinol Metab* 96(4): 1129–1135 available from: PM:21289247

Harvey S, Lavelin I and Pines M (2002) Growth hormone (GH) action in the brain: Neural expression of a GH-response gene. *J Mol Neurosci* 18(1–2): 89–95 available from: PM:11931354

Hoeflich A, Wu M, Mohan S et al. (1999) Overexpression of insulin-like growth factor-binding protein-2 in transgenic mice reduces postnatal body weight gain. *Endocrinology* 140(12): 5488–5496 available from: PM:10579311

Hojvat S, Baker G, Kirsteins L and Lawrence AM (1982) Growth hormone (GH) immunoreactivity in the rodent and primate CNS: Distribution, characterization and presence posthypophysectomy. *Brain Res* 239(2): 543–557 available from: PM:7093701

Holmes CS, Karlsson JA and Thompson RG (1985) Social and school competencies in children with short stature: Longitudinal patterns. *J Dev Behav Pediatr* 6(5): 263–267 available from: PM:4066961

Holmes CS, Thompson RG and Hayford JT (1984) Factors related to grade retention in children with short stature. *Child Care Health Dev* 10(4): 199–210 available from: PM:6206962

Hynes MA, Van Wyk JJ, Brooks PJ, D'Ercole AJ, Jansen M and Lund PK (1987) Growth hormone dependence of somatomedin-C/insulin-like growth factor-I and insulin-like growth factor-II messenger ribonucleic acids. *Mol Endocrinol* 1(3): 233–242 available from: PM:3453890

Johansson JO, Larson G, Andersson M et al. (1995) Treatment of growth hormone-deficient adults with recombinant human growth hormone increases the concentration of growth hormone in the cerebrospinal fluid and affects neurotransmitters. *Neuroendocrinology* 61(1): 57–66 available from: PM:7537355

Kadotani H, Hirano T, Masugi M et al. (1996) Motor discoordination results from combined gene disruption of the NMDA receptor NR2A and NR2C subunits, but not from single disruption of the NR2A or NR2C subunit. *J Neurosci* 16(24): 7859–7867 available from: PM:8987814

Kodl CT, Franc DT, Rao JP et al. (2008) Diffusion tensor imaging identifies deficits in white matter microstructure in subjects with type 1 diabetes that correlate with reduced neurocognitive function. *Diabetes* 57(11): 3083–3089 available from: PM:18694971

Kranzler JH, Rosenbloom AL, Martinez V and Guevara-Aguirre J (1998) Normal intelligence with severe insulin-like growth factor I deficiency due to growth hormone receptor deficiency: A controlled study in a genetically homogeneous population. *J Clin Endocrinol Metab* 83(6): 1953–1958 available from: PM:9626125

Lai Z, Roos P, Zhai O et al. (1993) Age-related reduction of human growth hormone-binding sites in the human brain. *Brain Res* 621(2): 260–266 available from: PM:8242339

Lai ZN, Emtner M, Roos P and Nyberg F (1991) Characterization of putative growth hormone receptors in human choroid plexus. *Brain Res* 546(2): 222–226 available from: PM:2070259

Laron Z (1984) Laron-type dwarfism (hereditary somatomedin deficiency): A review. *Ergeb Inn Med Kinderheilkd* 51: 117–150 available from: PM:6317375

Laron Z and Klinger B (1994) Laron syndrome: Clinical features, molecular pathology and treatment. *Horm Res* 42(4–5): 198–202 available from: PM:7868073

Lassarre C, Hardouin S, Daffos F, Forestier F, Frankenne F and Binoux M (1991) Serum insulin-like growth factors and insulin-like growth factor binding proteins in the human fetus. Relationships with growth in normal subjects and in subjects with intrauterine growth retardation. *Pediatr Res* 29(3): 219–225 available from: PM:1709729

Lijffijt M, van Dam PS, Kenemans JL et al. (2003) Somatotropic-axis deficiency affects brain substrates of selective attention in childhood-onset growth hormone deficient patients. *Neurosci Lett* 353(2): 123–126 available from: PM:14664916

Lobie PE, Garcia-Aragon J, Lincoln DT, Barnard R, Wilcox JN and Waters MJ (1993) Localization and ontogeny of growth hormone receptor gene expression in the central nervous system. *Dev Brain Res* 74(2): 225–233 available from: PM:8403384

Lynch CD, Lyons D, Khan A, Bennett SA and Sonntag WE (2001) Insulin-like growth factor-1 selectively increases glucose utilization in brains of aged animals. *Endocrinology* 142(1): 506–509 available from: PM:11145617

McClelland JL and Goddard NH (1996) Considerations arising from a complementary learning systems perspective on hippocampus and neocortex. *Hippocampus* 6(6): 654–665 available from: PM:9034852

Milner B and Penfield W (1955) The effect of hippocampal lesions on recent memory. *Tran Am Neurol Assoc* (80th Meeting) 42–48 available from: PM:13311995

Morsing E, Asard M, Ley D, Stjernqvist K and Marsal K (2011) Cognitive function after intrauterine growth restriction and very preterm birth. *Pediatrics* 127(4): e874–e882 available from: PM:21382944

Mustafa A, Adem A, Roos P and Nyberg F (1994) Sex differences in binding of human growth hormone to rat brain. *Neurosci Res* 19(1): 93–99 available from: PM:8008239

Netchine I, Azzi S, Houang M et al. (2009) Partial primary deficiency of insulin-like growth factor (IGF)-I activity associated with IGF1 mutation demonstrates its critical role in growth and brain development. *J Clin Endocrinol Metab* 94(10): 3913–3921 available from: PM:19773405

Ni W, Rajkumar K, Nagy JI and Murphy LJ (1997) Impaired brain development and reduced astrocyte response to injury in transgenic mice expressing IGF binding protein-1. *Brain Res* 769(1): 97–107 available from: PM:9374277

Ozdinler PH and Macklis JD (2006) IGF-I specifically enhances axon outgrowth of corticospinal motor neurons. *Nat Neurosci* 9(11): 1371–1381 available from: PM:17057708

Penfield W and Milner B (1958) Memory deficit produced by bilateral lesions in the hippocampal zone. *AMA: Arch Neurol Psychiatry* 79(5): 475–497 available from: PM:13519951

Pulford BE, Whalen LR and Ishii DN (1999) Peripherally administered insulin-like growth factor-I preserves hindlimb reflex and spinal cord noradrenergic circuitry following a central nervous system lesion in rats. *Exp Neurol* 159(1): 114–123 available from: PM:10486180

Reinhardt RR and Bondy CA (1994) Insulin-like growth factors cross the blood-brain barrier. *Endocrinology* 135(5): 1753–1761 available from: PM:7525251

Russo VC, Gluckman PD, Feldman EL and Werther GA (2005) The insulin-like growth factor system and its pleiotropic functions in brain. *Endocr Rev* 26(7): 916–943 available from: PM:16131630

Scheepens A, Moderscheim TA and Gluckman PD (2005) The role of growth hormone in neural development. *Horm Res* 64(Suppl 3): 66–72 available from: PM:16439847

Scheepens A, Sirimanne E, Beilharz E et al. (1999) Alterations in the neural growth hormone axis following hypoxic-ischemic brain injury. *Mol Brain Res* 68(1–2): 88–100 available from: PM:10320786

Schmithorst VJ, Wilke M, Dardzinski BJ and Holland SK (2005) Cognitive functions correlate with white matter architecture in a normal pediatric population: A diffusion tensor MRI study. *Hum Brain Mapp* 26(2): 139–147 available from: PM:15858815

Siemensma EP, Tummers-de Lind van Wijngaarden RF, Festen DA et al. (2012) Beneficial effects of growth hormone treatment on cognition in children with Prader-Willi syndrome: A randomized controlled trial and longitudinal study. *J Clin Endocrinol Metab* 97(7): 2307–2314 available from: PM:22508707

Silha JV, Gui Y, Mishra S, Leckstrom A, Cohen P and Murphy LJ (2005) Overexpression of gly56/gly80/gly81-mutant insulin-like growth factor-binding protein-3 in transgenic mice. *Endocrinology* 146(3): 1523–1531 available from: PM:15550509

Sonntag WE, Bennett C, Ingram R et al. (2006) Growth hormone and IGF-I modulate local cerebral glucose utilization and ATP levels in a model of adult-onset growth hormone deficiency. *Am J Physiol Endocrinol Metab* 291(3): E604–E610 available from: PM:16912061

Sonntag WE, Lynch C, Thornton P, Khan A, Bennett S and Ingram R (2000) The effects of growth hormone and IGF-1 deficiency on cerebrovascular and brain ageing. *J Anat* 197(Pt 4): 575–585 available from: PM:11197531

Stabler B, Siegel PT, Clopper RR, Stoppani CE, Compton PG and Underwood LE (1998) Behavior change after growth hormone treatment of children with short stature. *J Pediatr* 133(3): 366–373 available from: PM:9738718

Steinhausen HC and Stahnke N (1976) Psychoendocrinological studies in dwarfed children and adolescents. *Arch Dis Child* 51(10): 778–783 available from: PM:188386

Steinhausen HC and Stahnke N (1977) Negative impact of growth-hormone deficiency on psychological functioning in dwarfed children and adolescents. *Eur J Pediatr* 126(4): 263–270 available from: PM:590279

Tillmann V, Tang VW, Price DA, Hughes DG, Wright NB and Clayton PE (2000) Magnetic resonance imaging of the hypothalamic-pituitary axis in the diagnosis of growth hormone deficiency. *J Pediatr Endocrinol Metab* 13(9): 1577–1583 available from: PM:11154153

Turnley AM, Faux CH, Rietze RL, Coonan JR and Bartlett PF (2002) Suppressor of cytokine signaling 2 regulates neuronal differentiation by inhibiting growth hormone signaling. *Nat Neurosci* 5(11): 1155–1162 available from: PM:12368809

van Dam PS (2005) Neurocognitive function in adults with growth hormone deficiency. *Horm Res* 64(Suppl 3): 109–114 available from: PM:16439853

van Pareren YK, Duivenvoorden HJ, Slijper FSM, Koot HM, Hokken-Koelega ACS (2004) Intelligence and psychosocial functioning during long-term growth hormone therapy in children born small for gestational age. *J Clin Endocrinol Metab* 89(11): 5295–5302 available from: PM:15531473

Walenkamp MJ, van der Kamp HJ, Pereira AM et al. (2006) A variable degree of intrauterine and postnatal growth retardation in a family with a missense mutation in the insulin-like growth factor I receptor. *J Clin Endocrinol Metab* 91(8): 3062–3070 available from: PM:16757531

Wang X and Michaelis EK (2010) Selective neuronal vulnerability to oxidative stress in the brain. *Front Aging Neurosci* 2: 12 available from: PM:20552050

Webb EA, O'Reilly MA, Clayden JD et al. (2012) Effect of growth hormone deficiency on brain structure, motor function and cognition. *Brain* 135(Pt 1): 216–227 available from: PM:22120144

Werther GA, Russo V, Baker N and Butler G (1998) The role of the insulin-like growth factor system in the developing brain. *Horm Res* 49(Suppl 1): 37–40 available from: PM:9554468

Winkler T, Sharma HS, Stalberg E, Badgaiyan RD, Westman J and Nyberg F (2000) Growth hormone attenuates alterations in spinal cord evoked potentials and cell injury following trauma to the rat spinal cord. An experimental study using topical application of rat growth hormone. *Amino Acids* 19(1): 363–371 available from: PM:11026507

Woods KA, Camacho-Hubner C, Savage MO and Clark AJ (1996) Intrauterine growth retardation and postnatal growth failure associated with deletion of the insulin-like growth factor I gene. *N Engl J Med* 335(18): 1363–1367 available from: PM:8857020

Ye P, Li L, Richards RG, DiAugustine RP and D'Ercole AJ (2002) Myelination is altered in insulin-like growth factor-I null mutant mice. *J Neurosci* 22(14): 6041–6051 available from: PM:12122065

5
NEUROENDOCRINE DISORDERS OF SALT AND WATER BALANCE

Joseph A Majzoub

Introduction

Paediatric neuroendocrine disorders of salt and water balance are uncommon but important causes of morbidity and mortality. Most often they either arise independently from genetic or neoplastic causes, or occur subsequent to accidental or surgical trauma (Maghnie et al. 2000). This chapter focuses upon genetic causes, but notes other aetiologies for completeness. In most patients with central diabetes insipidus, a definitive diagnosis can eventually be made (Di lorgi et al. 2014), either upon initial presentation following a comprehensive evaluation (in ~28% of cases), or after continued evaluation over many years (in ~96% of cases). It is therefore useful to understand the pathophysiology and differential diagnosis of central diabetes insipidus in children.

Physiology of water balance

The posterior pituitary, or the neurohypophysis, secretes the nonapeptide hormone arginine vasopressin (AVP), also known as antidiuretic hormone (ADH). Vasopressin controls water homeostasis, and disorders of vasopressin secretion and action lead to clinically important derangements in water metabolism. Osmotic sensor and effector pathways control the regulation of vasopressin release, whereas volume homeostasis is determined largely through the action of the renin–angiotensin–aldosterone system, with contributions from both vasopressin and the natriuretic peptide family. The human vasopressin gene consists of three exons. The first exon encodes the 19-amino-acid signal peptide, followed by the vasopressin nonapeptide, which is followed by a 3-amino-acid protease cleavage site leading into the first nine amino acids of neurophysin II. After interruption of the coding region by an intron, the second exon continues with neurophysin coding sequences. The third exon completes the sequence of the neurophysin and is followed by coding information for an additional 39-amino-acid glycopeptide (copeptin) whose function is unclear.

Expression of the vasopressin gene occurs in the hypothalamic paraventricular and supraoptic nuclei. The magnocellular components of each of these nuclei are the primary neuronal populations involved in water balance, with vasopressin synthesised in these areas carried by means of axonal transport to the posterior pituitary, its primary site of storage and release into the systemic circulation.

The blood concentration of plasma vasopressin increases in response to increasing plasma tonicity. Normally, at a serum osmolality of less than 280mOsm/kg, plasma vasopressin concentration is at or below 1pg/mL, whereas above 283mOsm/kg—the normal threshold for vasopressin release—plasma vasopressin concentration increases in proportion to plasma osmolality, up to a maximum concentration of about 20pg/mL at a blood osmolality of approximately 320mOsm/kg. The sensation of thirst occurs at an osmolality approximately 10mOsm/kg higher than that for vasopressin release. Thus, water balance is regulated in two ways: (1) vasopressin secretion stimulates water reabsorption by the kidney, thereby reducing future water loss; and (2) thirst stimulates water ingestion, thereby restoring previous water loss.

Separate from osmotic regulation, vasopressin is secreted in response to alterations in intravascular volume. Afferent baroreceptor pathways arising from the right and left atria and the aortic arch (carotid sinus) are stimulated by increasing intravascular volume and stretch of vessel walls, and they send signals through the vagus and glossopharyngeal nerves, respectively, to the brainstem nucleus tractus solitarius. The pattern of vasopressin secretion in response to volume as opposed to osmotic stimuli is markedly different. Although minor changes in plasma osmolality above 280mOsm/kg evoke linear increases in plasma vasopressin, substantial alteration in intravascular volume is required for alteration in vasopressin output. No change in vasopressin secretion is seen until blood volume decreases by approximately 8%. With intravascular volume deficits exceeding 8%, vasopressin concentration increases exponentially. When blood volume decreases by approximately 25%, vasopressin concentrations increase to 20- to 30-fold above normal, vastly exceeding those required for maximal antidiuresis.

Modulation of water balance occurs through the action of vasopressin on V2 receptors located primarily in the renal collecting tubule. Vasopressin-induced increases in intracellular cyclic AMP mediated by the V2 receptor trigger a complex pathway of events resulting in increased permeability of the collecting duct to water and efficient water transit across an otherwise minimally permeable epithelium. Insertion of the water channels causes up to 100-fold increase in water permeability of the apical membrane, allowing water movement along its osmotic gradient into the hypertonic inner medullary interstitium from the tubule lumen and excretion of a concentrated urine. The molecular analysis of the water channels has revealed a family of related proteins, designated aquaporins, that differ in their sites of expression and pattern of regulation (Knepper 1994). Each protein consists of a single polypeptide chain with six membrane-spanning domains. Although functional as monomers, they are believed to form homotetramers in the plasma membrane. Aquaporin-2 is expressed primarily within the collecting duct. Studies with immunoelectron microscopy have demonstrated large amounts of aquaporin-2 in the apical plasma membrane and subapical vesicles of the collecting duct, consistent with the 'membrane shuttling' model of water channel aggregate insertion into the apical membrane after vasopressin stimulation.

Diabetes insipidus

AETIOLOGY, PATHOGENESIS AND CLINICAL FEATURES

Neuroendocrine causes of hypernatraemia are due to an inability to secrete adequate amounts of vasopressin (central diabetes insipidus). Hypernatraemia due to mutations in the renal vasopressin receptor, AVPR2, causing X-linked nephrogenic diabetes insipidus, or in the renal aquaporin 2 water channel, aquaporin 2, causing autosomal recessive nephrogenic diabetes insipidus, is reviewed elsewhere (Babey et al. 2011) (Table 5.1).

Monogenic causes

Familial, autosomal dominant central diabetes insipidus is usually manifest within the first half of the first decade of life (Pedersen et al. 1985) up to 9 years of age (Siggaard et al. 2005). Vasopressin secretion, initially normal, gradually declines until diabetes

TABLE 5.1

Causes of hypernatraemia

Excess salt ingestion: Fabricated or induced illness
Hypernatraemic Dehydration
Diabetes insipidus

Central
Congenital

Mutations in arginine vasopressin: dominant, recessive
Wolfram (DIDMOAD) syndrome: Mutations in *WFS1* and *WFS2*
Midline forebrain abnormalities: septo-optic dysplasia, holoprosencephaly, cleft palate
Mutations in genes implicated in hypothalamo-pituitary development such as *FGF8* and *ARNT2*

Acquired

Traumatic brain injury
Neoplasia – astrocytoma, craniopharyngioma, germinoma, optic glioma, pinealoma
Haematological malignancies, e.g. leukaemia
Langerhans ell histiocytosis
Lymphocytic histiocytosis
Sarcoidosis
ROHHAD/ROHHADNET syndrome
Infection, e.g. meningococcal, group B streptococcal, cryptococcal, listeria, toxoplasmosis, congenital cytomegalovirus

Nephrogenic
Congenital
Mutations in arginine vasopressin receptor type 2, aquaporin 2

Acquired

Polycystic kidney disease
Hypercalcaemia
Lithium toxicity
Hypokalaemia
Post-obstructive polyuria
Sickle cell disease
Sjogren syndrome
Bartter syndrome
Drugs, e.g. amphotericin B, orlistat, ifosfamide, ofloxacin, vaptanes

---

insipidus of variable severity ensues. Patients respond well to vasopressin replacement therapy. The disease has a high degree of penetrance, but may be of variable severity within a family (Os et al. 1985), and may spontaneously improve in middle age (Toth et al. 1984; Os et al. 1985). Approximately 70 different oligonucleotide mutations in the vasopressin structural gene have been found to cause the disease (http://omim.org/entry/192340). Most mutations are in the neurophysin portion of the vasopressin precursor, except for six in either the signal peptide or vasopressin peptide regions of the gene, or due to deletion of the entire gene. In vitro functional studies of these mutations suggest a correlation between functional disruption and disease severity (Christensen et al. 2004a, 2004b, 2004c; Siggaard et al. 2005). This suggests that neurophysin has a valuable function, possibly in the proper intracellular sorting or packaging of vasopressin into secretory granules. There are no disease-causing mutations in the copeptin region of the vasopressin precursor. This suggests either that this region has a low mutation rate, or more likely that it does not serve a critical function in vasopressin biology. Two families, with either a missense mutation within the vasopressin peptide region (proline→leucine at amino acid 7) of the gene (Willcutts et al. 1999), causing markedly reduced biological activity, or deletion of the entire AVP gene (Christensen et al. 2013), have been reported. Diabetes insipidus in these families is transmitted with an autosomal recessive pattern. This indicates that haploinsufficiency is not the basis for the autosomal dominant nature of the disease in families with the more common mutations in the neurophysin region of the gene. Rather, the abnormal gene product may interfere with the processing and secretion of the product of the normal allele (Ito et al. 1999), or cause neuronal degeneration and cell death (Ito and Jameson 1997). In support of this, mutant vasopressin precursors impair the secretion of the normal protein in cell models (Ito et al. 1999), and in a transgenic mouse model of the disease, a progressive loss of hypothalamic vasopressin-containing neurons occurs as the mice develop diabetes insipidus (Russell et al. 2003). Heterozygous mice with a mutation (p.C67X) in the vasopressin gene known to cause autosomal dominant familial neurohypophyseal diabetes insipidus in humans developed diabetes insipidus by 2 months of age. They were found to have retention of the precursor of vasopressin within the neurons and the induction of an endoplasmic reticulum chaperone protein, BiP (Russell et al. 2003).

Vasopressin deficiency is also associated with Wolfram (DIDMOAD) syndrome, consisting of diabetes insipidus, diabetes mellitus, optic atrophy and deafness (Grosse Aldenhovel et al. 1991; Thompson et al. 1989; Farmer et al. 2013). One mutant gene causing this syndrome complex was localised to human chromosome 4p16 by polymorphic linkage analysis (Collier et al. 1996) and subsequently isolated (Inoue et al. 1998). The Wolfram syndrome gene, *WFS1*, encodes an 890-amino-acid tetrameric transmembrane protein that primarily localises to the endoplasmic reticulum. It is thought to function as a calcium channel or regulator of a calcium channel (Osman et al. 2003; Riggs et al. 2005). In addition, mutations in a second gene, *WFS2*, which is located on chromosome 4q22 and encodes Miner1, also cause Wolfram syndrome. Miner1 regulates sulphydryl redox status, the unfolded protein response and Ca^{2+} homeostasis (Wiley et al. 2013).

Developmental, syndromic and structural causes

Midline brain anatomic abnormalities such as septo-optic dysplasia (SOD)/optic nerve hypoplasia (ONH) with agenesis of the corpus callosum (Masera et al. 1994), the Kabuki syndrome (Tawa et al. 1994), holoprosencephaly (Van Gool et al. 1990) and familial pituitary hypoplasia with absent stalk (Yagi et al. 1994) may be associated with central diabetes insipidus. These patients need not have external evidence of craniofacial abnormalities (Van Gool et al. 1990). Monogenic causes of some of these abnormalities have been found and may overlap. Mutations in *SHH, ZIC2, SIX3, TGIF, PTCH, GLI2* and *TDGF1* have been described in patients with holoprosencephaly (Dubourg et al. 2007). SOD/ONH can be caused by mutations in *HESX1* (Di Iorgi et al. 2009) in a minority of patients (Reynaud et al. 2006), although none of the patients with *HESX1* mutations actually manifests diabetes insipidus. There is genetic overlap between SOD/ONH and patients with Kallmann syndrome and combined pituitary hormone deficiencies (CPHDs), with mutations in *FGFR1, FGF8* and *PROKR2* contributing to approximately 8% of patients with a combination of SOD and CPHD (Raivio et al. 2012; Reynaud et al. 2012). *LHX3* and *LHX4* mutations do not cause diabetes insipidus, and although *LHX4* mutations are associated with pituitary stalk interruption syndrome (Tajima et al. 2007), *LHX3* mutations are not; they generally lead to a small anterior pituitary with no abnormality of the posterior pituitary (Sobrier et al. 2012). In most cases of pituitary stalk interruption syndrome associated with diabetes insipidus, no genetic cause is found (Lamine et al. 2012). Mutations in *LHX2* are unlikely in patients with diabetes insipidus and ocular hypoplasia (Perez et al. 2012). Recently, mutations in *ARNT2* have been described in association with thyroid-stimulating hormone, adrenocorticotropic hormone and probable somatostatin deficiencies and diabetes insipidus (Webb et al. 2013; also see Chapter 2 by Alatzoglou and Dattani).

Traumatic insults

Central diabetes insipidus is most commonly due to trauma to the hypothalamic-pituitary region, usually following surgical treatment for neoplasms including craniopharyngiomas or astrocytomas located in this area. Curiously, isolated high-dose radiation therapy to the hypothalamic-pituitary region has never been found to cause central diabetes insipidus, whereas it is a common cause of anterior pituitary hormonal deficits. Because vasopressin is carried directly to the posterior pituitary via magnocellular axonal transport, it may be that radiation affects hypothalamic-releasing hormone function by interruption of the portal-hypophyseal circulation to the anterior pituitary, which is absent from the vasopressin circuitry. Vasopressin axons travelling from the hypothalamus to the posterior pituitary terminate at various levels within the stalk and gland. Since surgical interruption of these axons can result in retrograde degeneration of hypothalamic neurons, lesions closer to the hypothalamus will affect more neurons and cause greater permanent loss of hormone secretion. Not infrequently, a 'triple phase' response is seen. Although the exact incidence of this phenomenon remains unknown, in a small study nearly one in three children who underwent surgery for a craniopharyngioma developed it (Finken et al. 2011). Following surgery, an initial phase of transient diabetes insipidus is observed, lasting ½ to 2 days, and possibly due to oedema in the area interfering with normal vasopressin secretion. If significant vasopressin cell destruction has occurred, this is often followed by a second phase of increased vasopressin release and hyponatremia, which may last up to 10 days, due to the unregulated release of vasopressin by dying neurons. A third phase of permanent diabetes insipidus may follow if more than 90% of vasopressin cells are destroyed. Usually, a prolonged second phase response foreshadows significant permanent diabetes insipidus in the final phase of this response.

Neoplasms

Germinomas and pinealomas typically arise near the base of the hypothalamus where vasopressin axons converge before their entry into the posterior pituitary and for this reason are among the most common primary brain tumours associated with diabetes insipidus. Germinomas causing the disease can be very small (Ono et al. 1992; Tarng and Huang 1995) and undetectable by magnetic resonance imaging (MRI) for several years following the onset of polyuria (Appignani et al. 1993). For this reason, quantitative measurement of the β subunit of human chorionic gonadotropin, often secreted by germinomas and pinealomas, and regularly repeated MRI scans should be performed in children with idiopathic or unexplained diabetes insipidus. Empty sella syndrome, possibly due to unrecognised pituitary infarction, can be associated with diabetes insipidus in children (Hung and Fitz 1992). Craniopharyngiomas and optic gliomas can also cause central diabetes insipidus when very large, although this is more often a postoperative complication of the treatment for these tumours (Di Iorgi et al. 2014; Werny et al. 2015).

Central diabetes insipidus is a rare complication associated with acute myelogenous leukemia (AML) (Cull et al. 2013). Most of these patients have monosomy of chromosome 7, and additionally may have chromosome 3q21q26/EVI-1 gene rearrangements. The pathogenesis is unknown, and is usually not associated with leukaemic infiltration of the hypothalamic-pituitary region, although this is occasionally the cause (Foresti et al. 1992). The diabetes insipidus responds to vasopressin analogue treatment. Infiltration of the pituitary stalk can also occur with medullary carcinoma of the thyroid (Santarpia et al. 2009).

Infiltrative, autoimmune and infectious diseases

Langerhans cell histiocytosis and lymphocytic hypophysitis are the most common types of infiltrative disorders causing central diabetes insipidus. Approximately 10% of patients with histiocytosis will have diabetes insipidus. These patients tend to have more serious, multisystem disease for longer periods of time than those without diabetes insipidus (Dunger et al. 1989; Grois et al. 1995), and anterior pituitary deficits often accompany posterior pituitary deficiency (Broadbent et al. 1993). MRI characteristically shows thickening of the pituitary stalk (Tien et al. 1990).

Lymphocytic infundibuloneurohypophysitis may account for over one-half of patients with 'idiopathic' central diabetes insipidus (Imura et al. 1993; Hamnvik et al. 2010). This entity may be associated with other autoimmune diseases (Paja et al. 1994). Image analysis discloses an enlarged pituitary and thickened stalk (Koshiyama et al. 1994), and biopsy of the posterior pituitary reveals lymphocytic infiltration of the gland, stalk and magnocellular hypothalamic nuclei (Kojima et al. 1989). A necrotising form of this entity has been described which also causes anterior pituitary failure and responds to steroid treatment (Ahmed et al. 1993). Diabetes insipidus can also be associated with pulmonary granulomatous diseases (Rossi et al. 1994) including sarcoidosis (Lewis et al. 1987).

In 2008, a syndrome with rapid-onset obesity with hypothalamic dysfunction, hypoventilation and autonomic dysregulation (ROHHAD) associated with central diabetes insipidus has been described (Bougneres et al. 2008). It is often associated with the presence of a neural tumour such as a paraganglioma, in which case it is termed ROHHADNET. Children with ROHHAD may present after infancy with rapid weight gain followed by alveolar hypoventilation, autonomic nervous system dysregulation and cardiorespiratory arrest. Its cause is not solely genetic, for it has been reported to occur discordantly in monozygotic twins (Patwari et al. 2011).

Infections involving the base of the brain – such as meningococcal (Christensen and Bank 1988), Group B streptococcal, cryptococcal, listeria (Sloane 1989) and toxoplasmosis (Brandle et al. 1995) – meningitis, congenital cytomegalovirus infection (Mena et al. 1993) and nonspecific inflammatory disease of the brain (Watanabe et al. 1994) can cause central diabetes insipidus. The disease is often transient, suggesting that it is due to inflammation rather than destruction of vasopressin-containing neurons.

INVESTIGATIONS

In children, it must first be determined whether pathologic polyuria or polydipsia (exceeding $2L/m^2/day$) is present. If present, the following should be obtained: serum osmolality; serum concentrations of sodium, potassium, glucose, calcium and blood urea nitrogen; and urinalysis, including measurement of urine osmolality, specific gravity and glucose concentration. A serum osmolality greater than 300mOsm/kg, with urine osmolality less than 300mOsm/kg, establishes the diagnosis of diabetes insipidus. If serum osmolality is less than 270mOsm/kg, or urine osmolality is greater than 600mOsm/kg, the diagnosis of diabetes insipidus is unlikely.

If, on initial screening, the patient has a serum osmolality less than 300mOsm/kg, but the intake/output record at home suggests significant polyuria and polydipsia that cannot be attributed to primary polydipsia (i.e., the serum osmolality is greater than 270mOsm/kg), the patient should undergo a water deprivation test to establish a diagnosis of diabetes insipidus and to differentiate central from nephrogenic causes. After a maximally tolerated overnight fast (based on the outpatient history), the child is admitted to the outpatient testing centre in the early morning of a day when an 8- to 10-hour test can be carried out, and the child is deprived of water (Richman et al. 1981). Physical signs (weight, postural pulse and blood pressure) and biochemical parameters (serum and urine osmolality, serum sodium, urine specific gravity) are measured. If at any time during the test, the urine osmolality exceeds 1 000mOsm/kg, or 600mOsm/kg and is stable over 1 hour, the patient does not have diabetes insipidus. If at any time the serum osmolality exceeds 300mOsm/kg and the urine osmolality is less than 600mOsm/kg, the patient likely has diabetes insipidus. If the serum osmolality is less than 300mOsm/kg and the urine osmolality is less than 600mOsm/kg, the test should be continued unless vital signs disclose hypovolemia. A common error is to stop a test too soon, based on the amount of body weight lost, before either urine osmolality has plateaued above 600mOsm/kg or a serum osmolality above 300mOsm/kg has been achieved. Unless the serum osmolality increases above the threshold for vasopressin release, a lack of vasopressin action (as inferred by a non-concentrated urine) cannot be deemed pathologic. If the diagnosis of diabetes insipidus is made, aqueous vasopressin (Pitressin, $1U/m^2$) should be given subcutaneously. If the patient has central diabetes insipidus, urine volume should fall and osmolality should at least double during the next hour, compared with the value before vasopressin therapy. If there is less than a twofold increase in urine osmolality after vasopressin administration, the patient probably has nephrogenic diabetes insipidus. Patients with a family history of X-linked nephrogenic diabetes insipidus can be evaluated for the disorder in the prenatal or perinatal period by DNA sequence analysis, thus allowing therapy to be initiated without delay (Bichet 1994).

The water deprivation test should be sufficient in most patients to establish the diagnosis of diabetes insipidus and to differentiate central from nephrogenic causes. Plasma vasopressin concentrations may be obtained during the test, although they are rarely needed for diagnostic purposes in children, and an immunoassay for copeptin, the carboxy-terminus of the vasopressin precursor, has been developed which may replace the measurement of vasopressin in the evaluation of diabetes insipidus. Copeptin is more stable than vasopressin, and blood concentrations of the two peptides are highly correlated (Christ-Crain and Fenske 2016). As an alternative to the water deprivation test, the infusion of hypertonic saline while monitoring urine osmolality is a more rapid, although more invasive, method to diagnose diabetes insipidus (Robertson 1995; Maghnie et al. 1998). It may be more suitable in a young child who cannot tolerate the lengthy period of fasting often required for a water deprivation test. After the patient urinates, 3% NaCl is administered intravenously for 120min. Plasma sodium, vasopressin and osmolality, and urinary osmolality are measured at 0, 30, 60, 90, and 120min. Urine osmolality should increase once serum osmolality rises over 295mOsm/kg/$H_2$0.

MRI is not very helpful in distinguishing central diabetes insipidus from nephrogenic diabetes insipidus (Papapostolou et al. 1995). Normally, the posterior pituitary is seen as an area of enhanced brightness in T1-weighted images after administration of gadolinium (Moses et al. 1992). The posterior pituitary 'bright spot' is diminished or absent in both forms of diabetes insipidus, presumably because of decreased vasopressin synthesis in central, and increased vasopressin release in nephrogenic, disease (Halimi et al. 1988; Maghnie et al. 1992; Moses et al. 1992). In primary polydipsia, the bright spot is normal, probably because vasopressin accumulates in the posterior pituitary during chronic water ingestion (Moses et al. 1992), whereas it is decreased in syndrome of inappropriate antidiuresis, presumably because of increased vasopressin secretion (Papapostolou et al. 1995). Dynamic, fast-frame, MRI analysis has allowed estimation of blood flow to the posterior pituitary (Maghnie et al. 1994). With this technique, both central and nephrogenic diabetes insipidus are associated with delayed enhancement in the area of the neurohypophysis (Sato et al. 1993).

Treatment of central diabetes insipidus
In the outpatient setting, treatment of central diabetes insipidus in older children should begin with oral desmopressin (des-amino D-arginine AVP, DDAVP) at bedtime and the dose

increased to the lowest amount that gives an antidiuretic effect (Oiso et al. 2013). Oral DDAVP in doses of 25–300 micrograms every 8 to 12 hours is reported to be highly effective and safe in children (Williams et al. 1986; Stick and Betts 1987). If the dose is effective, but has too short a duration, it should be increased further or a second, morning dose should be added. Patients should escape from the antidiuretic effect for at least 1 hour before the next dose, to ensure that any excessive water will be excreted. Otherwise, water intoxication may occur.

Vasopressin therapy coupled with excessive fluid intake (usually greater than $1L/m^2/$ day as discussed subsequently) can result in unwanted hyponatraemia. Because neonates and young infants receive all of their nutrition in liquid form, the obligatory high oral fluid requirements for this age ($3L/m^2$/day), combined with vasopressin treatment, are likely to lead to this dangerous complication (Crigler 1976). In infants, oral tablet and intranasal liquid desmopressin are not only difficult to administer accurately, but also their use is associated with significant fluctuations in the serum sodium concentrations. Such neonates may be better managed with fluid therapy alone. A reduced solute load diet will aid in this regard. Human milk is best for this purpose ($75mOsm/kg$ H_2O), whereas cow's milk is the worst ($230mOsm/kg$ H_2O). For example, in an infant with diabetes insipidus with a fixed urine osmolality of $100mOsm/kg$ H_2O, 300mL of urine per day is required to excrete the amount of solute consumed in human milk, whereas 900mL of urine per day is required to excrete the higher amount of solute consumed in cow's milk. The Similac PM 60/40 formula has a renal solute load of $92mOsm/kg$ H_2O. Additionally, supplementation with free water may be needed depending on the severity of the diabetes insipidus. Options such as 20–30mL of supplemental free water for every 120–160mL of formula or dilution of the formula with free water have been used. Alternatively, thiazide (chlorthiazide, 5–10mg/kg/dose, twice or thrice daily) (Rivkees et al. 2007) and/or amiloride diuretics may be added to facilitate renal proximal tubular sodium and water reabsorption (Jakobsson and Berg 1994) and thereby decrease oral fluid requirements. This therapy may be accompanied by a mild degree of dehydration. More recently, parenteral desmopressin (0.02–0.08mcg/dose given once or twice daily) has been administered subcutaneously in infants with good results, although this is not approved by the United States Food and Drug Administration (Blanco et al. 2006). Parenteral desmopressin was originally formulated at a concentration of 4mcg/mL, to be used at a dose of 0.3mcg/kg/dose to treat haemorrhage diatheses such as haemophilia A and von Willebrand's disease type 1. Thus, care must be taken if it is used at 1/40 to 1/4 of this dose to treat infants with diabetes insipidus. In older children on more calorie-dense solid diets, the use of short-acting agents such as AVP (Pitressin), or longer-acting desmopressin, will decrease fluid needs while minimising the possible occurrence of hyponatraemia.

Hyponatraemia
Aetiology, pathogenesis and clinical features
Virtually all causes of hyponatraemia in children are associated with an elevated blood concentration of vasopressin. In the vast majority of these, the elevation in AVP is appropriate, since it follows a decrease in blood volume, usually due to dehydration associated with another illness

TABLE 5.2
Causes of hyponatraemia

Systemic dehydration, e.g. gastroenteritis

Decreased 'effective' intravascular volume, e.g. congestive heart failure, cirrhosis, nephrotic syndrome, positive pressure mechanical ventilation,[1] severe burns (Potts and May 1986), lung disease (broncho-pulmonary dysplasia (Kojima et al. 1990) [in neonates]), cystic fibrosis with obstruction (Stegner et al. 1986) and severe asthma

Syndrome of inappropriate antidiuresis due to encephalitis, brain tumour, head trauma or psychiatric disease, in the postictal period after generalised seizures; after prolonged nausea, pneumonia or AIDS

Drugs, e.g. carbamazepine, chlorpropamide, vinblastine, vincristine and tricyclic antidepressants

Primary or secondary adrenal insufficiency

Des-amino D-arginine arginine vasopressin treatment

Nephrogenic syndrome of inappropriate anti-diuresis due to activating mutations of *AVP2R*

Salt loss due to diuretic therapy, polycystic kidney disease, gastroenteritis, cystic fibrosis, cerebral salt-wasting, congenital adrenal hyperplasia (with secondary increase in AVP)

---

[1] Zanardo et al. (1989).

such as gastroenteritis. Inappropriate vasopressin excess is one of the least common causes of hyponatraemia in children, except after vasopressin administration for treatment of diabetes insipidus. The one cause of hyponatraemia associated with suppressed blood concentrations of vasopressin is activating mutations in *AVPR2,* the renal vasopressin receptor (Table 5.2).

Systemic dehydration
Systemic dehydration (water in excess of salt depletion) initially results in hypernatraemia, hyperosmolality and activation of vasopressin secretion. As dehydration progresses, hypo-volaemia and/or hypotension become major stimuli for vasopressin release, much more potent than hyperosmolality. This effect, by attempting to preserve volume, decreases free water clearance further and may lead to water retention and hyponatraemia, if water replace-ment in excess of salt is given. In many cases, hyponatraemia caused by intravascular volume depletion is evident from physical and laboratory signs such as decreased skin turgor, low central venous pressure, haemoconcentration and elevated blood urea nitrogen levels. The diagnosis may be subtle. Many patients with gastroenteritis who present with mild hypona-traemia and elevated plasma vasopressin concentrations (Neville et al. 2005) have these on the basis of systemic dehydration rather than the syndrome of inappropriate antidiuresis (SIAD), and benefit from volume expansion rather than fluid restriction (Neville et al. 2006). More generally, most hospitalised paediatric patients with hyponatraemia benefit from isotonic rather than hypotonic fluid replacement, suggesting that the underlying cause of the electrolyte disturbance is dehydration (Freedman and Geary 2013).

Decreased 'effective' intravascular volume
A decrease in 'effective' intravascular volume occurs in congestive heart failure, cirrhosis, nephrotic syndrome, positive pressure mechanical ventilation (Zanardo et al. 1989), severe

burns (Potts and May 1986), lung disease (bronchopulmonary dysplasia (Kojima et al. 1990) [in neonates]), cystic fibrosis with obstruction (Stegner et al. 1986) and severe asthma (Iikura et al. 1989). This occurs because of impaired cardiac output, an inability to keep fluid within the vascular space or impaired blood flow into the heart. As with systemic dehydration, in an attempt to preserve intravascular volume, water and salt excretion by the kidney is reduced; and decreased barosensor stimulation results in a compensatory, appropriate increase in vasopressin secretion, leading to an antidiuretic state and hyponatraemia (O'Rahilly 1985).

Syndrome of inappropriate antidiuresis
SIAD is uncommon in children (Sklar et al. 1985; Judd et al. 1987). It can occur with encephalitis, brain tumour (Tang et al. 1991), head trauma (Padilla et al. 1989) or psychiatric disease (Goldman et al. 1988) in the postictal period after generalised seizures (Meierkord et al. 1994) – and after prolonged nausea (Edwards et al. 1989), pneumonia (Dhawan et al. 1992) or AIDS (Tang et al. 1993). Impaired free water clearance can result from alteration in vasopressin release, increased vasopressin effect at the same plasma vasopressin concentration or vasopressin-independent changes in distal collecting tubule water permeability. Common drugs that result in hyponatraemia (although not always with increased AVP secretion) include carbamazepine (Van Amelsvoort et al. 1994), chlorpropamide (Weissman et al. 1971), vinblastine (Zavagli et al. 1988), vincristine (Escuro et al. 1992) and tricyclic antidepressants (Liskin et al. 1984). Second-generation sulfonylurea agents, including glyburide, are not associated with SIAD (Moses et al. 1973). SIAD is the cause of the hyponatraemic second phase of the triple-phase response seen after hypothalamic-pituitary surgery. Hyponatraemia with elevated vasopressin secretion is found in up to 35% of patients 1 week after transsphenoidal pituitary surgery (Olson et al. 1995). The mechanism is most likely retrograde neuronal degeneration with cell death and vasopressin release. Secondary adrenal insufficiency causing stimulation of vasopressin release (Oelkers 1989) may also play a role, since hyponatremia most commonly follows the removal of adrenocorticotropin hormone-secreting corticotroph adenomas (Sane et al. 1994). In the vast majority of children with SIAD, the cause is the excessive administration of vasopressin, whether to treat central diabetes insipidus (Koskimies and Pylkkanen 1984) or, less commonly, haemorrhage disorders (Smith et al. 1989) or, most uncommonly, following DDAVP therapy for enuresis.

Several unrelated infants with mutations in the vasopressin V2 receptor that presented with severe hyponatraemia in the first months of life heralded a new genetic cause of hyponatraemia (Feldman et al. 2005). The first two infants described had missense mutations at codon 137 that converted arginine to cysteine or leucine and led to constitutive activation of the V2 receptor with appropriately suppressed plasma AVP concentration. This genetic disorder has been termed nephrogenic syndrome of inappropriate antidiuresis (NSIAD). It remains unclear what portion of isolated early onset chronic SIAD results from activating mutations of the V2 receptor, though the incidence is likely to be very low. Interestingly, this same codon is also the site of a loss-of-function mutation (p.R137H) which led to X-linked nephrogenic diabetes insipidus (Morello and Bichet 2001). A total of 16 patients with NSIAD have been reported (Vandergheynst et al. 2012).

Investigation of hyponatraemia

In evaluating the cause of hyponatraemia, one should first determine whether the patient is dehydrated and hypovolaemic. This is usually evident from the physical examination (decreased weight, skin turgor, central venous pressure) and laboratory data (high blood urea nitrogen, renin, aldosterone, uric acid). With a decrease in the glomerular filtration rate, proximal tubular reabsorption of sodium and water will be high, leading to a urinary sodium value less than 10mEq/L. Patients with decreased 'effective' intravascular volume from congestive heart failure, cirrhosis, nephrotic syndrome or lung disease will present with similar laboratory data but will also have obvious signs of their underlying disease, which often includes peripheral oedema. Patients with primary salt loss will also appear volume depleted. If the salt loss is from the kidney (e.g. diuretic therapy or polycystic kidney disease), the urine sodium concentration will be elevated, as may urine volume. Salt loss from other regions (e.g. the gut in gastroenteritis or the skin in cystic fibrosis) will cause urine sodium to be low, as in other forms of systemic dehydration. Cerebral salt wasting is encountered with central nervous system insults and results in high-serum ANP concentrations, leading to high-urine sodium and urine excretion. Cerebral salt wasting is a rare event and its very existence has been questioned (Rivkees 2008). Salt-losing congenital adrenal hyperplasia is associated with hyperkalaemia and primary hypocortisolaemia.

Treatment of hyponatraemia

Patients with systemic dehydration and hypovolaemia should be rehydrated with salt-containing fluids such as normal saline or lactated Ringer solution. Because of activation of the renin-angiotensin-aldosterone system, the administered sodium will be avidly conserved and a water diuresis will quickly ensue as volume is restored and vasopressin concentrations fall (Kamel and Bear 1993). Under these conditions, caution must be taken to prevent too rapid a correction of hyponatraemia, which may itself result in brain damage.

Hyponatraemia caused by a decrease in effective plasma volume from cardiac, hepatic, renal or pulmonary dysfunction is more difficult to reverse. The most effective therapy is the least easily achieved: treatment of the underlying systemic disorder. In general, patients with hyponatraemia caused by salt loss require ongoing supplementation with sodium chloride and fluids. This treatment contrasts to that of SIAD, in which water restriction without sodium supplementation is the mainstay.

Precautions in the emergency treatment of hyponatraemia

Most children with hyponatraemia develop the disorder gradually, are asymptomatic and should be treated with water restriction alone. The development of acute hyponatraemia, or a serum sodium concentration below 120mEq/L, may be associated with lethargy, psychosis, coma or generalised seizures, especially in younger children. Acute hyponatraemia causes cell swelling owing to the entry of water into cells, which can lead to neuronal dysfunction from alterations in the ionic environment or to cerebral herniation because of the encasement of the brain in the cranium. If present for more than 24 hours, cell swelling triggers a compensatory decrease in intracellular organic osmolytes, resulting in the partial restoration of normal cell volume in chronic hyponatraemia (Videen et al. 1995). The proper emergency treatment of cerebral dysfunction depends on whether the hyponatremia is acute or chronic (Ayus and Arieff 1993). In all cases, water restriction should be instituted. If hyponatraemia is acute, and therefore probably not associated with a decrease in intracellular organic osmolyte concentration, rapid correction with hypertonic 3% sodium chloride administered intravenously may be indicated. If hyponatraemia is chronic, hypertonic saline treatment must be undertaken with caution, because it may result in both cell shrinkage and the associated syndrome of central pontine myelinolysis (Sterns et al. 1986). This syndrome, affecting the central portion of the basal pons as well as other brain regions, is characterised by axonal demyelination, with sparing of neurons. It becomes evident within 24 to 48 hours after too rapid correction of hyponatraemia, has a characteristic appearance by computed tomography and MRI and often causes irreversible brain damage (Ayus et al. 1987). If hypertonic saline treatment is undertaken, the serum sodium concentration should be raised only high enough to cause an improvement in mental status, and in no case faster than 0.5mEq/L/hr or 12mEq/L/day (Ayus and Arieff 1993). In the case of systemic dehydration, the increase in serum sodium level may occur very rapidly using this regimen. The associated hyperaldosteronism will cause avid retention of the administered sodium, leading to rapid restoration of volume and suppression of vasopressin secretion and resulting in a brisk water diuresis and an increase in the serum sodium concentration (Kamel and Bear 1993). In patients with hyponatraemia secondary to primary adrenal insufficiency, the incremental replacement of glucocorticoid may blunt the otherwise rapid rise in sodium that occurs with glucocorticoid treatment (Yoshioka et al. 2012).

Acute treatment of hyponatraemia due to SIAD is only indicated if cerebral dysfunction is present. In that case, treatment is dictated by the duration of hyponatraemia and the extent of cerebral dysfunction. Because patients with SIAD have volume expansion, salt administration is not very effective in raising the serum sodium because it is rapidly excreted in the urine due to suppressed aldosterone and elevated atrial natriuretic peptide concentrations. Chronic SIAD is best treated by chronic oral fluid restriction. Oral urea has been effectively used to treat adult patients with chronic SIAD by virtue of its ability to induce an effective osmotic diuresis. This therapy was also demonstrated to be safe and effective in four children with chronic SIAD, including two with mutations in the vasopressin V2 receptor (Vandergheynst et al. 2012). Specific non-peptide V2 receptor antagonists (vaptans) have also been developed for use in subacute or chronic SIAD due to inappropriate increased vasopressin secretion (Decaux et al. 2008; Robertson 2011). The aquaretic effects of the vaptans, after either parental or oral administration, have a rapid onset of action, exert peak effects within a few hours and subside within 24 hours (Decaux et al. 2008; Robertson 2011). The primary adverse effect from these agents is inflammation at infusion sites, though rises in serum sodium above rates recommended to prevent myelinolysis have also been found (Robertson 2011). Very limited experience with vaptans has been reported in children, though they have been used to promote hydration during chemotherapy with malignancy-associated SIAD (Rianthavorn et al. 2008). These agents have not been effective in treating activating mutations of the V2 receptor (Decaux 2007), although low-dose urea has been useful (Vandergheynst et al. 2012). Because the predictability of hypertonic saline administration for acute, severe forms of SIAD is greater than that of vaptans, hypertonic saline infusion for symptomatic hyponatraemia due to inappropriate vasopressin secretion remains the recommended intervention (Robertson 2011). Of note, some of these V2 receptor antagonists facilitate the proper transport of loss-of-function V2 receptor mutants to the cell surface (Cheong et al. 2007).

Conclusion

Disorders of salt and water balance can be associated with considerable morbidity and mortality. The causes include congenital and acquired disorders. Correction of the disorders needs to take into account the underlying cause, the rate of progression of electrolyte abnormalities and the degree of abnormality. Correction must always be meticulous, and should involve simple manoeuvres such as replacement of salt or water, but there may be a role for careful use of pharmacotherapy, for example, use of DDAVP in central diabetes insipidus and the vaptans in SIAD. It is also important to investigate children with electrolyte imbalance carefully, for example, the use of brain/pituitary MRI in children with central diabetes insipidus.

REFERENCES

Ahmed SR, Aiello DP, Page R, Hopper K, Towfighi J and Santen RJ (1993) Necrotizing infundibulo-hypophysitis: A unique syndrome of diabetes insipidus and hypopituitarism. *J Clin Endocrinol Metab* 76: 1499–1504.

Appignani B, Landy B and Barnes P (1993) MR in idiopathic central diabetes insipidus of childhood. *AJNR: Am J Neuroradiol* 14: 1407–1410.

Ayus JC and Arieff AI (1993) Pathogenesis and prevention of hyponatremic encephalopathy. [Review]. *Endocrinol Metab Clin North Am* 22: 425–446.

Ayus JC, Krothapalli RK and Arieff AI (1987) Treatment of symptomatic hyponatremia and its relation to brain damage. A prospective study. [Review]. *N Engl J Med* 317: 1190–1195.

Babey M, Kopp P and Robertson GL (2011) Familial forms of diabetes insipidus: Clinical and molecular characteristics. *Nat Rev Endocrinol* 7: 701–714.

Bichet DG (1994) Molecular and cellular biology of vasopressin and oxytocin receptors and action in the kidney. [Review]. *Curr Opin Nephrol Hypertens* 3: 46–53.

Blanco EJ, Lane AH, Aijaz N, Blumberg D and Wilson TA (2006) Use of subcutaneous DDAVP in infants with central diabetes insipidus. *J Pediatr Endocrinol Metab* 19: 919–925.

Bougneres P, Pantalone L, Linglart A, Rothenbuhler A and Le Stunff C (2008) Endocrine manifestations of the rapid-onset obesity with hypoventilation, hypothalamic, autonomic dysregulation, and neural tumor syndrome in childhood. *J Clin Endocrinol Metab* 93: 3971–3980.

Brandle M, Vernazza PL, Oesterle M and Galeazzi RL (1995) [Cerebral toxoplasmosis with central diabetes insipidus and panhypopituitarism in a patient with AIDS]. [German]. *Schwei Med Wochenschr* 125: 684–687.

Broadbent V, Dunger DB, Yeomans E and Kendall B (1993) Anterior pituitary function and computed tomography/magnetic resonance imaging in patients with Langerhans cell histiocytosis and diabetes insipidus. *Med Pediatr Oncol* 21: 649–654.

Cheong HI, Cho HY, Park HW, Ha IS and Choi Y (2007) Molecular genetic study of congenital nephrogenic diabetes insipidus and rescue of mutant vasopressin V2 receptor by chemical chaperones. *Nephrology* 12: 113–117.

Christ-Crain M and Fenske W (2016) Copeptin in the diagnosis of vasopressin-dependent disorders of fluid homeostasis. *Nat Rev Endocrinol* 12: 168–176.

Christensen C and Bank A (1988) Meningococcal meningitis and diabetes insipidus. *Scand J Infect Dis* 20: 341–343.

Christensen JH, Kvistgaard H, Knudsen J et al. (2013) A novel deletion partly removing the AVP gene causes autosomal recessive inheritance of early-onset neurohypophyseal diabetes insipidus. *Clin Genet* 83: 44–52.

Christensen JH, Siggaard C, Corydon TJ et al. (2004a) Differential cellular handling of defective arginine vasopressin (AVP) prohormones in cells expressing mutations of the AVP gene associated with autosomal dominant and recessive familial neurohypophyseal diabetes insipidus. *J Clin Endocrinol Metab* 89: 4521–4531.

Christensen JH, Siggaard C, Corydon TJ et al. (2004b) Impaired trafficking of mutated AVP prohormone in cells expressing rare disease genes causing autosomal dominant familial neurohypophyseal diabetes insipidus. *Clin Endocrinol* 60: 125–136.

Christensen JH, Siggaard C, Corydon TJ et al. (2004c) Six novel mutations in the arginine vasopressin gene in 15 kindreds with autosomal dominant familial neurohypophyseal diabetes insipidus give further insight into the pathogenesis. *Eur J Hum Genet* 12: 44–51.

Collier DA, Barrett TG, Curtis D et al. (1996) Linkage of Wolfram syndrome to chromosome 4p16.1 and evidence for heterogeneity. *Am J Hum Genet* 59: 855–863.

Crigler JF Jr (1976) Commentary: On the use of pitressin in infants with neurogenic diabetes insipidue. *J Pediatr* 88: 295–296.

Cull EH, Watts JM, Tallman MS et al. (2013) Acute myeloid leukemia presenting with panhypopituitarism or diabetes insipidus: A case series with molecular genetic analysis and review of the literature. *Leuk Lymphoma* 55: 2125–2129.

Decaux G (2007) V2-antagonists for the treatment of hyponatraemia. *Nephrol Dial Transplant: Official Publication of the European Dialysis and Transplant Association – European Renal Association* 22: 1853–1855.

Decaux G, Soupart A and Vassart G (2008) Non-peptide arginine-vasopressin antagonists: The vaptans. *Lancet* 371: 1624–1632.

Dhawan A, Narang A and Singhi S (1992) Hyponatraemia and the inappropriate ADH syndrome in pneumonia. *Ann Trop Paediatr* 12: 455–462.

Di Iorgi N, Maria Allegri AE, Napoli F et al. (2014) Central diabetes insipidus in children and young adults: Etiological diagnosis and long – Term outcome of idiopathic cases. *J Clin Endocrinol Metab* 99: 1264–1272.

Di Iorgi N, Secco A, Napoli F, Calandra E, Rossi A and Maghnie M (2009) Developmental abnormalities of the posterior pituitary gland. *Endocr Dev* 14: 83–94.

Dubourg C, Bendavid C, Pasquier L, Henry C, Odent and S David V (2007) Holoprosencephaly. *Orphanet J Rare Dis* 2: 8.

Dunger DB, Broadbent V, Yeoman E, Seckl JR, Lightman SL and Grant DB (1989) The frequency and natural history of diabetes insipidus in children with Langerhans-cell histiocytosis. *N Engl J Med* 321: 1157–1162.

Edwards CM, Carmichael J, Baylis PH and Harris AL (1989) Arginine vasopressin – A mediator of chemotherapy induced emesis? *Br J Can* 59: 467–470.

Escuro RS, Adelstein DJ and Carter SG (1992) Syndrome of inappropriate secretion of antidiuretic hormone after infusional vincristine. *Cleve Clin J Med* 59: 643–644.

Farmer A, Ayme S, de Heredia ML et al. (2013) EURO-WABB: An EU rare diseases registry for Wolfram syndrome, Alstrom syndrome and Bardet-Biedl syndrome. *BMC Pediatr* 13: 130.

Feldman BJ, Rosenthal SM, Vargas GA et al. (2005) Nephrogenic syndrome of inappropriate antidiuresis. *N Engl J Med* 352: 1884–1890.

Finken MJ, Zwaveling-Soonawala N, Walenkamp MJ, Vulsma T, van Trotsenburg AS and Rotteveel J (2011) Frequent occurrence of the triphasic response (diabetes insipidus/hyponatremia/diabetes insipidus) after surgery for craniopharyngioma in childhood. *Horm Res Paediatr* 76: 22–26.

Foresti V, Casati O, Villa A, Lazzaro A and Confalonieri F (1992) Central diabetes insipidus due to acute monocytic leukemia: Case report and review of the literature. [Review]. *J Endocrinol Invest* 15: 127–130.

Freedman SB and Geary DF (2013) Bolus fluid therapy and sodium homeostasis in paediatric gastroenteritis. *J Paediatr Child Health* 49: 215–222.

Goldman MB, Luchins DJ and Robertson GL (1988) Mechanisms of altered water metabolism in psychotic patients with polydipsia and hyponatremia. *N Engl J Med* 318: 397–403.

Grois N, Flucher-Wolfram B, Heitger A, Mostbeck GH, Hofmann J and Gadner H (1995) Diabetes insipidus in Langerhans cell histiocytosis: Results from the DAL-HX 83 study. *Med Pediatr Oncol* 24: 248–256.

Grosse Aldenhovel HB, Gallenkamp U and Sulemana CA (1991) Juvenile onset diabetes mellitus, central diabetes insipidus and optic atrophy (Wolfram syndrome)–neurological findings and prognostic implications. *Neuropediatrics* 22: 103–106.

Halimi P, Sigal R, Doyon D, Delivet S, Bouchard P and Pigeau I (1988) Post-traumatic diabetes insipidus: MR demonstration of pituitary stalk rupture. *J Comput Assist Tomogr* 12: 135–137.

Hamnvik OP, Laury AR, Laws ER Jr and Kaiser UB (2010) Lymphocytic hypophysitis with diabetes insipidus in a young man. *Nat Rev Endocrinol* 6: 464–470.

Hung W and Fitz CR (1992) The primary empty-sella syndrome and diabetes insipidus in a child. *Acta Paediatr* 81: 459–461.

Iikura Y, Odajima Y, Akazawa A, Nagakura T, Kishida M and Akimoto K (1989) Antidiuretic hormone in acute asthma in children: Effects of medication on serum levels and clinical course. *Allergy Proc* 10: 197–201.

Imura H, Nakao K, Shimatsu A et al. (1993) Lymphocytic infundibuloneurohypophysitis as a cause of central diabetes insipidus. *N Engl J Med* 329: 683–689.

Inoue H, Tanizawa Y, Wasson J et al. (1998) A gene encoding a transmembrane protein is mutated in patients with diabetes mellitus and optic atrophy (Wolfram syndrome). *Nat Genet* 20: 143–148.

Ito M and Jameson JL (1997) Molecular basis of autosomal dominant neurohypophyseal diabetes insipidus. Cellular toxicity caused by the accumulation of mutant vasopressin precursors within the endoplasmic reticulum. *J Clin Invest* 99: 1897–1905.

Ito M, Yu RN and Jameson JL (1999) Mutant vasopressin precursors that cause autosomal dominant neurohypophyseal diabetes insipidus retain dimerization and impair the secretion of wild-type proteins. *J Biol Chem* 274: 9029–9037.

Jakobsson B and Berg U (1994) Effect of hydrochlorothiazide and indomethacin treatment on renal function in nephrogenic diabetes insipidus. *Acta Paediatr* 83: 522–525.

Judd BA, Haycock GB, Dalton N and Chantler C (1987) Hyponatraemia in premature babies and following surgery in older children. *Acta Paediatr Scand* 76: 385–393.

Kamel KS and Bear RA (1993) Treatment of hyponatremia: A quantitative analysis. [Review]. *Am J Kidney Dis* 21: 439–443.

Knepper MA (1994) The aquaporin family of molecular water channels. *Proc Natl Acad Sci USA* 91: 6255–6258.

Kojima H, Nojima T, Nagashima K, Ono Y, Kudo M and Ishikura M (1989) Diabetes insipidus caused by lymphocytic infundibuloneurohypophysitis. *Arch Pathol Lab Med* 113: 1399–1401.

Kojima T, Fukuda Y, Hirata Y, Matsuzaki S and Kobayashi Y (1990) Changes in vasopressin, atrial natriuretic factor, and water homeostasis in the early stage of bronchopulmonary dysplasia. *Pediatr Res* 27: 260–263.

Koshiyama H, Sato H, Yorita S et al. (1994) Lymphocytic hypophysitis presenting with diabetes insipidus: Case report and literature review. [Review]. *Endocr J* 41: 93–97.

Koskimies O and Pylkkanen J (1984) Water intoxication in infants caused by the urine concentration test with the vasopressin analogue (DDAVP). *Acta Paediatr Scand* 73: 131–132.

Lamine F, Kanoun F, Chihaoui M et al. (2012) Unilateral agenesis of internal carotid artery associated with congenital combined pituitary hormone deficiency and pituitary stalk interruption without HESX1, LHX4 or OTX2 mutation: A case report. *Pituitary* 15(Suppl 1): S81–S86.

Lewis R, Wilson J and Smith FW (1987) Diabetes insipidus secondary to intracranial sarcoidosis confirmed by low-field magnetic resonance imaging. *Magn Reson Med* 5: 466–470.

Liskin B, Walsh BT, Roose SP and Jackson W (1984) Imipramine-induced inappropriate ADH secretion. *J Clin Psychopharmacol* 4: 146–147.

Maghnie M, Bossi G, Klersy C, Cosi G, Genovese E and Arico M (1998) Dynamic endocrine testing and magnetic resonance imaging in the long-term follow-up of childhood Langerhans cell histiocytosis. *J Clin Endocr Metab* 83: 3089–3094.

Maghnie M, Cosi G, Genovese E et al. (2000) Central diabetes insipidus in children and young adults. *N Engl J Med* 343: 998–1007.

Maghnie M, Genovese E, Arico M, Villa A, Beluffi G and Campani R (1994) Evolving pituitary hormone deficiency is associated with pituitary vasculopathy: Dynamic MR study in children with hypopituitarism, diabetes insipidus, and Langerhans cell histiocytosis. *Radiology* 193: 493–499.

Maghnie M, Villa A, Arico M et al. (1992) Correlation between magnetic resonance imaging of posterior pituitary and neurohypophyseal function in children with diabetes insipidus. *J Clin Endocrinol Metab* 74: 795–800.

Masera N, Grant DB, Stanhope R and Preece MA (1994) Diabetes insipidus with impaired osmotic regulation in septo-optic dysplasia and agenesis of the corpus callosum. *Arch Dis Child* 70: 51–53.

Meierkord H, Shorvon S and Lightman SL (1994) Plasma concentrations of prolactin, noradrenaline, vasopressin and oxytocin during and after a prolonged epileptic seizure. *Acta Neurolog Scand* 90: 73–77.

Mena W, Royal S, Pass RF, Whitley RJ and Philips JB (1993) Diabetes insipidus associated with symptomatic congenital cytomegalovirus infection. *J Pediatr* 122: 911–913.

Morello JP and Bichet DG (2001) Nephrogenic diabetes insipidus. *Ann Rev Physiol* 63: 607–630.

Moses AM, Clayton B and Hochhauser L (1992) Use of T1-weighted MR imaging to differentiate between primary polydipsia and central diabetes insipidus [comment] [see comments]. *AJNR: Am J Neuroradiol* 13: 1273–1277.

Moses AM, Numann P and Miller M (1973) Mechanism of chlorpropamide-induced antidiuresis in man: Evidence for release of ADH and enhancement of peripheral action. *Metabolism* 22: 59–66.

Neville KA, Verge CF, O'Meara MW and Walker JL (2005) High antidiuretic hormone levels and hyponatremia in children with gastroenteritis. *Pediatrics* 116: 1401–1407.

Neville KA, Verge CF, Rosenberg AR, O'Meara MW and Walker JL (2006) Isotonic is better than hypotonic saline for intravenous rehydration of children with gastroenteritis: A prospective randomised study. *Arch Dis Child* 91: 226–232.

O'Rahilly S (1985) Secretion of antidiuretic hormone in hyponatraemia: Not always 'inappropriate'. *Br Med J (Clinical Research Ed.)* 290: 1803–1804.

Oelkers W (1989) Hyponatremia and inappropriate secretion of vasopressin (antidiuretic hormone) in patients with hypopituitarism [see comments]. *N Engl J Med* 321: 492–496.

Oiso Y, Robertson GL, Norgaard JP and Juul KV (2013) Clinical review: Treatment of neurohypophyseal diabetes insipidus. *J Clin Endocrinol Metab* 98: 3958–3967.

Olson BR, Rubino D, Gumowski J and Oldfield EH (1995) Isolated hyponatremia after transsphenoidal pituitary surgery. *J Clin Endocrinol Metab* 80: 85–91.

Ono N, Kakegawa T, Zama A et al. (1992) Suprasellar germinomas; relationship between tumour size and diabetes insipidus. *Acta Neurochir* 114: 26–32.

Os I, Aakesson I and Enger E (1985) Plasma vasopressin in hereditary cranial diabetes insipidus. *Acta Med Scand* 217: 429–434.

Osman AA, Saito M, Makepeace C, Permutt MA, Schlesinger P and Mueckler M (2003) Wolframin expression induces novel ion channel activity in endoplasmic reticulum membranes and increases intracellular calcium. *J Biol Chem* 278: 52755–52762.

Padilla G, Leake JA, Castro R, Ervin MG, Ross MG and Leake RD (1989) Vasopressin levels and pediatric head trauma. *Pediatrics* 83: 700–705.

Paja M, Estrada J, Ojeda A, Ramon y Cajal S, Garcia-Uria J and Lucas T (1994) Lymphocytic hypophysitis causing hypopituitarism and diabetes insipidus, and associated with autoimmune thyroiditis, in a non-pregnant woman. *Postgrad Med J* 70: 220–224.

Papapostolou C, Mantzoros CS, Evagelopoulou C, Moses AC and Kleefield J (1995) Imaging of the sella in the syndrome of inappropriate secretion of antidiuretic hormone. *J Intern Med* 237: 181–185.

Patwari PP, Rand CM, Berry-Kravis EM, Ize-Ludlow D and Weese-Mayer DE (2011) Monozygotic twins discordant for ROHHAD phenotype. *Pediatrics* 128: e711–e715.

Pedersen EB, Lamm LU, Albertsen K et al. (1985) Familial cranial diabetes insipidus: A report of five families. Genetic, diagnostic and therapeutic aspects. *Q J Med* 57: 883–896.

Perez C, Dastot-Le Moal F, Collot N et al. (2012) Screening of LHX2 in patients presenting growth retardation with posterior pituitary and ocular abnormalities. *Eur J Endocrinol* 167: 85–91.

Potts FL and May RB (1986) Early syndrome of inappropriate secretion of antidiuretic hormone in a child with burn injury. *Ann Emerg Med* 15: 834–835.

Raivio T, Avbelj M, McCabe MJ et al. (2012) Genetic overlap in Kallmann syndrome, combined pituitary hormone deficiency, and septo-optic dysplasia. *J Clin Endocrinol Metab* 97: E694–E699.

Reynaud R, Gueydan M, Saveanu A et al. (2006) Genetic screening of combined pituitary hormone deficiency: Experience in 195 patients. *J Clin Endocrinol Metab* 91: 3329–3336.

Reynaud R, Jayakody SA, Monnier C et al. (2012) PROKR2 variants in multiple hypopituitarism with pituitary stalk interruption. *J Clin Endocrinol Metab* 97: E1068–E1073.

Rianthavorn P, Cain JP and Turman MA (2008) Use of conivaptan to allow aggressive hydration to prevent tumor lysis syndrome in a pediatric patient with large-cell lymphoma and SIADH. *Pediatr Nephrol* 23: 1367–1370.

Richman RA, Post EM, Notman DD, Hochberg Z and Moses AM (1981) Simplifying the diagnosis of diabetes insipidus in children. *Am J Dis Child* 135: 839–841.

Riggs AC, Bernal-Mizrachi E, Ohsugi M et al. (2005) Mice conditionally lacking the Wolfram gene in pancreatic islet beta cells exhibit diabetes as a result of enhanced endoplasmic reticulum stress and apoptosis. *Diabetologia* 48: 2313–2321.

Rivkees SA (2008) Differentiating appropriate antidiuretic hormone secretion, inappropriate antidiuretic hormone secretion and cerebral salt wasting: The common, uncommon, and misnamed. *Curr Opin Pediatr* 20: 448–452.

Rivkees SA, Dunbar N and Wilson TA (2007) The management of central diabetes insipidus in infancy: Desmopressin, low renal solute load formula, thiazide diuretics. *J Pediatr Endocrinol Metab* 20: 459–469.

Robertson GL (1995) Diabetes insipidus. *Endocrinol Metab Clin North Am* 24: 549–572.

Robertson GL (2011) Vaptans for the treatment of hyponatremia. *Nat Rev Endocrinol* 7: 151–161.

Rossi GP, Pavan E, Chiesura-Corona M, Rea F, Poletti A and Pessina AC (1994) Bronchocentric granulomatosis and central diabetes insipidus successfully treated with corticosteroids. *Eur Respir J* 7: 1893–1898.

Russell TA, Ito M, Yu RN, Martinson FA, Weiss J and Jameson JL (2003) A murine model of autosomal dominant neurohypophyseal diabetes insipidus reveals progressive loss of vasopressin-producing neurons. *J Clin Invest* 112: 1697–1706.

Sane T, Rantakari K, Poranen A, Tahtela R, Valimaki M and Pelkonen R (1994) Hyponatremia after trans-sphenoidal surgery for pituitary tumors. *J Clin Endocrinol Metab* 79: 1395–1398.

Santarpia L, Gagel RF, Sherman SI, Sarlis NJ, Evans DB and Hoff AO (2009) Diabetes insipidus and pan-hypopituitarism due to intrasellar metastasis from medullary thyroid cancer. *Head Neck* 31: 419–423.

Sato N, Ishizaka H, Yagi H, Matsumoto M and Endo K (1993) Posterior lobe of the pituitary in diabetes insipidus: Dynamic MR imaging. *Radiology* 186: 357–360.

Siggaard C, Christensen JH, Corydon TJ et al. (2005) Expression of three different mutations in the arginine vasopressin gene suggests genotype-phenotype correlation in familial neurohypophyseal diabetes insipidus kindreds. *Clin Endocrinol* 63: 207–216.

Sklar C, Fertig A and David R (1985) Chronic syndrome of inappropriate secretion of antidiuretic hormone in childhood. *Am J Dis Child* 139: 733–735.

Sloane AE (1989) Transient diabetes insipidus following listeria meningitis. *Ir Med J* 82: 132–134.

Smith TJ, Gill JC, Ambruso DR and Hathaway WE (1989) Hyponatremia and seizures in young children given DDAVP. *Am J Hematol* 31: 199–202.

Sobrier ML, Brachet C, Vie-Luton MP et al. (2012) Symptomatic heterozygotes and prenatal diagnoses in a nonconsanguineous family with syndromic combined pituitary hormone deficiency resulting from two novel LHX3 mutations. *J Clin Endocrinol Metab* 97: E503–E509.

Stegner H, Caspers S, Niggemann B and Commentz J (1986) Urinary arginine-vasopressin (AVP) excretion in cystic fibrosis (CF). *Acta Endocrinolog Suppl* 279: 448–451.

Sterns RH, Riggs JE and Schochet SS Jr (1986) Osmotic demyelination syndrome following correction of hyponatremia. *N Engl J Med* 314: 1535–1542.

Stick SM and Betts PR (1987) Oral desmopressin in neonatal diabetes insipidus. *Arch Dis Child* 62: 1177–1178.

Tajima T, Hattori T, Nakajima T, Okuhara K, Tsubaki J and Fujieda K (2007) A novel missense mutation (P366T) of the LHX4 gene causes severe combined pituitary hormone deficiency with pituitary hypoplasia, ectopic posterior lobe and a poorly developed sella turcica. *Endocr J* 54: 637–641.

Tang TT, Whelan HT, Meyer GA, Strother DR, Blank EL and Camitta BM (1991) Optic chiasm glioma associated with inappropriate secretion of antidiuretic hormone, cerebral ischemia, nonobstructive hydrocephalus and chronic ascites following ventriculoperitoneal shunting. *Childs Nerv Syst* 7: 458–461.

Tang WW, Kaptein EM, Feinstein EI and Massry SG (1993) Hyponatremia in hospitalized patients with the acquired immunodeficiency syndrome (AIDS) and the AIDS-related complex. *Am J Med* 94: 169–174.

Tarng DC and Huang TP (1995) Diabetes insipidus as an early sign of pineal tumor. *Am J Nephrol* 15: 161–164.

Tawa R, Kaino Y, Ito T, Goto Y, Kida K and Matsuda H (1994) A case of Kabuki make-up syndrome with central diabetes insipidus and growth hormone neurosecretory dysfunction. *Acta Paediatr Jpn* 36: 412–415.

Thompson CJ, Charlton J, Walford S et al. (1989) Vasopressin secretion in the DIDMOAD (Wolfram) syndrome. *Q J Med* 71: 333–345.

Tien RD, Newton TH, McDermott MW, Dillon WP and Kucharczyk J (1990) Thickened pituitary stalk on MR images in patients with diabetes insipidus and Langerhans cell histiocytosis. *AJNR: Am J Neuroradiol* 11: 703–708.

Toth EL, Bowen PA and Crockford PM (1984) Hereditary central diabetes insipidus: Plasma levels of antidiuretic hormone in a family with a possible osmoreceptor defect. *Can Med Assoc J* 131: 1237–1241.

Van Amelsvoort T, Bakshi R, Devaux CB and Schwabe S (1994) Hyponatremia associated with carbamazepine and oxcarbazepine therapy: A review. [Review]. *Epilepsia* 35: 181–188.

Van Gool S, de Zegher F, de Vrie LS, Vanderschueren-Lodeweyckx M, Casaer P and Eggermont E (1990) Alobar holoprosencephaly, diabetes insipidus and coloboma without craniofacial abnormalities: A case report. *Eur J Pediatr* 149: 621–622.

Vandergheynst F, Brachet C, Heinrichs C and Decaux G (2012) Long-term treatment of hyponatremic patients with nephrogenic syndrome of inappropriate antidiuresis: Personal experience and review of published case reports. *Nephron Clin Pract* 120: c168–c172.

Videen JS, Michaelis T, Pinto P and Ross BD (1995) Human cerebral osmolytes during chronic hyponatremia. A proton magnetic resonance spectroscopy study. *J Clin Invest* 95: 788–793.

Watanabe A, Ishii R, Hirano K et al. (1994) Central diabetes insipidus caused by nonspecific chronic inflammation of the hypothalamus: Case report. *Surg Neurol* 42: 70–73.

Webb EA, AlMutair A, Kelberman D et al. (2013) ARNT2 mutation causes hypopituitarism, post-natal microcephaly, visual and renal anomalies. *Brain: J Neurol* 136: 3096–3105.

Weissman PN, Shenkman L and Gregerman RI (1971) Chlorpropamide hyponatremia: Drug-induced inappropriate antidiuretic-hormone activity. *N Engl J Med* 284: 65–71.

Werny D, Elfers C, Perez FA, Pihoker C and Roth CL (2015) Pediatric central diabetes insipidus: Brain malformations are common and few patients have idiopathic disease. *J Clin Endocrinol Metab* 100: 3074–3080.

Wiley SE, Andreyev AY, Divakaruni AS et al. (2013) Wolfram Syndrome protein, Miner1, regulates sulphydryl redox status, the unfolded protein response, and Ca^{2+} homeostasis. *EMBO Mol Med* 5: 904–918.

Willcutts MD, Felner E and White PC (1999) Autosomal recessive familial neurohypophyseal diabetes insipidus with continued secretion of mutant weakly active vasopressin. *Hum Mol Genet* 8: 1303–1307.

Williams TD, Dunger DB, Lyon CC, Lewis RJ, Taylor F and Lightman SL (1986) Antidiuretic effect and pharmacokinetics of oral 1-desamino-8-D-arginine vasopressin. 1. Studies in adults and children. *J Clin Endocrinol Metab* 63: 129–132.

Yagi H, Nagashima K, Miyake H et al. (1994) Familial congenital hypopituitarism with central diabetes insipidus. *J Clin Endocrinol Metab* 78: 884–889.

Yoshioka K, Minami M, Fujimoto S, Yamaguchi S, Adachi K and Yamagami K (2012) Incremental increases in glucocorticoid doses may reduce the risk of osmotic demyelination syndrome in a patient with hyponatremia due to central adrenal insufficiency. *Intern Med* 51: 1069–1072.

Zanardo V, Ronconi M, Ferri N and Zacchello G (1989) Plasma arginine vasopressin, diuresis, and neonatal respiratory distress syndrome. *Padiatr Padol* 24: 297–302.

Zavagli G, Ricci G, Tataranni G, Mapelli G and Abbasciano V (1988) Life-threatening hyponatremia caused by vinblastine. *Med Oncol Tumor Pharmacother* 5: 67–69.

6
THE HYPOTHALAMIC-PITUITARY-THYROID AXIS: ANATOMY AND PHYSIOLOGY

Mary-Jane Brassill, Apostolos I Gogakos, John G Logan, Julian A Waung and Graham R Williams

Introduction

Thyroid hormones act as key homeostatic regulators in all tissues and exert their effects during fetal development and postnatal growth and in adulthood. It is, therefore, critical to maintain circulating thyroid hormone concentrations within the physiological reference range and this is achieved by the hypothalamic-pituitary-thyroid (HPT) axis.

Anatomy of the hypothalamic-pituitary-thyroid axis

The hypothalamus and pituitary gland function as a tightly regulated unit, exerting control over several endocrine glands including the thyroid. Development of the hypothalamus and pituitary is coordinated, and their anatomy and blood supply are essential for physiological function of the HPT axis.

In the early human embryo, the prosencephalon (forebrain) divides to form the telencephalon, consisting largely of the cerebral hemispheres, and the diencephalon, comprising the third ventricle and its surrounding structures. During the sixth week of gestation, the hypothalamus emerges from the ventro-lateral wall of the diencephalon. The hypothalamus is located initially at the rostral end of the neural tube and progressively occupies a more caudal position as development proceeds. Ultimately, it lies at the base of the brain, below the third ventricle and above the optic chiasm and pituitary gland.

An evagination of the ventral hypothalamus gives rise to the posterior pituitary gland (neurohypophysis) and the pituitary stalk. The anterior pituitary (adenohypophysis) arises from Rathke's pouch, an invagination of oral ectoderm, and is identifiable in humans at 4–5 weeks' gestation. The pituitary gland sits outside the dura mater at the base of the skull within the sella turcica of the sphenoid bone (Fig 6.1a). The pituitary is confined laterally by the cavernous sinuses and superiorly by the optic chiasm, from which it is separated by a layer of dura called the diaphragma sella. The hypothalamus and pituitary are connected by the pituitary stalk that passes posterior to the optic chiasm through an opening in the dura. A functionally mature hypothalamic-pituitary unit is present in humans by 20 weeks of gestation (Melmed et al. 2011).

The hypothalamus contains two different types of neurosecretory neurones, magnicellular and parvicellular, which are clustered in 11 hypothalamic nuclei. The peptide hormones oxytocin and vasopressin are secreted by magnicellular neurons and transported directly down their axons, which terminate in the posterior pituitary. The axons of parvicellular neurones project to the median eminence of the hypothalamus. Parvicellular neurones secrete the neuropeptides thyrotropin-releasing hormone (TRH), growth hormone–releasing hormone, corticotropin-releasing hormone, gonadotropin-releasing hormone, somatostatin and dopamine. These hormones are transported from the median eminence to the anterior pituitary via the hypothalamic-pituitary portal system. TRH-secreting neurons are located in the medial region of the hypothalamic paraventricular nuclei. TRH is a tripeptide synthesised from a 242 amino acid precursor containing six copies of TRH (Low 2011).

The five cell types of the anterior pituitary are classified based on the hormones they secrete: somatotrophs secrete growth hormone; lactotrophs secrete prolactin; corticotrophs secrete adrenocorticotrophic hormone; gonadotrophs secrete follicle-stimulating hormone and luteinizing hormone, and thyrotrophs secrete thyroid-stimulating hormone (TSH). The differentiation and proliferation of these distinct cell types from a common lineage occur in a specific order under the control of a number of transcription factors and signalling molecules. The development of thyrotrophs, along with somatotrophs and lactotrophs, is dependent on the transcription factor Pit1. The interaction of a further transcription factor, GATA2, with Pit1 is essential for the development of thyrotrophs. Thyrotrophs comprise 5% or fewer of adenohypophyseal cells and are typically located in the anteromedial part of the anterior pituitary (Melmed et al. 2011).

Blood supply to the hypothalamus and pituitary
The median eminence of the hypothalamus receives an arterial blood supply from the superior hypophyseal arteries, which branch from the internal carotid arteries. Here they form a capillary plexus ultimately resulting in long portal veins that descend along the pituitary stalk and drain into a further capillary network in the anterior pituitary. This hypothalamic-hypophyseal portal system allows hypothalamic hormones to be delivered to the anterior pituitary rapidly, and in large concentrations, and is crucial to the function of the hypothalamic-pituitary axis. Venous drainage from the anterior pituitary, the route by which adenohypophyseal hormones reach the systemic circulation, is via the superior and inferior petrosal sinuses that drain to the jugular bulb and internal jugular vein. The pituitary stalk and posterior pituitary are supplied directly by the inferior hypophyseal arteries, branches of the internal carotid arteries (Crossman 2009).

Embryology and anatomy of the thyroid gland
The thyroid gland is located in the neck anterior to the trachea, below the thyroid cartilage, and extending inferiorly to the fifth or sixth tracheal ring. It consists of two lobes connected in their lower thirds by the isthmus (Fig 6.1b). The thyroid lies posterior to the infrahyoid muscles and medial to the sternocleidomastoid muscles. It is fixed to the underlying tracheal

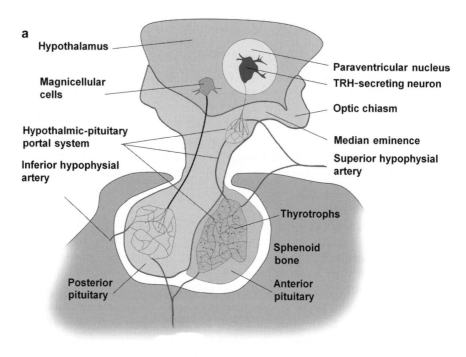

a
- Hypothalamus
- Magnicellular cells
- Hypothalmic-pituitary portal system
- Inferior hypophysial artery
- Paraventricular nucleus
- TRH-secreting neuron
- Optic chiasm
- Median eminence
- Superior hypophysial artery
- Thyrotrophs
- Sphenoid bone
- Posterior pituitary
- Anterior pituitary

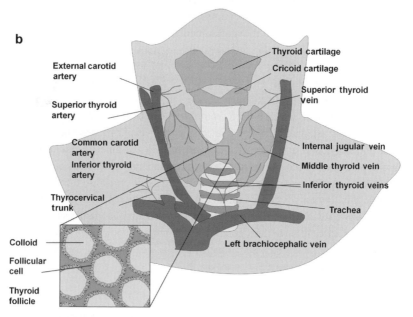

b
- Thyroid cartilage
- External carotid artery
- Cricoid cartilage
- Superior thyroid vein
- Superior thyroid artery
- Common carotid artery
- Internal jugular vein
- Inferior thyroid artery
- Middle thyroid vein
- Inferior thyroid veins
- Thyrocervical trunk
- Trachea
- Colloid
- Left brachiocephalic vein
- Follicular cell
- Thyroid follicle

Figure 6.1. Pituitary and thyroid gland anatomy and blood supply: (a) thyrotropin-releasing hormone (TRH) secreting neurons are clustered in the paraventricular nucleus within the hypothalamus. TRH is transported from the median eminence to the anterior pituitary via the hypothalamic-pituitary portal system. Thyrotrophs within the anterior pituitary secrete thyroid-stimulating hormone (TSH) into the systemic circulation. (b) The thyroid gland is located in the neck anterior to the trachea, below the thyroid cartilage. The major blood supply comes from paired superior and inferior thyroid arteries. Venous drainage from the thyroid gland is via the superior, middle, and inferior thyroid veins. The functional unit of the thyroid gland, responsible for the synthesis and storage of thyroid hormones (TH), is the thyroid follicle, formed by a layer of thyroid follicular cells surrounding a lumen.

cartilage by a thickening of fascia called the posterior suspensory ligament of Berry. The thyroid synthesises thyroid hormone and calcitonin in two distinct cell types, which derive from different embryological structures. Thyroid follicular cells, which synthesise thyroid hormone, are derived from the endoderm while neuroendocrine parafollicular C cells are responsible for calcitonin synthesis and derive from the ultimobranchial bodies, which in turn derive from the fourth pharyngeal pouch.

The first visible sign of thyroid follicular cell development is a thickening of the foregut endoderm in the ventral pharynx, which is referred to as the thyroid anlage. This occurs at embryonic day 20–22 (E20–22) in humans. Proliferation of the thyroid anlage forms the thyroid bud, which then begins to migrate into the underlying mesenchyme and down towards the trachea by E24. The foramen cecum is a small hole at the base of the tongue, which marks the site of origin of the thyroid anlage in the pharyngeal floor before closing later in development. As it descends, the thyroid bud remains connected to the foramen cecum by a narrow channel called the thyroglossal duct. This is resorbed by E30–40 when the connection with the pharynx is lost. Thyroid cells proliferate and expand laterally as the developing gland migrates, forming the early thyroid lobes. The thyroid lobes expand and the gland finally obtains its characteristic shape with the lateral lobes connected by the narrow isthmus. Thyroid migration in humans is complete by E45–50 and fusion with the ultimobranchial bodies occurs by E60.

The functional unit of the thyroid gland, responsible for the synthesis and storage of thyroid hormone, is the thyroid follicle, formed by a layer of thyroid follicular cells surrounding a lumen. The first evidence of follicle formation occurs at E70 with distinct, small follicles recognisable throughout the gland. Terminal differentiation of thyroid follicular cells only occurs once the gland has completed migration and follicles have begun to form. Parafollicular cells, which secrete calcitonin, are found scattered in the interfollicular spaces and make up 10% or less of the total thyroid mass. Iodine uptake and thyroid hormone synthesis are initiated between 10 and 14 weeks of gestation, but the onset of physiological amounts of thyroid hormone production and release into the circulation occur only by 16–18 weeks of gestation, when a fully mature thyroid gland has developed (Hoyes and Kershaw 1985; Santisteban 2012).

Blood supply to the thyroid gland
The thyroid gland receives an abundant blood supply with a flow rate estimated at 5ml/g of thyroid tissue per minute. The major blood supply comes from paired superior and inferior thyroid arteries. The superior thyroid arteries branch from the external carotid arteries and enter the thyroid lobes at the upper poles. The inferior thyroid arteries branch from the

thyrocervical trunk of the brachiocephalic arteries and enter the lower poles of the thyroid lobes posteriorly. Up to 10% of humans have a fifth artery, the thyroidea ima, which typically arises from the brachiocephalic trunk and supplies the isthmus. Venous drainage is via the superior, middle and inferior thyroid veins. The superior and middle veins drain into the internal jugular vein while the inferior veins anastomose together prior to draining into the left brachiocephalic vein (Standring 2009).

Thyroid hormone synthesis

Thyroid hormones are low molecular weight molecules that comprise two iodinated tyrosine moieties joined by an ether linkage. Thyroid hormone biosynthesis, storage and release consist of a series of well-orchestrated steps within the thyroid follicular cell. The whole process is dependent on the nutritional availability of iodide and tightly regulated by TSH, and involves a series of sequential steps shown in Figure 6.2.

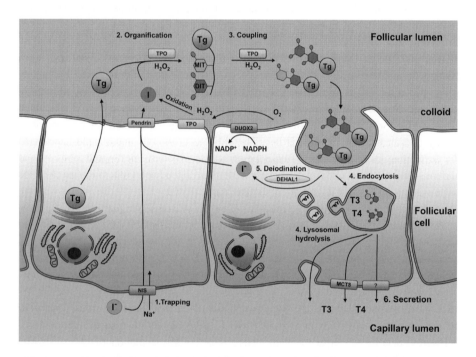

Figure 6.2. Thyroid hormone synthesis is a stepwise biosynthetic process that involves: (1) active uptake of iodide across the basement membrane into the thyroid cell (trapping), (2) H_2O_2 dependent iodination of tyrosine residues in thyroglobulin by TPO (organification), (3) coupling of iodotyrosines within thyroglobulin to form the iodothyronines T3 and T4, (4) endocytosis of thyroglobulin from the lumen, hydrolysis in lysosomes and release of iodothyronines and iodotyrosines, (5) deiodination of iodotyrosines within the thyroid cell and reuse of the iodide (6) secretion of thyroid hormones into circulation. Tg: Thyroglobulin, NIS: Sodium-iodide symporter, TPO: Thyroid peroxidase, DUOX2: Dual oxidase 2, DEHAL1: iodotyrosine dehalogenase 1, MIT: monoiodotyrosine, DIT: diiodotyrosine, MCT8: monocarboxylate transporter 8, I⁻ : iodide, I: iodine.

The sodium-iodide symporter (NIS) mediates the uptake of iodide from the circulation into the thyroid gland. NIS is a 643 amino acid protein that co-transports iodide (I^-) and sodium (Na^+) across the basolateral membrane of thyroid follicular cells. Iodide transport is dependent on an electrochemical gradient generated by the membrane Na^+/K^+ ATPase and results in intracellular concentrations of iodide that are 20- to 40-fold higher than in plasma. Iodide accumulation and consequent organification are regulated predominantly by TSH and iodide availability. High levels of iodide block further hormone synthesis via an autoregulatory process known as the Wolff–Chaikoff effect, which involves down-regulation of NIS expression (Dohan et al. 2003).

Organification of iodide and the formation of iodothyronines take place at the luminal surface of the apical membrane of thyroid follicular cells, and these processes are facilitated by combined actions of three major glycoproteins, thyroglobulin, thyroid peroxidase (TPO) and dual oxidase-2 (DUOX2). Iodide transport across the apical membrane into the follicular lumen is not yet fully characterised, but an iodide transporter, pendrin, is thought to have a role. Mutations in *SLC26A4*, encoding pendrin and causing Pendred syndrome, result in impaired iodide organification and variable degrees of hypothyroidism (Taurog 2000; Bizhanova and Kopp 2010).

Thyroglobulin is a large glycoprotein synthesised in thyroid follicular cells that functions as a highly specialised scaffold for the synthesis and storage of thyroid hormone. Thyroglobulin comprises two identical 2749 amino acid subunits each with 66 tyrosine residues, many of which are used for hormonogenesis. Iodination of tyrosine residues results in the formation of 3-iodotyrosine (monoiodotyrosine, MIT) and 3,5-diiodotyrosine (DIT). TPO catalyses both the prior oxidation of iodide to iodine, an essential step required for iodination, as well as the incorporation of iodine into tyrosine (organification). Both reactions require H_2O_2, which is generated and supplied to the follicular lumen by the 1527 amino acid transmembrane protein DUOX2 (Taurog 2000).

Finally, TPO also catalyses coupling of two suitably located iodotyrosine residues to form iodothyronines. 3,5,3'-L-triiodothyronine (T3) is formed by coupling of MIT and DIT residues, while 3,5,3',5'-L-tetraiodothyronine (thyroxine, T4) results from the coupling of two DIT residues. At this stage the newly formed iodothyronines are stored as colloid in the follicular lumen and remain attached to the thyroglobulin molecule until secretion is required (Taurog 2000). TSH stimulation causes thyroglobulin to be absorbed from the lumen back into the thyroid follicular cell by micro- and macro-pinocytosis. The iodinated thyroglobulin-containing vesicles are then fused with lysosomes containing proteases, resulting in hydrolysis of thyroglobulin and production of T4 and lesser amounts of T3, MIT and DIT. Iodotyrosine dehalogenase 1 then deiodinates MIT and DIT and the resulting iodide is recycled for further hormone synthesis (Moreno and Visser 2010).

The secretion of T4 and T3 into circulation is not yet fully understood. Release by the fusion of the thyroid hormone–containing vesicles with the basolateral membrane is one option, while transporter-mediated secretion via membrane transporters is also a possibility. The monocarboxylate transporter-8 (MCT8) has been considered as one candidate that may play a role in thyroid hormone secretion (Di Cosmo et al. 2010).

Circulation of thyroid hormones

Thyroid hormones are hydrophobic molecules and binding to plasma proteins is essential for their circulation in the bloodstream and delivery to target organs. Thyroxine-binding globulin (TBG), transthyretin (TTR, previously known as thyroxine-binding prealbumin) and albumin are the major plasma thyroid hormone transporters. Other minor carriers include lipoproteins and immunoglobulins. Protein binding facilitates the presence of a large circulating thyroid hormone pool with a 7-day half-life that ensures uniform and constant availability of thyroid hormone in target tissues independent of physiological variation in hormone production or demand. The total binding capacity of these carrier proteins is so high that only tiny fractions of thyroid hormone circulate unbound or free (0.03% of T4 and 0.3% of T3). The free hormones are available for entry and action in target cells and are thus defined as the biologically active fraction of thyroid hormones (Benvenga 2005).

TBG is a liver-derived 395 amino acid glycoprotein with a single binding site for thyroid hormone. Although it has the lowest plasma concentration among the thyroid hormone protein transporters (15mg/l), its high affinity for T4 results in it binding about 70% of circulating thyroid hormone. Plasma TTR is produced in the liver; however, it can also be synthesised in peripheral sites, including choroid plexus, and so TTR is the major thyroid hormone transport protein in cerebrospinal fluid. TTR consists of four identical 127 amino acid subunits, has a plasma concentration of 250mg/l and binds 10% of circulating T4. Its binding affinity for T4 is almost 10-fold greater than for T3. Albumin is by far the most abundant plasma transporter (40g/l), but has multiple low affinity binding sites for thyroid hormone and thus accounts for transport of only 15% of circulating T4 and T3 (Refetoff et al. 1996; Benvenga 2005).

Genetic variation, pathophysiological abnormalities or exogenous factors can cause fluctuations in the concentrations or binding affinities of these proteins, resulting in changes in total T4 and T3 levels. However, free T4 and free T3 concentrations, which determine thyroid hormone availability and action in target tissues, remain unaffected. Considering that most thyroid hormone in plasma is bound to TBG, variation in its concentration is of greater importance relative to variations of TTR or albumin. Inherited TBG deficiency is an X-linked recessive trait caused by a single base mutation in the *TBG* gene. The subsequent TBG deficiency may be partial, due to decreased T4 affinity and protein stability, or may result in complete lack of TBG. Oestrogens (pregnancy, tumours, estrogen therapy) cause decreased metabolic clearance of TBG and consequent increased plasma TBG concentrations (Benvenga 2005). In systemic illness, both T4-binding activity and levels of TBG decrease resulting in lower total thyroid hormone concentrations. Certain drugs can also affect the TBG concentration (androgens, glucocorticoids), or competitively inhibit T4 binding (salicylates, frusemide, heparin). TBG concentrations are also reduced in carbohydrate-deficient glycoprotein syndromes. Increased TTR levels may be present in patients with pancreatic or hepatic tumours due to ectopic production, while mutations in the *TTR* gene can be associated with both increased and decreased T4-binding affinity. *TTR* mutations can also cause amyloidosis as a result of the deposition of insoluble TTR fibrils in nerves or the heart (Benvenga 2005). Familial dysalbuminaemic hyperthyroxinaemia is an autosomal dominant condition in which albumin exhibits increased T4-binding affinity (Petitpas et al. 2003). In this situation, some free T4 assays may falsely report high free T4 concentrations, leading to misdiagnosis of hyperthyroidism in normal individuals.

Feedback regulation of the hypothalamic-pituitary-thyroid axis

Circulating thyroid hormone concentrations are maintained within a narrow reference range by activity of a classic endocrine negative feedback loop mediated by the HPT axis (Fig 6.3a).

TRH is secreted from the hypothalamus and stimulates anterior pituitary thyrotrophs to release TSH, the major regulator of thyroid hormone production. TSH acts on the G-protein coupled TSH receptor on the thyroid follicular cell membrane to activate cyclic adenosine monophosphate (AMP) and stimulate synthesis and secretion of thyroid hormone. Thyroid hormones act directly via nuclear T3 receptors in the hypothalamus and pituitary to repress *TRH* and *TSH* gene expression and inhibit their synthesis and secretion, thereby completing the negative feedback loop.

Control of thyrotropin-releasing hormone synthesis, secretion and action by thyroid hormones

TRH is a tripeptide (pyroglutamyl-histidyl-proline-amide) modified from a prohormone (pre-proTRH) by two convertases that are regulated by thyroid hormone. TRH is expressed in multiple tissues but the source that regulates TSH secretion is from parvocellular neurons within the paraventricular nucleus of the hypothalamus.

T3 negatively regulates TRH action at several levels. It inhibits both the transcription of *TRH* (Segerson et al. 1987; Sugrue et al. 2010) and the post-translational modification of TRH protein (Perello et al. 2006). Thyroid hormone receptors (THRs) are highly expressed in the paraventricular nucleus and mediate T3-dependent negative feedback of the HPT axis. Humans with mutations in the *THRB* gene, encoding THRβ, develop central resistance to thyroid hormone, and THRβ knockout mice have impaired regulation of both TRH and TSH expression (Abel et al. 2001).

TRH is degraded rapidly within the central nervous system by a tanycyte cell-surface ectoenzyme, pyroglutamyl peptidase II (PPII) that utilises TRH as a highly specific substrate. PPII expression is stimulated by T3 and this mechanism also contributes to negative feedback control of TRH concentrations by thyroid hormone (Costa-e-Sousa and Hollenberg 2012). Furthermore, T3 regulates TRH action by inhibiting expression of TRH receptor 1 (TRHR1), the specific thyrotroph cell membrane receptor through which TRH acts to stimulate TSH release.

Control of thyroid-stimulating hormone synthesis and secretion by thyroid hormones

TSH is a heterodimeric glycoprotein hormone composed of two subunits: an α subunit that is common to TSH, luteinizing hormone, follicle-stimulating hormone and human chorionic gonadotropin, and a TSH-specific β subunit. TSH binds to the thyroid follicular cell membrane TSH receptor and stimulates synthesis and release of thyroid hormone via a G-protein-coupled cell-signalling pathway that requires activation of cyclic AMP. There is a physiological inverse linear relationship between the serum-free T4 concentration and the logarithmic transformed concentration of TSH. The TSH concentration is thus a highly sensitive indicator of thyroid status. Nevertheless, the circulating TSH concentration is subject to pulsatile and circadian variations, with peak secretion occurring during the night in humans. This circadian variation is not influenced by circulating thyroid hormone concentrations and is preserved in primary hypothyroidism, although its physiological importance in the maintenance of thyroid hormone homeostasis is unclear (Roelfsema et al. 2010).

Transcription of both α and β subunits of TSH is regulated by TRH and thyroid hormone. TRH acts at the thyrotroph cell membrane in the anterior pituitary to stimulate TSH expression via second messenger signalling pathways, whilst T3 acts in the nucleus to inhibit *TSH* gene transcription directly. Although transcriptional regulation is the most important mechanism by which TSH is regulated, TRH is also required for post-translational glycosylation of TSH and is essential for its full physiological activity (Beck-Peccoz et al. 1985). Thus, TRH knockout mice have an elevated serum TSH concentration due to abnormal glycosylation, half-life and bioactivity of the secreted TSH peptide. Administration of TRH to some patients with central hypothyroidism results in increased TSH production and bioactivity, whilst patients with resistance to thyroid hormone due to mutations of *THRB* encoding TRβ also secrete inappropriate concentrations of TSH with abnormal glycosylation and increased bioactivity (Persani et al. 1994).

Thyroid hormone action

Although serum-free thyroid hormone concentrations are subject to negative feedback control and maintained within the physiological reference range, thyroid hormone action in target cells is controlled locally via regulation of hormone uptake and metabolism, and by regulation of THR expression and function.

Thyroid hormone transporters

Because of their lipophilic properties, thyroid hormones were considered to enter target cells by passive diffusion, but by the late 1970s, it was apparent that membrane transporter proteins are required. More than 20 transporters have been identified with the ability to transfer iodothyronine derivatives into the cytoplasm. In 2011, it has been shown that free thyroid hormones enter target cells via energy-dependent, stereospecific and saturable mechanisms mediated by iodothyronine-specific transporters including MCT8, MCT10 and the Na^+-independent organic anion transporter protein 1c1 (OATP1c1), as well as by less specific transporter proteins including the L-type amino acid transporters LAT1 and LAT2 (Visser et al. 2011).

The best characterised transporter, MCT8, is expressed in most thyroid hormone target tissues including the heart, liver, kidney, skeleton, thyroid and brain. Mutations of *SLC16A2*, encoding MCT8, result in Allan–Herndon–Dudley syndrome, a severe X-linked psychomotor retardation syndrome that presents in early childhood with developmental delay and lack of speech development, and results from defective neuronal T3 entry causing abnormal T3 action and metabolism. Affected boys have a characteristically elevated serum T3 concentration with reduced T4 and reverse T3 concentrations but inappropriately normal or modestly elevated TSH (Zung et al. 2011).

MCT10 shares 49% homology with MCT8 and facilitates transport of both T3 and T4 into cells, but with a preference for T3. MCT10 is expressed predominantly at the basolateral cell membrane in various tissues including the kidney, placenta, muscle, liver and intestine. In 2012, it was suggested that MCT10 may be the main thyroid hormone transporter in growth plate chondrocytes (Abe et al. 2012) in which it is expressed at far higher levels than MCT8. This finding may explain in part why boys with Allan–Herndon–Dudley syndrome have normal linear growth.

By contrast, the T4-specific transporter OATP1c1 has a more restricted tissue distribution with high levels of expression in capillary endothelial cells throughout the central nervous system. OATP1c1 is likely to be the principal transporter mediating passage of thyroid hormone across the blood–brain barrier.

Iodothyronine deiodinases
Although T4 circulates in peripheral blood at a 4- to 5-fold higher concentration than T3, it has a 100-fold lower affinity for the nuclear THR, and thus T4 is considered to be a pro-hormone that must be converted to the biologically active hormone T3.

The iodothyronine deiodinases are three selenoenzymes that activate or inactivate thyroid hormones (Fig 6.3b). The type 2 deiodinase (DIO2) catalyses efficient removal of an outer ring iodine atom from T4 and generates T3. By contrast, the type 3 enzyme (DIO3) efficiently inactivates T3, or prevents activation of T4, by catalysing removal of an inner ring iodine to generate 3,3'-diiodothyronine (T2) or 3,3',5'-triiodothyronine (reverse T3, rT3), respectively. The type 1 deiodinase (DIO1), however, is relatively inefficient and catalyses removal of inner or outer ring iodine atoms in equimolar proportions to generate T3, rT3 or T2 depending on the substrate. Most circulating T3 is derived from T4 by the actions of DIO1 in liver and kidney, although the physiological role of DIO1 remains unknown and DIO2 activity in skeletal muscle also probably contributes to the circulating T3 pool. Nevertheless, the primary function of DIO2 is to determine the intracellular concentration of T3 and level of saturation of the nuclear THR. Its low Michaelis constant (K_m) enables efficient local generation of T3 at times of T4 deprivation and DIO2 is thought to protect vital structures from periods of hypothyroidism. By contrast, the inactivating DIO3 enzyme prevents TH access to specific tissues and reduces THR saturation at critical times during embryogenesis and development, thus protecting tissues from the detrimental effects of thyrotoxicosis (Bianco 2011; Williams and Bassett 2011). Because DIO2 and DIO3 have similar affinities for substrate (10-9M), it is thought their relative levels of expression control the intracellular concentration of T3 and its availability to nuclear THRs.

Consistent with this hypothesis, expression of DIO2 and DIO3 is frequently regulated reciprocally in temporal and tissue-specific patterns. Thus, during fetal development, high levels of DIO3 activity in the placenta, uterus and fetal liver protect developing tissues from exposure to inappropriate levels of T3 and facilitate cell proliferation. At birth, DIO3 activity declines rapidly and expression of DIO2 in T3-responsive tissues increases. This 'developmental switch' triggers T3-dependent cell differentiation and organ maturation and is essential for normal postnatal growth and development.

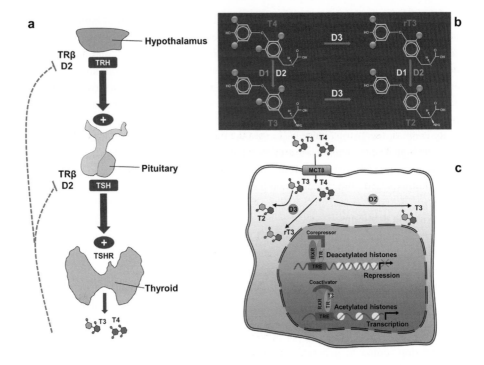

Figure 6.3. The HPT axis and thyroid hormone action (a), Thyrotropin-releasing hormone (TRH) is synthesised in the hypothalamus and stimulates secretion of thyroid stimulating hormone (TSH) from the anterior pituitary. TSH binds to the TSH receptor (TSHR) in thyroid follicular cells to stimulate synthesis and secretion of thyroid hormones (T4 and T3). In the hypothalamus and pituitary the type 2 deiodinase enzyme (D2) converts T4 to the active hormone T3, which acts via thyroid hormone receptor (TR) β to inhibit TRH and TSH expression (b), Within the target cell D2 converts T4 to T3. Alternatively, type 3 deiodinase enzyme (D3) irreversibly inactivates T3 and T4 by generating reverse diiodothyronine (T2) or reverse T3 (rT3), respectively (c), Thyroid hormones are transported actively into cells by cell membrane transporters including monocarboxylate transporter-8 (MCT8). The balance of activities of the D2 and D3 enzymes determines the intracellular concentration of T3 and its availability to the nuclear TR. The TR is present in the nucleus and binds thyroid hormone response elements (TRE) as a dimer with retinoid X receptor (RXR). In the absence of T3, corepressor proteins interact with TRs resulting in histone deacetylation and repression of target gene transcription. Following T3 binding to the TR, corepressors are released and coactivator proteins interact resulting in histone acetylation and transcriptional activation.

Thyroid hormone receptors

The major actions of T3 are mediated by two nuclear receptors, TRα and TRβ, which act as high-affinity T3-inducible transcription factors (Cheng et al. 2010) (Fig 6.3). The *THRA* and *THRB* genes encode the TRα1, TRβ1 and TRβ2 isoforms, which contain DNA and ligand-binding domains and act as fully functional T3 receptors. In addition, there are several isoforms of unknown physiological function that include the widely expressed TRα2 variant, which lacks T3-binding activity.

THRs are localised in the nucleus constitutively and bind to thyroid hormone response elements located in the promoter regions of T3 target genes even in the absence of hormone (Cheng et al. 2010). In the absence of hormone, unliganded THRs interact with co-repressor proteins including silencing mediator of retinoid and THR and nuclear receptor co-repressor, which possess histone deacetylase activity. Deacetylation of histones results in packing of chromatin in a compact configuration, leading to repression of gene expression. Thus, recruitment of co-repressor by THRs induces silencing of T3 target genes in the absence of hormone. Subsequently, entry of T3 into the nucleus and binding to the THR results in de-repression of gene transcription and hormone-dependent activation of target gene expression. This is achieved by a conformational change in the THR following T3 binding that releases co-repressor and results in recruitment of co-activator proteins, including steroid receptor co-activator-1 and other proteins with histone acetyl transferase activity. Acetylation of histones induces an open chromatin configuration that allows the transcription machinery and RNA polymerase access to the T3 target gene promoter, resulting in T3-dependent activation of gene expression.

TRα1 and TRβ1 are expressed widely but their relative concentrations differ during development and in adulthood due to tissue-specific and temporo-spatial regulation. Expression of TRβ2 is restricted to the hypothalamus and pituitary, where it mediates T3-dependent negative feedback regulation of TRH and TSH, and also to the cochlea and retina where it regulates timing of the onset of hearing and colour vision. Studies of mice with deletion or mutations of the *THRA* and *THRB* genes have identified tissue-specific functions for TRα and TRβ. Thus, T3 actions are mediated predominantly by TRα1 in the brain, heart, skeleton and gastro-intestinal tract and by TRβ1 in the hypothalamus, pituitary, liver and lung, whereas T3 responses in other tissues such as skeletal muscle and adipose tissue are mediated by both THR isoforms.

These studies have revealed the physiological complexity of thyroid hormone action and led to recent understanding that circulating thyroid status, as reflected by circulating thyroid hormone and TSH concentrations, does not necessarily provide an accurate indication of thyroid status in individual T3-responsive target tissues.

REFERENCES

Abe S, Namba N, Abe M, Fujiwara M, Aikawa T and Kogo M (2012) Monocarboxylate transporter 10 functions as a thyroid hormone transporter in chondrocytes. *Endocrinology* 153(8): 4049–4058.

Abel ED, Ahima RS, Boers ME, Elmquist JK and Wondisford FE (2001) Critical role for thyroid hormone receptor beta2 in the regulation of paraventricular thyrotropin-releasing hormone neurons. *J Clin Invest* 107(8): 1017–1023.

Beck-Peccoz P, Amr S, Menezes-Ferreira MM, Faglia G and Weintraub BD (1985) Decreased receptor binding of biologically inactive thyrotropin in central hypothyroidism. Effect of treatment with thyrotropin-releasing hormone. *N Engl J Med* 312(17): 1085–1090.

Benvenga S (2005) Thyroid hormone transport proteins and the physiology of hormone binding. In: Braverman LE Utiger RD (eds) *Werner & Ingbar's The Thyroid*. Philadelphia, PA: Lippincott Williams & Wilkins, 97–109.

Bianco AC (2011) Minireview: Cracking the metabolic code for thyroid hormone signaling. *Endocrinology* 152(9): 3306–3311.

Bizhanova A and Kopp P (2010) Genetics and phenomics of Pendred syndrome. *Mol Cell Endocrinol* 322(1–2): 83–90.

Cheng SY, Leonard JL and Davis PJ (2010) Molecular aspects of thyroid hormone actions. *Endocr Rev* 31(2): 139–170.

Costa-e-Sousa RH and Hollenberg AN (2012) Minireview: The neural regulation of the hypothalamic-pituitary-thyroid axis. *Endocrinology* 153(9): 4128–4135.

Crossman AR (2009) Diencephalon. In: Standring S (ed) *Gray's Anatomy*. Edinburgh: Churchill Livingstone, 311–324.

Di Cosmo C, Liao XH, Dumitrescu AM, Philp NJ, Weiss RE and Refetoff S (2010) Mice deficient in MCT8 reveal a mechanism regulating thyroid hormone secretion. *J Clin Invest* 120(9): 3377–3388.

Dohan O, De la Vieja A, Paroder V, Riedel C, Artani M, and Reed M (2003) The sodium/iodide symporter (NIS): Characterization, regulation, and medical significance. *Endocr Rev* 24(1): 48–77.

Hoyes AD and Kershaw DR (1985) Anatomy and development of the thyroid gland. *Ear Nose Throat J* 64(7): 318–333.

Low MJ (2011) Neuroendocrinology. In: Melmed S, Polonsky KS, Larsen PR Kronenberg KM (eds) *Williams Textbook of Endocrinology*. Philadelphia, PA: Elsevier, 103–174.

Melmed S, Kleinberg D and Ho K (2011) Pituitary physiology and diagnostic evaluation. In: Melmed S, Polonsky KS, Larsen PR Kronenberg KM, (eds) *Williams Textbook of Endocrinology*. Philadelphia, PA: Elsevier, 175–228.

Moreno JC and Visser TJ (2010) Genetics and phenomics of hypothyroidism and goiter due to iodotyrosine deiodinase (DEHAL1) gene mutations. *Mol Cell Endocrinol* 322(1–2): 91–98.

Perello M, Friedman T, Paez-Espinosa V, Shen X, Stuart RC and Nillni EA (2006) Thyroid hormones selectively regulate the posttranslational processing of prothyrotropin-releasing hormone in the paraventricular nucleus of the hypothalamus. *Endocrinology* 147(6): 2705–2716.

Persani L, Asteria C, Tonacchera M, Vitti P, Krishna V and Chatterjee K (1994) Evidence for the secretion of thyrotropin with enhanced bioactivity in syndromes of thyroid hormone resistance. *J Clin Endocrinol Metab* 78(5): 1034–1039.

Petitpas I, Petersen CE, Ha CE, Bhattacharya AA, Zunszain PA and Ghuman J (2003) Structural basis of albumin-thyroxine interactions and familial dysalbuminemic hyperthyroxinemia. *Proc Natl Acad Sci USA* 100(11): 6440–6445.

Refetoff S, Murata Y, Mori Y, Janssen OE, Takeda K and Hayashi Y (1996) Thyroxine-binding globulin: Organization of the gene and variants. *Horm Res* 45(3–5): 128–138.

Roelfsema F, Pereira AM, Adriaanse R, Endert E, Fliers E and Romijn JA (2010) Thyrotropin secretion in mild and severe primary hypothyroidism is distinguished by amplified burst mass and Basal secretion with increased spikiness and approximate entropy. *J Clin Endocrinol Metab* 95(2): 928–934.

Santisteban P (2012) Development of the hypothalamic-pituitary-thyroid axis. In: Braverman LE Cooper DS (eds) *Werner & Ingbar's The Thyroid: A Fundamental and Clinical Text*. Philadelphia, PA: Lippincott Williams & Wilkins, 26–45.

Segerson TP, Kauer J, Wolfe HC, Mobtaker H, Wu P and Jackson IM (1987) Thyroid hormone regulates TRH biosynthesis in the paraventricular nucleus of the rat hypothalamus. *Science* 238(4823): 78–80.

Standring S (2009) Neck. In: Standring S (ed) *Gray's Anatomy*. Edinburgh: Churchill Livingstone, 435–466.

Sugrue ML, Vella KR, Morales C, Lopez ME and Hollenberg AN (2010) The thyrotropin-releasing hormone gene is regulated by thyroid hormone at the level of transcription in vivo. *Endocrinology* 151(2): 793–801.

Taurog A (2000) Hormone synthesis: Thyroid iodine metabolism. In: Braverman LE Utiger RD (eds) *Werner & Ingbar's The Thyroid*. Philadelphia, PA: Lippincott Williams & Wilkins, 61–85.

Visser WE, Friesema EC and Visser TJ (2011) Minireview: Thyroid hormone transporters: The knowns and the unknowns. *Mol Endocrinol* 25(1): 1–14.

Williams GR and Bassett JH (2011) Deiodinases: The balance of thyroid hormone: Local control of thyroid hormone action: Role of type 2 deiodinase. *J Endocrinol* 209(3): 261–272.

Zung A, Visser TJ, Uitterlinden AG, Rivadeneira F and Friesema EC (2011) A child with a deletion in the monocarboxylate transporter 8 gene: 7-year follow-up and effects of thyroid hormone treatment. *Eur J Endocrinol* 165(5): 823–830.

7
DISORDERS OF THE HYPOTHALAMO-PITUITARY-THYROID AXIS

Tim Cheetham and Ramesh Srinivasan

Introduction

Thyroid hormones play a critical role in brain development. One of the major successes of paediatric endocrinology has been the introduction of the newborn blood spot screening programme for congenital hypothyroidism (CHT). This has led to the virtual elimination of CHT with its attendant mental impairment in participating nations. The recognition that endemic cretinism can be easily alleviated by iodine supplementation has also changed the lives of many for the better. This chapter addresses various causes of thyroid hormone deficiency or lack of action, all of which have the potential to impair neurological development.

Central hypothyroidism

Central hypothyroidism can be defined as hypothyroidism arising because of insufficient thyroid-stimulating hormone production (TSH deficiency or TSHD) in the context of an otherwise normal thyroid gland. It may reflect underlying pituitary pathology (secondary hypothyroidism) or a hypothalamic defect (tertiary hypothyroidism).

AETIOLOGY

TSHD may occur in isolation or, more commonly, as part of combined pituitary hormone deficiency (CPHD) (Table 7.1). The established genetic causes of isolated TSHD are defects in the thyrotropin-releasing hormone receptor (TRHR) (Collu et al. 1997) or TSH subunit (TSHβ) genes (Bonomi et al. 2001) and the recently identified syndrome where loss of function mutations of the Ig superfamily 1 (IGSF1) results in an X-linked syndrome that is characterised by central hypothyroidism, variable prolactin deficiency and macro-orchidism in adolescents and adults (Sun et al. 2012). Affected males may also have delayed puberty, transient growth hormone deficiency and an elevated BMI. Some female carriers may also have central hypothyroidism (Joustra et al. 2013). There are a number of established causes of TSH deficiency in the context of CPHD (including mutations in *POU1F1*, *PROP 1*, *SOX3*, *HESX1*, *LHX3* and *LHX4*). (Please see Chapter 2.)

Acquired causes of TSHD include central nervous system (CNS) tumours and CNS tumour treatment with surgery or radiotherapy. Surgery for diseases such as craniopharyngioma will frequently result in CPHD including TSHD. Abnormal TSH production

TABLE 7.1

Recognised causes of central hypothyroidism in childhood

Genetic defects

Pituitary-specific transcription factor defects such as *POU1F1*, *PROP1 SOX3*, *GLI2*, *LHX3*, *LHX4* or *HESX1* mutations can be associated with multiple pituitary hormone deficiencies

Mutations in the TSHβ subunit gene

Inactivating mutation in the thyrotropin-releasing hormone receptor gene

Loss of function mutations of *IGSF1*

Tumours or associated surgery

Pituitary adenoma, craniopharygioma, meningioma, germinoma

Cystic mass lesions – Rathke cysts, arachnoidal cysts, colloid cysts and epidermoid cysts

Iatrogenic

Radiation induced (e.g. following treatment of central nervous system tumours)

Trauma (head injury)

Vascular

Haemorrhage, ischemia, aneurysm

Autoimmune disease

Polyglandular autoimmune disease

Lymphocytic hypophysitis

Inflammatory

Infections such as bacterial abscess, tuberculosis, toxoplasmosis, fungal disease

Infiltrative

Langerhans cell histiocytosis, lymphoma, sarcoidosis

Drug related

Somatostatin therapy, dopamine

TSH, thyroid-stimulating hormone.

following radiotherapy for childhood brain tumours reflects altered thyrotropin-releasing hormone (TRH) release but is not usually profound in childhood. Other hypothalamo-pituitary axes are affected by radiotherapy to a greater degree. Radiation-induced TRH, and hence TSH, deficiency can, nevertheless, develop following radiation doses in excess of 30Gy, with a long-term cumulative frequency of 3%–6% when the pituitary is exposed to doses up to 50Gy.

There is a qualitative dimension to TSHD in central hypothyroidism because glycosylation modulates biological activity. TSH detected by immunoassay may be non-glycosylated and hence have impaired bioactivity (Horimoto et al. 1995; Persani 2012). This may explain why TSH concentrations in central hypothyroidism (which may be present in the non-glycosylated state) are not closely related to thyroid hormone concentrations.

TSHD may be a transient phenomenon, for example, in infants born to mothers with hyperthyroidism or following the treatment of Graves hyperthyroidism with antithyroid drug (ATD) when TSH concentrations can also remain low in the presence of reduced thyroid hormone. Transient TSH suppression may also occur in association with intercurrent illness.

INCIDENCE

The incidence of isolated TSHD determined from neonatal screening programmes for CHT depends upon the strategy used and whether cases at the milder end of the phenotypic spectrum are detected. The incidence based on a programme measuring TSH and FT4 in Japan was 1 in 160 000 (Asakura et al. 2002) but a strategy that included the measurement of thyroid-binding globulin (TBG) revealed a much higher incidence of 1 in 16 000 in Western Europe (Lanting et al. 2005; Kempers et al. 2006). Isolated central hypothyroidism has been reported to be a relatively common finding in short, slowly growing children with approximately one-third of a group of children with a height more than 2SD below the mean found to have subtle abnormalities of TSH release in association with a FT4 in the lower third of the normal range (Rose 1995).

CLINICAL FEATURES

In spite of the potential severity of the clinical picture, infants with CPHD do not necessarily present in the early neonatal period (Van Tijn et al. 2008). Thyroid function should be checked in any infant with symptoms suggestive of CPHD such as hypoglycaemia, prolonged jaundice (particularly conjugated hyperbilirubinaemia) or microphallus. Feeding difficulties, lethargy, poor weight gain and cold, pale skin should also prompt testing. Features of isolated TSHD may be relatively subtle but there may also be a classic neonatal hypothyroid phenotype, for example, in the case of biallelic TSHβ mutations. Late treatment can be associated with neurodevelopmental problems, particularly in those infants at the more severe end of the biochemical spectrum.

INVESTIGATIONS

The diagnosis of TSHD requires the identification of low plasma-free T3 and T4 concentrations together with low or 'inappropriately' normal TSH concentrations. Laboratories that only measure TSH concentrations when thyroid function is requested will not identify cases of central hypothyroidism. TSH concentrations in CPHD can be paradoxically mildly elevated, which may reflect impaired biological activity with retained immunoreactivity, although hypothalamic somatostatin deficiency could be a contributing factor. The TRH test as a means of investigating infants with suspected central hypothyroidism has both advocates and detractors (Mehta et al. 2003; Van Tijn et al. 2008). A normal (type 0) response is illustrated in Figure 7.1 together with a compromised response (type 2 response) and an exaggerated, delayed TSH response (type 3). A type 1 response is the pattern seen in primary thyroid pathology. Advocates of the TRH test argue that a type 3 response is helpful because it is frequently associated with CPHD and the lack of a rise in thyroid hormone concentrations during the test may also point to an underlying axis abnormality. It is important to highlight the fact that a normal 'type 0' response does not exclude CHT and it can be argued that TRH testing adds little to serial thyroid function tests (Mehta et al. 2003).

A more extensive assessment of TSH production above and beyond TRH testing has also been described. TSH is produced in a circadian pattern with a surge overnight, and

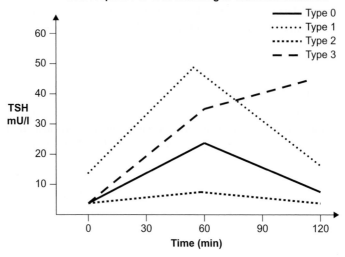

Figure 7.1. Illustration of typical pattern of thyroid-stimulating hormone (TSH) response to thyrotropin-releasing hormone (TRH) following its administration in primary and secondary disorders of the hypothalamo-pituitary axis.

blunting of this TSH rise may be associated with relatively low FT4 concentrations (Rose 2010) and suggest an underlying abnormality of TSH production.

TREATMENT

The treatment for TSHD is thyroxine with the objective of elevating the plasma FT4 concentration into the upper part of the appropriate age-related normal range (Slawik et al. 2007). TSH cannot be used as a guide to therapy and will typically become unrecordable in instances where it has been mildly elevated or normal (see text above). Other pituitary hormones should be evaluated in patients with central hypothyroidism, especially assessment of the hypothalamic-pituitary-adrenal axis to exclude hypocortisolism. If present, this should be treated prior to initiating thyroid hormone replacement. Growth hormone deficiency may mask subclinical forms of TSHD and thyroid function should be checked in the months following initiation of growth hormone replacement therapy (Behan et al. 2011). Children with short stature, slow growth and blunted TSH responses and 'low–normal' FT4 concentrations may grow more quickly on T4 supplementation (Rose 1995).

PROGNOSIS

The view that central hypothyroidism is less severe than primary CHT is not necessarily the case with untreated, severe primary CHT and severe, secondary CHT, both being associated with long-term neurodevelopmental sequelae. The prognosis of TSHD beyond infancy will depend upon the underlying cause.

Primary hypothyroidism

Impaired thyroid hormone generation by the thyroid gland will result in an increase in TRH and TSH production. The primary thyroid pathology may be congenital or acquired (Table 7.2) but, depending upon circumstances, such as tissue thyroid hormone requirement and metabolism, the impact on the HPT axis may change with age and maturity.

Primary congenital hypothyroidism

CHT (Léger et al. 2014) is one of the commonest preventable causes of learning difficulties and can be defined as a disorder of thyroid hormone generation in early life that reflects abnormal thyroid gland development (dysgenesis) or function (dyshormonogenesis). From a biochemical perspective, severe CHT is characterised by low thyroid hormone concentrations and an elevated TSH, although significant endogenous thyroid hormone production may result in a FT4 that is within normal limits for the population in association with an elevated TSH. CHT is best viewed as a clinical and biochemical spectrum. At the severe end of the spectrum are infants with thyroid agenesis, no significant thyroid hormone production and a markedly elevated TSH as a consequence of impaired feedback. At the mild end of the spectrum is the infant with a subtle abnormality of gland development with thyroid hormone concentrations within the local reference range in the presence of a mildly elevated TSH. Infants at the mild end of the spectrum are more likely to have a normally sited gland and include a greater proportion of preterm infants (Corbetta et al. 2009; Mengreli et al. 2010). Tissue thyroid hormone requirement changes with time, and infants with unequivocal abnormalities of thyroid hormone generation due to an underlying dyshormonogenesis can occasionally have normal thyroid gland function in later life when tissue requirements can presumably be met more easily (Hoste et al. 2010). There are a number of other well-recognised causes of transient hypothyroidism in early life. These include drugs that interfere with the HPT axis and iodine exposure with associated impaired thyroid hormone generation (Wolff–Chiakoff effect).

TABLE 7.2
Principal causes of primary hypothyroidism

Congenital hypothyroidism
• Dysgenesis; agenesis, ectopia, hypoplasia
• Inborn error of thyroid synthesis (dyshormonogenesis)
• Secondary to maternal antibody transfer

Acquired hypothyroidism
• Autoimmune thyroid disease (Hashimoto thyroiditis)
• Other causes of primary thyroid damage, e.g. cystinosis
• Iatrogenic:
  Post-radioiodine for hyperthyroidism
  Irradiation for non-thyroid tumour (e.g. medulloblastoma)
• Iodine deficiency
• Drugs:
  Antithyroid drugs: propylthiouracil, carbimazole, methimazole
  Others: anticonvulsants, lithium, amiodarone, aminosalicylic acid, interferon alpha

The incidence of CHT is 1 in 2000–4000 births with females being affected twice as commonly as males. A reduction in neonatal screening cut-off values has resulted in an increase in the number of infants diagnosed with CHT (Deladoey et al. 2011), although there is evidence to suggest that the incidence may be rising independently of the change in screening practice. Abnormal thyroid function at the milder end of the spectrum tends to have a more equal sex incidence, suggesting a different pathogenesis in many of these infants. The incidence of CHT may be higher in preterm infants although many reported abnormalities of thyroid function are transient and reflect the fact that these infants are more likely to have been unwell than term infants and hence exposed to medication and environmental factors such as topical iodine, which can interfere with thyroid hormone generation.

AETIOLOGY

CHT may be due to an abnormally sited or absent thyroid gland (dysgenesis) or a failure of hormone generation because of a defect in the enzyme activity involved in thyroid hormone synthesis (dyshormonogenesis). In iodine sufficient countries, 85% of CHT at the moderate to severe end of the spectrum is due to thyroid dysgenesis and 10%–15% of cases can be attributed to dyshormonogenesis. The precise nature of the subtle thyroid gland dysfunction in many infants at the milder end of the spectrum is unclear.

PATHOGENESIS

Thyroid dysgenesis

Thyroid dysgenesis presents in three major forms: ectopy, athyreosis and hypoplasia. Ectopy accounts for two-thirds of CHT due to thyroid dysgenesis. In these cases a thyroid remnant is found along the normal pathway of the thyroglossal duct, the route taken by the developing thyroid as it descends from the base of the tongue to its final location in the neck. Athyreosis refers to the complete absence of thyroid tissue and in hypoplasia the gland is normally sited but small or a hemithyroid. The cause of most cases of thyroid dysgenesis is unknown although environmental factors may be important (Pearce et al. 2011). Genetic defects have been identified in a minority of cases with mutations in genes such as *PAX8*, *TTF-2*, *NKX2.1* and *NXK2.5*.

Dyshormonogenesis

Hereditary defects in virtually all the steps of thyroid hormone biosynthesis and secretion have been described and account for 10%–15% of permanent CHT. These are generally transmitted in an autosomal recessive manner, although they are occasionally autosomal dominant. If untreated, they may lead to a goitre because of ongoing TSH stimulation.

CLINICAL FEATURES

Infants at the severe end of the spectrum may have feeding difficulties, sleepiness, constipation and prolonged jaundice. The examination in many infants may be unremarkable but infants with very low thyroid hormone concentrations have a characteristic facies with a flat nasal bridge, a large posterior fontanelle, macroglossia, a distended abdomen with umbilical hernia, bradycardia and hypotonia with delayed reflexes. The skin may be cool and mottled in appearance. The fact that the phenotype is not more profound in early life reflects thyroid hormone transfer from mother. Approximately 50% of circulating thyroid hormone is maternally derived, and it is this thyroid hormone transfer that provides some protection to the infant with no functioning thyroid tissue. Where this does not occur (e.g. if mother is also hypothyroid), then the infant can be markedly unwell with problems such as respiratory distress.

INVESTIGATIONS

Thyroid status is best assessed by measuring TSH and thyroid hormone (FT4 and FT3) concentrations. The aetiology of CHT can be established more precisely by isotope scanning, ultrasonography and measurement of thyroglobulin. A knee X-ray will reveal absent femoral epiphyses in up to 54% of children, particularly those at the more severe end of the phenotypic spectrum.

Genetic analysis can be undertaken in children with an in situ gland suggestive of a dyshormonogenesis. Candidate genes include thyroid peroxidase, thyroglobulin, *DUOX2* and *TSHR*. Establishing a more precise diagnosis is useful because it may help to determine the likelihood of further children being affected (one in four in the case of dyshormonogenesis) and because it can clarify whether the underlying defect is likely to be permanent. This information can also be used to guide management because infants with agenesis are likely to require more thyroid hormone replacement and may also be at greater risk of other problems such as impaired hearing.

SCREENING

Many countries have screening programmes for CHT. The screening strategy may involve the identification of an elevated TSH, low free T4 concentrations or a combination of the two parameters. All programmes have advantages and disadvantages that reflect issues of test sensitivity, specificity and cost. Most programmes identify elevated TSH concentrations although the more refined TSH assays have tended to be associated with lower screening thresholds even though the benefits from treating marginally elevated TSH concentrations are unclear.

TREATMENT

The overall goal of therapy is to ensure that children have growth and mental development that are as close as possible to their genetic potential. Levothyroxine (L-thyroxine) is the treatment of choice. Although triiodithyronine (T3) is the biologically active form of the hormone, most T3 in the brain is formed from local deiodination of T4 and so T3 replacement is not usually required. The recommended initial L-thyroxine dose is 10–15mcg/kg per day (LaFranchi 2011) for infants at the more severe end of the spectrum. In term infants, this amounts to an average of 37.5 to 50mcg per day. Thyroxine tablets or solution but not suspensions should be used. There is a relationship between the time taken for TSH to normalise and neurodevelopmental outcome. It is important to closely monitor these infants and adjust the L-thyroxine dose frequently until the desired level is achieved.

Plasma T3 and FT4 concentrations reach the normal range a few days after thyroxine treatment is started but it can take several weeks for TSH to normalise. Larger doses are required to normalise TSH concentrations in some children with CHT when compared to other forms of hypothyroidism, suggesting a degree of pituitary thyroid hormone resistance in some children. This has been linked to a period of relative hypothyroxinaemia in utero.

Normalising TSH concentrations may sometimes require relatively high circulating FT4 concentrations, reflecting the fact that the thyroid gland produces both T4 and T3. The question of what TSH threshold warrants intervention with thyroxine therapy is unknown.

PROGNOSIS

Prior to the newborn infants screening era, the diagnosis of CHT was made after the development of clinical manifestations with studies reporting an inverse relationship between the age of diagnosis and IQ outcome. The advent of newborn infants screening programmes has allowed earlier detection and treatment of infants with CHT with a much-improved neurocognitive outcome. The factors affecting outcome include the severity of the underlying hypothyroidism, the timing of therapy and the dose of thyroxine. Even when diagnosed and treated early, neuro-development may not be entirely normal, presumably reflecting the degree of thyroid hormone deficiency in utero. There also appears to be an association between suboptimal treatment in the first two to three years of life, as reflected by elevated TSH concentrations, and outcome. Hence these patients need close monitoring throughout early life.

Acquired hypothyroidism

INCIDENCE

Acquired primary hypothyroidism is the most common endocrine disease. The prevalence of hypothyroidism in the general population ranges from 3.8% to 4.6%. The Whickham survey in the north-east of England demonstrated an annual incidence of hypothyroidism of 4.1 per 1000 in women and 0.6 per 1000 in men (Vanderpump et al. 1995).

AETIOLOGY

In Western countries, the most common cause of primary hypothyroidism is autoimmune thyroid disease. Iodine deficiency remains an important cause in many parts of the world. Other causes of primary hypothyroidism include treatments such as thyroidectomy, radiotherapy and radioiodine therapy.

AUTOIMMUNE THYROID DISEASE – CLINICAL FEATURES

In atrophic thyroid disease, the gland is destroyed with little in the way of preceding phenotypic clues, whilst in classic Hashimoto disease, a goitre may be present and there is residual thyroid function at the time of diagnosis. The clinical features associated with severe, atrophic hypothyroidism include tiredness, weight gain, dry skin, cold intolerance, constipation, muscle weakness, puffiness around the eyes and slow growth with short stature (Table 7.3). Long-standing thyroid gland failure can result in pituitary enlargement

TABLE 7.3
Clinical features of hypothyroidism in children

Symptoms
Lethargy
Cold intolerance
Constipation
Dry skin
Hair loss
Muscle weakness
Short stature
Weight gain
Menstrual irregularity

Signs
Goitre
Myxoedematous facies
Bradycardia
Cool peripheries
Delayed relaxation of deep tendon reflexes
Hip discomfort/limp secondary to slipped femoral capital epiphysis
Delayed/late puberty
Macroorchidism
Cystic ovarian enlargement
Visual field defects secondary to TSH pseudotumour (rare)

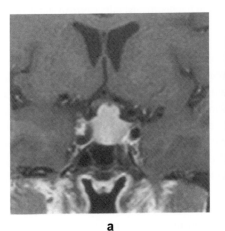 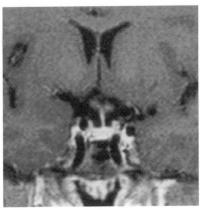

a   b

Figure 7.2. Thyrotrope hyperplasia (thyroid-stimulating hormone pseudotumour) in long-standing primary (autoimmune) hypothyroidism before (a) and after (b) one year of thyroxine.

('pseudotumour') with a risk of optic nerve compression (Fig 7.2), slipped capital femoral epiphysis (Fig 7.3) and ovarian/gonadal enlargement. The goitre in Hashimoto will frequently be associated with fluctuating thyroid hormone generation rather than profound thyroid gland failure.

95

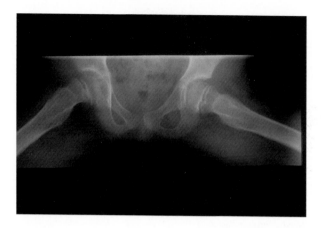

Figure 7.3. Slipped capital femoral epiphysis seen in long-standing hypothyroidism.

INVESTIGATION

Overt primary hypothyroidism is diagnosed biochemically with a serum TSH concentration above the reference range and a low free T4. If the TSH is raised but free T4 is in the normal range, then this is sometimes referred to as subclinical hypothyroidism or hyperthyrotropi-naemia. It is important to be aware of potential confounders and of particular note is the increased TSH concentration seen in patients with hypocortisolaemia. Cortisol status needs to be considered in all patients with a mildly elevated TSH. The biochemistry in Hashimoto disease can change quickly with rapid changes in TSH in the absence of intervention.

The population reference range of TSH will depend on the nature of the population sampled. Steps to exclude occult thyroid dysfunction and individuals where there is a family history of thyroid dysfunction will result in a tighter reference range. The variation in TSH concentrations within an individual is narrower than the variation in the general population. Hence a TSH level within the population reference range may still be abnormal for the individual in question. It is thought that genetic factors play a part in influencing the thyroid set point in the individual. This is supported by studies showing associations between TSH and common variations in different genes, including *PDE8B* and *TSHR* (Medici et al. 2011).

TREATMENT

The aim of the treatment of hypothyroidism is to render the patient 'euthyroid' with a normal TSH. L-thyroxine is the treatment of choice for the hypothyroid patient. It has a 7-day half-life, allowing daily dosing. Serum TSH is the most straightforward way of assessing replacement but can take weeks to normalise. It is recommended that the TSH is measured 6–8 weeks after initiation of, or following a change in, L-thyroxine dose. Monitoring will reflect factors such as patient age and growth rate but should be at least 6 monthly prior to the attainment of final adult height. In the majority of individuals, there is little or no benefit from adding triiodothyronine to L-thyroxine.

PROGNOSIS

The outlook for a child diagnosed with primary (acquired) hypothyroidism is excellent. Thyroid dysfunction is associated with alterations in cardiovascular and renal physiology (creatinine levels may be elevated at diagnosis) but these largely correct on therapy.

Hashimoto encephalopathy

Hashimoto encephalopathy is an uncommon syndrome of steroid responsive encephalopathy of presumed autoimmune origin. The condition has also been referred to as steroid-responsive encephalopathy associated with autoimmune thyroiditis syndrome.

AETIOLOGY

Despite the link to autoimmune thyroid disease, the pathogenesis of Hashimoto encephalopathy is still unclear. Many patients are euthyroid and hence the mechanism is not closely linked to low thyroid hormone concentrations or raised TRH or TSH. An autoimmune process, potentially involving the cerebral microvasculature, has been postulated and autopsy studies demonstrate lymphocytic infiltration of the CNS.

INCIDENCE

The incidence of Hashimoto encephalopathy in young people is unknown and the number of reported cases in childhood and adolescence is less than 50. In the population as a whole, the prevalence is believed to be around 2 per 100 000. It is likely that the disorder is significantly underdiagnosed. Most reported cases are female.

CLINICAL FEATURES

The clinical presentation of Hashimoto encephalopathy is highly variable and may occur over weeks or months, sometimes with a relapsing and remitting course. The neurological manifestations are diverse but include altered consciousness, confusion, seizures, myoclonus, involuntary movements, neuropsychiatric disturbance and cognitive decline.

INVESTIGATION

The diagnosis of Hashimoto encephalopathy should be considered in patients presenting with any unexplained neuropsychiatric picture or encephalopathy. High titres of antibodies to antigens, notably peroxidase but also thyroglobulin and the thyrotropin receptor, are required to make the diagnosis. The CSF is usually abnormal with high protein concentrations. The exclusion of toxic, metabolic and infectious causes of encephalopathy with neuroimaging and CSF examination is crucial.

TREATMENT AND PROGNOSIS

Treatment with systemic corticosteroids is frequently successful, although relapse may occur if this treatment is ceased abruptly. Steroid unresponsive patients have been treated with azathioprine, IV immunoglobulins or plasmapheresis (Ferracci et al. 2004), although the true impact of these interventions is unclear because of the small numbers of patients involved. Thyroid hormone replacement is appropriate in the context of biochemical hypothyroidism.

Thyrotoxicosis
Thyroid hormone excess or thyrotoxicosis is relatively uncommon in paediatric practice with an incidence in the United Kingdom that is around 1 in 100 000 under the age of 16 years.

AETIOLOGY
Thyrotoxicosis in children and adolescents is usually due to autoimmune thyroid disease. The severity and natural history will depend upon the nature of the autoimmune response and in particular whether stimulating thyroid receptor antibodies (sTRAb) are present. Patients without sTRAb may still have thyrotoxicosis but this will typically be of shorter duration (hashitoxicosis). In classic Graves hyperthyroidism the TRAb titre will be elevated. Thyrotoxicosis in the fetus or neonatal period is usually due to the transplacental passage of TRAb from mothers with active or treated Graves disease. The disorder will resolve within the first months' of life as the antibody titre falls. Rarer causes of thyrotoxicosis in children include activating mutations of *TSHR*, in which case there may be a family history of thyrotoxicosis. Thyrotoxicosis is also a recognised feature of McCune–Albright syndrome where somatic mutations in the Gs alpha subunit of the TSHr can result in thyroid hormone excess.

CLINICAL FEATURES
Features in childhood and adolescence are outlined in Table 7.4 and include weight loss, hyperphagia, heat intolerance and emotional liability. These diverse features can result in referral to a range of subspecialists including gastroenterologists (loose stools), cardiologists (palpitations, heart murmur) and psychiatrists. Clinicians need to be aware of the features of McCune–Albright syndrome.

INVESTIGATION
TSH concentrations will be suppressed. FT4 can be normal but is usually elevated along with FT3. In classic Graves hyperthyroidism, the TRAb titre will be raised and isotope scans will demonstrate uniform uptake in an enlarged gland. Hashimoto disease can also lead to short periods of thyroid hormone excess as outlined above. This will not typically be associated with antibodies to the TSH receptor and isotope imaging will tend to show patchy rather than uniformly enhanced uptake. In Graves hyperthyroidism, the ratio of FT4 to FT3 is typically less than 3 and greater than 3 in hashitoxicosis.

TREATMENT
Relatively subtle thyroid dysfunction in a patient who is well does not necessarily require treatment immediately and patients can be monitored whilst the underlying explanation for thyroid hormone excess and hence the likely natural history of the disorder are established. Treatment of autoimmune thyrotoxicosis is with ATD such as carbimazole or methimazole.

TABLE 7.4
Clinical features of thyrotoxicosis

Symptoms
Anxiety
Palpitations
Weight loss
Increased appetite
Sweating
Diarrhoea
Heat intolerance
Irritability
Headache

Signs
Goitre
Tremor
Tachycardia
Heart murmur (e.g. mitral valve prolapse)
Warm, moist hands
Proximal muscle weakness
Premature fusion of cranial sutures
Tall stature
Splenomegaly
Exophthalmos (Fig 7.4)
Skin pigmentation (McCune–Albright syndrome).

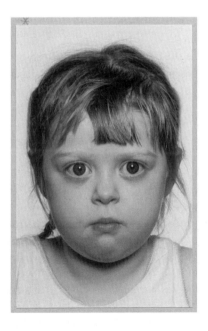

Figure 7.4. Exophthalmos in a child with Graves disease.

Beta-blockade may be appropriate whilst thyroid hormone concentrations are elevated. Propylthiouracil is not routinely recommended in paediatric practice because of the risk of liver failure. ATD can be used in isolation and titrated according to thyroid gland function or as part of a block and replace regimen where endogenous thyroxine production is abolished and then thyroxine added in a replacement dose. The advantage of the titration approach is the reduced risk of side effects, although block and replace regimen may be associated with greater biochemical stability and fewer hospital appointments (Schenk et al. 2012). Several months may elapse before TSH levels rise, presumably because of the lengthy period of preceding hypothalamo-pituitary suppression.

Thyrotoxicosis due to antibody transfer from mother in the neonatal period can be managed with a combination of iodine, beta-blockade and ATD, which can be titrated and then weaned as the disease abates.

PROGNOSIS

Most children with Graves disease will relapse after a 2- to 3-year course of ATD therapy, although remission rates may be as high as 50% with prolonged therapy (Leger et al. 2012). Those most likely to relapse will have a more profound phenotype at presentation. Young age and male sex are also risk factors. Those relapsing can return to ATD or undergo ablation with radioiodine or surgery. If surgery is chosen, then the preferred operation is total thyroidectomy because of the risk of relapse if the surgeon conducts a partial thyroidectomy and does not remove sufficient functioning thyroid tissue. Children with activating mutations of *TSHR* or with McCune–Albright syndrome require surgery or, in older children/ adolescents, radioiodine, as definitive treatment.

Thyroid hormone resistance

Thyroid hormone resistance (RTH) is a disorder where end-organ insensitivity to thyroid hormone typically results in abnormal hypothalamo-pituitary feedback.

INCIDENCE

RTH is rare with an incidence of around 1 in 40 000 in the case of TRβ-mediated RTH (see below).

PATHOGENESIS

There are two principal thyroid hormone receptors, TRα and TRβ, encoded by two genes (*THRA* and *THRB*). Mutations in either of these two genes result in RTH. The clinical picture in RTH is largely explained by the differing tissue distributions of the respective receptors with TRα the predominant subtype in bone, the gastrointestinal tract, cardiac and skeletal muscle and the CNS. TRβ is most abundant in the hypothalamus, pituitary, liver and kidney. The most common cause of RTH (RTH β) reflects heterozygous *THRB* gene mutations, although homozygous mutations have also been reported (Ferrara et al. 2012). Recently mutations in the *THRA* gene causing RTH due to an abnormal TRα receptor (RTH α) have been described and linked to a characteristic clinical picture (Bochukova et al. 2012; Moran et al. 2013, 2014).

INVESTIGATION

The biochemical picture in RTH β typically involves a raised thyroid hormone concentration (FT4 and FT3) but a TSH concentration that is normal or mildly elevated. The biochemistry in RTH α is more subtle with a normal TSH, low or low normal FT4 and normal FT3. However, the ratio of free thyroxine to free triiodothyronine is low (Bochukova et al. 2012).

CLINICAL FEATURES

The phenotype in RTH β is highly variable and the child can be asymptomatic or present with goitre and features of hyperthyroidism including hyperphagia. Homozygous mutations in *THRB* result in a particularly severe hyperthyroid phenotype with goitre and tachycardia. Patients with RTH α have a phenotype that is characterised by short stature, skeletal disproportion with short limbs, macrocephaly, delayed bone development and dentition, constipation, neurodevelopmental retardation and motor incoordination. The patient described by Bochukova and colleagues had slow, monotonous speech, but with no receptive or expressive deficit (Bochukova et al. 2012). Neuropsychological assessment showed impairments in selected cognitive domains with a visuoperceptual reasoning score on the 3rd centile (using the Wechsler Intelligence Scale for Children), and a working memory score on the 4th centile with verbal comprehension in the 32nd centile.

TREATMENT

The treatment of RTH β is challenging and controversial with little in the way of effective pharmacological intervention for many symptomatic patients, although a combination of ATD (to reduce thyroid hormone concentrations) and the T3 analogue 3,5,3'-triiodothyroacetic acid to reduce pituitary TSH production has been used in severe cases. Administration of supra-physiological doses of L-thyroxine may be beneficial in cases where the thyroid gland has been removed or ablated. There is some evidence to suggest that patients with mutations of the *THRA* gene may benefit from thyroxine therapy (Moran et al. 2013, 2014).

PROGNOSIS

Patients with RTH β may have a compromised bone mineral density and increased cardiovascular risk. Few adults with RTH α have been described but the phenotype is likely to include a placid affect with chronic constipation.

Thyroid hormone transporters

The intracellular actions of thyroid hormone are dependent on their being first transported into the cell by monocarboxylate transporter 8 (MCT8) and related thyroid hormone transporters. Mutations of MCT8 result in an X-linked disorder (Allan–Herndon–Dudley syndrome) characterised by profound developmental delay, truncal hypotonia, poor head control and paroxysmal dyskinesia. Investigations typically show elevated T3 concentrations, low rT3 and T4 with a slightly elevated TSH (Jansen et al. 2008).

Conclusion

Disorders of the hypothalamo-pituitary-thyroid axis are relatively common and the clinical picture extremely diverse. New disease entities are steadily being recognised and the biochemical 'signature' of these conditions can be relatively subtle. Clinicians may need to be particularly vigilant if a connection between phenotype and thyroid status is to be made. Implementing more widespread screening for CHT and optimising iodine status in childhood remain key challenges in this field of medicine.

REFERENCES

Asakura Y, Tachibana K, Adachi M, Suwa S and Yamagami Y (2002) Hypothalamo-pituitary hypothyroidism detected by neonatal screening for congenital hypothyroidism using measurement of thyroid-stimulating hormone and thyroxine. *Acta Paediatr* 91(2): 172–177.

Behan LA, Monson JP and Agha A (2011) The interaction between growth hormone and the thyroid axis in hypopituitary patients. *Clin Endocrinol (Oxf)* 74(3): 281–288.

Bochukova E, Schoenmakers N, Agostini M et al. (2012) A mutation in the thyroid hormone receptor alpha gene. *N Engl J Med* 366(3): 243–249.

Bonomi M, Proverbio MC, Weber G, Chiumello G, Beck-Peccoz P and Persani L (2001) Hyperplastic pituitary gland, high serum glycoprotein hormone alpha-subunit, and variable circulating thyrotropin (TSH) levels as hallmark of central hypothyroidism due to mutations of the TSH-beta gene. *J Clin Endocrinol Metab* 86(4): 1600–1604.

Collu R, Tang J, Castagné J et al. (1997) A novel mechanism for isolated central hypothyroidism: Inactivating mutations in the thyrotropin-releasing hormone receptor gene. *J Clin Endocrinol Metab* 82(5): 1561–1565.

Corbetta C, Weber G, Cortinovis F et al. (2009) A 7-year experience with low blood TSH cutoff levels for neonatal screening reveals an unsuspected frequency of congenital hypothyroidism (CH). *Clin Endocrinol* 71: 739–745.

Deladoey J, Ruel J, Giguere Y and Van Vliet G (2011) Is the incidence of congenital hypothyroidism really increasing? A 20-year retrospective population-based study in Quebec. *J Clin Endocrinol Metab* 96(8): 2422–2429.

Ferracci F, Bertiato G and Moretto G (2004) Hashimoto encephalopathy: Epidemiologic data and pathogenetic considerations. *J Neurol Sci* 217: 165–168.

Ferrara AM, Onigata K, Ercan O, Woodhead H, Weiss RE and Refetoff S (2012) Homozygous thyroid hormone receptor -gene mutations in resistance to thyroid hormone: Three new cases and review of the literature. *J Clin Endocrinol Metab* 97(4): 1328–1336.

Horimoto M, Nishikawa M, Ishihara T, Yoshikawa N, Yoshimura M and Inada M (1995) Bioactivity of thyrotropin (TSH) in patients with central hypothyroidism: Comparison between in vivo 3, 5, 3'-triiodothyronine response to TSH and in vitro bioactivity of TSH. *J Clin Endocrinol Metab* 80(4): 1124–1128.

Hoste C, Rigutto S, Van Vliet G, Miot F and De Deken X (2010) Compound heterozygosity for a novel hemizygous missense mutation and a partial deletion affecting the catalytic core of the H2O2-generating enzyme DUOX2 associated with transient congenital hypothyroidism. *Hum Mutat* 31(4): E1304–E1319.

Jansen J, Friesema EC, Kester MH, Schwartz CE and Visser TJ (2008) Genotype-phenotype relationship in patients with mutations in thyroid hormone transporter MCT8. *Endocrinology* 149(5): 2184–2190.

Joustra SD, Schoenmakers N, Persani L et al. (2013) The IGSF1 deficiency syndrome: Characteristics of male and female patients. *J Clin Endocrinol Metab* 98(12): 4942–4952.

Kempers MJ, Lanting CI, van Heijst AF et al. (2006) Neonatal screening for congenital hypothyroidism based on thyroxine, thyrotropin, and thyroxine-binding globulin measurement: Potentials and pitfalls. *J Clin Endocrinol Metab* 91(9): 3370–3376.

LaFranchi SH (2011) Approach to the diagnosis and treatment of neonatal hypothyroidism. *J Clin Endocrinol Metab* 96(10): 2959–2967.

Lanting CI, van Tijn DA, Gerard Loeber J, Vulsma T, de Vijlder JJM and Verkerk PH (2005) Clinical effectiveness and cost-effectiveness of the use of the thyroxine/thyroxine-binding globulin ratio to detect congenital hypothyroidism of thyroidal and central origin in a neonatal screening program. *Pediatrics* 116: 168–173.

Leger J, Gelwane G, Kaguelidou F, Benmerad M, Alberti C and the French Childhood Graves' (2012) Disease Study Group. Positive impact of long-term antithyroid drug treatment on the outcome of children with Graves' disease: National Long-Term Cohort Study. *J Clin Endocrinol Metab* 97: 110–119.

Léger J, Olivieri A, Donaldson M et al. (2014) ESPE-PES-SLEP-JSPE-APEG-APPES-ISPAE; Congenital Hypothyroidism Consensus Conference Group. European Society for Paediatric Endocrinology consensus guidelines on screening, diagnosis, and management of congenital hypothyroidism. *J Clin Endocrinol Metab* 99(2): 363–384.

Medici M, van der Deure WM, Verbiest M et al. (2011) A large-scale association analysis of 68 thyroid hormone pathway genes with serum TSH and FT4 levels. *Eur J Endocrinol* 164(5): 781–788.

Mehta A, Hindmarsh PC, Stanhope RG, Brain CE, Preece MA and Dattani MT (2003) Is the thyrotropin-releasing hormone test necessary in the diagnosis of central hypothyroidism in children. *J Clin Endocrinol Metab.* 88(12): 5696–5703.

Mengreli C, Kanaka-Gantenbein C, Girginoudis P et al. (2010) Screening for congenital hypothyroidism: The significance of threshold limit in false-negative results. *J Clin Endocrinol Metab* 95: 4283–4290.

Moran C, Agostini M, Visser WE et al. (2014) Resistance to thyroid hormone caused by a mutation in thyroid hormone receptor (TR)1 and TR2: Clinical, biochemical, and genetic analyses of three related patients. *Lancet Diabetes Endocrinol* 2: 619–626. doi: 10.1016/S2213-8587(14)70111-1.

Moran C, Schoenmakers N, Agostini M et al. (2013) An adult female with resistance to thyroid hormone mediated by defective thyroid hormone receptor. *J Clin Endocrinol Metab* 98(11): 4254–4261.

Pearce MS, McNally RJ, Day J, Korada SM, Turner S and Cheetham TD (2011 May) Space-time clustering of elevated thyroid stimulating hormone levels. *Eur J Epidemiol* 26(5): 405–411.

Persani L (2012) Clinical review: Central hypothyroidism: Pathogenic, diagnostic, and therapeutic challenges. *J Clin Endocrinol Metab* 97(9): 3068–3078.

Rose SR (1995) Isolated central hypothyroidism in short stature. *Pediatr Res* 38(6): 967–73.

Rose SR (2010) Improved diagnosis of mild hypothyroidism using time-of-day normal ranges for thyrotropin. *J Pediatr* 157(4): 662–667.

Schenk D, Donaldson M Cheetham T (2012) Which antithyroid drug regimen in paediatric Graves' disease? *Clin Endocrinol (Oxf)* 77(6): 806–807.

Slawik M, Klawitter B, Meiser E et al. (2007) Thyroid hormone replacement for central hypothyroidism: A randomized controlled trial comparing two doses of thyroxine (T4) with a combination of T4 and triiodothyronine. *J Clin Endocrinol Metab* 92(11): 4115–4122.

Sun Y, Bak B, Schoenmakers N et al. (2012) Loss-of-function mutations in IGSF1 cause an X-linked syndrome of central hypothyroidism and testicular enlargement. *Nat Genet* 44(12): 1375–1381.

Van Tijn DA, de Vijlder JJ and Vulsma T (2008) Role of the thyrotropin-releasing hormone stimulation test in diagnosis of congenital central hypothyroidism in infants. *J Clin Endocrinol Metab* 93(2): 410–419.

Vanderpump MP, Tunbridge WM, French JM et al. (1995) The incidence of thyroid disorders in the community: A twenty-year follow-up of the Whickham Survey. *Clin Endocrinol (Oxf)* 43(1): 55–68.

8
IMPACT OF THYROID DISORDERS ON NEUROLOGICAL FUNCTION

Joanne F Rovet

Introduction

Thyroid hormone is essential for normal brain development and subsequent brain function. During gestation and infancy, thyroid hormone serves to regulate transcription of critical genes for essential neurobiological processes such as neurogenesis and myelination and it accomplishes this via regionally specific thyroid hormone receptors with unique ontogenetic schedules. Subsequently, thyroid hormone plays a critical role in neurotransmission and associated cognitive activities (e.g. attention, speed of processing). These various effects appear to differ in developing versus mature brain. Consequently, to ensure normal neurologic and neuropsychologic abilities, it is necessary to maintain adequate levels of thyroid hormone throughout development. Since paediatric hypothyroidism and thyrotoxicosis each involve abnormal concentrations of thyroid hormone, it is not surprising that children affected by these disorders show cognitive and behavioural abnormalities. In this chapter, I will review the current state of knowledge on outcome following both disorders, although the evidence is far greater for hypothyroid than for hyperthyroid childhood disorders.

Hypothyroidism

Hypothyroidism refers to the conditions arising from thyroid hormone insufficiency and can be congenital or acquired in origin. Congenital hypothyroidism begins during gestation or following birth, whereas acquired hypothyroidism typically appears from mid-childhood onwards, although a few patients presenting in infancy have been described (Foley et al. 1994). It is now also recognised that a number of environmental factors ranging from excess iodine due to radio-contrast and antiseptic solutions in the neonatal nursery to thyroid-disrupting chemicals such as flame-retardants, dioxins and polychlorinated biphenyls can perturb the infantile and juvenile thyroid systems, thus contributing to thyroid hormone insufficiency.

CONGENITAL HYPOTHYROIDISM
Epidemiology, etiology and clinical features
The two main forms of congenital hypothyroidism are primary hypothyroidism or central hypothyroidism. Primary congenital hypothyroidism, which affects ~1 in 2500 newborn infants (Harris and Pass 2007), is due to either dysgenesis (e.g. atopia, ectopia, hypoplasia,

hemithyroid) or dyshormonogenesis of the thyroid gland. Among the sporadically occurring dysgenetic forms, the athyreotic etiology is the most severe beginning in utero. In contrast, the ectopic etiology, which is the most common, is typically the mildest since it allows some partial thyroid function postnatally until the gland is eventually depleted. Several gene mutations (e.g. *TTF1*, *TTF2*, *PAX8*) have been associated with the different dysgenetic etiologies but are seen in only a minority of patients (Van Vliet 2003). In contrast, thyroid dyshormonogenesis arises from one of many gene defects in each step of the metabolic pathway for thyroid hormone production from initial iodine uptake to triiodothyronine (T3) and thyroxine (T4) release from the thyroid colloid. These defects can occur in families. Central hypothyroidism, which occurs in 1 in 20 000–25 000 births, can be idiopathic or familial in origin and is associated with a variety of gene mutations (viz., *TSHβ*, *TRH-R*, *POU1FI/PIT1*, *PROP1*, *HESX1*, *SOX3*, *LHX3*, *LHX4*) (Alexopoulou et al. 2004) as well as the newly described *IGSF1* deficiency (Sun et al. 2012), all of which contribute to differing degrees of congenital hypothyroidism severity and different ages of onset (neonatal vs. infantile).

Until a generation ago, congenital hypothyroidism was the world's leading cause of major intellectual impairment. Because of the late onset of the most evident clinical signs and symptoms (e.g. jaundice, hypothermia, constipation), affected children were typically not diagnosed until 2 to 3 months of age and thus underwent significant brain damage by the time treatment was given. Generally, treatment past the third month of life led to frank and severe intellectual delay, whereas earlier treatment led to a lesser degree of impairment and selective learning disabilities. In addition, late treated congenital hypothyroidism was associated with a number of significant neurobehavioural and neurological as well as ophthalmologic sequelae.

Newborn infant screening: types and pitfalls
Beginning in the late 1970s and 1980s, statewide or regional newborn infant screening programmes were implemented in Europe, North America, Australia, and many parts of the developing world allowing for earlier diagnosis and a far shorter period of thyroid hormone insufficiency than before. The two main screening approaches have involved assaying for either thyroid-stimulating hormone (TSH) elevations or low T4 concentrations, although a few jurisdictions screen for both hormones. However with each protocol, a few children can be missed: TSH screening does not find patients with central hypothyroidism who have normal TSH concentrations despite low T4 while T4 screening programmes miss patients with T4 concentrations at the lowest end of the normal range, due to TSH compensation and partially functioning ectopic glands.

In children identified by newborn infant screening, the period of hypothyroidism extends from late gestation, especially in those with thyroid aplasia, until treatment takes effect (~1–2 months of age). Duration reflects both initial disease severity and the initial dosage, and while a higher starting dose usually optimises outcome, it may also be associated with behavioural irregularities in a few children. Over the years, a number of improvements have been seen in the congenital hypothyroidism screening process as well as management guidelines.

Outcome following newborn infant screening: global findings

Since the implementation of newborn infant screening, a number of research teams have followed positively identified patients, some into adulthood. In several studies, investigations have involved detailed and elaborate examination of multiple facets of outcome that are affected by early thyroid hormone insufficiency. This includes attention, visual processing, memory and specific behavioural and motor sequelae. Recently with the advent of advanced neuroimaging techniques to study children's brains directly, several groups have been using such techniques to elucidate the impact of early thyroid hormone loss on specific neural systems.

Follow-up studies of patients with congenital hypothyroidism identified by screening can be classified according to the diagnostic and treatment protocols used at the time of identification. In 'first-generation studies', treatment usually occurred at 3–4 weeks (e.g. 27 days in Quebec, 28 days in Greece, 29 days in the Netherlands) and doses of L-thyroxine were relatively low (e.g. 5–10g/kg/day) (Heyerdahl and Oerbeck 2003); our programme at the time treated at ~17 days age (see Rovet 1989 for a review). Studies from this era reported IQ levels within the normal range but significantly below expectations and below those of sibling controls. A meta-analysis of seven studies reported an IQ difference of 6.3 points (Derksen-Lubsen and Verkerk 1996) that was maintained into adolescence (Rovet 1999) and adulthood (Kempers et al. 2006; Oerbeck et al. 2003). Lowest scores were usually from the most severe cases (due to athyrosis) or those with lowest starting doses and the longest times to achieve euthyroidism. Although patients with 'second-wave' congenital hypothyroidism evidenced a smaller IQ decline at ~4 points (Rovet, 2005), the most severe of these cases still had significant IQ reductions regardless of treatment age, implying in utero effects. A recent Swiss report on optimally treated adolescents from both screening eras indicated that IQ was 10 points below controls, with 52% and 21% of congenital hypothyroidism and 14% and 4% of controls respectively scoring 1 and 2 standard deviation (SD) below population norms, and needing special education services or special schooling (Dimitropoulos et al. 2009). Third-generation studies involve cohorts born after the publication of guidelines by the American Academy of Pediatrics (1993) and the European Pediatric Society (Gruters et al. 1994), which recommended a starting dose of 10–15µg/kg/day as well as individualising doses to severity of hypothyroidism (LaFranchi 2011). These guidelines led to a much earlier time of achieving euthyroidism (3 days for T4 and 2 weeks for TSH). Findings from our group on 5-year-olds born 1996–2000 indicate that IQ still remains low relative to controls (Rovet 2005) through to adolescence (Wheeler et al. 2011). In the Netherlands, where different cohorts of children have been directly compared, results have shown that only milder later-generation patients are fully improved, despite the superior treatment of all children relative to first-generation patients (Kempers et al. 2007; van der Sluijs Veer et al. 2012). Persisting deficits in more severe cases likely reflect their thyroid hormone inadequacy in utero and in the first few weeks of life.

Outcome following newborn infant screening: specific findings

In addition to reduced IQ, children with congenital hypothyroidism experience a variety of sensory, motor, cognitive and behavioural weaknesses (Rovet and Daneman 2003). These include (a) hearing and vision impairments; (b) weak motor skills and clumsiness; (c) delayed speech acquisition; (d) visual, visuomotor and visuospatial deficits and (e) attention and memory difficulties. Within each cognitive domain, some specific abilities are more affected than others (e.g. focusing versus inhibiting attention and associative memory vs. face recognition). Generally, deficits in the visual domain reflect in utero hypothyroidism, whereas those in language and memory areas reflect duration of postnatal hypothyroidism. Executive function abilities are usually spared, unless treatment is delayed.

Sensory and motor deficits. About 20% of children with congenital hypothyroidism are reportedly at risk for a hearing deficit, mostly a sensorineural hearing loss in the high frequency range (Rovet et al. 1996). In adults, a study from France on a large cohort reported 9.5% with self-reported hearing impairments versus 2.5% of controls, which was highly significant (Leger et al. 2011). Visual deficits include reduced contrast sensitivity (Mirabella et al. 2005) and reduced colour vision in the blue–yellow range (Borkowski, unpublished findings). Likewise, as many as 50% of adults with congenital hypothyroidism indicate vision problems (Leger et al. 2011).

Various motor deficits have also been observed in children and adults with congenital hypothyroidism (Rovet 2003). These deficits include reduced strength and balance, increased clumsiness and difficulty with throwing. A study examining cerebellar function reported that patients with congenital hypothyroidism had no abnormalities on indices of dysmetria, dysdiadochokinesia or motor timing (Kooistra et al. 1994). Recent studies show an association between age at TSH normalisation and postural control (Gauchard et al. 2006). On indices of fine motor functioning, we observed that children with congenital hypothyroidism show difficulties in visuomotor integration and manual dexterity, reflecting time of diagnosis (Rovet 2003).

Language difficulties. Children with congenital hypothyroidism, particularly those with athyreosis, are at risk for speech and language deficits (Bargagna et al. 2000). Delayed speech acquisition is evident up to 3 years of age, after which children surprisingly show catch-up. Comprehensive language testing has revealed weak expressive and receptive skills, particularly word knowledge, whereas grammar tends to be unaffected, a finding that continues until adulthood (Oerbeck et al. 2003). In addition, 5- to 7-year-olds from a first-generation cohort were reported to have weaknesses in auditory processing (Rovet et al. 1996) while difficulties in the language domain were associated with time to normalisation (Rovet 1992) and biochemical severity of disease at birth (Alvarez et al. 2004).

Visuospatial difficulties. A hallmark finding in congenital hypothyroidism research is the patients' reduced Performance IQ relative to Verbal IQ, signifying selective difficulty in the visuospatial processing domain. Specifically, children with congenital hypothyroidism have difficulty manipulating mental images, locating objects in space, forming block constructions and solving visual puzzles (Leneman et al. 2001; Salerno et al. 2002). These deficits, which are associated with initial disease severity and suggest a prenatal origin, continue to be evident in third-generation patients and predict difficulty in everyday visuospatial activities, such as sense of direction (Simic et al. 2013).

Attention difficulties. Attention may also be compromised in children with congenital hypothyroidism, particularly their ability to focus and sustain attention in contrast to their abilities when inhibiting, shifting and dividing attention, which are unaffected (Rovet and Hepworth 2001; Rovet 2003). Specific deficits in attention reflect both initial disease severity (Kooistra et al. 1996) and abnormal concurrent thyroid hormone concentrations at the time of testing (Rovet and Alvarez 1996).

Memory difficulties. Memory is also an area of particular vulnerability in both children and adults with congenital hypothyroidism (Rovet 2003; Oerbeck et al. 2005). Memory weaknesses include shorter memory spans and difficulty remembering locations and forming associations (Song et al. 2001). Parents report that their children have increased difficulty on a variety of everyday memory skills, particularly remembering where things are put (Wheeler et al. 2011). A recent study of autobiographical memory from our lab has indicated children with congenital hypothyroidism have less rich memories of their own past experiences (Willoughby et al. 2013) and are less accurate than peers in recall a common staged event in which all participated (Willoughby et al., unpublished results).

Academic difficulties. On tests of achievement, siblings and classmates were seen to outperform children with congenital hypothyroidism (Rovet and Ehrlich 2000) and this effect continued into adulthood (Oerbeck et al. 2003). Generally, arithmetic is more affected than reading, although children who manifest auditory processing difficulties are slow in learning to read (Rovet and Ehrlich 2000). In addition, children with congenital hypothyroidism are at increased risk of learning difficulties, particularly in the nonverbal domain and are more likely than siblings or other controls to have received special education (Rovet 2003). School success was correlated with initial dosage of thyroxine.

A population-based study of patients with congenital hypothyroidism from the original French screening programme has shown increased delay at school was associated with severity of congenital hypothyroidism at diagnosis, low treatment levels and long time to achieve normality (Leger et al. 2011). These effects led to a reduced likelihood of graduating from high school, particularly in males. As adults, fewer of the patients were in the highest socioeconomic category and employed full-time while more were still living with parents than were controls. In our experience, however, many patients, particularly those with the mildest congenital hypothyroidism forms who had received early and optimal treatment, do achieve considerable success and a substantial number has graduated with advanced post-secondary and professional degrees (Rovet, unpublished findings).

Behavioural difficulties. Increased behavioural difficulty has been described in children with congenital hypothyroidism while the specific manifestations vary with age. In infants temperament difficulties including heightened arousal and sensitivity to environmental stimuli are seen (Rovet et al. 1984). Older children with congenital hypothyroidism show increased introversion, anxiety, social immaturity and conduct problems, all of which are correlated with a higher starting dose (Rovet and Ehrlich 1995). Among adolescents, especially females, increased levels of withdrawal, anxiety/depression, thought and attention problems and aggression were described (Tinelli et al. 2003) but no associated risk factors were found. An analysis of different congenital hypothyroidism age groups showed that primary-school-age children (6–10 years) were most likely to exhibit behavioural problems; however, as these results were unrelated to initial disease severity or hormonal or treatment values in the first year, authors attributed these effects to parents' increased anxiety about coping with congenital hypothyroidism and about the child's future outcome (Bisacchi et al. 2011).

Among adults with congenital hypothyroidism, reduced self-esteem and quality of life have been described. Compared with the general population, patients with congenital hypothyroidism report fewer daily activities, decreased vitality, more depressed moods, increased anxiety and less engagement in social activities (Oerbeck et al. 2005; van der Sluijs Veer et al. 2008; Leger et al. 2011). Moreover, the Dutch study showed that these effects were greater for females than for males (van der Sluijs Veer et al. 2008). In contrast, the French study showed that neonatal congenital hypothyroidism characteristics, hypothyroidism at time of survey and other associated health impairments predicted different dimensions of perceived quality of life (Leger et al. 2011) while the Norwegian study failed to find an association between early high treatment levels and later behavioural outcome (Oerbeck et al. 2005) as observed in children (Rovet and Ehrlich 1995). Notably, all of the adult studies are based on first-generation patients and these effects may be minimised when younger later cohorts reach adulthood.

Neuroimaging evidence
To date, only a few studies have examined the effects of congenital hypothyroidism on brain structure and function. An EEG study reported that patients treated past 30 days of life had slower somatosensory but not auditory evoked potentials than those treated earlier (Weber et al. 2000). Similarly, we reported slow P300 latencies in recognising visual repetitions of stimuli than controls (Hepworth et al. 2006). Autopsy findings of late-treated patients with congenital hypothyroidism have shown extensive neuropathology with frontal and parietal lobe atrophy and delayed myelination. In contrast, unpublished MRI findings from our group on 10- to 16-year-olds belonging to a 'second-generation' congenital hypothyroidism cohort indicate no overall increase in incidental findings but the congenital hypothyroidism group showed more abnormalities in the sellar region than controls (16.7% vs. 7.9%) and 3 out of 30 patients had evidence of a calcar avis cyst, previous stroke or callosal abnormality (Rachmiel et al., unpublished data). In these, as well as third-generation patients, we have additionally observed reductions in hippocampal and caudate size (Wheeler et al. 2011) and abnormal hippocampal functioning, reflecting increased activation when remembering object pairs, locations and past personal events (Wheeler et al. 2012), which may signify greater hippocampal engagement when remembering the same information. A group from Italy which used functional magnetic resonance imaging (fMRI) to study the neuroanatomic substrates of visual processing in children with congenital hypothyroidism found they

were less likely than controls to use parietal regions and more likely to use frontal, suggesting atypical brain activation (Blasi et al. 2008).

Outcome following a delayed diagnosis of congenital hypothyroidism
Children who experience a delayed diagnosis of congenital hypothyroidism because of medical or laboratory error usually score about 2SD below their parents and siblings in IQ and exhibit marked deficiencies in language development, especially receptive language development, and attention, memory and executive function skills. Additionally in this author's experience, these children are at risk for severe psychopathology including obsessive-compulsive disorder, attention-deficit hyperactivity disorder, Asperger-like features, severe anxiety disorder and oppositional-defiant disorder, and they are unable to function independently in adulthood. As children, they require extensive professional services (e.g. speech therapy, physiotherapy, occupational therapy) and special class placements.

Central hypothyroidism
Limited evidence exists on children with central hypothyroidism as a separate entity. However, a study from the Netherlands on five such children (identified via T4 screening) treated in a timely fashion showed they had varying severity of initial hypothyroidism from mild to moderate (but not severe); their IQs were midway between those of the mild and moderate thyroidal congenital hypothyroidism groups but above the severe thyroidal group (Kempers et al. 2007). Additionally, motor skills of children with central hypothyroidism were subnormal and similar to those in the severe thyroidal congenital hypothyroidism group. In my limited experience with similar children diagnosed clinically, by TSH screening, at about 2 months of age, a mild IQ reduction (~1SD) and attention, math and sensorimotor problems were noted. One boy diagnosed at 2 months of age following a dramatic neonatal course showed stronger verbal than nonverbal skills, slightly compromised linguistic skills (all in the normal range), but strong verbal memory, secure and happy adjustment, good social skills, and strong athletic ability (Rovet, 2003).

Summary of congenital hypothyroidism
Findings on children with congenital hypothyroidism identified via newborn infants screening and treated early in life show far less cognitive morbidity than those diagnosed clinically. However, given the brief pre- and perinatal periods of thyroid hormone deficiency of children identified by screening, they are at risk for mild IQ reductions and subtle cognitive, neuromotor and behavioural deficits. Contributory factors are the etiology of congenital hypothyroidism and its severity at diagnosis, the age at treatment onset and initial dose levels. One factor, however, that has received little attention so far is the adequacy of the maintenance dose, especially as the frequency of thyroid hormone testing between medical visits may be as long as 1 year in older children, who may be experiencing a growth spurt and pubertal onset during this interval. Furthermore, very little is known about transitioning to adulthood and the impact of fluctuations in thyroid hormone levels, including the possibility of increased thyroid hormone resistance over time as observed by some adult endocrinologists (Kempers et al. 2005).

ACQUIRED HYPOTHYROIDISM

Epidemiology and clinical features

Acquired hypothyroidism affects as many as 1%–2% of young people and is more common in those above age 10 years, and in females than males (see Chapter 2.2). Although rare in infants, acquired hypothyroidism has been described in several infant cases (Foley et al. 1994). The most common etiology of acquired hypothyroidism is Hashimoto thyroiditis, the reason for which remains unknown. Although acquired hypothyroidism may also be drug-induced, children seldom consume the medications of concern, such as amiodarone and lithium carbonate. The diagnostic features of acquired hypothyroidism are growth deceleration with delayed skeletal maturity and pubertal onset, changes in body shape, coarsening of facial features, constipation, coldness, dry skin and muscle weakness. Typically, however, the onset of acquired hypothyroidism is insidious taking months or even years before a diagnosis is made. Brain MRIs as part of the diagnostic work-up sometimes reveal an enlarged sella turcica.

Because of the high risk of severe behavioural problems following aggressive treatment of children (particularly adolescents) with acquired hypothyroidism, a titrated dosing schedule has been recommended for attaining euthyroidism (Rovet et al. 1993). Following initiation of therapy, a small proportion of children may also experience visual impairment and severe headaches due to papilloedema and pseudotumour cerebri.

Neuropsychological and neuropsychiatric outcome following acquired hypothyroidism

Patients with acquired hypothyroidism seldom show the severe mental deficiency seen in late-treated congenital hypothyroidism. In the hypothyroid state, adolescents with acquired hypothyroidism are reportedly very well behaved and high achievers at school, possibly due to their pliant behaviour and reduced activity levels. However, the less commonly seen toddlers and preschoolers may show regression of intellectual and motor milestones and engage in frequent severe temper tantrums and increased irritability (Foley et al. 1994; Joergensen et al. 2005).

One of the remarkable features of acquired hypothyroidism is the appearance of severe psychiatric symptoms prior to (Bhatara et al. 1993) or following treatment of hypothyroidism (Rovet et al. 1993), as described in a few case examples. Notably, this observation has also been reported in adults, including a case of murder ascribed to myxedema madness. Bhatara et al. (2004) described an adolescent male with severe psychotic symptoms (obsessions with auditory hallucinations and aggressive tendencies) aggravated surreptitiously by acquired hypothyroidism, which was diagnosed during initial hospitalisation for psychosis and ameliorated only when euthyroidism was achieved. For a period of 10 years, this boy was followed and had several further hospitalisations after having voluntarily discontinued either his antipsychotics or his thyroxine. On thyroxine alone or antipsychotics alone, his symptoms continued and optimisation occurred only when he received an SSRI, respiridone and L-T4 (Bhatara et al. 2004). Likewise, a 12-year-old girl with newly diagnosed acquired hypothyroidism and pre-existing attention-deficit–hyperactivity disorder (ADHD) treated with psychostimulants developed an obsessive-compulsive disorder after being given L-T4 for her acquired hypothyroidism. She was recommended a course

111

of antidepressants along with current therapies of ADHD and acquired hypothyroidism (Bhatara and Sankar 1999).

In contrast, some children develop problems *after* diagnosis and treatment for acquired hypothyroidism. We described three teenagers treated for long-standing acquired hypothyroidism (2–3 years), who each demonstrated severe *de novo* behavioural abnormalities once treated (typically aggressively) (Rovet et al. 1993). The first was a 13-year-old female honours student who premorbidly demonstrated superior mathematical and artistic abilities, but after treatment was failing at school, unable to concentrate and acquire new information, and had erratic drawing skills. The second, a 12-year-old male honours student with no signs of hyperactivity or major behaviour problems, developed acute psychosis and absence epilepsy right after thyroxine treatment. He subsequently showed severe concentration, organisation and behavioural difficulties and was failing at school. The third was a 16-year-old male who sexually assaulted an older neighbour following treatment and subsequently suffered significant school and behavioural problems.

To assess the commonality of these problems and associated risk factors, a prospective study of 23 newly diagnosed pediatric patients with acquired hypothyroidism tested prior to therapy and 6, 12, and 24 months post-treatment was conducted (Rovet et al. 1993). Considerable variability was observed with 17% developing *de novo* behavioural problems (temper tantrums, moodiness, aggression, irritability), and 17% developing attention problems. However, 22% also improved showing a better attitude and increased energy levels. Although this group showed no overall change in intelligence, 26% did exhibit a significant decline, 26% a significant improvement and the rest remained constant. In contrast, after 2 years, the entire group showed declines in visuomotor skills and a mild decline in achievement, with a third of the group failing to make any gains in reading or arithmetic over this period. Those with the worst outcome had the most severe and longest standing hypothyroidism and also achieved their euthyroidism very rapidly after having received high dosages of thyroid hormone. However, none of these patients was as severely affected as the three clinical cases described above.

Summary of acquired hypothyroidism

Before age 3, acquired hypothyroidism is associated with permanent behavioural and learning problems. In contrast, acquired hypothyroidism past age 3 is associated with adverse effects reflecting severe learning and memory deficits as well as attention and new behavioural problems primarily after initiation of therapy, especially if it precedes a prolonged period of hypothyroidism. The coexistence of severe psychiatric disorders and acquired hypothyroidism or the aggravation of psychiatric problems following initiation of L-T4 signifies the need for consultation with child psychiatrists who have a special interest in child psychopharmacology when treating atypical presentations of acquired hypothyroidism.

Thyrotoxicosis

Despite considerable animal evidence showing that excess thyroid hormone is disruptive for normal brain development (Lauder 1979), very little is known about the neurologic consequences of thyrotoxicosis in children.

Follow-up studies of neonatal thyrotoxicosis report suboptimal outcome (Hollingsworth and Mabry 1976). In one study, nine patients with neonatal hyperthyroidism successfully treated were studied at an average follow-up interval of 3.5 years (range = 5 months to 10 years) (Daneman and Howard 1980). Despite normal thyroid function in all when subsequently tested, the majority showed varying degrees of intellectual impairment or developmental delay. All also had craniosynostosis and prominent frontal bossing of varying degrees. Six of the patients showed intellectual impairment and/or severe cognitive disabilities while the one child with the least degree of craniosynostosis had superior outcome. Overall, these findings were attributed to the effects of the early excess thyroid hormone on brain development.

A prospective study was conducted on nine children aged 12 years with newly diagnosed hyperthyroidism (Alvarez et al. 1996). They were assessed prior to and one year after onset of therapy. Initially, they showed reduced intelligence (particularly nonverbal intelligence) and poor attention with attentional problems reflecting difficulties in disengaging and shifting focus. Most results returned to normal after one year. There were no effects of the hyperthyroidism on their anxiety, which in fact was lower than controls. These results were interpreted as signifying a direct impact of thyrotoxicosis on brain function that subsides when thyroid hormone concentrations return to normal and suggest the need to closely monitor children with thyrotoxicosis to optimise their levels of attention.

According to Bhatara and Sankar (1999), as many as 10% of patients with thyrotoxicosis may acquire new psychiatric symptoms and deteriorating school performance, which can in fact antedate their hyperthyroidism diagnosis by as much as one year. Frequently observed symptoms are hyperactivity, anxious dysphoria, irritability and poor attention that typically abate following treatment for hypothyroidism. One dramatic case was a 4-year-old boy who developed increased aggressive and fire-setting behaviours that were associated with thyrotoxicosis following ingestion of ground beef contaminated with bovine thyroid tissue (Bhatara et al. 1995). Authors stress the need to consider hyperthyroidism in children with newly acquired behavioural problems that fit this profile.

Given the limited body of evidence and profound effects of thyrotoxicosis, further study of this population from a psychological perspective is clearly warranted.

Conclusion

Pediatric thyroid disorders are notable for their direct association with multiple aspects of cognitive and behavioural functioning that differ from those seen in thyroid disease of adult origin. These findings are likely due to the impact of thyroid hormone loss or excess on the developing and continually changing fetal, neonatal and pediatric brain. The findings on children with congenital hypothyroidism indicate that it is essential to (a) diagnose and treat these patients optimally and as soon after birth as possible in order to reduce the risk of significant brain damage and (b) manage them closely and continuously throughout childhood and adolescence. Because a few children may be missed by each of the screening methods or because of errors at various steps of the screening program, it is incumbent for all physicians to be prudent of the possibility of congenital hypothyroidism in clinical diagnosis. The findings on acquired hypothyroidism indicate that severe behavioural problems may follow therapy and suggest the need to slowly titrate the dose level, particularly if the hypothyroidism was long-standing. As acquired hypothyroidism can also occur in infants, whose brains are as vulnerable to a lack of thyroid hormone as in congenital hypothyroidism, it is critical that physicians be aware of this possibility when seeing a child with growth failure or unexplained decline in neurodevelopment. Finally in hyperthyroidism, it is important that physicians be aware of the cognitive and behavioural difficulties that can precede diagnosis and that some difficulties may persist despite treatment. Given the close association between treated patients and mental illness, particularly during adolescence, it is also important that psychiatrists perform thyroid function tests as part of the diagnostic work-up for specific psychiatric problems, particularly when past history is negative.

REFERENCES

Alexopoulou O, Beguin CI, de Nayer P and Maiter D (2004) Clinical and hormonal characterics of central hypothyroidism at diagnosis and during follow-up in adult patients. *Europ J Endocrinol* 150: 1–8.

Alvarez M, Carvajal F, Renon A et al. (2004) Differential effect of fetal, neonatal and treatment variables on neurodevelopment in infants with congenital hypothyroidism. *Horm Res* 61: 17–20.

Alvarez M, Guell R, Chong D and Rovet J (1996) Attentional processing in hyperthyroid children before and after treatment. *J Pediatr Endocrinol Metab* 9: 447–454.

American Academy of Pediatrics Section on Endocrinology and Committee on Genetics and American Thyroid Association Committee on Public Health (1993) Newborn screening for congenital hypothyroidism: Recommended guidelines. *Pediatrics* 91: 1203–1209.

Bargagna S, Canepa G, Costagli C et al. (2000) Neuropsychological follow-up in early-treated congenital hypothyroidism: A problem-oriented approach. *Thyroid* 10: 243–249.

Bhatara VS, Alshari MG, Warhol P, McMillin JM and Bhatara A (2004) Co-existent hyperthyroidism, psychosis, and severe obsessions in an adolescent: A 10-year follow-up. *J Child Adolesc Psychopharm* 14: 315–323.

Bhatara VS, McMillin JM and Bandettini F (1993) Behavioral manifestations of hypothyroidism versus thyroxine effects. *J Pediatr* 123: 840–841.

Bhatara VS, McMillin JM and Kummer M (1995) Aggressive behavior and fire-setting in a 4-year-old boy associated with ingestion of ground beef contaminated with bovine thyroid tissue: A case report and review of neuropsychiatric findings in pediatric thyrotoxicosis. *J Child Adolesc Psychopharm* 5: 255–271.

Bhatara VS and Sankar R (1999) Neuropsychiatric aspects of pediatric thyrotoxicosis. *Ind J Pediatr* 66: 277–284.

Bisacchi N, Bal MP, Nardi L et al. (2011) Psychological and behavioural aspects in children and adolescents with congenital hypothyroidism diagnosed by neonatal screening: Comparison between parents' and children's perceptions. *Euro J Endocrinol* 164: 269–276.

Blasi V, Logaretti R, Giovanettoni C et al. (2008) Decreased parietal cortex activity during mental rotation in children with congenital hypothyroidism. *Neuroendocrinology* 89: 56–65.

Daneman D and Howard NJ (1980) Neonatal thyrotoxicosis: intellectual impairment and craniosynostosis in later years. *J Pediatr* 97: 257–259.

Derksen-Lubsen G and Verkerk PH (1996) Neuropsychologic development in early-treated congenital hypothyroidism: Analysis of literature data. *Pediatr Res* 39: 561–566.

Dimitropoulos A, Molinari L, Etter K et al. (2009) Children with congenital hypothyroidism: Long-term intellectual outcome after early high-dose treatment. *Pediatr Res* 65: 242–248.

Foley TP, Abbassi V, Copeland KC and Draznin MB (1994) Hypothyroidism caused by chronic autoimmune thyroiditis in very young infants. *New Engl J Med* 330: 466–468.

Gauchard GC, Deviterne D, Leheup B and Perrin PP (2006) Effect of age at thyroid stimulating hormone normalization on postural control in children with congenital hypothyroidism. *Dev Med Child Neurol* 46: 107–113.

Grüters A, Delange F, Giovannelli G et al. (1994) Guidelines for neonatal screening programs for congenital hypothyroidism. European Society for Pediatric Endocrinology Working Group on Congenital Hypothyroidism. *Horm Res* 41: 1–2.

Harris KB and Pass KA (2007) Increase in congenital hypothyroidsm in New York State and in the United States. *Mol Genet Metab* 91: 268–277.

Hepworth S, Pang E and Rovet J (2006) Word and face recognition in children with congenital hypothyroidism: An event-related potential study. *J Clin Exper Neuropsychol* 28: 509–527.

Heyerdahl S and Oerbeck B (2003) Congenital hypothyroidism: Developmental outcome in relation to levothyroxine treatment variables. *Thyroid* 13: 1029–1038.

Hollingsworth DR and Mabry CC (1976) Congenital graves disease. Four familial cases with long-term follow-up and perspective. *Am J Dis Child* 130: 148–155.

Joergensen JV, Oerbeck B, Jebsen P, Hyerdahl S and Kase BF (2005) Severe hypothyroidism due to atrophic thyroiditis from second year of life influenced developmental outcome. *Acta Paediatr* 94: 1049–1054.

Kempers MJ, van der Sluijs Veer L, Nijhuis van der Sanden MWG et al. (2006) Intellectual and motor development of young adults with congenital hypothyroidism diagnosed by neonatal screening. *J Clin Endo Metab* 91: 418–424.

Kempers MJE, van der Sluijs Veer L, Nijhuis van der Sanden MWG et al. (2007) Neonatal screening for congenital hypothyroidism in The Netherlands: Cognitive and motor outcome at 10 years of age. *J Clin Endo Metab* 92: 919–924.

Kempers MJE, van Trotsenburg ASP, van Tijn DA et al. (2005) Disturbance of the fetal thyroid hormone state has long-term consequences for treatment of thyroidal and central congenital hypothyroidism. *J Clin Endocrinol Metab* 90: 4094–4100.

Kooistra L, Laane C, Vulsma T, Schellekens JM, Van der Meere JJ and Kalverboer AF (1994) Motor and cognitive development in children with congenital hypothyroidism: A long-term evaluation of the effects of neonatal treatment. *J Pediatr* 124: 903–909.

Kooistra L, Van der Meere JJ, Vulsma T and Kalverboer AF (1996) Sustained attention problems in children with early treated congenital hypothyroidism. *Acta Paediatr* 85: 425–429.

LaFranchi SH (2011) Approach to the diagnosis and treatment of neonatal hypothyroidism. *J Clin Endo Metab* 96: 2959–2967.

Lauder JJ (1979) Granule cell migration in developing rat cerebellum. Influence of neonatal hypo- and hyperthyroidism. *Dev Biol* 79: 105–115.

Leger J, Ecosse E, Roussey M, Lanoe JL and Larroque B (2011) Subtle health impairment and socioeducational attainment in young adult patients with congenital hypothyroidism diagnosed by neonatal screening: A longitudinal population-based cohort study. *J Clin Endo Metab* 96: 1771–1782.

Leneman M, Buchanan L and Rovet J (2001) "Where" and "what" visuospatial processing in adolescents with congenital hypothyroidism. *J Intern Neuropsychol Soc* 7: 556–562.

Mirabella G, Westall CA, Asztalos E, Perlman K, Koren G and Rovet J (2005) Development of contrast sensitivity in infants with prenatal and neonatal thyroid hormone insufficiencies. *Pediatr Res* 57: 902–907.

Oerbeck B, Sundet K, Kase BF and Heyerdahl S (2003) Congenital hypothyroidism: Influence of disease severity and L-thyroxine treatment on intellectual, motor, and school-associated outcomes in young adults. *Pediatrics* 112: 923–930.

Oerbeck B, Sundet K, Kase BF and Heyerdahl S (2005) Congenital hypothyroidism: No adverse effects of high dose thyroxine treatment on adult memory, attention, and behaviour. *Arch Dis Child* 90: 132–713.

Rovet JF (1999) Long-term neuropsychological sequelae of early treated congenital hypothyroidism: effects in adolescence. *Acta Paediatrica Scandinavica*, 88(Suppl 432): 1–8.

Rovet J (2003) Congenital hypothyroidism: Persisting deficits and associated factors. *Child Neuropsychol* 8:150–162.

Rovet J (2005) Congenital hypothyroidism: Treatment and outcome. *Curr Opin Endocrinol Diabetes* 12: 42–52.

Rovet J and Alvarez M (1996) Thyroid hormone and attention in congenital hypothyroidism. *J Pediatr Endocrinol Metab* 9: 63–66.

Rovet J and Daneman D (2003) Congenital hypothyroidism: A review of current diagnostic and treatment practices in relation to neuropsychologic outcome. *Pediatr Drugs* 5: 141–149.

Rovet J, Daneman D and Bailey J (1993) Adverse psychological consequences of thyroxine therapy for juvenile acquired hypothyroidism. *J Pediatr* 122: 543–549.

115

Rovet JF and Ehrlich RM (1995) Long-term effects of L-thyroxine therapy for congenital hypothyroidism. *J Pediatr* 126: 380–386.

Rovet J and Ehrlich RM (2000) The psychoeducational characteristics of children with early-treated congenital hypothyroidism. *Pediatrics* 105: 515–522.

Rovet JF and Hepworth S (2001) Attention problems in adolescents with congenital hypothyroidism: A multicomponential analysis. *J Intern Neuropsychol Soc* 7: 734–744.

Rovet J, Walker W, Bliss B, Buchanan L and Ehrlich R (1996) Long-term sequelae of hearing impairment in congenital hypothyroidism. *J Pediatr* 128: 776–783.

Rovet JF (1989) Neuropsychological outcome and risk factors following neonatal screening for congenital hypothyroidism: A review of 23 studies. *Proceedings of the 7th National Neonatal Screening Symposium*. New Orleans, LA, 48–56.

Rovet JF (1992) Neurodevelopmental outcome in infants and preschool children following newborn screening for congenital hypothyroidism. *J Pediatr Psychol* 17: 187–213.

Rovet JF, Westbrook D and Ehrlich RM (1984) Neonatal thyroid deficiency: Early temperamental and cognitive characteristics. *J Am Acad Child Adolesc Psychiatry* 23: 10–22.

Salerno M, Militerni R, Bravaccio C et al. (2002) Effect of different starting doses of levothyroxine on growth and intellectual outcome at four years of age in congenital hypothyroidism. *Thyroid* 12: 45–52.

Simic N, Khan S and Rovet J (2013) Visuospatial, visuoperceptual, and visuoconstructive abilities in congenital hypothyroidism. *J Intern Neuropsychol Soc,* resubmitted.

Song SI, Daneman D and Rovet J (2001) The influence of etiology and treatment factors on intellectual outcome in congenital hypothyroidism. *J Dev Behav Pediatr* 22: 376–384.

Sun Y, Bak B, Schoenmakers N et al. (2012) Loss-of-function mutations in IGSF1 cause a novel X-linked syndrome of central hypothyroidism and testicular enlargement. *Nature Genetics* 44: 1375–1381.

Tinelli F, Costagli C, Bargagna S, Marcheschi M, Parrini B and Perelli V (2003) Behavioural disorders in adolescents with early-treated congenital hypothyroidism. *Func Neurol* 18: 161–164.

Van Der Sluijs Veer L, Kempers MJE, Last BF, Vulsma T and Grootenhuis MA (2008) Quality of life, developmental milestones, and self-esteem of young adults with congenital hypothyroidism diagnosed by neonatal screening. *J Clin Endo Metab* 93: 2654–2661.

Van Der Sluijs Veer L, Kempers MJE, Maurice-Stam H, Last BF, Vulsma T and Grootenhuis MA (2012) Health-related quality of life and self-worth in 10-year old children with congenital hypothyroidism diagnosed by neonatal screening. *Child Adolesc Psychiatr Ment Health* 6: 1–10.

Van Vliet G (2003) Development of the thyroid gland: Lessons from congenitally hypothyroid mice and men. *Clin Genet* 63: 445–455.

Weber G, Mora S, Prina-Cerai LM et al. (2000) Cognitive function and neurophysiological evaluation in early-treated hypothyroid children. *Neurol Sci* 21: 307–314.

Wheeler SM, McAndrews MP, Sheard ED and Rovet JF (2012) Visuospatial associative memory and hippocampal functioning in congenital hypothyroidism. *J Int Neuropsychol Soc* 18: 49–56.

Wheeler SM, Willoughby KA and Rovet J (2011) Hippocampal size and memory functioning in children and adolescents with congenital hypothryoidism. *J Clin Endo Metab* 96: e1427–e1434 (abstract JCEM 2011 96: 2927).

Willoughby KA, McAndrews MP and Rovet J (2013) Effects of early thyroid hormone deficiency on children's autobiographical memory performance. *J Int Neuropsychol Soc* 19: 419–429.

9
THE ROLE OF THE HYPOTHALAMUS IN NORMAL WEIGHT REGULATION

Simon M Luckman

Introduction

Human physiology is organised to maintain constancy in a number of critical parameters: for example, body temperature and plasma glucose concentrations. The hypothalamus plays a key role in homeostasis by its ability to measure these parameters and by collating this with information from peripheral sensors (e.g. skin thermal sensors or glucosensors in the hepatic portal vein). Neurones in the preoptic or the ventromedial regions of the hypothalamus respond to temperature or glucose, respectively, depending on deviation from the desired level. The error signals are corrected by activating behavioural, autonomic or neuroendocrine counter-regulatory responses. If we are cold, our body induces shivering and releases thyroid hormone and we also put on more clothes. When hot, we perspire, our superficial blood vessels dilate and we seek the shade. We tend to think about these homeostatic mechanisms in terms of control theory, and we learn the analogy of how temperature in our homes is regulated by a thermostat. It is true that the hypothalamus appears to act like both a thermostat and a glucostat, to regulate around genetically defined set points. We cannot afford for either body temperature or plasma glucose concentrations to stray beyond defined ranges or the whole of our body metabolism grinds to a halt and we can die. Do we, however, regulate body weight precisely within a determined range? This is a point of debate. Individual experience suggests that, even though our food intake and the amount of exercise we do can vary greatly from day to day, we tend to have a fairly constant body weight over extended periods. But is this the same kind of homeostatic regulation as for temperature or glucose? If body weight is critically determined, why do humans display such variation? Fundamentally, if we are defending a body-weight set point, why are we facing an obesity epidemic?

In this chapter, we will review the organisation of the hypothalamus, concentrating on elements of sensory and motivational input, on the foci of integration and on the generators of regulatory output. This will be based necessarily on knowledge gleaned from studying rodent models, but this has often been validated through human genetics and pathophysiology (see Chapter 10 by Farooqi).

The importance and the basic structure of the hypothalamus

The major axiom for life is that an organism has to survive long enough to reproduce, and survival requires the controlled management of available energy. Multi-cellular organisms evolved simple nervous networks to control behavioural reflexes and enhance their ability to find and ingest food. Parts of the network condensed to form a central nervous system which enabled reflexes to be integrated with sensory information from around the body and from the external environment. This basic format still exists in humans, with the brainstem sensing signals from the gut and implementing motor responses. At the head of the brainstem is the body's master endocrine and metabolic coordinator: the hypothalamus.

The importance of the hypothalamus to body-weight regulation was appreciated by the early twentieth century when it was realised that the obesity of Frohlich syndrome was associated with the interference of pituitary tumours with the overlying brain rather than dysfunction of the pituitary itself. Then, in the 1940s, more direct evidence was achieved through the seminal lesioning experiments of Hetherington and Ranson. They found that bilateral electrolytic lesions confined to the ventromedial region of the rat hypothalamus caused hyperphagia and weight gain. By contrast, similar bilateral lesions to the lateral hypothalamus, at the same antero-posterior level, caused unrestrained weight loss. The 'dual centre' theory of weight regulation, with the hypothalamus being the custodian of the 'set point', has had a troubled existence for many years, though the anatomical basis of this theory was demonstrated to have some validity following advances in molecular physiology and genetics during the late twentieth century (Elmquist et al. 1999).

The human hypothalamus is only about the size of an almond and it lies at the base of the brain. It receives ascending connections from the brainstem and descending con-nections from limbic forebrain structures involved in motivation and emotion. The hypo-thalamus surrounds the third cerebral ventricle and so can be divided grossly into periventricular, medial and lateral regions in the transverse (coronal) plane. Bidirectional connections with the brainstem and with higher cortical structures are made via fibres coursing through the lateral zone (notably in the medial forebrain bundle), and via the fornix, a bundle of fibres that separates the medial and lateral regions. In the antero-posterior orientation, the hypothalamus can be divided also into preoptic (named according to its position in front of the chiasm of the optic nerves in the base of the brain), anterior, tuberal (connected to the infundibulum and pituitary gland) and mammillary regions (Fig 9.1).

The hypothalamus has anatomically distinct, bilateral clusters of neurons (nuclei), lying either side of the third ventricle. Closest to the ventricle are the periventicular, supraoptic, paraventricular and arcuate/infundibular nuclei, all of which contain neuroen-docrine output neurones. These cells project directly either to the posterior pituitary to release hormones into the circulation or to the median eminence to release their hormones into the pituitary portal system and, thus, regulate the anterior pituitary gland. The neuro-endocrine outputs of the hypothalamus play an indirect role in body-weight regulation, for example, through the controlled release of growth hormone from the pituitary and gluco-corticoids from the adrenal gland and thyroid hormone, each of which can greatly affect body composition. However, the arcuate nucleus also contains two populations of non-neuroendocrine neurones, to which we will return later, as they are critically involved in body-weight regulation (neurones that produce either neuropeptide Y [NPY] or

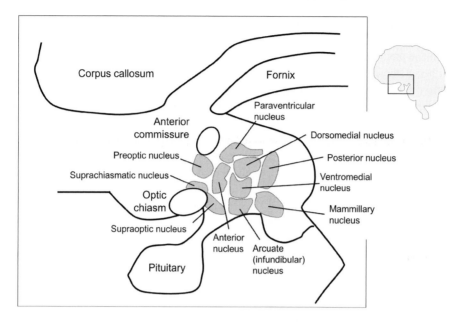

Figure 9.1. Diagrammatic parasagittal section through the human hypothalamus to show the arrangement of anatomical nuclei (see inset for scale). Major tracts (white matter) are marked (corpus callosum, fornix and optic chiasm). Hypothalamic nuclei, shaded grey, are anatomical rather than functional units.

proopiomelanocortin [POMC]). The medial region of the hypothalamus contains distinct nuclei, all involved, to some degree, in motivated behaviours: the medial preoptic, anterior, paraventricular, ventromedial and premammillary nuclei. Of particular note are segments of the ventromedial and paraventricular nuclei which control output to the autonomic nervous system and to brainstem areas controlling ingestive behaviour. Also, interspersed between the nuclei of the periventricular and medial hypothalamus are poorly defined, interconnected groups of cells that have been identified in rodents as belonging to a visceromotor pattern generator, including in the dorsomedial nucleus and in five small groups in the preoptic area (Thompson and Swanson 2003). Finally, the lateral portion of the hypothalamus is the least anatomically defined in terms of nuclei, and is very much an extension of brainstem structures involved in overall state of behaviour and arousal. For example, populations of neurones here, containing the peptide orexin (also called hypocretin), are involved not only in sleep–wake cycles, but also in attending to low plasma glucose concentrations (Sakurai and Mieda. 2011).

The peptide revolution
Before the molecular revolution in biology and the development of transgenic mouse models, unveiling the workings of the hypothalamus was an arduous affair, based largely on lesioning or time-consuming tracing studies, both invariably affecting unidentified and multiple cell types. A key discovery, the identification of leptin as the product of the obese

gene (Zhang et al. 1994), coincided with the harnessing of recombinant DNA technology, and has led to an acceleration of our understanding of anatomy and function. Leptin is a hormone produced by white adipose tissue and is secreted in proportion to the amount of fat being stored in this tissue. Its major function is to signal that the body has sufficient energy to allow successful growth and reproduction, functions that will stall if fat stores are depleted. The first two downstream mediators of leptin's effects to be described were neurones in the hypothalamic arcuate nucleus that produce NPY (Mercer et al. 1996) and POMC (Cheung et al. 1997), which have opposing effects on energy balance (Fig 9.2; Seeley and Woods 2003). POMC is the precursor for a number of peptides, including α-melanocyte-stimulating hormone which acts on downstream targets possessing melano-cortin receptors to reduce energy intake (feeding) and to facilitate energy expenditure. Many of these targets also possess NPY receptors, which act oppositely to increase energy intake and reduce expenditure. Interestingly, NPY neurones also produce agouti-related peptide (Agrp), which is an antagonist at melanocortin receptors, as well as the fast, inhibitory transmitter, γ-aminobutyric acid. These three trans-neuronal messengers in one cell type all affect energy balance, but across different time frames (Krashes et al. 2013).

Arcuate NPY and POMC neurones are critical for body-weight regulation, and their identification has led to the development of a number of molecular tools that have allowed their selective manipulation. This facilitated a massive growth in our understanding of the functioning of these two, model leptin-sensitive neurones, though there has been a rather slower appreciation of the importance of other central regulatory mechanisms. This will be balanced with time, and it is important to bear in mind that our knowledge of wider hypo-thalamic function is still very limited, as has been exemplified in an elegant series of transgenic mouse experiments. Knowing the identity of arcuate neurones that respond to leptin allowed the generation of conditional transgenic mice in which leptin receptors are knocked out selectively in POMC-containing cells (Balthasar et al. 2004). This mouse is hyperphagic, has a low rate of metabolism, and has a mildly obese phenotype. This is a beautiful demonstration of the importance of POMC neurones in mediating some of the effects of leptin. However, the same experimenters instead then knocked out leptin receptors only in neurones of the hypothalamic ventromedial nucleus, and produced a similarly obese mouse (Dhillon et al. 2006). This proves that a population of as yet unidentified neurones in the ventromedial nucleus is equally as important a target for the actions of leptin to regulate body weight. Interestingly, if the two mice are bred together, their offspring are additively heavier, but they are still not as obese as mice which lack all of their leptin receptors. Thus, we still need to identify many more regulatory pathways.

Since the 1990s, when the revolution in identifying peptides and their receptors began, the black box of the hypothalamus is slowly being filled with the regulators of metabolism. The evidence for some is greater than others, but the peptides produced by hypothalamic neurones, for which there is clear evidence for a role in energy homeostasis, are indicated in Figure 9.2. Needless to say, this picture will have evolved further by the time this book is published. Mouse conditional transgenics has been further boosted recently by the development of pharmaco- and opticogenetics, whereby distinct populations of neurones can be activated selectively *in vivo* or *in vitro* to map connections in the brain. Thus, for example,

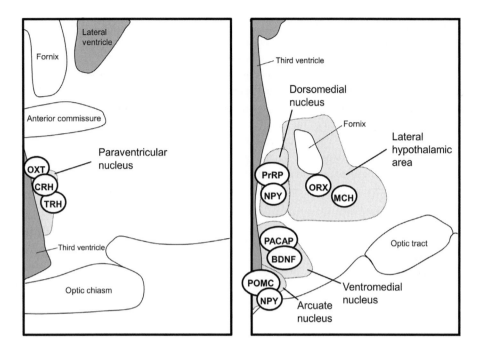

Figure 9.2. Diagrammatic coronal (frontal) sections through the anterior and tuberal levels of the hypothalamus to indicate the main hypothalamic nuclei involved in weight regulation (shaded light grey). The hypothalamus is split symmetrically by the third ventricle which lies at the midline (darker grey). Clear fibre tracts are visible, such as the anterior commissure (which crosses the midline at the anterior level), the fornix and the optic nerves. Two major regions involved in detecting and integrating energy signals are the arcuate and ventromedial nuclei. Major output nuclei from the hypothalamus, which connect with neuroendocrine, autonomic and behavioural effectors, include the dorsomedial and paraventricular nuclei. For each nucleus, peptidergic markers for neurones which have been shown to have a clear role in energy homeostasis in humans or experimental rodents have been indicated. BDNF, brain-derived neurotrophic factor; CRH, corticotrophin-releasing hormone; MCH, melanin-concentrating hormone; NPY, neuropeptide Y; ORX, orexin/hypocretin; OXT, oxytocin; PACAP, pituitary adenylate cyclase-activating polypeptide; POMC, proopiomelanocortin; PrRP, prolactin-releasing hormone; TRH, thyrotrophin-releasing hormone.

opticogenetics has been used to show that NPY/Agrp neurons in the arcuate nucleus produce most of their effect to increase feeding by inhibiting three independent anorexigenic neurones: POMC neurones in the arcuate nucleus, oxytocin neurones in the paraventricular nucleus and calcitonin gene-related peptide neurones in the hindbrain parabrachial nucleus (Atasoy et al. 2012; Carter et al. 2013). Although experimental manipulation of rodent models is leading the revolution, anatomy and function are largely conserved between mammalian species. This is borne out by the similar phenotypes between single-gene mutations in humans and transgenic knock-out mice (Farooqi and O'Rahilly 2008). This allows us to make confident assumptions about human physiology based on the study of laboratory rodents.

Integrating signals of energy status

A primary function of the hypothalamus is to sense metabolic signals from the whole body (Fig 9.3). As mentioned, the amount of circulating leptin is a direct measure of adiposity and, therefore, an indication of stored energy and fitness to undergo reproduction and/or growth. Leptin has a permissive effect on the excitability of different types of hypothalamic neurone, allowing the excitation of some and inhibition of others. This may be facilitated by longer-term modification of the circuitry itself. Recent studies have indicated a neuro-trophic action of leptin, to change the synaptic connectivity of key hypothalamic neurones (Bouret et al. 2004). The important signalling function of leptin, however, is that its absence will promote a build-up of fat stores by priming the hypothalamus to increase energy intake (feeding) and decrease energy expenditure. The corollary of this is that increased leptin,

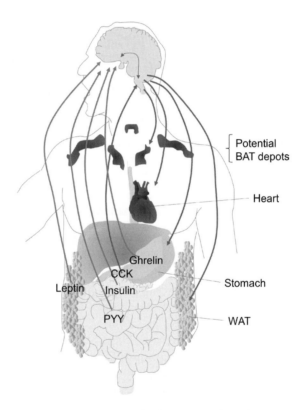

Figure 9.3. Representation of functional signalling between peripheral tissues and the hypothalamus, including from the stomach, intestine, pancreas, liver, heart, white and brown adipose tissue. Blue and green arrows denote that signals are carried by the nervous system or by hormones, respectively. Cholecystokinin released by the duodenum activates ascending sensory fibres in the vagus nerve. Peripheral tissues are regulated by sympathetic and parasympathetic branches of the autonomic nervous system. The double-headed arrow denotes bidirectional neural communication between the hypothalamus and caudal brainstem/spinal cord. CCK, cholecystokinin; BAT, brown adipose tissue; PYY, peptide YY; WAT, white adipose tissue.

often mimicked experimentally by injection of supra-physiological doses of the hormone, has the opposing effects. This has led to two erroneous suppositions: that leptin is a satiety factor and that its physiological role is to guard against obesity. First, the circulating levels of leptin do not change appreciably in association with meals. Second, obese humans have high concentrations of circulating leptin, but rapidly become insensitive to its actions. The human biology of leptin will be considered in greater depth elsewhere (see Chapter 10 by Farooqi). Insulin is also secreted in proportion to adiposity, and has somewhat similar hypothalamic effects as leptin over the midterm to longer term.

As well as determining the levels of energy stored in adipose tissue, the hypothalamus is able to detect readily available energy in the form of nutrients. While evidence is now emerging for the ability of hypothalamic neurones to respond to circulating lipids and amino acids, it has been well documented for half a century that certain specialised neurones in the ventromedial and lateral regions of the hypothalamus are exquisitely sensitive to very small changes in glucose (Burdakov et al. 2005). This probably reflects the importance of this nutrient as an energy source, particularly for the brain. While meal-to-meal plasma glucose ranges from 5mM to 8mM, even when maximal after a meal, hypothalamic levels probably peak at around 2.5mM. However, the specialised glucose-sensing neurones are sensitive at around 0.2mM. This suggests that an important function may be to protect against hypoglycaemia. Certainly, the fact that they are neurons means that they can react much more rapidly than peripheral systems to acute hypoglycaemic challenges. Some glucose-excited neurones, whose firing rate is positively correlated with glucose concentrations, may use similar glucose-sensing apparatus as pancreatic β-cells (including a low-affinity hexokinase and an adenosine triphosphate [ATP]-sensitive potassium channel which closes to allow depolarisation). The mechanism by which glucose-inhibited neurons (whose firing rate is inversely correlated with glucose) are affected is much less understood though a number of theories have been proposed (Burdakov et al. 2005). Glucose-excited neurons include those that contain POMC or melanin-concentrating hormone, while glucose-inhibited neurons include those that contain NPY or orexin (in the arcuate nucleus and lateral hypothalamus; Figs 9.2 and 9.4). The neurons in the ventromedial nucleus, which are particularly critical for the counter-regulatory response to hypoglycaemia, may include glucose-inhibited neurons that contain pituitary adenylate cyclase-activating peptide (PACAP).

All eukaryotic cells possess molecular mechanisms that sense available energy, which are dependent on the normal intracellular metabolism of specific nutrients. A lack of nutrients and the consequent low cellular energy levels are detected as an increase in the ratio of adenosine monophosphate to ATP (AMP:ATP). This activates AMP-dependent phosphokinase (AMPK), leading to an increase in activities promoting ATP synthesis and decreasing activities utilising it (Hardie et al. 2012). Thus, when the AMP:ATP ratio is high, tissues are stimulated to take up glucose and fatty acids, and to increase their catabolism. Interestingly, AMPK is also activated in hypothalamic neurons by orexigenic signals such as Agrp or the gut-produced hormone, ghrelin, but inhibited by leptin and insulin, providing a direct link between cellular and whole-body metabolism. By contrast, another protein kinase, the mammalian version of 'target of rapamycin' (mTOR), has opposing

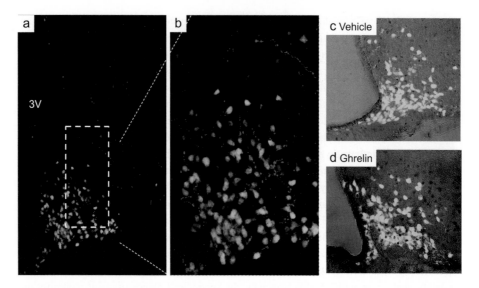

Figure 9.4. (a) Fluorescently labelled NPY neurones in the arcuate nucleus of a transgenic *Npy*-GFP mouse in which the *Npy* gene promoter drives the expression of green fluorescent protein and (b) increased magnification of the same photomicrograph. The section has been dual labelled to demonstrate orexin-containing neuronal fibres intermingling with the NPY neurones and (c) section from a similar mouse given a systemic, control injection of isotonic saline. The section has been dual labelled for the cellular activity marker, c-Fos, and (d) a mouse given a systemic injection of the gut-derived hormone, ghrelin. NPY neurones have been activated, as demonstrated by the induction of c-Fos (black cell nuclei). 3V, third cerebral ventricle. (A colour version of this figure can be seen in the plate section at the end of the book.)

cellular effects. Adequate supplies of cellular energy increase the kinase activity of mTOR, which initiates anabolic activity. In neurons of the hypothalamus, mTOR is also activated by insulin or leptin signalling, together promoting reductions in food intake (Woods et al. 2008). Thus, hypothalamic neurons have evolved the ability to integrate intracellular molecular signals, with sensitivity to metabolic hormones and other neuronal inputs, and to summate this information into electrical signals which are transmitted to effector systems.

Connecting the hypothalamus with gut function

The major determinant of body weight in humans is the amount of food eaten. Therefore, the hypothalamus needs to sense this energy input. Once food enters the mouth, the processes of chewing, swallowing and moving it along the gastrointestinal tract occur automatically and are controlled by a series of brainstem reflexes in response to sensory stimulation from the ingested nutrients. As food is digested, nutrient components (fats, proteins and carbohydrates) are sensed by specialised enteroendocrine cells which are dispersed throughout the gut mucosa. These cells release hormones, such as cholecystokinin (CCK), glucagon-like peptide (GLP-1), peptide YY (PYY) and ghrelin (Field et al. 2008). Each of these hormones can act in a paracrine fashion, including the activation of sensory endings of the vagus nerve. Vagal afferents from the gut to the brain terminate almost exclusively in the caudal brainstem, where information is modified before motor signals are sent back down to the gut to control digestion. Importantly, many mammals, including humans, eat in discrete meals. Thus, as food enters the digestive system, feedback sensory information begins the process of satiation which acts to terminate the meal. The feed-forward mechanisms of digestion and the feed-back mechanisms of satiation are controlled entirely and autonomously by the caudal brainstem and do not require projections to the rest of the brain. Indeed, newborn infants, in which the reciprocal connections with the forebrain have yet to fully develop, or experimental animals, in which these connections have been severed, will ingest food until a natural level of satiety is reached.

The autonomous regulators of eating need to be integrated with higher brain circuits in order to take into account other factors such as the levels of both immediate (mainly glucose) and stored (mainly fat) energy sources already available in the body. This information is collated by the hypothalamus, which may be viewed as sitting at the head of the brainstem. CCK is the archetypal satiety factor. It activates vagal reflexes in the brainstem to control the digestion, particularly of fats, by slowing gastric emptying and by causing the release of bile. To integrate gut signals, the hypothalamus receives ascending neuronal input indirectly from the gastrointestinal tract via the caudal brainstem and the medial forebrain bundle. The main hypothalamic nuclei to receive this information are the arcuate, ventromedial and paraventricular nuclei, and the main output nuclei to send information back down to the caudal brainstem are the dorsomedial and paraventricular nuclei. Compared with the dorsomedial nucleus, the components of which are mostly unknown, the paraventricular nucleus is relatively well described. Neurons which contain corticotrophin-releasing hormone and thyrotrophin-releasing hormone project mainly to the median eminence to control pituitary hormone secretion, but additional descending projections can have regulatory effects on gut function. However, oxytocin-containing neurons in the paraventricular nucleus seem especially important in controlling gut function. Furthermore, they may, along with descending neurons from the dorsomedial nucleus and other parts of the hypothalamic visceromotor pattern generator, affect output from the brainstem motor nuclei which control eating.

As well as acting locally in the gut, some of the enteroendocrine hormones reach sufficient concentrations in the systemic blood circulation to behave as true endocrine hormones, with remote target organs. Classically, GLP-1 has an incretin effect on the pancreas to enhance insulin secretion. Experimental administration of GLP-1 to humans causes a decrease in food intake. This, however, may be mainly due to nausea-inducing effects on the brainstem. PYY is produced by enteroendocrine cells along the length of the intestine, whereas ghrelin production is confined mainly to the stomach. Although both PYY and ghrelin can stimulate local vagal afferents, they can also travel in the circulation to access the arcuate nucleus of the hypothalamus. Here the two hormones have opposing effects on NPY neurones. Ghrelin activates NPY neurones and downstream pathways to increase the hypothalamic drive to eat, whereas PYY has the opposing effect. Ghrelin is the only enteroendocrine hormone that can induce feeding, so unsurprisingly its release increases before a meal, unlike most enteroendocrine hormones which are secreted after a meal to aid digestion and initiate satiation.

Integrating motivational and social cues: what makes us eat?

Physiological and social evolution in humans has led to us eating and sharing food within meals. This provides the time and means to gather, prepare and invariably cook our food. The period of satiety between meals also allows for the effective digestion and assimilation of nutrients. The latter is the reason for the satiety mechanisms provided by the brainstem and hypothalamus: to curtail individual meals, not to protect against over-eating. The importance of environmental factors in affecting the amount of food we eat and ultimately our body weight is becoming clearer with the appearance of the modern epidemic in obesity and though we will return to this at the end of this chapter, here we can only briefly mention how they impact on the hypothalamus.

When, where and how much we eat depend not only on homeostatic need, but also on choice, which itself is dependent on previous experience. Our experience of food can provide extreme emotions, which can be fixed in memory, and that are believed to potentiate future beneficial stimuli and suppress harmful ones. All aspects of the eating experience (taste, smell, social context, etc.) are integrated by the limbic cortices, notably the orbitofrontal and cingulate, and memories are stored in the amygdala and hippocampal formation. Positive emotions are often associated with the reward value of a particular food, and this is especially strong for sweet and fatty foods. Cognitive processing provides strong motivational drive to eat energy-dense foods and may have evolved to maximise foraging efficiency and energy assimilation. Each facet of reward, including hedonic value (how much we like the food), incentive salience (how much we want a type of food) and memory are affected by our nutritional state – food tastes better when we are hungry! It is becoming clear that energy-signalling hormones (leptin, insulin and ghrelin) can interact directly with limbic structures (Shin et al. 2009). However, there is also connectivity between these structures and the energy-regulatory circuits in the hypothalamus. For example, there are projections from the amygdala directly to NPY neurones in the arcuate nucleus (DeFalco et al. 2001). Furthermore, the main reward outputs from the limbic forebrain, which act to engage relevant motivational behaviour (i.e. eating), are channelled to the lateral hypothalamus via the nucleus accumbens. This channel is bidirectional and the energy-sensing orexin neurons of the lateral hypothalamus project to limbic structures to affect reward seeking (Harris et al. 2005).

Does the hypothalamus regulate energy expenditure?

Thus, there are extremely powerful motivational drives to eat food. If we take in more energy than we expend, then the excess has to go somewhere (fat storage), and in many cases this can lead to obesity. However, as stated at the start of this chapter, it is a common experience of most people that their weight remains stable over long periods. This suggests that by opposing any excess in energy intake, in order to maintain body-weight balance, we also regulate our energy expenditure. Indeed, most of the hormones that act on the hypothalamus have dual effects on energy intake and expenditure if given experimentally in high doses. This does not mean that we regulate energy expenditure for homeostasis.

Energy expenditure occurs because we have a basal metabolic rate that maintains tissue function (the heavier we are, the higher our metabolic rate), and because we need to move around and do work. We also need to keep warm, which we can achieve by modifying our behaviour or by shivering. Small mammals, such as experimental mice, are very heavily dependent on another method to maintain their body temperature, which is called non-shivering, adaptive thermogenesis. Cold temperatures are detected by both peripheral sensors and neurons in the preoptic region of the hypothalamus (Morrison et al. 2008). The information is further integrated by one of the major output regions of the hypothalamus, the dorsomedial nucleus, which sends information to the midbrain and ultimately to pre-ganglionic sympathetic neurons in the spinal cord. The latter are responsible for activating specialised brown adipose tissue. Brown adipose contrasts with white adipose, in that they have opposing primary functions to expend and store fat, respectively. Sympathetic activation of brown adipose tissue induces the uncoupling of oxidative phosphorylation in mitochondria so that energy does not convert ADP to ATP, but is instead dissipated as heat. The smaller the mammal, the more developed brown adipose appears, and in humans its existence is noticeable in newborn infants. However, in recent years the prevalence of brown adipose tissue in adult humans has been found to be correlated with two important factors: environmental temperature and leanness (Nedergaard and Cannon 2010). It is understandable that living in cold climates might promote brown adipose tissue development in adults. But, are lean people thin as a result of having more active brown adipose?

This is an interesting concept, not least because thermogenesis can also be turned on by 'energy-dense' foods. So-called diet-induced thermogenesis is measurable in both experimental rodents and in humans after individual meals, and is particularly robust following the ingestion of foods high in fat and carbohydrates. After an initial rapid induction following a change to a high-energy diet, thermogenesis then decreases sharply, which suggests that it is not an actively regulated mechanism to control body weight. However, if the animal remains on such a diet, thermogenesis then starts increasing again with the development of obesity. It is likely that it is, therefore, dependent on levels of adiposity, and it can be induced experimentally by the injection of leptin. Importantly, both cold stimulation and leptin engage the same central circuitry including the dorsomedial nucleus of the hypothalamus and its outputs. The dorsomedial neurones which integrate information to induce thermogenesis have yet to be characterised fully, though there is emerging evidence for two populations containing either NPY or prolactin-releasing peptide (Dodd et al. 2014). Questions remain whether diet-induced thermogenesis is truly adaptive and specifically evolved as a mechanism to control body weight, rather than simply being a response to obesity. An interesting hypothesis was put forward by the discoverers of diet-induced thermogenesis (Rothwell and Stock 1986). Assuming that obesity is maladaptive, then animals may only eat excessive amounts of food if it is poor in certain nutrients, such as protein. In order to get sufficient protein, excess fat and carbohydrate has to be absorbed also, which will lead to obesity unless the excess is utilised through adaptive thermogenesis.

Is our body weight set or does it settle?

We have seen in this chapter that the hypothalamus is a master regulator of energy balance, capable of modulating the relevant parameters: intake, expenditure and storage. But, we are left with an underlying problem: Does the hypothalamus control body weight *per se*, and if so, does it defend a set point? There are good arguments to suggest so. It is notoriously difficult to reduce body weight by dieting or exercising. Our bodies appear to grudgingly adapt to the new lifestyle, but as soon as we revert to our normal habits, so does our weight. There are similar examples of where temporary over-nutrition leads to increased weight, which then reverts once normal dietary habits are resumed. Despite these well-catalogued examples, on average our weight tends to climb inexorably as we get older, plus undeniably we are witnessing an obesity epidemic. Exponents of the set point theory point out that we appear to defend a new, higher level, because further perturbations will again result in changes in energy intake and expenditure (e.g. Keesey and Hirvonen 1997). However, if weight is not maintained at a genetically defined constant (or at least within strict bounds, as temperature), then can it really be termed a set point? It would be alarmingly dangerous if our body temperature set point gradually crept up over time.

An alternative to set point is settling point. The basis of this is that, if our energy intake is perturbed within certain limits, then our energy expenditure adapts passively, but in proportion to the change in body weight. Gradually, weight settles at a new level. Take as an example a man in energy balance and with a stable body weight. Assume that his daily energy intake is 2500kcal and that this is matched by 2500kcal/day expenditure. If he suddenly goes on a diet and reduces his intake by 500kcal, he is no longer taking in enough energy to maintain the demands of his body, and he loses weight as energy stores are depleted. He will suffer from hunger and/or lethargy, but if he maintains the diet, his body weight reduces. A lower tissue mass requires less energy to sustain it, so the difference between his intake and expenditure gets smaller (until both are at 2000kcal/day) and he settles at a new body weight. If he then stops his diet, his energy intake will now be in excess of that required to maintain the lower weight, which will gradually increase along with greater energy demand until balance is reached again. The importance of this model is that while the amount of food eaten has been actively altered independent of body weight, energy expenditure changes passively in proportion to body weight.

A current model for body-weight regulation incorporates aspects of both set point and settling point theories (reviewed by Speakman et al. 2011). In this model there is a broad range within which body weight settles, which allows for wide human variation, and this changes with age and status. The level at which settling occurs is affected to some extent by a series of homeostatic mechanisms which control metabolic parameters, for example, plasma glucose concentrations or the energy expenditure required to maintain body temperature. However, the main determinants of settling point are environmental factors: the society we live in, our habits, religion, the availability and quality of food, the choices we make and so on. These environmental factors should not be underestimated as they are causally responsible for the growing epidemic in obesity. The settling range is broad if compared, for example, to the narrow range within which we maintain our body temperature. However, at the extremes of the range, powerful physiological mechanisms are engaged to bring body weight back within the 'safe zone'. This has been termed the dual intervention point model, and it rephrases the crucial set point question: Is there a genetically determined range? If so, then the question becomes, what are the evolutionary pressures to set the lower and higher intervention points?

There are very good reasons for responding strongly at the lower intervention point: to prevent starvation and to maintain the capacity for growth and reproduction. Powerful physiological mechanisms, operated by the hypothalamus, are in place to combat excessive weight loss. It is less clear why a higher intervention point exists or, indeed, if one is required. Most of the problems of being overweight are secondary to the development of cardiovascular disease, arthritis or diabetes. However, there are some direct consequences of carrying too much weight, such as reduced mobility, problems related to finding food or a mate or escaping from predators. As humans evolved into social animals, living in groups, acquiring food collectively and protecting themselves from predation, the positive evolutionary pressures to maintain the higher intervention point may have relaxed. This can lead to genetic drift, whereby certain useful genes become modified in some individuals by mutation, because their function is no longer critical to survival. These individuals may no longer have a defined upper limit to their body weight, and the interaction of their genes in an obesogenic environment could explain why only they become obese.

REFERENCES

Atasoy D, Betley JN, Su HH and Sternson SM (2012) Deconstruction of a neural circuit for hunger. *Nature* 488: 172–177.

Balthasar N, Coppari R, McMinn J et al. (2004) Leptin receptor signaling in POMC neurons is required for normal body weight homeostasis. *Neuron* 42: 983–991.

Bouret SG, Draper SJ and Simerly RB (2004) Trophic action of leptin on hypothalamic neurons that regulate feeding. *Science* 304: 108–110.

Burdakov D, Luckman SM and Verkhratsky A (2005) Glucose-sensing neurons of the hypothalamus. *Philos Trans R Soc Lond B Biol Sci* 360: 2227–2235.

Carter ME, Soden ME, Zweifel LS and Palmiter RD (2013) Genetic identification of a neural circuit that suppresses appetite. *Nature* 503: 111–114.

Cheung CC, Clifton DK and Steiner RA (1997) Proopiomelanocortin neurons are direct targets for leptin in the hypothalamus. *Endocrinology* 138: 4489.

DeFalco J, Tomishima M, Liu H et al. (2001) Virus-assisted mapping of neural inputs to a feeding center in the hypothalamus. *Science* 291: 2608–2613.

Dhillon H, Zigman JM, Ye C et al. (2006) Leptin directly activates SF1 neurons in the VMH, and this action by leptin is required for normal body-weight homeostasis. *Neuron* 49: 191–203.

Dodd GT, Worth AA, Nunn N et al. (2014) The thermogenic effect of leptin is dependent on a distinct population of prolactin-releasing peptide (PrRP) neurons in the dorsomedial hypothalamus. *Cell Metab* 20: 639–649.

Elmquist JK, Elias CF and Saper CB (1999) From lesions to leptin: Hypothalamic control of food intake and body weight. *Neuron* 22: 221–232.

Farooqi IS and O'Rahilly S (2008) Mutations in ligands and receptors of the leptin-melanocortin pathway that lead to obesity. *Nat Clin Pract Endocrinol Metab* 4: 569–577.

Field BC, Chaudhri OB and Bloom SR (2008) Bowels control brain: Gut hormones and obesity. *Nat Rev Endocrinol* 6: 444–453.

Hardie DG, Ross FA and Hawley SA (2012) AMPK: A nutrient and energy sensor that maintains energy homeostasis. *Nat Rev Mol Cell Biol* 13: 251–262.

Harris GC, Wimmer M and Aston-Jones G (2005) A role for lateral hypothalamic orexin neurons in reward seeking. *Nature* 437: 556–559.

Keesey RE and Hirvonen MD (1997) Body weight set-points: Determination and adjustment. *J Nutr* 127: 1875S–1883S.

Krashes MJ, Shah BP, Koda S and Lowell BB (2013) Rapid versus delayed stimulation of feeding by the endogenously released AgRP neuron mediators GABA, NPY, and AgRP. *Cell Metab* 18: 588–595.

Mercer JG, Hoggard N, Williams LM, Lawrence CB, Hannah LT and Trayhurn P (1996) Localization of leptin receptor mRNA and the long form splice variant (Ob-Rb) in mouse hypothalamus and adjacent brain regions by in situ hybridization. *FEBS Lett.* 387: 113.

Morrison SF, Nakamura K and Madden CJ (2008) Central control of thermogenesis in mammals. *Exp Physiol* 93: 773–797.

Nedergaard J and Cannon B (2010) The changed metabolic world with human brown adipose tissue: Therapeutic visions. *Cell Metab* 11: 268–272.

Rothwell NJ and Stock MJ (1986) Whither brown fat? *Biosci Rep* 6: 3–18.

Sakurai T and Mieda M (2011) Connectomics of orexin-producing neurons: Interface of systems of emotion, energy homeostasis and arousal. *Trends Pharmacol Sci* 32: 451–462.

Seeley RJ and Woods SC (2003) Monitoring of stored and available fuel by the CNS: Implications for obesity. *Nat Rev Neurosci* 4: 901–909.

Shin AC, Zheng H and Berthoud HR (2009) An expanded view of energy homeostasis: Neural integration of metabolic, cognitive, and emotional drives to eat. *Physiol Behav* 97: 572–580.

Speakman JR, Levitsky DA, Allison DB et al. (2011) Set points, settling points and some alternative models: Theoretical options to understand how genes and environments combine to regulate body adiposity. *Dis Model Mech* 4: 733–745.

Thompson RH and Swanson LW (2003) Structural characterization of a hypothalamic visceromotor pattern generator network. *Brain Res Rev* 41: 153–202.

Woods SC, Seeley RJ and Cota D (2008) Regulation of food intake through hypothalamic signaling networks involving mTOR. *Annu Rev Nutr* 28: 295–311.

Zhang Y, Proenca R, Maffei M, Barone M, Leopold L and Friedman JM (1994) Positional cloning of the mouse obese gene and its human homologue. *Nature* 372: 425–432.

10
GENETIC CHILDHOOD OBESITY SYNDROMES

I Sadaf Farooqi

Introduction

Traditionally, patients affected by genetic forms of obesity were identified as a result of their association with developmental delay, dysmorphic features and/or other developmental abnormalities, that is, a pattern of clinical features which represented a recognisable syndrome. However, the identification of genetic disorders that disrupt the hypothalamic leptin-melanocortin signalling pathway has led to the recognition that obesity is the predominant presenting feature in a significant subset of individuals. Based on case series of patients with genetic obesity syndromes, childhood onset of obesity (before the age of 10 years) is a consistent feature. For purposes of clinical assessment, it remains useful to categorise the genetic obesity syndromes (Fig 10.1) as those with dysmorphism and/or developmental delay and those without these features; however, in some cases the spectrum of clinical features can be quite variable.

Clinical history, examination and investigation

The assessment of severely obese children and adults should be directed at screening for potentially treatable endocrine and neurological conditions and identifying genetic conditions so that appropriate genetic counselling, and in some cases, treatment can be instituted. A careful family history to identify potential consanguineous relationships, the presence of other family members with severe early onset obesity and the ethnic and geographical origin of family members should be taken. The history and examination can then guide the appropriate use of diagnostic tests.

Prader–Willi syndrome

Prader–Willi syndrome (PWS) is the most common obesity syndrome (estimated prevalence of about 1 in 25 000). Key clinical features include hypotonia and failure to thrive in infancy, intellectual disability, short stature, hyperphagic obesity and hypogonadotropic hypogonadism (Goldstone 2004). Children with PWS have reduced lean body mass and increased fat mass, abnormalities that resemble those seen in growth hormone deficiency; growth hormone treatment decreases body fat, and increases linear growth, muscle mass, fat oxidation and energy expenditure (Carrel and Allen 2001). Plasma concentrations of the stomach-derived hormone ghrelin are markedly elevated in children and adults with PWS

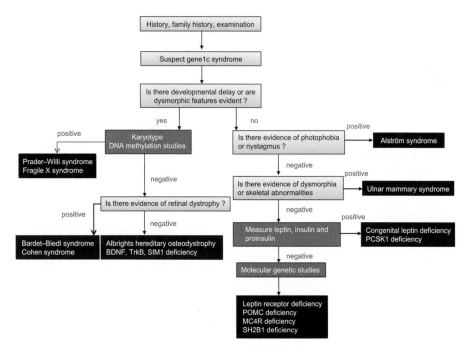

Figure 10.1. A diagnostic approach to genetic obesity syndromes.

compared to patients who are obese and patients with other genetic obesity syndromes. The significance of this finding and its possible role in the pathogenesis of hyperphagia in these patients are unknown.

PWS is caused by the deletion of a critical segment on the paternally inherited copy of chromosome 15q11.2-q12, or loss of the entire paternal chromosome 15 with presence of two maternal copies (uniparental maternal disomy). Most chromosomal abnormalities in PWS occur sporadically. Deletions account for 70%–80% of cases; the majority are interstitial deletions, many of which can be visualised by karyotype analysis. There are distinct differences in DNA methylation of the parental alleles, and DNA methylation can be used as a reliable postnatal diagnostic tool in PWS. Small deletions encompassing only the HBII-85 family of small nucleolarRNAs have been reported in association with the cardinal features of PWS including obesity (de Smith et al. 2009; Sahoo et al. 2008), suggesting that these noncoding RNAs and the genes they regulate may be important in the aetiology of PWS.

Albright hereditary osteodystrophy
Mutations in *GNAS1* that decrease expression or function of Gs alpha protein result in Albright hereditary osteodystrophy (AHO), which is an autosomal dominant disorder. Maternal transmission of *GNAS1* mutations leads to classical AHO (characterised by short stature, obesity, skeletal defects and impaired olfaction) plus resistance to several hormones

(e.g. parathyroid hormone) that activate Gs in their target tissues (pseudohypoparathyroidism type IA), while paternal transmission leads only to AHO (pseudopseudohypoparathyroidism).

Some patients with *GNAS1* mutations may present with obesity without all the features. Studies in both mice and humans demonstrate that *GNAS1* is imprinted in a tissue-specific manner, being expressed primarily from the maternal allele in some tissues and bi-allelically in other tissues; thus multi-hormone resistance occurs only when Gs (alpha) mutations are inherited maternally (Weinstein et al. 2002).

Bardet–Biedl syndrome

Bardet–Biedl syndrome (BBS) is a rare (prevalence <1/100, 000), autosomal recessive disease characterised by obesity, learning disability, dysmorphic extremities (syndactyly, brachydactyly or polydactyly), retinal dystrophy or pigmentary retinopathy, hypogonadism and structural abnormalities of the kidney or functional renal impairment. BBS is a genetically heterogeneous disorder that is now known to map to at least 16 loci, with mutations in more than 1 locus sometimes required for complete expression of the phenotype. Many BBS genes appear to affect proteins localised to the basal body, a key element of the monocilium thought to be important for intercellular sensing in mammalian cells including neurons (Ansley et al. 2003). Other disorders of ciliary function, for example, Alström syndrome (retinal dystrophy, severe insulin resistance, deafness) and Carpenter syndrome, are also associated with obesity. The link between ciliary function and obesity remains unclear although studies in mice have suggested that leptin signalling and ciliary dysfunction may be linked (Seo et al. 2009).

Brain-derived neurotrophic factor and tropomycin-related kinase B deficiency

We have reported a small number of children with severe hyperphagia and obesity, impaired short-term memory, hyperactivity and learning disability who have mutations or chromosomal deletions that disrupt brain-derived neurotrophic factor (BDNF) or its tyrosine kinase receptor tropomycin-related kinase B (TrkB) (Yeo et al. 2004; Gray et al. 2006). Yanovski and colleagues showed that in patients with WAGR syndrome, a subset of deletions on chromosome 11p.12 which encompass the BDNF locus was associated with early onset obesity (Han et al. 2008). Given the severe developmental phenotype of these patients, it is not surprising that mutations seem to arise *de novo* and as such should be considered where both parents are of normal weight and IQ.

Single-minded 1 deficiency

Single-minded 1 (SIM1) is a basic helix-loop-helix transcription factor involved in the development and function of the paraventricular nucleus of the hypothalamus. Obesity has been reported in a patient with a balanced translocation disrupting SIM1 (Holder et al. 2000) and in multiple severely obese patients with heterozygous loss of function mutations. SIM1 variants with reduced activity co-segregate with obesity in extended family studies in a dominant manner with variable penetrance. Patients with SIM1 deficiency are hyperphagic with evidence of autonomic dysfunction (characterised by low systolic blood pressure) as seen in melanocortin 4 receptor (MC4R) deficiency, which suggests that some aspects of the clinical phenotype can be explained by altered melanocortin signalling (see below). However, many *SIM1* mutations carriers have speech and language delay and exhibit neurobehavioural abnormalities including autistic-type behaviours. These features are not recognised features of MC4R deficiency but show some overlap with the behavioural phenotypes seen in PWS. As the hyperphagia of *SIM1* haplo-insufficient mice is partly ameliorated by the central administration of oxytocin (Kublaoui et al. 2008), a neurotransmitter involved in the modulation of emotion and social interaction, impaired oxytocinergic signalling is one possible mechanism implicated in the obesity and behavioural phenotype seen in SIM1 deficiency.

Obesity without developmental delay

Severe childhood-onset obesity can result from genetic defects involving the leptin-melanocortin pathway (Fig 10.2). Leptin is an adipocyte-derived hormone whose circulating concentrations correlate closely with fat mass, and which signals through the long isoform of the leptin receptor (LEPR) to regulate energy homeostasis. Leptin stimulates the expression of pro-opiomelanocortin (POMC) in the arcuate nucleus of the hypothalamus. POMC is extensively post-translationally modified to generate the melanocortin peptides (ACTH and alpha, beta, gamma melanocyte-stimulating hormone [MSH]), which in turn activate melanocortin receptors in the skin (MC1R) to modulate pigmentation, in the adrenal gland (MC2R) to

HYPOTHALAMUS

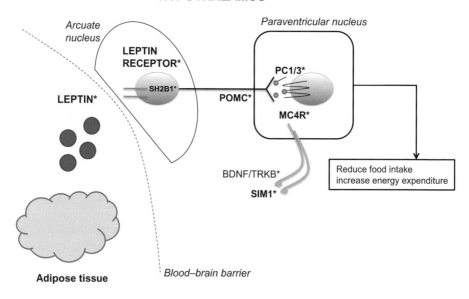

Figure 10.2. Schematic of the hypothalamic leptin-melanocortin pathway. * indicates genetic obesity syndromes. SH2B1, Src homology 2 B adapter protein 1; POMC, proopiomelanocortin; MC4R, melanocortin 4 receptor; BDNF, brain-derived neurotrophic factor; TRKB, tyrosine kinase receptor tropomycin-related kinase B; SIM1, single-minded 1.

regulate glucocorticoid synthesis and in the brain (MC3 and MC4R) to reduce energy intake and increase expenditure. In parallel, leptin inhibits pathways that stimulate food intake (orexigenic), effects that are mediated by neurons expressing the melanocortin antagonist agouti-related protein and neuropeptide Y (NPY); NPY can suppress the expression of POMC. These two sets of primary leptin-responsive neurons project to second-order neurons, expressing the MC4R in the paraventricular nucleus of the hypothalamus and other brain regions.

Leptin and leptin receptor deficiency

Additional homozygous frameshift, nonsense, and missense *LEPR* mutations have been identified in approximately 2%–3% of severely obese patients from consanguineous families (Holder et al. 2000; Han et al. 2008). *LEPR* mutations have been found in some non-consanguineous families, where both parents were unrelated but carried rare heterozygous alleles that result in a loss of function (Han et al. 2008).

Serum leptin is a useful test in patients with severe early onset obesity as an undetectable serum leptin is highly suggestive of a diagnosis of congenital leptin deficiency. It is plausible that mutations in the *LEP* gene could result in a bio-inactive form of the hormone in the presence of apparently appropriate leptin concentrations, and indeed, such a case has recently been reported in Wabitsch et al. (2015).

Serum leptin concentrations are appropriate for the degree of obesity in patients with leptin receptor deficiency and as such an elevated serum leptin concentration is not necessarily a predictor of leptin receptor deficiency (Han et al. 2008). However, in some patients, particular *LEPR* mutations which result in abnormal cleavage of the extracellular domain of LEPR (which can then act as a leptin-binding protein) are associated with markedly elevated leptin concentrations (Gray et al. 2006; Kublaoui et al. 2008).

CHARACTERISTIC CLINICAL FEATURES SEEN IN LEPTIN AND LEPTIN RECEPTOR DEFICIENCY

The clinical phenotypes associated with leptin and leptin receptor deficiencies are broadly similar (Huszar et al. 1997; Haqq et al. 2003; Han et al. 2008). Patients are born of normal birth weight but exhibit rapid weight gain in the first few months of life resulting in severe obesity (mean body mass index [BMI] standard deviation score [BMI SDS]: 5.8–7.8). Patients often have a distinctive clinical appearance with excessive amounts of subcutaneous fat over the trunk and limbs. Body composition measurements have shown that these disorders are characterised by the preferential deposition of fat mass; indeed the mean percentage body fat among homozygous carriers of *LEP* mutations is very high at 58% (compared with 45% for equally obese children of the same age [Han et al. 2008]).

In the clinical history, early development is usually normal. The most notable feature is intense hyperphagia with food-seeking behaviour and aggressive behaviour when food is denied. In the research setting, measurements of energy intake at *ad libitum* test meals reveal the extent of hyperphagia with food intake 3–5 times that of children of the same age, with both an increase in hunger and impaired satiety seen after meals of fixed quantity and composition (Weinstein et al. 2002). Increased food-seeking behaviour continues into later life in the adults (Huszar et al. 1997). Children with leptin deficiency have marked abnormalities of T cell number and function (Weinstein et al. 2002), consistent with high rates of childhood infection and a high reported rate of childhood mortality from infection (Huszar et al. 1997). In those who survive, obesity continues into adult life with hepatic steatosis (Farooqi et al. 2007b) and hyperinsulinaemia, consistent with the severity of obesity. Some adults have developed type 2 diabetes in the third to fourth decade of their life (Sahoo et al. 2008).

Serum leptin is a useful test in patients with severe early onset obesity as an undetectable serum leptin is highly suggestive of a diagnosis of congenital leptin deficiency due to homozygous loss of function mutations in the gene encoding leptin. Serum leptin concentrations are appropriate for the degree of obesity in patients with leptin receptor deficiency and as such an elevated serum leptin concentration is not necessarily a predictor of leptin receptor deficiency (Farooqi et al. 2007b). Approximately 1% of patients with severe childhood onset obesity from consanguineous families may have leptin mutations; 2%–3% may have mutations in the leptin receptor. Leptin receptor mutations have been found in some non-consanguineous families, where both parents are unrelated but happen to carry rare alleles in heterozygous form.

The clinical phenotypes associated with congenital leptin and leptin receptor deficiencies are similar. Children with leptin and leptin receptor deficiency are born of normal birth weight but exhibit rapid weight gain in the first few months of life, resulting in severe obesity (Farooqi et al. 2002) characterised by intense hyperphagia with food-seeking behaviour and aggressive behaviour when food is denied. While measurable changes in resting metabolic rate or total energy expenditure have not been demonstrated, abnormalities of sympathetic nerve function in adults who are leptin deficient suggest that autonomic dysfunction may contribute to the obesity phenotype observed. Leptin and leptin receptor deficiency are associated with hypothalamic hypothyroidism; additionally normal pubertal development does not occur in adults with leptin or leptin receptor deficiency, with biochemical evidence of hypogonadotropic hypogonadism. However, there is some evidence for the delayed but spontaneous onset of menses in some adults with leptin and leptin receptor deficiency. Children with leptin and leptin receptor deficiency have normal linear growth in childhood and normal insulin-like growth factor-1 concentrations. However, the final height of adults is reduced due to the absence of a pubertal growth spurt.

Although leptin deficiency appears to be rare, it is entirely treatable with daily subcutaneous injections of recombinant human leptin (Farooqi et al. 2002) which is currently available to patients on a named patient basis in a small number of centres around the world (Fig 10.3). The major effect of leptin treatment is on food intake, with normalisation of hyperphagia and enhanced satiety (Farooqi et al. 1999, 2002). Importantly, leptin also has permissive effects on the development of puberty and if given in early childhood permits appropriate linear growth.

Disorders affecting pro-opiomelanocortin and its processing
Children who are homozygous or compound heterozygous for mutations in the *POMC* gene present in neonatal life with an adrenal crisis due to ACTH deficiency, as POMC is a precursor of ACTH in the pituitary. They require long-term corticosteroid replacement (Krude

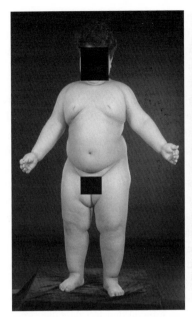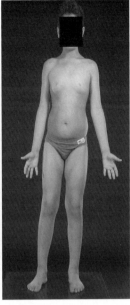

Figure 10.3. A 3-year-old boy with congenital leptin deficiency, weighing 42kg before (left) and 32kg after (right) four years of treatment with recombinant leptin therapy.

et al. 2003). Such children have pale skin and white Caucasians often have red hair due to the lack of MSH function at melanocortin 1 receptors in the skin. Although red hair may be an important diagnostic clue in patients of Caucasian origin, its absence in patients originating from other ethnic groups should not result in this diagnostic consideration being excluded as children from different ethnic backgrounds may have a less obvious phenotype such as dark hair with red roots. POMC deficiency results in hyperphagia and early onset obesity due to loss of melanocortin signalling at the MC4R. The clinical features are comparable to those reported in patients with mutations in the receptor for POMC-derived ligands, MC4R (see below). Selective melanocortin receptor agonists are in clinical trials and may be feasible therapies for such patients in the future.

Proprotein convertase subtilisin/kexin type 1 and 2 deficiency
Proprotein convertases are a family of serine endoproteases that cleave inactive pro-peptides into biologically active peptides (Seidah 2011). Proprotein convertase subtilisin/kexin type 1 and 2 (PCSK1 and PCSK2) are expressed in neuroendocrine tissues where they cleave prohormones including POMC, pro-thyrotrophin-releasing hormone, proinsulin, proglucagon, and pro-gonadotrophin-releasing hormone to release biologically active peptides. Compound heterozygous or homozygous mutations in the *PCSK1* gene, which encodes PC1/3, cause small bowel enteropathy and patients may present in neonatal life/early infancy with persistent diarrhoea requiring parenteral feeding. Other important clinical

features include hypoglycaemia and complex neuroendocrine effects (including diabetes insipidus) due to a failure to process a number of prohormones. Hyperphagia and severe obesity tend to become apparent by 2–3 years of age (Jackson et al. 1997, 2003).

Melanocortin 4 receptor deficiency

MC4R deficiency is the most common genetic form of obesity, and assessment of the sequence of *MC4R* is increasingly seen as a necessary part of the clinical evaluation of the severely obese child. The prevalence of pathogenic *MC4R* mutations has varied from 0.5%–2.5% of people with a BMI>30kg/m^2 in UK and European populations to 5% in patients with severe childhood obesity (Farooqi et al. 2003; Stutzmann et al. 2008). Given the large number of potential influences on body weight, it is perhaps not surprising that both genetic and environmental modifiers will have important effects on the severity of obesity associated with *MC4R* mutations in some pedigrees. Most patients have heterozygous mutations; co-dominance, with modulation of expressivity and penetrance of the phenotype, is the most appropriate descriptor for the mode of inheritance. Homozygous mutations in *MC4R* have been identified in children from consanguineous families.

The clinical features of *MC4R* deficiency include hyperphagia in early childhood. Alongside the increase in fat mass, patients with *MC4R* deficiency also have an increase in lean mass and a marked increase in bone mineral density; thus they often appear 'big-boned' (Farooqi et al. 2003). They exhibit accelerated linear growth, which may be a consequence of disproportionate early hyperinsulinaemia and effects on pulsatile growth hormone secretion, which is retained in adults with *MC4R* deficiency in contrast to common forms of obesity (Martinelli et al. 2011). Reduced sympathetic nervous system activity in patients with *MC4R* deficiency is likely to explain the lower prevalence of hypertension and lower systolic and diastolic blood pressures seen in adults (Greenfield et al. 2009). Thus, central melanocortin signalling appears to play an important role in the regulation of blood pressure and its coupling to changes in weight.

Several studies have now shown that adolescents and adults with heterozygous *MC4R* mutations do respond to Roux-en-Y bypass surgery (Hatoum et al. 2012). As most patients are heterozygotes with one functional allele intact, it is possible that small molecule *MC4R* agonists or pharmacological chaperones which improve receptor trafficking to the cell surface might be appropriate treatments for this disorder. A number of compounds are under development and one is likely to be in phase 2 clinical trials in the near future.

As complete loss-of-function *MC4R* mutations are associated with a more severe form of obesity than partial loss-of-function mutations (Farooqi et al. 2003), modulation of melanocortinergic tone has been the focus of drug development strategies for some time. However, despite promising pre-clinical studies, the first generation of *MC4R* agonists were small molecules that failed, primarily because of safety issues, particularly increases in blood pressure. Loss of function *MC4R* mutations are associated with a reduced prevalence of hypertension, low systolic blood pressure, lower urinary noradrenaline excretion and reduced peripheral nerve sympathetic nervous system activation, revealing that *MC4R* expressing neurons represent a key circuit linking changes in weight with changes in blood pressure (Greenfield et al. 2009). More recently, a potent melanocortin receptor agonist,

RM-493, has been administered as part of a phase 1b proof-of-concept clinical trial in obese patients, including one cohort of patients with heterozygous loss of function mutations in *MC4R*, where there was promising weight loss after four weeks. If this compound moves forward, this may be one of the first examples of a personalised medicine approach for treating obesity in people with a genetically characterised subtype of obesity.

SRC homology 2 B adapter protein 1 deficiency

Severe obesity without developmental delay is associated with a significantly increased burden of rare, typically singleton copy number variants (deletions/duplications) (Wheeler et al. 2013). Deletion of a 220-kb segment of 16p11.2 is associated with highly penetrant familial severe early onset obesity and severe insulin resistance (Bochukova et al. 2010). This deletion includes a small number of genes, one of which is *SH2B1* (Src homology 2 B adapter protein 1), known to be involved in leptin and insulin signalling. These patients gain weight in the first years of life, with hyperphagia and fasting plasma insulin concentrations that are disproportionately elevated compared to age- and obesity-matched controls. Several mutations in *SH2B1* have also been reported in association with early onset obesity, severe insulin resistance and behavioural abnormalities including aggression (Doche et al. 2012).

Kinase suppressor of RAS2 deficiency

To date, most of the genetic obesity syndromes are characterised by hyperphagia as a major driver of the obesity. We recently identified multiple mutations in the gene-encoding KSR2 (kinase suppressor of Ras2), where in addition to increased food-seeking behaviour in childhood, we found that basal metabolic rate (BMR) was significantly less than predicted BMR. In the presence of normal thyroid function and in the absence of other explanations for reduced BMR, our findings indicate that mutations in *KSR2* represent a novel genetic influence on basal metabolic rate. Clinical reports suggested that some *KSR2* mutation carriers experienced marked weight loss in childhood when prescribed the antidiabetic drug metformin (for severe insulin resistance). We found that the reduced basal level of fatty acid oxidation seen with the *KSR2* mutations was completely rescued in all cases by the addition of metformin to cells. Further work will be needed to see if these observations can be replicated in formal experimental clinical studies and to investigate the cellular mechanisms underlying these effects.

REFERENCES

Ansley SJ, Badano JL, Blacque OE et al. (2003) Basal body dysfunction is a likely cause of pleiotropic Bardet-Biedl syndrome. *Nature* 425: 628–633.

Bochukova EG, Huang N, Keogh J et al. (2010) Large, rare chromosomal deletions associated with severe early-onset obesity. *Nature* 463: 666–670.

Carrel AL and Allen DB (2001) Prader-Willi syndrome: How does growth hormone affect body composition and physical function? *J Pediatr Endocrinol Metab* 14(Suppl 6): 1445–1451.

de Smith AJ, Purmann C, Walters RG et al. (2009) A deletion of the HBII-85 class of small nucleolar RNAs (snoRNAs) is associated with hyperphagia, obesity and hypogonadism. *Hum Mol Genet* 18: 3257–3265.

Doche ME, Bochukova EG, Su HW et al. (2012) Human SH2B1 mutations are associated with maladaptive behaviors and obesity. *J Clin Invest* 122: 4732–4736.

Farooqi IS, Bullmore E, Keogh J, Gillard J, O'Rahilly S and Fletcher PC (2007a) Leptin regulates striatal regions and human eating behavior. *Science* 317: 1355.

Farooqi IS, Jebb SA, Langmack G et al. (1999) Effects of recombinant leptin therapy in a child with congenital leptin deficiency. *N Engl J Med* 341: 879–884.

Farooqi IS, Keogh JM, Yeo GS, Lank EJ, Cheetham T and O'Rahilly S (2003) Clinical spectrum of obesity and mutations in the melanocortin 4 receptor gene. *N Engl J Med* 348: 1085–1095.

Farooqi IS, Matarese G, Lord GM et al. (2002) Beneficial effects of leptin on obesity, T cell hyporesponsiveness, and neuroendocrine/metabolic dysfunction of human congenital leptin deficiency. *J Clin Invest* 110: 1093–1103.

Farooqi IS, Wangensteen T, Collins S et al. (2007b) Clinical and molecular genetic spectrum of congenital deficiency of the leptin receptor. *N Engl J Med* 356: 237–247.

Goldstone AP (2004) Prader-Willi syndrome: Advances in genetics, pathophysiology and treatment. *Trends Endocrinol Metab* 15: 12–20.

Gray J, Yeo GS, Cox JJ et al. (2006) Hyperphagia, severe obesity, impaired cognitive function, and hyperactivity associated with functional loss of one copy of the brain-derived neurotrophic factor (BDNF) gene. *Diabetes* 55: 3366–3371.

Greenfield JR, Miller JW, Keogh JM et al. (2009) Modulation of blood pressure by central melanocortinergic pathways. *N Engl J Med* 360: 44–52.

Han JC, Liu QR, Jones M et al. (2008) Brain-derived neurotrophic factor and obesity in the WAGR syndrome. *N Engl J Med* 359: 918–927.

Haqq AM, Farooqi IS, O'Rahilly S et al. (2003) Serum ghrelin levels are inversely correlated with body mass index, age, and insulin concentrations in normal children and are markedly increased in Prader-Willi syndrome. *J Clin Endocrinol Metab* 88: 174–178.

Hatoum IJ, Stylopoulos N, Vanhoose AM et al. (2012) Melanocortin-4 receptor signaling is required for weight loss after gastric bypass surgery. *J Clin Endocrinol Metab* 97: E1023–E1031.

Holder JL Jr, Butte NF and Zinn AR (2000) Profound obesity associated with a balanced translocation that disrupts the SIM1 gene. *Hum Mol Genet* 9: 101–108.

Huszar D, Lynch CA, Fairchild-Huntress V et al. (1997) Targeted disruption of the melanocortin-4 receptor results in obesity in mice. *Cell* 88: 131–141.

Jackson RS, Creemers JW, Farooqi IS et al. (2003) Small-intestinal dysfunction accompanies the complex endocrinopathy of human proprotein convertase 1 deficiency. *J Clin Invest* 112: 1550–1560.

Jackson RS, Creemers JW, Ohagi S et al. (1997) Obesity and impaired prohormone processing associated with mutations in the human prohormone convertase 1 gene [see comments]. *Nat Genet* 16: 303–306.

Krude H, Biebermann H, Schnabel D et al. (2003) Obesity due to proopiomelanocortin deficiency: Three new cases and treatment trials with thyroid hormone and ACTH4-10. *J Clin Endocrinol Metab* 88: 4633–4640.

Kublaoui BM, Gemelli T, Tolson KP, Wang Y and Zinn AR (2008) Oxytocin deficiency mediates hyperphagic obesity of Sim1 haploinsufficient mice. *Mol Endocrinol* 22: 1723–1734.

Martinelli CE, Keogh JM, Greenfield JR et al. (2011) Obesity due to melanocortin 4 receptor (MC4R) deficiency is associated with increased linear growth and final height, fasting hyperinsulinemia, and incompletely suppressed growth hormone secretion. *J Clin Endocrinol Metab* 96: E181–E188.

Sahoo T, del Gaudio D, German JR et al. (2008) Prader-Willi phenotype caused by paternal deficiency for the HBII-85 C/D box small nucleolar RNA cluster. *Nat Genet* 40: 719–721.

Seidah NG (2011) The proprotein convertases, 20 years later. *Methods in Mol Biol* 768: 23–57.

Seo S, Guo DF, Bugge K, Morgan DA, Rahmouni K and Sheffield VC (2009) Requirement of Bardet-Biedl syndrome proteins for leptin receptor signaling. *Hum Mol Genet* 18: 1323–1331.

Stutzmann F, Tan K, Vatin V et al. (2008) Prevalence of melanocortin-4 receptor deficiency in Europeans and their age-dependent penetrance in multigenerational pedigrees. *Diabetes* 57: 2511–2518.

Wabitsch M, Funcke JB, Lennerz B et al. (2015) Biologically inactive leptin and early-onset extreme obesity. *N Engl J Med* 372(1): 48–54.

Weinstein LS, Chen M and Liu J (2002) Gs(alpha) mutations and imprinting defects in human disease. *Ann NY Acad Sci* 968: 173–197.

Wheeler E, Huang N, Bochukova EG et al. (2013) Genome-wide SNP and CNV analysis identifies common and low-frequency variants associated with severe early-onset obesity. *Nat Genet* 45: 513–517.

Yeo GS, Connie Hung CC, Rochford J et al. (2004) A de novo mutation affecting human TrkB associated with severe obesity and developmental delay. *Nat Neurosci* 7: 1187–1189.

11
TREATMENT OF OBESITY

Terry Segal and Bhavni Shah

Introduction

Obesity is now a common childhood condition and is widely acknowledged as having become a global epidemic. There are well-recognised health consequences of childhood obesity, both during childhood and during adulthood, affecting physical health and psychological welfare.

Obesity is the excessive or abnormal accumulation of fat, to the degree that health may be impaired. It is a chronic condition of imbalance between appetite regulation and energy metabolism, controlled by numerous biological, social and psychological factors. The past 30 years have seen a significant rise in the prevalence of obesity in children and adolescents worldwide. Data from the Health Survey of England (2012) identified 16% of females and 17% of males aged 2–15 years as obese in 2011 but this has recently decreased to 14% for both sexe. Obesity in childhood is predictive of obesity in adulthood. The Foresight report (2003) predicts that 50% adults will be obese by 2050.

Whilst the adverse effects of obesity on health have long been known in adults, the complications and comorbidities associated with obesity are starting to be recognised in children and adolescents. Childhood obesity is also predictive of cardiovascular disease, diabetes, metabolic syndrome, cancer and osteoarthritis (Ho et al. 2013).

This chapter seeks to suggest an approach to the medical assessment and treatment of the obese child or young person, and associated comorbidities, although the treatment of this condition is no means straightforward.

Definition of obesity

The standard criterion for measuring obesity is by ascertaining the body fat composition which is best done by DEXA scan, or, as Baumgartner et al. (1991) have suggested, the four-compartment model (4C model) may be used in adults and results adjusted, using the Lohman equation (1989), against which other body composition techniques are evaluated, in children. The 4C model involves an independent assessment of body density, body water and bone. However, as these are costly, inconvenient and impractical, body mass index (BMI) is commonly used as a surrogate marker. Sometimes bioelectrical impedance is used in the assessment of overweight and obese children; however, this is not accurate in measuring body fat as reported by L'Abée C et al. (2010). Skinfold thickness can also be a useful adjunct clinically but can be inaccurate depending on experience.

BMI is a simple index of weight-for-height that is commonly used to classify overweight and obesity in adults. It is defined as a person's weight in kilograms divided by the square of his/her height in metres (kg/m^2). BMI levels correlate with body fatness (Johnson RK 2002) as well as concurrent health risks (Freedman et al. 2001).

In children, the relationship between BMI and body fatness varies with age and sex, as such growth reference centile charts are used to define underweight, normal healthy weight, overweight and obesity. It is important to be aware of the limitations of using BMI, as individuals with high muscle mass will also have a high BMI reading. BMI does not distinguish between excess fat, muscle or bone mass, nor does it provide information on the distribution of fat among individuals.

The cut-off points, used to define each of these categories, are set to capture varying risk levels and minimise over-diagnosis and under-diagnosis. When BMI is at ≤85th centile, body fat levels pose little risk, but at a BMI ≥95th centile, the risk is high. At a BMI between the 85th and 95th centiles, the health risks vary depending on the body composition, BMI trajectory, family history and other factors.

Child growth references

Many countries have their own population-specific thresholds for assessing BMI in children. The child growth reference most commonly used in the United Kingdom is the British 1990 growth reference (UK90). Other countries use the World Health Organisation (WHO) growth reference, Centers of Disease Control (CDC) growth reference and International Obesity Task Force (IOTF) thresholds. The IOTF cut-offs were not intended for clinical definition and were not intended to replace national reference ranges, but rather to provide a common set of definitions that researchers worldwide can use for comparative purposes (Tables 11.1 and 11.2).

Each of these use age- and sex-appropriate charts to determine weight status and are summarised below.

The UK90 (Cole et al. 1995) cut-offs are slightly lower than the clinical cut-offs and are similar to the WHO (WHO 2006), CDC (Kuczmarski RJ et al. 2000) and IOTF (Cole

TABLE 11.1
Clinical definitions of weight status based on UK90 Growth Reference

Description	Clinical assessment	Population monitoring
Severely underweight	≤0.4th centile	
Low weight	≤2nd centile	≤2nd centile
Healthy weight	>2–<91st centile	>2–<85th centile
Overweight	≥91st centile	≥85th centile
Clinically obese	≥98th centile	≥95th centile
Severely obese	≥99.6th centile	

Centile cut-offs based on the UK–Childhood and Puberty Close Monitoring BMI charts. (There are nine centiles and each one is two-thirds of a standard deviation score apart.)

TABLE 11.2
Variations in the different child growth references and their applicability

Reference criteria	Age	Population based on	Cut-offs	Clinical assessment	Population assessment
UK90	**0–23yrs**	UK only	**Underweight**	≤2nd centile	≤2nd centile
			Overweight	≥91st centile	≥85th centile
			Obese	≥98th centile	≥95th centile
WHO	**2–5yrs**	Brazil, Ghana, India, Norway, Oman and USA	**Underweight**	≤2nd centile	
			Overweight	≥97th centile	
			Obese	≥99.9th centile	
WHO	**5–19yrs**	Brazil, Ghana, India, Norway, Oman and USA	**Underweight**	<−2SD	<−2SD
			Overweight	>+1SD	>+1SD
			Obese	>+2SD	>+2SD
IOTF	**2–18yrs**	Brazil, Great Britain, Hong Kong, Netherlands, Singapore and USA	**Underweight**	n/a	<17kg/m^2
			Overweight		>25kg/m^2
			Obese		>30kg/m^2
CDC	**2–19yrs**	USA	**Underweight**	≤5th centile	≤5th centile
			Overweight	≥85th centile	≥85th centile
			Obese	≥95th centile	≥95th centile

CDC, Centers of Disease Control; IOTF, International Obesity Task Force; UK90, British 1990 growth reference; WHO, World Health Organization.

et al. 2012) growth references, therefore making it important to use the same thresholds when comparing data.

There are different cut-offs applied when monitoring populations and in clinical assessment. The population-monitoring thresholds are used mostly for published obesity and overweight prevalence figures, for example, those using Health Survey for England. The clinical cut-offs are recommended by NICE (National Institute for Health and Clinical Excellence) for use in clinical settings with individual children (www.noo.org.uk). This is clearly demonstrated by Lopes et al. (2012), showing the clinical applicability of the WHO criteria and the international comparability of the IOTF criteria. Heidari et al. (2013) showed that the CDC and IOTF were equally good markers of obesity and overweight screening in the adolescent population, a statement that Cole et al. had demonstrated whilst defining the IOTF criteria.

Classification and causes of obesity
COMORBIDITIES ASSOCIATED WITH OBESITY

Various diseases or conditions (comorbidities) may be associated with obesity in childhood. These are described below as well as investigations and treatment of the specific comorbidities, and are also summarised in Table 11.3 and 11.4.

TABLE 11.3
Classification of causes of obesity

Classification	Aetiology	Examples	Comment
Primary obesity	Multifactorial/lifestyle and polygenic factors in balance of calorie intake and energy expenditure	Primary or simple obesity	Accounts for 95% cases Characterised by tallness if origin in infancy
Genetic obesity	Genetic syndromes	Prader–Willi syndrome Laurence–Moon–Biedl syndrome Down syndrome Bloom syndrome Carpenter syndrome	Characterised by learning disability, short stature and dysmorphic features
	Monogenic obesity syndromes	Mutations in melanocortin receptor 4 (*MC4R*), leptin, leptin receptor, proopiomelanocortin (POMC), prohormone convertase I (*PCI*), KSR2, BDNF	See Chapter 10 Some have characteristic features, e.g. red hair in POMC, gastrointestinal abnormalities in PCI
Secondary obesity	Endocrine	Hypothalamic (secondary to surgery or occult tumour) ROHHAD/ROHHADNET Congenital/acquired hypopituitarism e.g. post-craniopharyngioma resection Hypogonadism Cushing syndrome Growth hormone deficiency Hypothyroidism Pseudohypoparathyroidism Hyperinsulinism	Hyperphagia Characteristic findings on history and examination
	Neurological	Hypothalamic tumours, learning difficulties, anti-epileptic medication, chronic neuromuscular disorders leading to inactivity	
	Iatrogenic	Exogenous: medications e.g. glucocorticoids Oestrogen Antipsychotics especially the second-generation antipsychotics	
	Behavioural	Hyperphagia 'Comfort eating'	

TABLE 11.4
Classification of complications of obesity

Metabolic

- Cardiovascular
  - Metabolic syndrome
  - Hypertension
  - Increased plasma glucose
  - Dyslipidaemia (low HDL, high triglycerides)
  - Left ventricular hypertrophy
- Endocrine
  - Insulin resistance
  - Type 2 diabetes
  - Thyroid disease
  - Hyperandrogenism
- Gastrointestinal
  - Non-alcoholic steatohepatitis (NAFLD)
  - Cholelithiasis (gallstones)
  - GORD
  - Constipation
- Renal
  - Focal segmental Glomeruloscleroisis[21]
  - Chronic kidney disease
- Genitourinary
  - Polycystic ovary syndrome
  - Menstrual abnormalities
  - Primary amenorrhoea
  - Early-onset puberty

Mechanical

- Pulmonary
  - Obstructive sleep apnoea
  - Pulmonary hypertension and RHF
- Musculoskeletal
  - Slipped capital femoral epiphysis
  - Blounts disease
  - Joint problems
- Central nervous system
  - pseudotumour cerebri
  - idiopathic intracranial hypertension

Psychological

- Psychological
- Low self-esteem
- Depression
- Anxiety
- Bullying
- Social marginalisation
- Negative body image

Cardiovascular risk factors and metabolic syndrome

The Expert Panel on Integrated Guidelines for Cardiovascular Health and Risk Reduction in Children and Adolescents has shown relationships of risk factors measured in adolescents (specifically low-density lipoprotein [LDL] cholesterol, non-high-density lipoprotein [HDL] cholesterol and serum apolipoproteins; obesity; hypertension; tobacco use; and diabetes) to measures of subclinical atherosclerosis in adulthood. In many of these studies, risk factors measured in childhood and adolescence were better predictors of the severity of adult atherosclerosis than were risk factors measured at the time of the subclinical atherosclerosis study. Their main recommendations are summarised in Table 11.5.

Being overweight as a child has also been associated with other cardiovascular risk factors in childhood or early adulthood (Craig et al. 2008; Logue and Sattar 2011).

Metabolic syndrome, also known as dysmetabolic syndrome, insulin-resistance syndrome or syndrome-X, comprises a constellation of cardiovascular risk factors including abdominal obesity and two of the following: elevated triglycerides, low HDL cholesterol,

TABLE 11.5
Expert Panel on Integrated Guidelines for Cardiovascular Health and Risk Reduction in Children and Adolescents: Summary Report

Condition-specific treatment recommendations for high-risk conditions

Rigorous age-appropriate education in diet, activity, smoking cessation for all

Specific therapy as needed to achieve blood pressure (BP), LDL cholesterol, glucose, and HbA1c goals indicated for each tier, as outlined in algorithm; timing individualised for each patient and diagnosis

Diabetes mellitus regardless of type:

For T1DM, intensive glucose management with frequent glucose monitoring/insulin titration to maintain optimal plasma glucose and HbA1c levels for age

For T2DM, intensive weight management and glucose control as needed to maintain optimal plasma glucose and HbA1c levels for age

Assess body mass index and fasting lipid concentrations: step 4 lifestyle management of weight and lipid concentrations for 6 months

If LDL goals are not achieved, consider statin therapy if age ≥10yrs to achieve tier 1 treatment goals for LDL cholesterol

Initial BP ≥90th centile: step 4 lifestyle management plus no added salt, increased activity for 6 months

If BP is consistently at the ≥95th centile for age/sex/height, initiate angiotensin-converting enzyme inhibitor therapy with a BP goal of <90th centile for sex/height or <120/80mm Hg, whichever is lower

hypertension, increased plasma glucose and insulin insensitivity. Additional metabolic risk factors include increased concentrations of serum apolipoprotein B, small dense LDL particles and plasminogen activator inhibitor 1.

Unfortunately there are no internationally accepted definitions for metabolic syndrome in children and adolescents, partly because of the effects of puberty on insulin sensitivity. The most cited definitions are those of the International Diabetes Federation 2007 (IDF) and National Cholesterol Education Program's Adult Treatment Panel III (NCEP ATP III) criteria, and the definition suggested by Weiss et al. (2013). The differences depend on cut-offs for lipids, blood pressure (BP) and waist circumference. Tavares (2014) reported that the prevalence of metabolic syndrome is higher using NCEP-ATPIII compared to IDF (40.4% and 24.6% in obese adolescents, respectively). Weiss et al. (2004) and Cook et al. (2003) report that the prevalence of metabolic syndrome in 12- to 19-year-olds in the United States is 4.2% and increases to 50% in the severely obese. There is a link between increased intra-abdominal-adipose tissue and the likelihood of developing metabolic syndrome.

Population-based data from the United States suggest that 22% of children and adolescents with BMI ≥98th centile have ≥2 risk factors in addition to their obesity, rising to 33% of those at the ≥99th centile (Freedman et al. 2007). Clinic-based data in UK children suggest that around 20%–25% of obese children and adolescents have two or more of the above risk factors in addition to obesity (Viner et al. 2005).

Glucose intolerance

Impaired glucose tolerance (IGT), impaired fasting glucose (IFG) and the progression to type 2 diabetes mellitus (T2DM) are the most serious complications of childhood obesity.

Obese children and adolescents affected by IGT, IFG (either of these are classified as pre-diabetes by the American Diabetes Association [ADA]) and T2DM are characterised by severe insulin insensitivity, which is associated with increased lipid accumulation in visceral compartments, liver and muscle, and by reduced sensitivity of β-cells of first- and second-phase insulin secretion.

The incidence of type 2 diabetes is increasing rapidly in line with the obesity epidemic. Pinhas-Hamiel et al. (2005) and Liese et al. (2006) estimated that as much as 45% of newly diagnosed diabetes in children is of type 2 rather than type 1. The incidence is highest in African American, Hispanic and Asian, and lowest in Caucasian, adolescents. Over the past decade, more children (some as young as 7 years) and adolescents are being diagnosed with this condition (Diabetes UK facts and stats 2014).

Picking up IFG/IGT (pre-diabetes) as well as diabetes in obese adolescents is important. The ADA currently recommends cut-offs of fasting glucose >7mmol/L and HbA1c >6.5%, or a 2-hour blood glucose post-OGTT (oral glucose tolerance test) >11.1mmol/L as positive for T2DM. IGT is diagnosed by a fasting glucose of 5.6–6.9mmol/L, and 2-hour post-OGTT blood glucose of 7.8–11.1mmol/L or an HbA1C of 5.7%. It must however be remembered that these cut-offs are derived from adult data.

Relative insulin insensitivity is normal in adolescence. There is little evidence in young people of therapeutic interventions that prevent progression from IGT/pre-diabetes to T2DM. Haemer et al. (2014) show that some children will normalise their glycaemic control without medication.

The ADA's Professional Practice Committee recommends that adults with pre-diabetes be referred to a programme targeting weight loss of 7% and increasing moderate physical activity to >150 minutes per week.

Studies in adolescents have also demonstrated an increase in insulin sensitivity with diet and exercise–induced weight loss (Steffen et al. 2003; Ebbeling et al. 2003) and resolution of pre-diabetes in multicomponent lifestyle programs (Savoye et al. 2007, 2014; Shaw et al. 2009).

Research on low glycaemic diets among adults and adolescents demonstrate improvement in insulin secretion and body composition without evidence of harm. An hour a day of moderate physical exercise is also recommended. Controversy surrounds the use of glucose-lowering medication to prevent the progression of pre-diabetes to diabetes.

Metformin, a biguanide, has been used to prevent progression of pre-diabetes to diabetes. Although its mechanism of action is not clearly understood, it decreases hepatic glucose production and also increases insulin sensitivity in peripheral tissues (Kirpichnikov et al. 2002). In obese adolescents, a meta-analysis including three small, short-term randomised trials of metformin in patients with insulin insensitivity found a reduction in BMI and fasting insulin with treatment (Quinn et al. 2010). Three other small randomised trials in normoglycemic obese children with elevated fasting insulin concentrations showed a reduction in fasting glucose and insulin (Freemark et al. 2001; Kay et al. 2001; Yanovski et al 2011). However, none of these studies lasted longer than 6 months. No studies have shown prevention of progression from pre-diabetes to diabetes in this age group, and longitudinal studies are required. In the absence of these studies, it is not uncommon for paediatric endocrinologists to attempt to treat pre-diabetes with metformin in clinical practice.

Hypertension

Systolic BP correlates with BMI. Lurbe et al. (2001) found that the relative risk of hypertension in obese children was 3.26 compared to non-obese children. The Framingham study in adults showed an increase of 6.5mmHg with every 10% increase in body weight.

The Fourth Report on the Diagnosis, Evaluation, and Treatment of High Blood Pressure in Children and Adolescents (the Fourth Report) recommends that BP should be assessed in children with appropriate sized cuffs and levels defined according to age, sex and height centiles. Elevated BP must be confirmed on repeated visits before characterising a child as having hypertension. If white-coat hypertension is suspected, ambulatory BP monitoring is recommended.

Stage 1 hypertension is diagnosed if diastolic or systolic BP is >95th centile for age, sex and height on three occasions, with pre-hypertension lying on the 90th centile. If there are conditions such as heart disease or diabetes, then treatment is considered in the pre-hypertension stage. For those identified as having stage 1 hypertension, weight loss and a dietary approach to stop hypertension (DASH) plan is recommended as well as increased physical activity. If comorbidities are present, anti-hypertensive medication may be started. Stage 2 hypertension is defined as BP >99th centile plus 5mmHg; end organ damage should be assessed with an echocardiogram to look for LVH, as well as comorbidities such as metabolic syndrome and diabetes. Other causes should be considered, but in this population, it is likely primary hypertension is caused by obesity, although Cushing syndrome needs to be considered. Weight reduction is the primary therapy for obesity-related hypertension with family intervention improving success. Treatment consists of attempted weight loss and DASH diet and exercise. Pharmacologic therapy, when indicated, should be initiated with a single drug. Acceptable drug classes for use in children include angiotensin-converting enzyme inhibitors, angiotensin-receptor blockers, beta-blockers, calcium channel blockers and diuretics. The goal for anti-hypertensive treatment in children should be a reduction of BP to <95th centile, unless concurrent conditions are present. In the latter case, BP should be lowered to <90th centile.

Hyperlipidaemia

Obesity in childhood is linked to hyperlipidaemia, and hence the increase in obesity has led to an increase in children and adolescents with lipid abnormalities. Between 12% and 17% of obese and overweight children and adolescents have lipid abnormalities (Jago et al. 2006).

The characteristic pattern observed consists of elevated serum LDL cholesterol and triglycerides and lowered HDL cholesterol levels. Central fat distribution, perhaps through its effect on insulin concentrations, appears to be an important mediating variable between lipid levels and obesity (Freedman et al. 1987, 1989, [Bogalusa Heart Study], Steinberger et al. 1995). Potential mechanisms are similar to those operative in adults. Increased free fatty acids produced by increased lipolysis in visceral adipocytes and hyperinsulinemia may promote hepatic triglyceride and LDL cholesterol synthesis.

A series of critical observational studies (Berenson et al. 1998; Bogalusa Heart Study 1998; and McGill et al. 2000) have demonstrated a clear correlation between lipoprotein disorders and the onset and severity of atherosclerosis in children, adolescents and young adults. Tracking of elevated lipid and lipoprotein concentrations from childhood into adulthood has been shown in many studies including the Bogalusa Heart Study. Therefore, identification of children with dyslipidemias by undertaking assessment of serum lipids and lipoproteins is imperative.

The NCEP provided cut-offs and guidelines in 1992 for lipid management in children and adolescents, and more recent evidence-based guidelines have been provided by the US National Heart Lung and Blood Institute (Integrated Guidelines for Cardiovascular Health and Risk Reduction in Children and Adolescents for Lipids and Lipoproteins). These addressed the association between dyslipidemia and atherosclerosis in childhood, lipid assessment in childhood and adolescence with tables of normative results provided, the dyslipidaemias, dietary treatment of dyslipidemia and medication therapy. Elevated lipid concentrations have been shown to respond to weight reduction following diet and physical activity regimens. A low fat and cholesterol diet is the next line in treatment of dyslipidaemia. If the lipid concentrations do not fall below suggested thresholds, then referral to a lipid specialist for consideration of cholesterol-lowering agents such as statins is recommended.

Adipokines and inflammation

Obesity induces local inflammation in adipose tissue. Adipokines, inflammatory mediators produced by adipose tissue, are secreted into the circulation; this local obesity-induced inflammation is conveyed to other sites in the body, such as cardiovascular tissue and circulating immune cells. Studies of circulating mediators showed greater concentrations of inflammatory mediators, including high-sensitivity C-reactive protein, leptin, Interleukin-6(IL-6) and IL-8, together with decreased concentrations of the insulin-sensitising adipokine, adiponectin and higher leucocyte numbers in obese children than in lean controls (Visser et al. 2001; Skinner et al. 2010; Tam et al. 2010b). Schipper et al. (2012) demonstrated that inflammatory mechanisms linking obesity to its metabolic and cardiovascular complications are already activated in childhood obesity. These inflammatory mediator clusters were associated with insulin resistance in obese and lean children. The activation of CD14[++] monocyte subsets, which is associated with increased development of atherosclerosis in obese adults, was also readily detected in obese children.

Polycystic ovary disease

In girls with a BMI >95th centile, there is a high association with hyperandrogenism (high testosterone and dehydroepiandrosterone sulphate) and hyperinsulinism, and hence a high risk of polycystic ovary syndrome (PCOS; McCartney et al. 2007). Hyperinsulinism is thought to be the driver in the association between obesity and development of PCOS (Rojas et al. 2014). Menstrual abnormalities may begin at adolescence.

PCOS can be diagnosed once other conditions have been excluded and more than two of the following are present: oligo-ovulation or anovulation (usually manifested as oligomenor-rhoea or amenorrhea), elevated concentrations of circulating androgens (hyperandrogenaemia) or clinical manifestations of androgen excess (hyperandrogenism) and polycystic ovaries, as defined by ultrasonography.

Treatments include weight loss and maintenance, and metformin to address insulin insensitivity. The combined oral contraceptive (COC) pill can be used with caution with a BMI of 30–39 and no other risk factors. If hypertension or type 2 diabetes is present, or if the patient smokes, COC should be avoided. Other commonly used treatments include flutamide or spironolactone for their antiandrogenic properties (Mastorakos 2006).

Respiratory problems

These include asthma, sleep apnoea and restrictive lung disease. Asthmatic children with obesity are characterised by poorer asthma control and an increased need for asthma medication (Frey et al. 2014). Obstructive sleep apnoea is becoming a significant problem with resultant end organ morbidities and increased use of healthcare resources (Tauman and Gozal 2011). It is six times more likely to affect obese children than lean children (Young et al. 2004). The prevalence is between 20% and 40% of obese children aged 3–14 years (Alonso-Alvarez et al. 2014). Gileles-Hillel et al. (2014) have also suggested a pro-inflammatory effect of obstructive sleep apnoea (OSA; Nanos study). OSA can also lead to right ventricular failure and pulmonary hypertension, if untreated. Additionally, poor sleep leads to poor academic performance, poor attention and enuresis. Neurocognitive deficits are common among obese children with sleep apnoea. The relationship between sleep apnoea and the obesity hypoventilation syndrome remains unclear. Hypoventilation may represent a long-term consequence as well as a cause of sleep apnoea. The high mortality reported among published cases of the obesity hypoventilation syndrome suggests that investigation and aggressive management are warranted.

In the presence of snoring, fatigue, morning headaches and difficulty in breathing, further detailed screening such as the Chervin Paediatric Sleep Questionnaire should be undertaken. Diagnosis is made through polysomnography. Adenotonsillectomy may or may not improve symptoms. Topical (nasal) steroids and/or anti-inflammatory agents may play a role in the non-surgical treatment of mild OSA. Continuous positive airway pressure (CPAP) and orthodontic interventions are treatment options for persisting OSA in children (Waters 2013).

In the obesity hypoventilation syndrome, ventilation is impaired due to excess fat on the chest and abdomen. It presents with similar symptoms to OSA. Polysomnography in these patients shows elevated CO_2 levels and raised haemoglobin and haematocrit concentrations on a full blood count. They usually require referral to the respiratory physician for CPAP.

Sleep problems

There appears to be a relationship between reduced sleep duration or deprivation and obesity due to several possible biological pathways including increased sympathetic activity, elevated cortisol and ghrelin concentrations, decreased leptin and growth hormone and/or IGT (Spiegel et al. 2004; Taheri et al. 2004). Hormonal changes may contribute to selection of calorie-dense food, excessive food intake, changes in energy expenditure and insulin insensitivity (Taheri 2006). Other potential mechanisms are effects of sleep deprivation on basal metabolic rate, thermic effect of food and non-exercise activity thermogenesis. Chen et al. (2012) performed a meta-analysis and provided more supportive data on the proposed biological mechanisms as well as supportive evidence of the relationship between sleep deprivation and obesity.

Gastrointestinal problems

Non-alcoholic fatty liver disease (NAFLD) is a clinico-pathologic entity defined as the presence of hepatic steatosis in individuals who drink little or no alcohol and represents a spectrum of liver disease ranging from bland steatosis to non-alcoholic steatohepatitis (NASH), a progressive form of liver disease that may lead to advanced fibrosis, cirrhosis and hepatocellular carcinoma in a subset of affected individuals. Serum alanine aminotransferase (ALT) and aspartate aminotransferase concentrations are usually elevated in association with obesity, and are markers of metabolic dysfunction and reduced insulin sensitivity. Obesity is the commonest cause of chronic liver disease in the United States (Loomba et al. 2009). There is an association with adverse cardiovascular health in adults and children. Abdominal ultrasound scans should be undertaken to make the diagnosis but cannot indicate the degree of fibrosis or inflammation. Liver biopsy is the standard criterion for diagnosis. A systematic review and meta-analysis by Musso et al. (2012) reported that ≥5% weight loss in adults improves steatosis and cardio-metabolic variables; a ≥7% weight loss also improves histological disease activity in NASH. A weight loss of 5kg on average results in a reduced ALT in children with NAFLD (Nobili 2007). Aerobic exercise should be implemented in lifestyle intervention, as it enhances whole body lipid oxidation, and improves steatosis and cardio-metabolic risk profile regardless of weight loss. For patients with NASH not responding to lifestyle intervention, pharmacological treatment should be considered.

Gallstones are found in 2% of obese children and are also seen in those with rapid and significant weight loss (Koebnick et al. 2012); gastroesophageal reflux and constipation are also exacerbated in obesity (Fishman et al. 2004).

Hormones and growth

Overweight children tend to be taller, have advanced bone ages and mature earlier than non-overweight children. Longitudinal studies of children who became overweight have shown that height gain accelerates or follows shortly after, excessive weight gain (Freedman et al. 2005).

Various endocrine disorders are associated with increased BMI. However, in those with growth hormone deficiency, hypopituitarism, hypothyroidism, hypothalamic disease, Cushing syndrome and pseudohypoparathyroidism, obesity is usually associated with short stature and a reduced height velocity.

Pubertal assessment (with a chaperone as is always good practice) is very important in the obese patient. Premature puberty is linked to elements of metabolic syndrome and PCOS and thus it is important to monitor these children as they mature (Ibanez et al. 2000).

On the other hand, both hyper- and hypogonadotrophic hypogonadism may be associated with excess weight gain.

Thyroid function
Hypothyroidism does not usually cause severe obesity, and patients may have goitre. In adults, thyroid hormone and thyroid-stimulating hormone (TSH) concentrations have been described as normal, elevated or reduced. In obese children, the most common abnormality is hyperthyrotropinemia. These changes are thought to be functional and do normalise with weight loss, and management of an elevated TSH is not usually necessary by treatment with thyroxine (Longhi and Radetti 2013).

Other complications of obesity
These include urinary incontinence, idiopathic intracranial hypertension (which has an increased prevalence of 15-fold with increasing obesity and can be associated with visual loss), orthopaedic complications including Blount disease and slipped capital femoral epiphysis and skin conditions such as acanthosis nigricans, skin tags, furunculosis and intertrigo.

Psychological comorbidities
There is evidence that childhood obesity impacts on self-esteem and quality of life (Griffiths et al. 2010). In adolescence, it has been associated with depression (Sjoberg et al. 2005), experience of bullying and stigma (Griffiths et al. 2006), which can also impact on their self-esteem. Some of these issues may, in turn, lead to under-achievement at school (Bromfield 2009). There is evidence that sexual and physical abuse increases the risk of severe obesity (Gustafson and Sarwer 2004). Depression may result from obesity or precipitate it. It is important to look for purging behaviour and related eating disorders.

Clinical assessment of the obese child/adolescent
The NICE guidance and the UK OSCA consensus statement on the assessment of obese children and adolescents for paediatricians advise that the following children be seen by paediatricians:

A. Children with BMI ≥98th centile who fulfill the following criteria: (i) the child or family are seeking help/treatment and (ii) the child has one or more risk factors for either possible underlying pathology or future morbidity.
B. Any child with extreme obesity. Those extremely obese should be referred regardless of additional risk factors. There are no currently agreed definitions for extreme obesity. It is suggested that any child with a BMI >3.5 standard deviation above the mean should be regarded as having extreme obesity, as this is equivalent at age 18 years to the adult definition of morbid obesity (BMI ≥40kg/m^2).

The initial assessment appointment with a child with obesity and his/her family includes a focus on establishing a rapport, identifying the degree of obesity, evaluating the underlying aetiologies contributing to the excess weight gain, screening for the presence of current and future risk of weight-related comorbidities, identification of modifiable lifestyle behaviours and assessment of patient and family engagement.

It should include a detailed history, clinical examination and appropriate investigations. Thereafter, it is important to work together with the family and other multidisciplinary team members to initiate an appropriate treatment plan.

It is very important to consider the environment in which this is undertaken. This includes offering appropriately sized furniture and equipment, and time alone with the young person.

History

When taking a history from an obese child or adolescent and their family, it is important, as usual in paediatric and adolescent medicine, to create a non-judgemental engagement with the young person and his or her family. It is important to explore their expectations of the appointment, in order to ensure a shared agenda for the consultation, and to engage the young person with obesity by talking about his or her skills and attributes before focusing on the weight.

Once a rapport is established, a full history is undertaken in order to ascertain the aetiology and comorbidities of obesity. Specific pointers in the history are highlighted in Table 11.6.

Clinical examination

Clinical examination is essential (see Table 11.7 for a summary). An accurate measurement of weight and height and BMI should be plotted on BMI centile chart, and BP should be taken. It is unclear whether waist circumference is helpful in the clinical situation. A waist circumference at assessment may be useful for assessing risk of comorbidity associated with central adiposity by comparison with published UK centiles (McCarthy et al. 2003). However, the clinical utility of change in waist circumference over time is unclear due to very poor reproducibility in clinical settings (Rudolph et al. 2007).

The OSCA does not recommend waist circumference to be used as a clinical marker of adiposity change in obese children. A full examination including pubertal assessment should be performed looking for any endocrine, neurodevelopmental or genetic causes and comorbidities.

Investigation of a child or an adolescent with body mass index >98th centile

This is a controversial area with little data to guide practice. The OSCA network suggests that the investigation for comorbidities should be routine but the investigation into causes of obesity should be performed in specific cases. In an obese child, assessment for comorbidities includes the routine measurement of fasting lipids and total cholesterol, glucose, insulin, HbA1C, liver function test for raised ALT, C-reactive protein and thyroid function tests plus additional blood tests as indicated above depending on history and examination. It is not routine to perform an oral glucose tolerance test but suggested if BMI >98th centile and >2 of the following are present: family history T2DM; ethnicity South Asian, middle-eastern, Hispanic or African; clinical signs of insulin insensitivity such as acanthosis nigricans or hyperinsulinaemia or dyslipidaemia; signs of PCOS; and extreme obesity. A pelvic ultrasound can be useful.

TABLE 11.6
Clinical history to ascertain causes and comorbidities

Weight history	Birth weight
	Weight trajectory. (obesity <6 months consider leptin signalling pathway defects)
	Precipitating events
	Previous interventions
	Recent weight loss or gain
	Level of physical activity
Dietary history	Hyperphagia? Night eating?
	Dietary – meals, snacks, take away, fruit and vegetables,
	Drinks: juice, high-energy/fizzy drinks
Developmental history	Birth – weight, type of delivery, gestational age
	Developmental milestones
	Intellectual ability and schooling
Past medical history	Previous illness, surgery or injury
Drug history	CNS surgery or illness
	Use of glucocorticoids, anti-psychotics and other weight-increasing medications
Family history	Consanguinity
Social history	Weight
	Type 2 diabetes, stroke, hypertension, cardiovascular disease, dyslipidaemia, obesity, sleep apnoea, PCOS, bariatric surgery, eating disorders
	Family stressors, e.g. bereavement, divorce
	Family support – accepting, sustaining and supporting change
	Is there social work support?
Mental health	Anxiety
	Anger and behavioural problems
	Depression
	Bullying
	Self-esteem
Menstrual history in girls	Regularity and dysmenorrhoea
Systems review generally and assess for comorbidities	Bones and joints
	Physical ability/disability
	Signs of sleep apnoea: difficulty breathing during sleep, snoring, morning headaches
	Fatigue
	Gastrointestinal: constipation, gastro-oesophageal reflux symptoms, vomiting, abdominal pain
	Genitourinary: enuresis
	CNS: headaches, visual disturbance
Sleep	Associations between lack of sleep and obesity
	Sleep: routine and amount of sleep
Screen time	Include television, social media, gaming, phone –
	do they sleep with phone on?
	Limit to 1–2 hours quality screen time
HEADS psychosocial screening tool (young person alone)	Explain confidentiality and then ask open non-judgemental questions about home, education, activities, friendships, school, drugs, alcohol, smoking, sexual relationships, mood including suicidal ideation
Motivation to change	Assess importance, confidence and priority of getting in charge of overweight

CNS, central nervous system; PCOS, polycystic ovary syndrome.

TABLE 11.7
The clinical assessment and investigations in a child >95th centile for body mass index

System	Features	Explanation	Investigations/referral/ treatment
General	Accurate weight and height measurement – plot body mass index (BMI) on age and sex-specific chart abdominal circumference – see text		
	BMI >95th centile – with short stature for family and low-height velocity	Endocrine disorders – e.g. hypothyroidism, growth hormone deficiency if short stature and/or low-height velocity	Refer to endocrinologist for further assessment – TFTs, early morning cortisol
			Midnight cortisol/ACTH
	Buffalo hump	Cushing syndrome/disease	Urinary-free cortisol Dexamethasone suppression
	Red hair	*POMC* mutation	
	Dysmorphic features, Small hands and feet	Genetic causes	
		e.g. Prader–Willi syndrome, pseudohypoparathyroidism or pseudopseudo-hypoparathyroidism	
			Refer to geneticist
			Calcium and phosphate
	Polydactyly, retinal dystrophy	Bardet-Biedl syndrome	Genetic testing
Vital signs	Elevated blood pressure (BP)	Hypertension	Systolic BP readings (>90th centile for age, sex and height on >3 occasions)
CNS	Visual disturbance (diplopia, VI nerve palsy)	Idiopathic intracranial hypertension	CT/MRI brain/pituitary and urgent referral to neurologist
	Difficulties with balance and coordination		
Eyes	Papilloedema	Idiopathic intracranial hypertension	Ophthalmology review
	VI cranial nerve paralysis	(pseudomotor cerebri)	
Throat/neck	Tonsillar hypertrophy	Risk of sleep apnoea	Chervin paediatric sleep questionnaire, Polysomnography
	Goitre	Thyroid disease	TFTs
Mouth	Dental health	Dental caries – High-sugar drinks	Dentist

(Continued)

TABLE 11.7
(Continued)

System	Features	Explanation	Investigations/referral/ treatment
Skin	Acanthosis nigricans (thickened darkened skin in neck and axilla)	Insulin insensitivity Type 2 diabetes mellitus	HbA1c, fasting glucose
	Acne	PCOS	Androgens (DHEAS, testosterone, androstenedione), FSH,
	Hirsutism		LH, SHBG, pelvic ultrasound scan (USS)
	Violacious striae	Cushing	
	Other striae	General obesity	Early morning and midnight cortisol
	Intertrigo	Skin infection under folds	
	Infections		Hygiene, antibiotics, dermatology referral
Abdominal	Hepatomegaly	NAFLD	ALT (usually twice above normal) i.e. >70 for liver USS – if >120 refer to
	Tenderness	Gallstones, GOR	hepatologist
			Abdominal USS
Cardiovascular	ECG – LVH	LVH RVH – Sleep apnoea associated RHF	Paediatric sleep questionnaire
Chest	Wheezing	Asthma	
	Gynaecomastia	Obesity related – peripheral aromatisation of oestrogen associated with body image and self-esteem as well as impact on PE at school	Breast surgeon and clinical psychologist
Extremities	Abnormal gait	SCFE	Orthopaedics and physiotherapy
	Limited hip range of movement	SCFE	
	Bowing of tibia	Blount disease	
Reproductive system	Tanner staging	Premature puberty	
	Undescended testes	Prader–Willi syndrome	Genetics for Ch15
	Apparent micropenis	May be normal – buried penis	
	PCOS		Adrenal androgens, FSH, LH, 17-OHP, SHBG, prolactin

ACTH, adrenocorticotropic hormone; POMC, proopiomelanocortin; TFTs, thyroid function tests; PCOS, polycystic ovary syndrome; DHEAS, dehydroepiandrosterone sulphate; FSH, follicle-stimulating hormone; LH, luteinizing hormone; GOR, gastro-oesophageal reflux; LVH, left ventricular hypertrophy; RVH, right ventricular hypertrophy; SCFE, slipped capital femoral epiphysis.

Treatment

Treatment in childhood and adolescent obesity is aimed at treating comorbidities and aiming to stop weight gain in a growing child, with a view to reducing weight.

There are several broad principles of conventional management: management of co-morbidities, family involvement, taking a developmentally appropriate approach, the use of a range of behaviour-modification techniques, long-term dietary change, increased physical activity, increase in sleep and decreased sedentary behaviours (Baur et al. 2011).

The treatment options progress from single modality, that is, dietitian alone, exercise alone, or multicomponent lifestyle change incorporating ideally a healthier diet, increased energy expenditure and reduction of sedentary behaviour. This usually involves a family approach as the whole family needs to be involved in lifestyle changes.

Specific comorbidities requiring treatment include those mentioned earlier in the chapter including hypercholesterolaemia, hyperlipidaemia, reduced insulin sensitivity and type 2 diabetes, orthopaedic comorbidities including knee pain, OSA, and psychological comorbidities such as depression and low self-esteem.

Note that prevention of obesity is important but will not be discussed here.

The studies of treatment modalities mentioned below have differing criteria for outcomes, for example, BMI/future cardiovascular risk.

McGovern et al. (2008) reviewed 61 interventions to treat childhood and adolescent obesity. Only 23% of these resulted in a significant decrease in adiposity. Most of these interventions were short term and follow-up data were, for the most part, not available. Statistically significant reduction in BMI was found with sibutramine (no longer licensed), orlistat and lifestyle interventions. The most recent Cochrane analysis of interventions to treat childhood and adolescent obesity reviewed 64 studies (Oude Luttikhuis et al. 2009). Only 12 of these studies lent themselves to pooled analyses. In general, most of the studies that were included in the pooled analyses achieved positive outcomes. Family-targeted behavioural lifestyle interventions seemed most effective, and combined diet, physical activity and behavioural interventions were suggested as promising areas for future efforts. Unfortunately, most of the studies included in this review were underpowered.

Recommendations for the future include larger-scale interventions with process and fidelity measures and cost/effectiveness analyses. The authors emphasise the need for including psychosocial mediators of behaviour change and building interventions based on psychosocial theory.

Exercise

Exercise prescriptions have been shown to be effective at reducing body fat. Based on the small number of short-term randomised trials currently available, an aerobic exercise prescription of 155–180 min/week at moderate to high intensity is effective for reducing body fat in overweight children/adolescents, but effects on body weight and central obesity are inconclusive (Atlantis et al. 2006). This is still lower than the 60 minutes a day recommended by the Physical Activity Guidelines Advisory Committee (2008).

Motivational interviewing
A systematic review and meta-analysis (Armstrong 2011) showed that motivational interviewing was associated with a greater reduction in body mass compared to controls (standardised mean difference = −0.51 [95% CI, −1.04, 0.01]). There was a significant reduction in body weight (kg) for those in the intervention group compared with those in the control group (weighted mean difference = −1.47kg [95% CI, −2.05, −0.88]). For the BMI outcome, the weighted mean difference was −0.25kg/m² (95% CI, −0.50, 0.01). Thus, motivational interviewing appears to enhance weight loss in overweight and obese patients.

Dietary interventions
The first specific review assessing dietary interventions found positive effects of interventions that included a dietary component (Collins et al. 2006, 2007).

Ho et al. (2012) conducted a review of randomised controlled trials including children and adolescents <18 years old that compared the effectiveness of lifestyle intervention programmes incorporating a nutrition or dietary component with no treatment or a waiting list control.

BMI and BMI z scores were used as weight loss outcomes, as well as body composition (% body fat). Cardiometabolic outcomes were also examined. Interventions that included diet therapy generally resulted in significant weight loss, at least in the short term. Limitations of these studies were found to be poor design or minimal follow-up. Details of the dietary intervention and adherence to it were poorly reported. There is therefore an urgent need for high-quality studies investigating the optimal dietary approach to management of paediatric overweight and obesity (Collins 2007).

Ho (2013) reviewed 15 studies assessing dietary interventions with or without exercise interventions, both of which resulted in weight loss and metabolic profile improvement. However, the addition of exercise to dietary intervention led to greater improvements in concentrations of high-density lipoprotein cholesterol (3.86 mg/dL; 95% CI, 2.70 to 4.63), fasting glucose (−2.16 mg/dL; 95% CI, −3.78 to −0.72) and fasting insulin (−2.75 μIU/mL; 95% CI, −4.50 to −1.00) over 6 months. The diet-only intervention caused greater reductions in concentrations of triglycerides and low-density lipoprotein cholesterol.

In the adult population, high-protein, low-carbohydrate diets and 5:2 diets are being trialed, with initial positive effects; however, initial evidence indicates that the optimal diet is one to which the patient can adhere.

There are quite detailed evidence-based dietary recommendations in the Expert Panel on Integrated Guidelines for Cardiovascular Health and Risk Reduction in Children and Adolescents, which include 2010 dietary guidelines for Americans and the NCEP paediatric panel report 1992.

These findings are echoed by the position paper for the Academy of Nutrition and Dietetics where Hoelscher et al. (2013) advocate systems-level approaches for the prevention and treatment of paediatric overweight and obesity that include the skills of registered dietitians, as well as environmental support across all sectors of society. This position paper provides guidance and recommendations for levels of intervention targeting overweight and obesity prevention and treatment from preschool age through to adolescence. Methods included a review of the literature from 2009 to April 2012, including the academy's 2009 evidence analysis of school-based reviews. Multicomponent interventions showed the greatest impact for primary prevention; secondary prevention and tertiary prevention/treatment should emphasise sustained family-based, developmentally appropriate approaches that include nutrition education, dietary counselling, parenting skills, behavioural strategies and physical-activity promotion.

Lifestyle interventions

Lifestyle interventions including a combination of diet, exercise and/or behaviour modification are an essential part of obesity management (NICE 2010; SIGN 2010; NHMRC 2003).

Several systematic reviews of the management of childhood obesity have been published, and these assessed lifestyle interventions, and found that they are efficacious on weight in the short and medium terms (McGovern et al. 2008; Whitlock et al. 2010; Kelly et al. 2011). The body of research reviewed suggests that lifestyle interventions incorporating a dietary component along with an exercise and/or behavioural therapy component are effective in treating childhood obesity and improving the cardio-metabolic outcomes under a wide range of conditions, at least up to 1 year (Ho et al. 2012).

NICE guidelines for lifestyle weight management services exist after assessing the evidence, for children aged 6–18 years. These guidelines advocate multicomponent lifestyle weight management programmes, which have been developed by, and include input from, a multidisciplinary team. The core components should include behaviour-change techniques, positive parenting skills training and a tailored plan to meet individual needs, appropriate to the child or young person's age, sex, ethnicity, cultural background, economic and family circumstances, any special needs and how obese or overweight they are. Help should be available to identify opportunities to become less sedentary and the aim should be to achieve the age-specific UK physical activity guidelines. Dietary changes that are age-appropriate, affordable, culturally sensitive and consistent with healthy-eating advice should be adopted.

Drugs/medication

Many anti-obesity drugs have been trialled and prescribed since amphetamines were first used in the 1950s, and ongoing studies are utilising improved understanding of gut-brain and fat-signalling pathways to develop new drug targets (Rodgers et al. 2012). Whilst many showed promising results, all but one were subsequently withdrawn from the UK market. Their central drug targets resulted in unacceptable side effects, and most recently, sibutramine was withdrawn following cardiac events in those with pre-existing heart disease (Scheen 2011). Only two drugs are currently used in adolescents in the United Kingdom, with only modest outcomes compared to bariatric surgery. Meta-analyses of randomised controlled trials show BMI changes of 1.42kg/m^2 with metformin (Park et al. 2009) and 0.83kg/m^2 with orlistat (Viner et al. 2010). Their use is currently limited, with high levels of discontinuation likely related to their side-effect profile and inadequate ongoing support (Viner et al. 2009).

Metformin has anorexigenic and weight-loss properties, decreases gastrointestinal glucose absorption and increases insulin sensitivity by increasing glucose uptake and

AMP-kinase-mediated oxidative glucose and lipid metabolism. As such, it is used in those with diabetes; its use in those with insulin insensitivity and 'pre-diabetes' is controversial and is usually initiated by endocrinologists. Its role in the treatment of polycystic ovarian syndrome is less controversial and it is commonly used for this indication.

Orlistat is the only licensed anti-obesity drug recommended in the United Kingdom (NICE Guidelines 2006). Few patients tolerate it and most self-terminate it due to the gastrointestinal sequelae (pain, bloating, nausea, diarrhoea and faecal incontinence) experienced after a meal containing moderate to high levels of fat. Those who benefit from it are likely to use it as an educational feedback tool to identify, and in future avoid, food items that are inconsistent with a low-fat diet. Good practice is to start on a low-fat diet with dietician support before trialing orlistat, and to take multivitamin supplements that contain fat-soluble vitamins.

Bariatric surgery

The BMI outcomes associated with bariatric surgery far exceed those of any other intervention currently available (Black et al. 2013). Bariatric surgery has predominantly been performed in adolescents, with much smaller numbers in younger children (Alqahtani et al. 2012). Only one randomised control trial has been performed to date, comparing 2-year outcomes of adjustable gastric band (AGB) to placebo (O'Brien et al. 2010). Two high-quality non-randomised longitudinal studies are ongoing, the Teenlabs (Inge et al. 2007) and AMOS (Olbers et al. 2012) consortia based in Midwest United States and Sweden, respectively. The long-term data associated with adolescent surgery are currently limited, with few data beyond 2 years. Current outcomes are comparable with those in adults, with meta-analysis of 1-year BMI outcomes showing the largest effect in Roux-en-y gastric bypass (RYGB), then sleeve gastrectomy and the least effect was observed with AGB ($-17. 2$, -14.5 and $-10.5kg/m^2$, respectively) (Black et al. 2013).

These procedures were initially considered to be effective simply as a result of calorie restriction; however, subsequent publications have demonstrated significant changes in hormonal and neural homeostatic mechanisms controlling hunger, satiety and glucose homeostasis, and RYGB is thought to have the largest effect not because of malabsorption and restriction, but because of these homeostatic changes involving gut hormones, vagal nerve, bile acids and the gut microbiome (Madsbad et al. 2014).

Mortality and morbidity appear low compared to adults, with no reported adolescent deaths to date (Black et al. 2013). The greatest concerns about morbidity are related to peri-operative anastomotic leaks after sleeve gastrectomy and RYGB, spontaneous late gastric perforations after AGB, strictures, and complications related to the combination of poor fat-soluble vitamin absorption after RYGB and poor compliance with vitamin supplementation.

The data supporting RYGB are strongest, in terms of both BMI outcomes and patient numbers and, as such, is increasingly the intervention of choice for adolescents. BMI thresholds of $35kg/m^2$ in those with obesity-related comorbidities such as type 2 diabetes and hypertension and $40kg/m^2$ in the remainder have been recommended by the majority of national bodies (NICE Guidelines, Brei and Mudd 2014). Despite this, there is ongoing controversy about the selection of patients, and which procedure they should undergo.

In summary, the role of the paediatrician or endocrinologist in relation to childhood and adolescent obesity is to make a diagnosis of the degree of obesity, determine any causal or contributing factors, identify comorbidities and advise on further investigation of possible causes or comorbidities. Treatment should be multicomponent when possible, involving dietary, exercise and behavioural components, and convenient for the young person and family. Medical treatment such as drugs or bariatric surgery should be discussed and offered where indicated. The young person should be followed regularly for development of comorbidities.

REFERENCES

ADA – Diagnostic criteria for T2DM.

Alqahtani AR, Antonisamy B, Alamri H, Elahmedi M and Zimmerman VA (2012) Laparoscopic sleeve gastrectomy in 108 obese children and adolescents aged 5 to 21 years. *Ann Surg* 256: 266–273.

Alonso-Álvarez ML, Cordero-Guevara JA, Terán-Santos J et al. (2014) Obstructive sleep apnea in obese community-dwelling children: The NANOS study. *Sleep* 37(5): 943–949.

Armstrong MJ, Mottershead TA, Ronksley PE, Sigal RJ, Campbell TS and Hemmelgarn BR (2011) Motivational interviewing to improve weight loss in overweight and/or obese patients: A systematic review and meta-analysis of randomized controlled trials. *Obes Rev.: An Official Journal of the International Association for the Study of Obesity* 12: 709–723. doi:10.1111/j.1467-789X.2011.00892.x

Atlantis E, Barnes EH and Singh MA (2006) Efficacy of exercise for treating overweight in children and adolescents: A systematic review. *Int J Obes* 30: 1027–1040.

Baumgartner RN, Heymsfield SB and Lichtman S (1991) Body composition in elderly people: Effect of criterion estimates on predictive equations. *Am J Clin Nutr* 53: 1345–1353.

Baur LA, Hazelton B and Shrewsbury VA (2011) Assessment and management of obesity in childhood and adolescence. *Nat Rev Gastroenterol Hepatol* 8(11): 635–45. doi:10.1038/nrgastro.2011.165

Black JA, White B, Viner RM and Simmons RK (2013) Bariatric surgery for obese children and adolescents: A systematic review and meta-analysis. *Obes Rev.*

Berenson GS, Srinivasan SR, Bao W et al. (1998) Association between multiple cardiovascular risk factors and atherosclerosis in children and young adults. The Bogalusa Heart Study. *Engl J Med* 338(23): 1650–6.

Brei MN and Mudd S (2014) Current guidelines for weight loss surgery in adolescents: A review of the literature. *J Pediatr Health Care: Official Publication of National Association of Pediatric Nurse Associates & Practitioners* 28: 288–294.

Bromfield PV (2009) Childhood obesity: Psychosocial outcomes and the role of weight bias and stigma. *Educational Psychology in Practice* 25: 193–209.

Bull FC and the Expert Working Groups (2010) Physical Activity Guidelines in the U.K.: Review and Recommendations. School of Sport, Exercise and Health Sciences, Loughborough University.

Chen X, Beydoun MA and Wang Y (2008) Is sleep duration associated with childhood obesity? A systematic review and meta-analysis 6 SEP 2012. North American Association for the Study of Obesity (NAASO).

Cole TJ, Freeman JV and Preece MA (1995) Body mass index reference curves for the UK, 1990. *Arch Dis Child* 73(1): 25–29.

Cole TJ and Lobstein T (2012) Extended international (IOTF) body mass index cut-offs for thinness, overweight and obesity. *Pediatr Obes* 7(4): 284–294.

Collins CE, Warren JM, Neve M, McCoy P and Stokes BJ (2006) Measuring effectiveness of dietetic interventions in child obesity: A systematic review of randomized trials. *Arch Pediatr Adolesc Med* 160(9): 906–922.

Collins CE, Warren JM, Neve M, McCoy P and Stokes BJ (2007) Systematic review of interventions in the management of overweight and obese children which include a dietary component. *Int J Evid-Based Healthc* 5(1): 2–53.

Cook S, Weitzman M, Auinger P, Nyugen M and Dietz WH (2003) Prevalence of metabolic syndrome phenotype in adolescents: Findings from the third National Health and Nutrition Examination Survey, 1988–1994. *Arch Pediatr Adol Med* 157: 821–827.

Craig LC, Love J, Ratcliffe B and McNeill G (2008) Overweight and cardiovascular risk factors in 4- to 18-year-olds. *Obes Facts* 1(5): 237–42. doi: 10.1159/000156720.

Diabetes UK facts and stats (2014).

Ebbeling CB, Leidig MM, Sinclair KB et al. (2003) A reduced-glycemic load diet in the treatment of adolescent obesity. *Arch Pediatr Adolesc Med* 157: 773–779.

Expert Panel on Integrated Guidelines for Cardiovascular Health and Risk Reduction in Children and Adolescents (2011) Expert Panel on Integrated Guidelines for Cardiovascular Health and Risk Reduction in Children and Adolescents: Summary Report. *Pediatrics* 128(Suppl 5): S213–S256. doi: 10.1542/peds.2009-2107C. Epub 2011 Nov 14.

Fagot-Campagna A, Pettitt DJ, Engelgau MM et al. (2000) Type 2 diabetes among North American children and adolescents: An epidemiologic review and a public health perspective. *J Pediatr* 136: 664–672.

Fishman L, Lenders C, Fortunato C, Noonan C and Nurko S (2004) Increased prevalence of constipation and fecal soiling in a population of obese children. *J Pediatr* 145: 253–254.

The Foresight report http://www.bis.gov.uk/foresight/MediaList/foresight/media%20library/BISPartners/Foresight/docs/obesity/~/media/BISPartners/Foresight/docs/obesity/0

Freedman DS, Kettel L, Serdula MK, Dietz WH, Srinivasan SR and Berenson GS (2005) The relation of childhood BMI to adult adiposity: The Bogalusa Heart Study. *Pediatrics* 115: 22–27.

Freedman DS, Khan LK, Dietz WH, Srinivasan SR and Breneson GS (2001) Relationship of childhood obesity to coronary heart disease risk factors in adulthood: The Bogalusa Heart Study. *Pediatrics* 108: 712–718.

Freedman DS, Srinivasan SR, Burke GL et al. (1987) Relation of body fat distribution to hyperinsulinemia in children and adolescents: The Bogalusa Heart Study. *Am J Clin Nutr* 46: 403–410.

Freedman DS, Srinivasan SR, Harsha DW et al. (1989) Relation of body fat patterning to lipid and lipoprotein concentrations in children and adolescents: The Bogalusa Heart Study. *Am J Clin Nutr* 50: 930–939.

Freedman DS1, Mei Z, Srinivasan SR, Berenson GS and Dietz WH (2007) Cardiovascular risk factors and excess adiposity among overweight children and adolescents: the Bogalusa Heart Study. *J Pediatr* 150(1): 12–17.e2.

Freemark M and Bursey D (2001) The effects of metformin on body mass index and glucose tolerance in obese adolescents with fasting hyperinsulinemia and a family history of type 2 diabetes. *Pediatrics* 107: E55.

Frey U, Latzin P, Usemann J, Maccora J, Zumsteg U and Kriemler S (2014) Asthma and obesity in children: Current evidence and potential systems biology approaches. *Allergy* 70: 26–40.

Gileles-Hillel A, Alonso-Álvarez ML, Kheirandish-Gozal L et al. (2014) Inflammatory markers and obstructive sleep apnea in obese children: the NANOS study. Mediators Inflamm. 2014(2014): 605280. doi: 10.1155/2014/605280.

Griffiths LJ, Wolke D, Page AS, Horwood JP (2006)ALSPAC Study Team. Obesity and bullying: different effects for boys and girls. *Arch Dis Child* 91(2): 121–5. Epub 2005 Sep 20.

Griffiths LJ, Parsons TJ and Hill AJ (2010) Self-esteem and quality of life in obese children and adolescents: a systematic review. *Int J Pediatr Obes* 5(4): 282–304. doi: 10.3109/17477160903473697.

Gustafson TB and Sarwer DB (2004) Childhood sexual abuse and obesity. *Obes Rev* 5: 129–135.

Haemer MA, Grow HM, Fernandez C et al. (2014) Addressing prediabetes in childhood obesity treatment programs: Support from research and current practice. *Child Obes* 10(4): 292–303. doi: 10.1089/chi.2013.0158. Epub 2014 Jul 23.

A Health survey for England 2012. – http://www.hscic.gov.uk/catalogue/PUB13218/HSE2012-Sum-bklet.pdf

Ho M, Garnett SP, Baur LA et al. (2012) Effectiveness of lifestyle interventions in child obesity: A systematic review with meta-analysis. *Obes Res Clin Pract* doi:10.1016/j.

Ho M, Garnett SP, Baur LA et al. (2013) Impact of dietary and exercise interventions on weight change and metabolic outcomes in obese children and adolescents: A systematic review and meta-analysis of randomized trials. *JAMA Pediatr* 167: 759–768.

Hoelscher DM, Kirk S, Ritchie L and Cunningham-Sabo L (2013) Position of the Academy of Nutrition and Dietetics: Interventions for the prevention and treatment of pediatric overweight and obesity. *J Acad Nutr Diet* 113: 1375–1394. doi:10.1016/j.jand.2013.08.004.

Ibanez L, Dimartino-Nardi J, Potau N and Seanger P (2000) Premature adrenarche – Normal variant or frontrunner of adult disease? *Endocr Rev* 21: 671–696.

Inge TH, Zeller M, Harmon C et al. (2007) Teen-Longitudinal Assessment of Bariatric Surgery: Methodological features of the first prospective multicenter study of adolescent bariatric surgery. *J Pediatr Surg* 42: 1969–1971.

Jago R, Harrell JS, McMurray RG, Edelstein S, El Ghormli L and Bassin S (2006) Prevalence of abnormal lipid and blood pressure values among an ethnically diverse population of eigth-grade adolescents and screening implications. *Pediatrics* 117: 2065–2073.

Johnson RK (2002) Dietary intake: How do we measure what people are really eating? *Obes Res* 10(Suppl 1): 63S–68S.

Kay JP, Alemzadeh R, Langley G et al. (2001) Beneficial effects of metformin in normoglycemic morbidly obese adolescents. *Metabolism* 50: 1457–1461.

Kelly KP and Kirschenbaum DS (2011) Immersion treatment of childhood and adolescent obesity: The first review of a promising intervention. *Obes Rev* 12(1): 37–49.

Kirpichnikov D, McFarlane SI and Sowers JR (2002) Metformin: An update. *Ann Intern Med* 137: 25–33.

Koebnick C, Smith N, Black MH et al. (2012) Pediatric obesity and gallstone disease. *J Pediatr Gastroenterol Nutr* 55(3):328–33. doi:10.1097/MPG.0b013e31824d256f.

Kuczmarski RJ, Ogden C, Grummer-Strawn L et al. (2000) *CDC Growth Charts: United States*. Advance Data Report No. 314. Vital and Health Statistics of the Centers for Disease Control and Prevention. National Center for Health Statistics, 2000.

L'Abée C, Visser GH, Liem ET, Kok DE, Sauer PJ and Stolk RP (2010) Comparison of methods to assess body fat in non-obese six to seven-year-old children. *Clin Nutr* 29(3): 317–322.

Liese AD, D'Agostino Jr RB, Hamman RF et al. (2006) The burden of diabetes mellitus amont US youth: Prevalence estimates form the SEARCH for Diabetes in Youth Study. *Pediatrics* 118: 1510–1518.

Logue J, Thompson L, Romanes F, Wilson DC, Thompson J, Sattar N; Guideline Development Group (2010) Management of obesity: Summary of SIGN guideline. *BMJ* 340: c154.

Logue J and Sattar N (2011) Childhood obesity: a ticking time bomb for cardiovascular disease? *Clin Pharmacol Ther* 90(1): 174–8. doi: 10.1038/clpt.2011.88.

Lohman TG (1989) Assessment of body composition in children. *Pediatric Exercise Science* 1: 19–30.

Longhi S and Radetti G Thyroid function and obesity. *J Clin Res Pediatr Endocrinol*.

Loomba R, Sirlin CB, Schwimmer JB and Lavine JE (2009) Advances in pediatric nonalcoholic fatty liver disease. *Hepatology* 50(4): 1282–1293.

Lopes HMS (2012) Diagnostic accuracy of CDC, IOTF and WHO criteria for obesity classification, in a Portuguese school-aged children population. Maestrado en Saúde Pública. Universidad do Porto. Facultade de Medicina. Instituto de Ciências Biomédicas Abel Salazar.

Lurbe E, Alvarez V and Redon J (2001) Obesity, body fat distribution and ambulatory blood pressure in children and adolescents. *J Clin Hypertens (Greenwich)* 3: 362–367.

Madsbad S, Dirksen C and Holst JJ (2014) Mechanisms of changes in glucose metabolism and bodyweight after bariatric surgery. *Lancet Diabetes Endocrinol* 2(2): 152–164.

Mastorakos G, Lambrinoudaki I and Creatsas G (2006) Polycystic ovary syndrome in adolescents: Current and future treatment options. *Pediatr Drugs* 8(5): 311–318.

McCarthy HD, Ellis SM and Cole TJ (2003) Central overweight and obesity in British youth aged 11–16 years: Cross sectional surveys of waist circumference. *BMJ* 326(7390).

McCartney CR, Blank SK, Prendergast KA et al. (2007) Obesity and sex steroid changes across puberty:evidence for marked hyperandrogenemia in pre and early pubertal obese girls. *J Clin Endocrinol Metab* 92: 430–436.

McGill HC Jr1, McMahan CA, Herderick EE et al. (2000) Origin of atherosclerosis in childhood and adolescence. *Am J Clin Nutr* 72(5 Suppl): 1307S–1315S.

McGovern L, Johnson JN, Paulo R et al. (2008) Clinical review: Treatment of pediatric obesity: A systematic review and meta-analysis of randomized trials. *J Clin Endocrinol Metab* 93(12): 4600–4605.

Musso G, Cassader M, Rosina F and Gambino R Impact of current treatments on liver disease, glucose metabolism and cardiovascular risk in non-alcoholic fatty liver disease (NAFLD): A systematic review and meta-analysis of randomised trials.

National Cholesterol Education Program (NCEP) Expert Panel on Detection, Evaluation, and Treatment of High Blood Cholesterol in Adults (Adult Treatment Panel III) (2002) Third Report of the National Cholesterol Education Program (NCEP) Expert Panel on Detection, Evaluation, and Treatment of High Blood Cholesterol in Adults (Adult Treatment Panel III) final report. *Circulation* 106(25): 3143–3421.

National Health and Medical Research Council (2003) *Clinical Practice Guidelines for the Management of Overweight and Obesity in Children and Adolescents*. Canberra, Australia.

NICE public health guidance 47 (2013) Managing overweight and obesity among children and young people: Lifestyle weight management services.

National Institute for Health and Clinical Excellence (2006) *NICE Clinical Guideline 43 Obesity: Guidance on the Prevention, Identification, Assessment and Management of Overweight and Obesity in Adults and Children.* London, UK: NICE (last updated in 2010).

Nobili V and Manco M (2007) Therapeutic strategies for pediatric non-alcoholic fatty liver disease: a challenge for health care providers. *World J Gastroenterol* 13(18): 2639–41.

O'Brien PE, Sawyer SM, Laurie C et al. (2010) Laparoscopic adjustable gastric banding in severely obese adolescents. A randomised trial. *JAMA* 303: 519–522.

Office of the Surgeon General (2010) *The Surgeon General's Vision for a Healthy and Fit Nation.* [pdf 840K]. Rockville, MD: U.S. Department of Health and Human Services.

Olbers T, Gronowitz E, Werling M et al. (2012) Two-year outcome of laparoscopic Roux-en-Y gastric bypass in adolescents with severe obesity: Results from a Swedish Nationwide Study (AMOS). *Int J Obes* 36: 1388–1395.

Oude Luttikhuis H, Baur L, Jansen H et al. (2009) Review interventions for treating obesity in children. *Cochrane Database Syst Rev* 1: CD001872.

Park MH, Kinra S, Ward KJ, White B and Viner RM (2009) Metformin for obesity in children and adolescents: A systematic review. *Diabetes Care* 32: 1743–1745.

Pinhas-Hamiel O and Zeitler P (2005) The global spread of type 2 diabetes mellitus in children and adolescents. *J Pediatr* 146: 693–700.

Quinn SM, Baur LA, Garnett SP and Cowell CT (2010) Treatment of clinical insulin resistance in children: A systematic review. *Obes Rev* 11: 722–730.

Rodgers RJ, Tschop MH and Wilding JP (2012) Anti-obesity drugs: Past, present and future. *Dis Model Mech* 5: 621–626.

Rojas J, Chávez M, Olivar L et al. Review article polycystic ovary syndrome, insulin resistance, and obesity: Navigating the pathophysiologic labyrinth.

Rudolf MC, Walker J and Cole TJ (2007) What is the best way to measure waist circumference? *Int J Pediatr Obes* 2(1): 58–61.

Savoye M, Caprio S, Dziura J et al. (2014) Reversal of early abnormalities in glucose metabolism in obese youth: Results of an intensive lifestyle randomized controlled trial. *Diabetes Care* 37: 317–324.

Savoye M, Shaw M, Dziura J et al. (2007) Effects of a weight management program on body composition and metabolic parameters in overweight children: A randomized controlled trial. *JAMA* 297: 2697–2704.

Scheen AJ (2011) Sibutramine on cardiovascular outcome. *Diabetes Care* 34(Suppl 2): S114–S119.

Schipper HS, Nuboer R, Prop S et al. (2012) Systemic inflammation in childhood obesity: Circulating inflammatory mediators and activated CD14++ monocytes. *Diabetologia* 55(10): 2800–2810. doi: 10.1007/s00125-012-2641-y. Epub 2012 Jul 18.

Scottish Intercollegiate Guidelines Network(SIGN) obesity management (2010).

Shaw M, Savoye M, Cali A et al. (2009) Effect of a successful intensive lifestyle program on insulin sensitivity and glucose tolerance in obese youth. *Diabetes Care* 32: 45–47.

Sjöberg RL, Nilsson KW and Leppert J (2005)Obesity, shame, and depression in school-aged children: a population-based study. *Pediatrics* 116(3): e389–92.

Skinner AC, Steiner MJ, Henderson FW and Perrin EM (2010) Multiple markers of inflammation and weight status: Cross-sectional analyses throughout childhood. *Pediatrics* 125: e801–e809.

Spiegel K, Leproult R, L'Hermite-Baleriaux M et al. (2004) Leptin levels are dependent on sleep duration: Relationships with sympathovagal balance, carbohydrate regulation, cortisol, and thyrotropin. *J Clin Endocrinol Metab* 89: 5762–5771.

Steffen LM, Jacobs DR Jr, Murtaugh MA et al. (2003) Whole grain intake is associated with lower body mass and greater insulin sensitivity among adolescents. *Am J Epidemiol* 158: 243–250.

Steinberger J, Moorehead C, Katch V and Rocchini AP (1995) Relationship between insulin resistance and abnormal lipid profile in obese adolescents. *J Pediatr* 126: 690–695.

Tavares Giannini D, Caetano Kuschnir MC and Szklo M (2013) Metabolic syndrome in overweight and obese adolescents: A comparison of two different diagnostic criteria. *Ann NY Acad Sci* 1281(1): 123–140. Published online 2013 Jan 28.

Taheri S (2006) The link between short sleep duration and obesity: We should recommend more sleep to prevent obesity. *Arch Dis Child* 91: 881–884.

Taheri S, Lin L, Austin D, Young T and Mignot E (2004) Short sleep duration is associated with reduced leptin, elevated ghrelin, and increased body mass index. *PLoS Med* 1: e62.

Tam CS, Clement K, Baur LA and Tordjman J (2010a) Obesity and low-grade inflammation: A paediatric perspective. *Obes Rev* 11: 118–126.

Tam CS, Garnett SP, Cowell CT et al. (2010b) IL-6, IL-8 and IL-10 levels in healthy weight and overweight children. *Horm Res Paediatr* 73: 128–134.

Tauman R and Gozal D (2011) Obstructive sleep apnea syndrome in children. *Expert Rev Respir Med* 5(3): 425–40. doi: 10.1586/ers.11.7.

Ther Clin Risk Manag. 2012; 8: 55–63. Published online 2012 Feb 2.

Viner RM, Segal TY, Lichtarowicz-Krynska E and Hindmarsh P (2005) Prevalence of the insulin resistance syndrome in obesity. *Arch Dis Child* 90(1):10–4.

Viner RM, Hsia Y, Neubert A and Wong IC (2009) Rise in antiobesity drug prescribing for children and adolescents in the UK: A population-based study. *Br J Clin Pharmacol* 68: 844–851.

Viner RM, Hsia Y, Tomsic T and Wong ICK (2010) Efficacy and safety of anti-obesity drugs in children and adolescents: Systematic review and meta-analysis. *Obes Rev* 11: 593–602.

Visser M, Bouter LM, McQuillan GM, Wener MH and Harris TB (2001) Low-grade systemic inflammation in overweight children. *Pediatrics* 107: E13.

Waters KA, Suresh S and Nixon GM (2013) Sleep disorders in children. *Med J Aust* 199(8): S31–S35.

Weiss R, Bremer AA and Lustig RH (2013) What is metabolic syndrome, and why are children getting it? *Ann NY Acad Sci* 1281: 123–140.

Weiss R, Dziura J, Burgert TS et al. (2004) Obesity and the metabolic syndrome in children and adolescents. *N Engl J Med* 350(23): 2362–2374.

Whitlock EP, O'Connor EA, Williams SB, Beil TL and Lutz KW (2010) Effectiveness of weight management interventions in children: A targeted systematic review for the USPSTF. *Pediatrics* 125(2).

Weiss R, Dziura J, Bunjert TS et al. (2011) Effects of metformin on body weight and body composition in obese insulin-resistant children: A randomized clinical trial. *Diabetes* 60: 477–485.

World Health Organization (2006) *WHO Child Growth Standards: Length/Height-for-Age, Weight-for-Age, Weight-for-Length, Weight-for-Height and Body Mass, Index-for-Age: Methods and Development.* Geneva: World Health Organization.

http://www.noo.org.uk/uploads/doc/vid_11601_A_simple_guide_to_classifying_BMI_in_children.pdf

Yanovski JA, Krakoff J, Salaita CG et al. (2011) Effects of metformin on body weight and body composition in obese insulin-resistant children: a randomized clinical trial. *Diabetes* 60(2): 477–85. doi: 10.2337/db10-1185.

Young T, Skatrud J and Peppard PE (2004) Risk factors for obstructive sleep apnea in adults. *JAMA* 291: 2013–2016.

12

LATE EFFECTS OF CANCER AND ITS TREATMENTS ON THE NEUROENDOCRINE SYSTEM

Wassim Chemaitilly and Charles A Sklar

Introduction

Endocrine complications can affect between 20% and 50% of childhood cancer survivors and often occur as therapy-related late effects (Diller et al. 2009). Individuals with central nervous system (CNS) tumours and those whose hypothalamus and/or pituitary was exposed to surgery or radiation are particularly at risk of hypothalamic and pituitary dysfunction. Tumoural expansion, surgical procedures and radiotherapy can all be associated with a variety of neuroendocrine abnormalities including both diminished and excessive hormone secretion (Gurney et al. 2003; Hows et al. 2006). Hypothalamic injury can also impact metabolism and appetite regulation, which in turn can significantly affect body composition (Table 12.1) (Sklar et al. 2000; Lustig et al. 2003b).

General overview

When caused by tumoural expansion in close proximity to the sellar region and/or by surgical treatments involving this area, hypothalamic-pituitary dysfunction generally involves multiple hormonal systems from the outset. Moreover, problems become clinically evident fairly quickly following the primary diagnosis or surgery. In contrast, hypothalamic-pituitary dysfunction following exposure to radiotherapy may not become evident for many years following the exposure. In addition, the threshold dose and the time course of hormone dysfunction vary for the different anterior pituitary hormones.

The nature and site of post-irradiation neuroendocrinopathies (purely neuronal vs. neurovascular, hypothalamic vs. pituitary) remain unclear (Spoudeas 2002). Only one published work specifically studied changes in hypothalamic blood flow following exposure to radiotherapy (Chieng et al. 1991). The authors, Chieng and colleagues, used single-photon emission CT imaging to study hypothalamic blood flow in 34 individuals (aged 30–65 years) treated with radiotherapy (fractionated regimen with 46–56Gy to the hypothalamic/pituitary area) for nasopharyngeal carcinoma 6 months to 5 years prior and compared their findings to those of four healthy comparison individuals. The authors reported significantly decreased hypothalamic blood flow in individuals treated with radiotherapy when compared to controls. There were no significant differences in hypothalamic blood flow among

TABLE 12.1

Summary of the most common neuroendocrine late effects with therapy-related risk factors, elements of clinical suspicion and screening tools

Function	Complication	Therapy-related risks	Relationship to time, dose to gland or organ when applicable	Laboratory studies
Linear growth	Growth hormone deficiency	Surgery	Damage to the pituitary by tumour expansion and/or surgery	Bone age
		Radiotherapy to hypothalamus or pituitary	Doses >30Gy, effect by 5 years after exposure; Doses 18–24Gy, effect may appear >10 years following exposure	Growth hormone stimulation test
Puberty	Central precocious puberty	Radiotherapy to hypothalamus or pituitary	Doses ≥18Gy, Girls <5 years old at exposure have a higher risk	Bone age, pelvic ultrasound scan; GnRH or GnRH agonist stimulation test
	Hypogonadotropic hypogonadism	Surgery	Damage to the pituitary by tumour expansion and/or surgery	Baseline luteinizing hormone, FSH
		Radiotherapy to hypothalamus or pituitary	Doses >30Gy; Decreased fertility (partial deficit?) 22–27Gy	GnRH stimulation test; Pelvic ultrasound scan; Estradiol (girls); Testosterone (boys)
Pituitary, other	ACTH deficiency	Surgery	Damage to the pituitary by tumour expansion and/or surgery	
		Radiotherapy to hypothalamus or pituitary	Doses >30Gy	Low-dose ACTH stimulation test
	TSH deficiency	Surgery	Damage to the pituitary by tumour expansion and/or surgery	TSH, free T4
		Radiotherapy to hypothalamus or pituitary	Doses > 30Gy	
Metabolism	Obesity	Surgery to hypothalamus	Large resections cause 'central obesity'	Fasting glucose, lipids, insulin concentrations
		Radiotherapy	Cranial radiotherapy	Oral glucose tolerance test

ACTH, adrenocorticotropic hormone; TSH, thyroid-stimulating hormone; FSH, follicle-stimulating hormone; GnRH, gonadotropin releasing hormone.

individuals treated with radiotherapy when they were grouped according to the time interval since exposure to cranial radiation (6 months vs. 1 year vs. 5 years). This was in contrast to a clear trend of worsening endocrine deficits with time in individuals exposed to radiotherapy. The authors concluded that the continued worsening of endocrine function despite stable vascular injury favours direct insult to the neurons as a mechanism for radiation-induced hypothalamic damage, although a possible impact of chronic ischemic changes could not be totally excluded (Chieng et al. 1991).

Several observations suggest a higher degree of hypothalamic versus pituitary sensitivity to radiotherapy (Schriock 1984; Constine et al. 1993). Exposure of the hypothalamic pituitary region to doses of radiation 50Gy and above can be associated with hyperprolactinemia. This is thought to be the result of the disruption within the hypothalamus of the dopaminergic pathways that normally inhibit prolactin release from the anterior pituitary (Constine et al. 1993). A higher degree of hypothalamic versus pituitary vulnerability to radiation was also described in regard to the growth hormone–releasing hormone (GHRH)–growth hormone axis. This was based on the observation of a suppressed growth hormone response to peripheral stimuli (such as insulin induced hypoglycemia) versus a better preserved growth hormone response to exogenous GHRH in certain individuals treated with radiotherapy. The lack of deficits, in the context of high-dose cranial radiotherapy, of certain hypothalamic neurohormones such as vasopressin does suggest, however, that differences in hypothalamic versus pituitary vulnerability to radiation may not be relevant to all hypothalamic-pituitary axes (Schriock 1984).

Growth hormone deficiency
Tumours developing close to the hypothalamus and/or pituitary gland such as craniopharyngiomas, germinomas, and optic nerve gliomas can cause growth hormone deficiency (GHD) as a direct anatomical insult or because of the surgery required to remove or reduce the size of these tumours. More commonly in childhood cancer survivors, GHD results from exposure of the hypothalamus-pituitary to radiation. GHD is the most common, and often the only, pituitary deficiency observed in survivors of childhood brain tumours and those with a history of exposure to cranial radiotherapy or total body irradiation (Chrousos et al. 1982; Sklar and Constine 1995; Heikens 1998; Laughton et al. 2008). In these individuals, the deficit occurs in a time- and dose-dependent fashion (Fig 12.1). The higher the dose of radiation and the longer the interval from treatment, the greater the risk (Clayton and Shalet 1991a; Merchant et al. 2011). GHD can be observed within 5 years when the dose exceeds 30Gy (Laughton et al. 2008). Following lower doses, such as 18Gy to 24Gy, GHD may not become evident for 10 or more years (Brennan et al. 1998). In contrast to individuals treated with hypothalamic-pituitary radiotherapy, GHD has been reported in relatively small numbers of individuals treated with chemotherapy alone and the effects of chemotherapy on growth hormone secretion (GHS) remain controversial (Bakker et al. 2004; Rose et al. 2004; van den Heijkant et al. 2011).

As in the general population, the diagnosis of GHD is based on the convergence of clinical (short stature or decreased growth velocity) and laboratory features (dynamic stimulation tests and plasma concentration of surrogate markers of GHS). However, certain

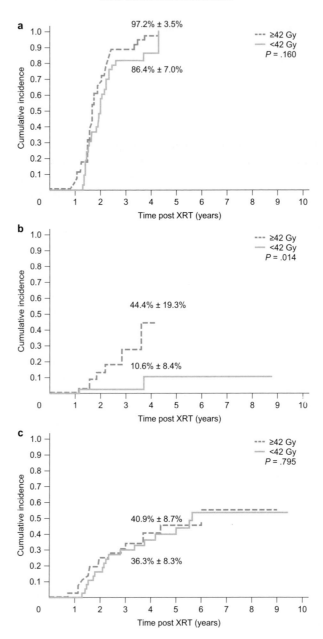

Figure 12.1. Pituitary deficits in survivors of childhood embryonal brain tumours after risk-adapted craniospinal and conformal primary-site irradiation and high-dose chemotherapy with stem-cell rescue on the SJMB-96 trial. Cumulative incidence of (a) growth hormone deficiency, (b) thyroid-stimulating hormone deficiency and (c) adrenocorticotropic hormone deficiency by hypothalamic radiation dose divided around the median (42Gy). XRT, radiation therapy. From Laughton et al. (2008). Reprinted with the permission of the American Society of Clinical Oncology.

elements deserve special attention in the context of childhood cancer survivors. Therapy-related non-endocrine factors can contribute to growth deceleration and compromised growth potential. For instance, high-dose radiotherapy to the spine can directly damage the vertebral growth plates and cause a skeletal dysplasia where the sitting height is more affected than the growth of the legs (Clayton and Shalet 1991b; Shalet et al. 1987; Brauner et al. 1993; Thomas et al. 1993). Conversely, individuals with severe obesity can sustain a normal linear growth rate despite having GHD in the context of accelerated weight gain (Iwayama et al. 2011). Concurrent central precocious puberty, a fairly common endocrine complication observed in individuals treated with hypothalamic-pituitary axis radiotherapy, can mask the clinical signs of GHD; individuals with GHD and central precocious puberty can present with seemingly normal linear growth rates, owing to inappropriately elevated levels of sex steroids.

The laboratory tools used to establish a diagnosis of GHD also need to be interpreted with caution in the context of childhood cancer survivors. Plasma insulin-like growth factor-1 (IGF-1) and IGF binding protein-3 (IGFBP-3), which are more stable than growth hormone levels and are widely used as surrogate markers of GHS in the general population, are not reliable in childhood cancer survivors with a history of hypothalamic-pituitary axis radiation exposure (Sklar et al. 1993; Weinzimer et al. 1999). Hence, when clinical suspicion is present, growth hormone stimulation testing should be offered even if IGF-1 and/or IGFBP-3 levels are within the normal range. Several secretagogues are used for growth hormone stimulation testing in children; these include arginine, clonidine, glucagon, insulin and L-dopa. Diagnosing GHD in children generally requires failing two growth hormone stimulation tests using two different secretagogues given difficulties with the reliability and reproducibility of these tests (Growth Hormone Research Society 2000). The criterion standard procedure for the diagnosis of GHD in adults is the insulin tolerance test (ITT) (Thorner et al. 1995; Biller et al. 2002; Finucane et al. 2008). Given the potential for adverse events associated with insulin-induced hypoglycemia, alternatives to the ITT have been explored (Growth Hormone Research Society 2000). The combination of GHRH and arginine (GHRH-Arg), a widely used test in adults suspected of GHD, has a lower sensitivity than the ITT in patients treated with craniospinal radiation, possibly because of an earlier onset of hypothalamic versus pituitary damage (Darzy et al. 2003; Ham et al. 2005). Other alternatives to the ITT include the glucagon provocative test (Conceicao et al. 2003).

Replacement therapy with human recombinant growth hormone (hGH) is proven to improve final height in survivors with childhood-onset GHD (Adan et al. 2000; Leung et al. 2002; Gleeson et al. 2003; Brownstein et al. 2004; Dai et al. 2004; Sanders et al. 2004; Bakker et al. 2007; Chemaitilly et al. 2007; Beckers et al. 2010; Ciaccio et al. 2010; Isfan et al. 2012). Initiation of replacement therapy at a younger bone age (and hence longer duration of replacement therapy) and higher doses of therapy positively correlated with a better final height outcome (Leung et al. 2002). Given the effects of radiotherapy on the vertebral growth plates and that of other comorbidities affecting growth (e.g. graft vs. host disease), the improvement in final height was limited in survivors exposed to spinal irradiation and more specifically in stem cell transplant survivors whose conditioning regimen included total body irradiation; it is nevertheless possible that final height outcomes would

TABLE 12.2

Suggested screening and management guidelines for neuroendocrine late-effects following cranial radiotherapy

	GH Deficiency*	Central Precocious Puberty	Hyper-prolactinemia	TSH Deficiency	LH/FSH Deficiency	ACTH Deficiency
1-Systematic Surveillance Modality						
History	Nutritional status	-	Libido, menstrual, galactorrhea	Hypothyroidism symptoms	Puberty, sexual function, menses, medications	Adrenal insufficiency symptoms
Physical	Height, weight, BMI, Tanner staging	Height, weight, BMI, Tanner staging	-	Height, weight, BMI, hair, skin, thyroid	Tanner staging	-
Laboratory screening	-	Consider testosterone AM level (m)†	Prolactin	TSH‡, Free T4	LH, FSH, estradiol(f), AM testosterone (m)	8 AM cortisol
2-Frequency of Screening						
Screening performed every	6 monthly until growth and puberty completed	Yearly until sexually mature	Yearly	Yearly	Baseline by age 14 y (m) or 13 y (f), then as clinically indicated. Yearly in males if hypothalamic /pituitary RT ≥ 30 Gy	Yearly if hypothalamic /pituitary RT ≥ 30 Gy
3-Intervention following Abnormal Screening Results						
Additional investigations	Bone age GH stimulation test	Bone age GnRH or GnRHa test	Assess gonadal function	-	Reproductive endocrine-fertility evaluation	Low-dose ACTH stimulation test
Treatment	Human recombinant GH for replacement-	Puberty suppression with GnRHa-	Dopamine receptor agonists	Levothyroxine for replacement	Sex-hormone replacement therapy	Hydrocortisone for replacement
Remarks	Specific guidelines needed for adults*	Frequent association with GH deficiency	Only in presence of symptoms	Dosing solely guided by Free T4 levels‡	-	Educate regarding stress dosing

*Recommendations pertain to *GH* deficiency in pediatric patients. Guidelines for the evaluation, screening and management of adult survivors with this condition need to be developed. m=males, f=females, GnRH agonist. † Consider in males with a history of exposure to gonadotoxic treatments including alkylating agents given the unreliability of testicular volume measurements.‡ TSH values can help differentiate central and primary forms of hypothyroidism at the time of diagnosis; they are not useful for the follow-up of patients with an established diagnosis of TSH deficiency.

172

have been even more impaired without hGH (Brownstein et al. 2004; Dai et al. 2004; Sanders et al. 2004; Bakker et al. 2007; Chemaitilly et al. 2007; Beckers et al. 2010; Ciaccio et al. 2010; Isfan et al. 2012). Screening and management guidelines for GHD were summarised in Table 12.2.

Safety concerns pertaining to the use of growth hormone in individuals with a history of malignancy are related to the known pro-mitogenic and proliferative effects of growth hormone and IGF-1. Large-scale studies assessing the long-term risks associated with the use of hGH in childhood cancer survivors have not shown an increase in the risk of recurrence of the primary disease or death following hGH replacement therapy (Swerdlow et al. 2000; Packer et al. 2001; Sklar et al. 2002). However, there are data to suggest a small increase in the risk of a secondary solid tumour, the most commonly observed being meningiomas (Sklar et al. 2002; Ergun-Longmire et al. 2006). In the initial report from the Childhood Cancer Survivor Study (CCSS) of a cohort of 13 222 participants, including 361 patients treated with hGH, 15 individuals treated with hGH developed second neoplasms, including 7 while on hGH. After adjustment for confounding factors, including age at diagnosis, sex, radiation and alkylating agent effects, exposure to hGH significantly increased the risk of second neoplasms (relative risk [RR] 3.21; 95% CI, 1.88–5.46; $p<.0001$) (Sklar et al. 2002). An updated CCSS report with nearly 3 years of additional follow-up continued to demonstrate that treatment with hGH was associated with an increased risk of second neoplasms (RR 2.15; 95% CI, 1.3–3.5). The investigators reported in total 20 cases of second neoplasms in survivors treated with growth hormone. Diagnoses included meningioma ($n=9$), osteosarcoma ($n=3$), soft tissue sarcoma ($n=2$), brain glioma ($n=2$), brain astrocytoma ($n=1$), papillary thyroid carcinoma ($n=1$), muco-epidermoid carcinoma of parotid ($n=1$) and colon adenocarcinoma ($n=1$). Among survivors not treated with hGH, 555 developed second neoplasms. The updated report included data on hGH dose and duration of therapy and neither was associated with the risk of developing a second neoplasm (Ergun-Longmire et al. 2006). Meningioma was the most common diagnosis among second neoplasms observed in individuals treated with hGH; all individuals who developed it were exposed to cranial radiotherapy, itself a known risk factor for meningioma (Paulino et al. 2009).

The relatively small number of events, the decrease in the relative risk with longer follow-up and the possibility of ascertainment bias related to a closer monitoring of individuals treated with hGH have nevertheless led some investigators to question the findings of the CCSS reports (Mackenzie et al. 2011). In a recent article by (Mackenzie et al. 2011) on 110 survivors of childhood and adult cancer treated with hGH and 110 matched non-hGH treated controls and followed in a single institution for a median of 14.5 years, individuals treated with hGH did not have a higher risk of developing second neoplasms than those not treated with hGH. Individuals were matched for cranial radiotherapy dose, age at primary diagnosis and duration of follow-up. In this study, five individuals treated with hGH developed second neoplasms (four meningioma, one malignant nerve sheath tumour) versus three individuals not treated with hGH (two meningioma, one oligodendroglioma). Of note, when considering the 41 matched pairs for childhood cancer survivors, five secondary tumours occurred among survivors versus two among the controls (a 2.5-fold difference)

(Mackenzie et al. 2011). This is similar to the magnitude of difference reported by the CCSS (Ergun-Longmire et al. 2006).

Cancer survivors treated with hGH may also be at higher risk of developing slipped femoral epiphyses compared with children treated with hGH for idiopathic GHD (Blethen and Rundle 1996). Beneficial effects on body composition, plasma lipids, bone mass and quality of life have supported the extension of the use of hGH to adults with hypopituitarism over the past few years (Bakker et al. 2004; Link et al. 2004; van den Heijkant et al. 2011). The safety and benefit of this practice in adult survivors of childhood cancers deserve further investigation (Murray et al. 2002; Mukherjee et al. 2005; Follin et al. 2006; van den Heijkant et al. 2011).

Disorders of luteinizing hormone and follicle-stimulating hormone
CENTRAL PRECOCIOUS PUBERTY

Central precocious puberty occurs following the premature activation of the hypothalamic-pituitary-gonadal axis (Sigurjonssdottir and Hayes 1968). Precocious puberty can lead to abnormally rapid skeletal maturation, with early fusion of the growth plates, hence contributing to the risk of adult short stature. In addition, a very early onset of puberty, and of menstrual activity in girls in particular, can be a source of psychosocial stress leading to adjustment difficulties.

The initiation of pubertal development is normally triggered by the increase in the pulsatile secretion of the hypothalamic neuropeptide gonadotropin-releasing hormone (GnRH) as a result of changes in the trans-synaptic and glial inputs to the GnRH-producing neurons (Ojeda et al. 2006). The balance between inhibitory influences (as exemplified by -aminobutyric acid [GABA] and opiod peptide–producing neurons) and excitatory input (as exemplified by kisspeptin and glutamic acid producing neurons or via changes in controlling glial cells) shifts in favour of the latter and activates the GnRH 'pulse generator'. The premature activation of the GnRH pulse generator in children with cancer as well as survivors of childhood cancer can be a consequence of the tumoural process itself (such as in individuals with hypothalamic hamartomas or optic nerve gliomas) or follow neuroendocrine disruptions caused by hypothalamic exposure to radiation. Hypothalamic-pituitary radiation across a wide spectrum of doses (18Gy to >35Gy) is associated with an increased risk of the development of central precocious puberty (Brauner et al. 1984; Constine et al. 1993; Oberfield et al. 1996; Chow et al. 2008; Armstrong et al. 2009). Risk factors associated with radiation-induced central precocious puberty include female sex, younger age at treatment and increased body mass index (BMI) (Ogilvy-Stuart and Shalet 1995; Oberfield et al. 1996).

Precocious puberty is a clinical diagnosis and relies on the observation of sustained pubertal development before the age of 8 years in girls and before the age of 9 years in boys (Sigurjonssdottir and Hayes 1968) (see Chapter 21). In boys, the measurement of the testicular volume, used to assess the onset of pubertal development in the general population, is not a reliable indicator of puberty in individuals who have been exposed to certain types of chemotherapeutic agents (e.g. alkylating agents, procarbazine, cisplatin) and/or direct testicular radiation. Treatment-induced testicular damage can cause the testes to be inappropriately small for a given stage of puberty. Thus, clinicians may need to rely on other indicators of early puberty (e.g. pubic hair, excessive linear growth, elevated morning testosterone concentration and advanced bone age) in at-risk boys. Gonadotropin secretion is best assessed using the GnRH or GnRH agonist stimulation tests.

The treatment of central precocious puberty in this population relies on the same class of agents used in the general population, namely GnRH agonists. The treatment of precocious puberty has been shown to improve final height outcomes, especially when contemporary regimens for growth hormone replacement are used concurrently to treat GHD, with better results in the absence of severe bone age advancement (Greulich and Pyle 1959; Thorner et al. 1995). Screening and management guidelines for central precocious puberty are summarised in Table 12.2.

LUTEINIZING HORMONE/FOLLICLE- STIMULATING HORMONE DEFICIENCY

Luteinizing hormone/follicle-stimulating hormone (FSH) deficiency can occur as a component of the multiple pituitary hormone deficiencies observed due to local tumoural growth and/or surgical treatment. It can also occur as a complication of hypothalamic-pituitary radiotherapy but is less frequently observed than central precocious puberty. It tends to occur following the exposure of the hypothalamus/pituitary to doses of radiation >30Gy (Sklar and Constine 1995; Byrne et al. 2004; Relander et al. 2006; Armstrong et al. 2009; Green et al. 2009). In female acute lymphoblastic leukaemia (ALL) survivors, 'subtle' defects of gonadotropin secretion following radiation doses in the 18–24Gy range have been described (Bath et al. 2001; Byrne et al. 2004). In a recent study, female survivors enrolled in the CCSS who received 22–27Gy of hypothalamic/pituitary irradiation were found to have decreased fertility compared to survivors not treated with hypothalamic/pituitary radiotherapy (Green et al. 2011); additional long-term follow-up data are needed to better understand the ultimate effect of these lower doses of radiation on fertility and gonadal function.

The clinical manifestations of luteinizing hormone/FSH deficiency the timing of its occurrence in regard to the individual's age and pubertal development. These manifestations include delayed or arrested puberty, primary or secondary amenorrhea in females and low testosterone-related symptoms in males. The diagnosis can be further corroborated by low sex steroid concentrations associated with low or inappropriately 'normal' luteinizing hormone and FSH concentrations. The treatment entails age-adjusted sex hormone replacement such as use of low-dose therapy for the induction of pubertal development in prepubertal individuals and full-dose sex hormone replacement therapies in postpubertal individuals (Viswanathan and Eugster 2011). Screening and management guidelines for luteinizing hormone/FSH deficiency are summarised in Table 12.2.

Corticotropin deficiency

Corticotropin (adrenocorticotropic hormone or ACTH) deficiency in childhood cancer survivors can be observed along with other pituitary deficiencies, as a result of local tumoural expansion or surgery or following high-dose (>30Gy) radiation (Rose et al. 2005; Laughton et al. 2008; Patterson et al. 2009). In a chart review of 88 patients treated for embryonal brain tumours with doses of craniospinal radiotherapy ranging from 23Gy to 40.5Gy, the cumulative incidence at 4 years of a diagnosis of ACTH deficiency was reported at 38±6% by Laughton et al. (2008) (Fig 12.1). In a report by Patterson et al. compiling data on 78 patients, including 53 exposed to hypothalamic-pituitary radiotherapy, ACTH deficiency was diagnosed in 17% of individuals exposed to less than 40Gy, and up to 50% in those exposed to doses ≥40Gy (Patterson et al. 2009). Symptoms and signs suggestive of ACTH deficiency include fatigue, nausea, vomiting, abdominal pain, hypotension, shock, unexplained clinical deterioration, vulnerability to infections and hypoglycemia. Given the life-threatening nature of adrenal insufficiency, individuals with known risk of ACTH deficiency should be screened upon their entry in long-term follow-up even if they do not have complaints suggestive of adrenal disease (Patterson et al. 2009). The diagnosis of ACTH deficiency requires dynamic testing; the most commonly used procedure is the low-dose ACTH stimulation test (Kazlauskaite et al. 2008; Chrousos et al. 2009). Screening for ACTH deficiency using 8 AM cortisol concentrations is problematic because of difficulties in defining adequate thresholds (9–15mcg/dL) and discrepancies with dynamic testing (Patterson et al. 2009). The treatment relies on replacement therapy with oral glucocorticoids. Screening and management guidelines for ACTH deficiency are summarised in Table 12.2.

Thyroid-stimulating hormone deficiency

Thyroid-stimulating hormone (TSH) deficiency, resulting in central hypothyroidism, can be observed along with other pituitary deficiencies as a result of local tumoural expansion or surgery or following the irradiation of the hypothalamic/pituitary area. It has been reported following doses of >30Gy to 40Gy (Sklar and Constine 1995; Rose et al. 1999; Schmiegelow et al. 2003; Laughton et al. 2008; Brabant et al. 2011). In the chart review of 88 patients by Laughton et al. (2008) mentioned above (Fig 12.1), the cumulative incidence at 4 years from diagnosis of TSH deficiency was reported at 23±8%. In a report by the British Childhood Cancer Survivor Study, up to 31% of individuals treated for a CNS abnormality reported being diagnosed with hypothyroidism. The questionnaire-based methodology used in this report did not allow, however, the distinction between primary and central etiologies (Brabant et al. 2011). The clinical symptoms associated with central hypothyroidism are generally subtle and non-specific but include fatigue, cold intolerance, low energy levels and menstrual irregularities in females. In children who have not completed growth, TSH deficiency may be associated with a decreased growth velocity. The diagnosis is based on finding a low free T4 concentration with a TSH concentration that is either low or inappropriately within the normal range. Subtle forms of 'hidden' central hypothyroidism may be additionally uncovered using dynamic testing (nocturnal TSH surge and response to thyroid releasing hormone) (Rose et al. 1999), but there is no consensus in respect of the clinical relevance of this diagnosis (Darzy and Shalet 2005). The treatment is based on replacement with levothyroxine with the dose being titrated against the concentration of free T4. Although optimal dose of replacement is not established, most clinicians aim to bring the free T4 concentration into the upper range of normal for age. Screening and management guidelines for TSH deficiency are summarised in Table 12.2.

Hyperprolactinemia

Hyperprolactinemia is often mild and reported as a fortuitous laboratory finding following high dose hypothalamic radiotherapy, above 50Gy (Constine et al. 1993). Rarely, it can disrupt normal hypothalamic-pituitary gonadal function and cause clinical hypogonadism (e.g. secondary amenorrhea). Screening and management guidelines for hyperprolactinemia are summarised in Table 12.2.

Overweight and obesity

Hypothalamus plays an important role in the regulation of food intake and energy balance. The arcuate nucleus, located within the hypothalamus, is a hub where peripheral signals pertaining to energy balance such as those mediated by leptin and insulin are sensed and integrated in order to allow the adjustment of food intake to the individual's needs. Complex interactions occurring within the hypothalamus between orexigenic factors, such as neuro-peptide Y and anorexigenic factors such as proopiomelanocortin are responsible for regulat-ing appetite, food intake and energy expenditure (Guyenet and Schwartz 2012; see Chapter 9). Hypothalamic injury and disruptions in the circuits regulating energy balance and food intake in the CNS may account for the fact that survivors who have sustained damage to this region as a result of tumour location, surgery or irradiation are more likely to be over-weight or obese than others. Survivors of childhood ALL treated with cranial radiotherapy and survivors of childhood brain tumours have indeed been shown to have the highest risk of being overweight or obese within the survivor population (Oeffinger et al. 2003; Lustig et al. 2003a, 2003b; Sklar et al. 2000; Garmey et al. 2008).

In a report from the CCSS comparing 1765 adult survivors of childhood ALL to 2565 siblings, cranial radiotherapy >20Gy, especially in females treated at a young age (<4 years), was significantly associated with obesity (i.e. BMI >30) (Oeffinger et al. 2003). Genetic predisposition also contributes to this risk (Ross et al. 2004; Armenian and Bhatia 2009). Other risk factors in the childhood ALL survivor population include sedentary lifestyle (Reilly et al. 1998) and GHD (Talvensaari et al. 1996). Resistance to leptin in ALL survivors treated with cranial radiotherapy was described as a possible mechanism for the observed insulin resistance, in both obese and non-obese individuals (Tonorezos et al. 2010).

Brain tumours developing near the sellar region and their treatments (e.g. surgery, radiation) can disrupt hypothalamic and pituitary functions and rapidly induce dramatic states of morbid 'central' obesity (Lustig et al. 2003a, 2003b). Hyperphagia, resulting from a hypothalamic insult and increased parasympathetic tone leading to hyperinsulinemia (the latter promoting fat storage), has been suggested as a contributing factor to obesity in these patients. It is with respect to that latter mechanism that treatment with octreotide has been tried in a small number of patients with hypothalamic obesity (Lustig et al. 2003a). Dex-troamphetamine has also been used with some success in order to control weight gain in patients with obesity related to hypothalamic injury (Mason et al. 2002).

Conclusion

Neuroendocrine complications are among the most common late effects affecting childhood cancer survivors. These complications, primarily arising in survivors of brain tumours and those with CNS exposure to radiotherapy, involve multiple endocrine systems and can have serious implications on the individual's long-term health. Early detection and treatment are key elements in improving the individual's well-being. It is therefore very important for childhood cancer survivors to receive long-term medical follow-up and surveillance. It is also very important for the medical providers caring for this population to recognise these complications, and to be mindful that many endocrine late effects may not manifest until many years after the completion of all cancer therapies.

REFERENCES

Adan L, Sainte-Rose C, Souberbielle JC, Zucker JM, Kalifa C and Brauner R (2000) Adult height after growth hormone (GH) treatment for GH deficiency due to cranial irradiation. *Med Pediatr Oncol* 34: 14–19.

Armenian SH and Bhatia S (2009) Chronic health conditions in childhood cancer survivors: is it all treatment-related-or do genetics play a role? *J Gen Intern Med* 24(Suppl 2): S395–S400.

Armstrong GT, Whitton JA, Gajjar A et al. (2009) Abnormal timing of menarche in survivors of central nervous system tumors. A report from the childhood cancer survivor study. *Cancer* 115: 2562–2570.

Bakker B, Oostdijk W, Bresters D, Walenkamp MJ, Vossen JM and Wit JM (2004) Disturbances of growth and endocrine function after busulfan-based conditioning for haematopoietic stem cell transplantation during infancy and childhood. *Bone Marrow Transplant* 33: 1049–1056.

Bakker B, Oostdijk W, Geskus RB, Stokvis-Brantsma WH, Vossen JM and Wit JM (2007) Growth hormone (GH) secretion and response to GH therapy after total body irradiation and haematopoietic stem cell transplantation during childhood. *Clin Endocrinol (Oxf)* 67: 589–597.

Bath LE, Anderson RA, Critchley HOD, Kelnar CJ and Wallace WH (2001) Hypothalamic pituitary- ovarian dysfunction after prepubertal chemotherapy and cranial irradiation for acute leukaemia. *Hum Reprod* 16: 1838–1844.

Beckers D, Thomas M, Jamart J et al. (2010) Adult final height after GH therapy for irradiation-induced GH deficiency in childhood survivors of brain tumors: The Belgian experience. *Eur J Endocrinol* 162: 483–490.

Biller BM, Samuels MH, Zagar A et al. (2002) Sensitivity and specificity of six tests for the diagnosis of adult GH deficiency. *J Clin Endocrinol Metab* 87: 2067–2079.

Blethen SL and Rundle AC (1996) Slipped capital femoral epiphyses in children treated with growth hormone. A summary of the National Cooperative Growth experience. *Horm Res* 46: 113–116.

Brabant G, Toogood AA, Shalet SM et al. (2011) Hypothyroidism following childhood cancer therapy – An under diagnosed complication. *Int J Cancer* 130: 1145–1150. doi: 10.1002/ijc.26086.

Brauner R, Czernichow P and Rappaport R (1984) Precocious puberty after hypothalamic and pituitary irradiation in young children. *N Engl J Med* 311: 920.

Brauner R, Fontoura M, Zucker JM et al. (1993) Growth and growth hormone secretion after bone marrow transplantation. *Arch Dis Child* 64: 458–463.

Brennan BM, Rahim A, Mackie EM, Eden OB and Shalet SM (1998) Growth hormone status in adults treated for acute lymphoblastic leukaemia in childhood. *Clin Endocrinol* 48: 777–783.

Brownstein CM, Mertens AC, Mitby PA et al. (2004) Factors that affect final height and change in height standard deviation scores in survivors of childhood cancer treated with growth hormone: A report from the Childhood Cancer Survivor Study. *J Clin Endocrinol Metab* 89: 4422–4427.

Byrne J, Fears TR, Mills JL et al. (2004) Fertility of long-term male survivors of acute lymphoblastic leukemia diagnosed during childhood. *Pediatr Blood Cancer* 42: 364–372.

Chemaitilly W, Boulad F, Heller G et al. (2007) Final height in pediatric patients after hyperfractionated total body irradiation and stem cell transplantation. *Bone Marrow Transplant* 40: 29–35.

Chieng PU, Huang TS, Chang CC, Chong PN, Tien RD and Su CT (1991) Reduced hypothalamic blood flow after radiation treatment of nasopharyngeal cancer: SPECT studies in 34 patients. *AJNR Am J Neuroradiol* 12: 661–665.

Chow EJ, Friedman DL, Yasui Y et al. (2008) Timing of menarche among survivors of childhood acute lymphoblastic leukemia: A report from the Childhood Cancer Survivor Study. *Pediatr Blood Cancer* 50: 854–858.

Chrousos GP, Kino T and Charmandari E (2009) Evaluation of the hypothalamic-pituitary – Adrenal axis function in childhood and adolescence. *Neuroimmunomodulation* 16: 272–283.

Chrousos GP, Poplack D, Brown T, O'Neill D, Schwade J and Bercu BB (1982) Effects of cranial radiation on hypothalamic-adenohypophyseal function: Abnormal growth hormone secretory dynamics. *J Clin Endocrinol Metab* 54: 1135–1139.

Ciaccio M, Guercio G, Vaiani E et al. (2010) Effectiveness of rhGH treatment on adult height in GH-deficient childhood survivors of medulloblastoma. *Horm Res Paediatr* 73: 281–286.

Clayton PE and Shalet SM (1991a) Dose dependency of time of onset of radiation-induced growth hormone deficiency. *J Pediatr* 118: 226–228.

Clayton PE and Shalet SM (1991b) The evolution of spinal growth after irradiation. *Clin Oncol* 3: 220–222.

Conceicao FL, da Costa e Silva A, Leal Costa AJ and Vaisman M (2003) Glucagon stimulation test for the diagnosis of GH deficiency in adults. *J Endocrinol Invest* 26: 1065–1070.

Constine LS, Woolf PD, Cann D et al. (1993) Hypothalamic pituitary dysfunction after radiation for brain tumors. *N Engl J Med* 328: 87–94.

Dai QY, Souillet G, Bertrand Y et al. (2004) Antileukemic and long-term effects of two regimens with or without TBI in allogeneic bone marrow transplantation for childhood acute lymphoblastic leukemia. *Bone Marrow Transplant* 34: 667–673.

Darzy KH, Aimaretti G, Wieringa G, Gattamaneni HR, Ghigo E and Shalet SM (2003) The usefulness of the combined growth hormone (GH)-releasing hormone and arginine stimulation test in the diagnosis of radiation-induced GH deficiency is dependent on the post-irradiation time interval. *J Clin Endocrinol Metab* 88: 95–102.

Darzy KH and Shalet SM (2005) Circadian and stimulated thyrotropin secretion in cranially irradiated adult cancer survivors. *J Clin Endocrinol Metab* 90: 6490–6497.

Diller L, Chow EJ, Gurney GJ et al. (2009) Chronic disease in the Childhood Cancer Survivor Study Cohort: A review of published findings. *J Clin Oncol* 27: 2339–2355.

Ergun-Longmire B, Mertens AC, Mitby P et al. (2006) Growth hormone treatment and risk of second neoplasm in the childhood cancer survivor. *J Clin Endocrinol Metab* 91: 3494–3498.

Finucane FM, Liew A, Thornton E, Rogers B, Tormey W and Agha A (2008) Clinical insights into the safety and utility of the insulin tolerance test (ITT) in the assessment of the hypothalamo-pituitary-adrenal axis. *Clin Endocrinol (Oxf)* 69: 603–607.

Follin C, Thilén U, Ahrén B and Erfurth EM (2006) Improvement in cardiac systolic function and reduced prevalence of metabolic syndrome after two years of growth hormone (GH) treatment in GH-deficient adult survivors of childhood-onset acute lymphoblastic leukemia. *J Clin Endocrinol Metab* 91: 1872–1875.

Garmey EG, Liu Q, Sklar CA et al. (2008) Longitudinal changes in obesity and body mass index among adult survivors of childhood acute lymphoblastic leukemia: A report from the Childhood Cancer Survivor Study. *J Clin Oncol* 26: 4639–4645.

Gleeson HK, Stoeter R, Ogilvy-Stuart AL, Gattamaneni HR, Brennan BM and Shalet SM (2003) Improvements in final height over 25 years in growth hormone (GH)-deficient childhood survivors of brain tumours receiving GH replacement. *J Clin Endocrinol Metab* 88: 3682–3689.

Green DM, Kawashima T, Stovall M et al. (2009) Fertility of female survivors of childhood cancer: a report from the Childhood Cancer Survivor Study. *J Clin Oncol* 27: 2677–2685.

Green DM, Nolan VG, Kawashima T et al. (2011) Decreased fertility among female childhood cancer survivors who received 22–27 Gy hypothalamic/ pituitary irradiation: A report from the Childhood Cancer Survivor Study. *Fertil Steril* 95: 1922–1927.

Greulich W and Pyle S (1959) *Radiographic Atlas of Skeletal Development of the Hand and Wrist,* 2nd edn. Stanford, CA: Stanford University Press.

Growth Hormone Research Society (2000) Consensus guidelines for the diagnosis and treatment of growth hormone (GH) deficiency in childhood and adolescence: Summary statement of the GH Research Society. *J Clin Endocrinol Metab* 85: 3990–3993.

Gurney JG, Kadan-Lottick NS, Packer RJ et al. (2003) Endocrine and cardiovascular late effects among adult survivors of childhood brain tumors: Childhood Cancer Survivor Study. *Cancer* 97: 663–673.

Guyenet SJ and Schwartz MW (2012) Regulation of food intake, energy balance and body fat mass: Implications for the pathogenesis and treatment of obesity. *J Clin Endocrinol Metab* 97: 745–755.

Ham JN, Ginsberg JP, Hendell CD and Moshang T Jr (2005) Growth hormone releasing hormone plus arginine stimulation testing in young adults treated in childhood with cranio-spinal radiation therapy. *Clin Endocrinol (Oxf)* 62: 628–632.

Heikens J, Michiels EM, Behrendt H, Endert E, Bakker PJ and Fliers E (1998) Long-term neuro-endocrine sequelae after treatment for childhood medulloblastoma. *Eur J Cancer* 34: 1592–1597.

Hows JM, Passweg JR, Tichelli A et al. (2006) Comparison of long-term outcomes after allogeneic hematopoietic stem cell transplantation from matched sibling and unrelated donors. *Bone Marrow Transplant* 38: 799–805.

Isfan F, Kanold J, Merlin E et al. (2012) Growth hormone treatment impact on growth rate and final height of patients who received HSCT with TBI or / and cranial irradiation in childhood. A report from the French Leukaemia Long-Term Follow-Up Study (LEA). *Bone Marrow Transplant* 47: 684–693.

Iwayama H, Kamijo T and Ueda N (2011) Hyperinsulinemia may promote growth without GH in children after resection of suprasellar brain tumors. *Endocrine* 40: 130–133.

Kazlauskaite R, Evans AT, Villabona CV et al. (2008) Corticotropin tests for hypothalamic-pituitary- adrenal insufficiency: A meta-analysis. *J Clin Endocrinol Metab* 93: 4245–4253.

Laughton SJ, Merchant TE, Sklar CA et al. (2008) Endocrine outcomes for children with embryonal brain tumors after risk adapted craniospinal and conformal primary-site irradiation and high-dose chemotherapy with stem cell rescue on the SJMB-96 trial. *J Clin Oncol* 26: 1112–1118.

Leung W, Rose SR, Zhou Y et al. (2002) Outcomes of growth hormone replacement therapy in survivors of childhood acute lymphoblastic leukemia. *J Clin Oncol* 20: 2959–2964.

Link K, Moëll C, Garwicz S et al. (2004) Growth hormone deficiency predicts cardiovascular risk in young adults treated for acute lymphoblastic leukemia in childhood. *J Clin Endocrinol Metab* 89: 5003–5012.

Lustig RH, Hinds PS, Ringwald-Smith K et al. (2003a) Octreotide therapy of pediatric hypothalamic obesity: A doubleblind, placebo-controlled trial. *J Clin Endocrinol Metab* 88: 2586–2592.

Lustig RH, Post SR, Srivannaboon K et al. (2003b) Risk factors for the development of obesity in children surviving brain tumors. *J Clin Endocrinol Metab* 88: 611–616.

Mackenzie S, Craven T, Gattamaneni HR, Swindell R, Shalet SM and Brabant G (2011) Long-term safety of growth hormone replacement after CNS irradiation. *J Clin Endocrinol Metab* 96: 2756–2761.

Mason PW, Krawiecki N and Meacham LR (2002) The use of dextroamphetamine to treat obesity and hyperphagia in children treated for craniopharyngioma. *Arch Pediatr Adolesc Med* 156: 887–892.

Merchant TE, Rose SR, Bosley C, Wu S, Xiong X and Lustig RH (2011) Growth hormone secretion after conformal radiation therapy in pediatric patients with localized brain tumors. *J Clin Oncol* 29: 4776–4780.

Mukherjee A, Tolhurst-Cleaver S, Ryder WD, Smethurst L and Shalet SM (2005) The characteristics of quality of life impairment in adult growth hormone (GH)-deficient survivors of cancer and their response to GH replacement therapy. *J Clin Endocrinol Metab* 90: 1542–1549.

Murray RD, Darzy KH, Gleeson HK and Shalet SM (2002) GH deficient survivors of childhood cancer: GH replacement during adult life. *J Clin Endocrinol Metab* 87: 129–135.

Oberfield SE, Soranno D, Nirenberg A et al. (1996) Age at the onset of puberty following high-dose central nervous system radiation therapy. *Arch Pediatr Adolesc Med* 150: 589–592.

Oeffinger KC, Mertens AC, Sklar CA et al. (2003) Obesity in adult survivors of childhood acute lymphoblastic leukemia: A report from the childhood cancer survivor study. *J Clin Oncol* 21: 1359–1365.

Ogilvy-Stuart AL and Shalet SM (1995) Growth and puberty after growth hormone treatment after irradiation for brain tumours. *Arch Dis Child* 73: 141–146.

Ojeda SR, Lomniczi A, Mastronardi C et al. (2006) Minireview: The neuroendocrine regulation of puberty: Is the time ripe for a systems biology approach? *J Clin Endocrinol Metab* 147: 1166–1174.

Packer RJ, Boyett JM, Janns AJ et al. (2001) Growth hormone replacement therapy in children with medulloblastoma: Use and effect on tumor control. *J Clin Oncol* 19: 480–487.

Patterson BC, Truxillo L, Wasilewski-Masker K, Mertens AC and Meacham LR (2009) Adrenal function testing in pediatric cancer survivors. *Pediatr Blood Cancer* 53: 1302–1307.

Paulino AC, Ahmed IM, Mai WY and Teh BS (2009) The influence of pretreatment characteristics and radiotherapy parameters on time interval to development of radiation-associated meningioma. *Int J Radiation Oncology Biol Phys* 75: 1408–1414.

Reilly JJ, Vetham JC, Ralston JM, Donaldson M and Gibson B (1998) Reduced energy expenditure in pre-obese children treated for acute lymphoblastic leukemia. *Pediatr Res* 44: 557–562.

Relander T, Gavallin-Stahl E, Garwicz S, Olsson AM and Willen M (2000) Gonadal and sexual function in men treated for childhood cancer. *Med Pediatr Oncol* 35: 52–63.

Rose SR, Danish RK, Kearney NS et al. (2005) ACTH deficiency in childhood cancer survivors. *Pediatr Blood Cancer* 45: 808–813.

Rose SR, Lustig RH, Pitukcheewanont P et al. (1999) Diagnosis of hidden central hypothyroidism in survivors of childhood cancer. *J Clin Endocrinol Metab* 84: 4472–4479.

Rose SR, Schreiber RE, Kearney NS et al. (2004) Hypothalamic dysfunction after chemotherapy. *J Pediatr Endocrinol Metab* 17: 55–66.

Ross JA, Oeffinger KC, Davies SM et al. (2004) Genetic variation in the leptin receptor gene and obesity in survivors of childhood acute lymphoblastic leukemia: A report from the Childhood Cancer Survivor Study. *J Clin Oncol* 22: 3558–3562.

Sanders JE, Guthrie KA, Hoffmeister PA, Woolfrey AE, Carpenter PA and Appelbaum FR (2004) Final adult height of patients who received hematopietic cell transplantation in childhood. *Blood* 105: 1348–1354.

Schmiegelow M, Feldt-Rasmussen U, Rasmussen AK, Poulsen HS and Muller J (2003) A population-based study of thyroid function after radiotherapy and chemotherapy for a childhood brain tumor. *J Clin Endocrinol Metab* 88: 136–140.

Schriock EA, Lustig RH, Rosenthal SM, Kaplan SL and Grumbach MM (1984) Effect of growth hormone (GH) –releasing hormone (GRH) on plasma GH in relation to magnitude and duration of GH deficiency in 26 children and adults with isolated GH deficiency or multiple pituitary hormone deficiencies: Evidence for hypothalamic GRH deficiency. *J Clin Endocrinol Metab* 58: 1043–1049.

Shalet SM, Gibson B, Swindell R and Pearson D (1987) Effects of spinal irradiation on growth. *Arch Dis Child* 62: 461–464.

Sigurjonssdottir T and Hayes A (1968) Precocious puberty: A report of 96 cases. *Am J Dis Child* 1115: 309–321.

Sklar CA and Constine LS (1995) Chronic neuro-endocrinological sequelae of radiation therapy. *Int J Radiat Oncol Biol Phys* 31: 1113–1120.

Sklar CA, Mertens AC, Mitby P et al. (2002) Risk of disease recurrence and second neoplasm in survivors of childhood cancer treated with growth hormone: A report from the Childhood Cancer Survivor Study. *J Clin Endocrinol Metab* 87: 3136–3141.

Sklar CA, Mertens AC, Walter A et al. (2000) Changes in body mass index and prevalence of overweight in survivors of childhood acute lymphoblastic leukemia: Role of cranial irradiation. *Med Pediatr Oncol* 35: 91–95.

Sklar C, Sarafoglou K and Whittam E (1993) Efficacy of insulin-like growth factor binding protein-3 (IGFBP-3) in predicting the growth hormone response to provocative testing in children treated with cranial irradiation. *Acta Endocrinol* 129: 511–515.

Spoudeas HA (2002) Growth and endocrine function after chemotherapy and radiotherapy in childhood. *Eur J Cancer* 38: 1748–1759.

Swerdlow AJ, Reddingius RE, Higgins CD et al. (2000) Growth hormone treatment of children with brain tumours and risk of tumour recurrence. *J Clin Endocrinol Metab* 85: 4444–4449.

Talvensaari KK, Lanning M, Tapanainen P and Knip M (1996) Long term survivors of childhood cancer survivors have an increased risk of manifesting the metabolic syndrome. *J Clin Endocrinol Metab* 81: 3051–3055.

Thomas BC, Stanhope R, Plowman PN and Leiper AD (1993) Growth following single fraction and fractionated total body irradiation for bone marrow transplantation. *Eur J Pediatr* 152: 888–892.

Thorner MO, Bengtsson BA, Ho KY et al. (1995) The diagnosis of growth hormone deficiency (GHD) in adults. *J Clin Endocrinol Metab* 80: 3097–3098.

Tonorezos ES, Vega LG, Sklar CA et al. (2010) Adipokines, body fatness and insulin resistance among survivors of childhood leukemia. *Pediatr Blood Cancer* 58: 31–36. doi: 10.1002/pbc.

van den Heijkant S, Hoorweg-Nijman G, Huisman J et al. (2011) Effects of growth hormone therapy on bone mass, metabolic balance and well-being in young adult survivors of childhood acute lymphoblastic leukemia. *J Pediatr Hematol Oncol* 33: e231–e38.

Viswanathan V and Eugster EA (2011) Etiology and treatment of hypogonadism in adolescents. *Pediatr Clin North Am* 58: 1181–1200.

Weinzimer SA, Homan SA, Ferry RJ and Moshang T (1999) Serum IGF-1 and IGFBP-3 concentrations do not accurately predict growth hormone deficiency in children with brain tumors. *Clin Endocrinol* 51: 339–345.

13
CRANIOPHARYNGIOMA

Hoong-Wei Gan, Juan Pedro Martinez-Barbera, Helen A Spoudeas and Mehul T Dattani

Introduction

First described in 1857 (Barkhoudarian and Laws 2013), craniopharyngiomas are benign non-gliomatous central nervous system (CNS) tumours (WHO classification grade I [World Health Organization 2000]) originating from embryonal tissue in the hypothalamo-pituitary region. Although their incidence is rare (1.1–1.7 cases/million/year [Bunin et al. 1998; Nielsen et al. 2011; Zacharia et al. 2012]), craniopharyngiomas are the commonest supra-sellar tumour in childhood (Warmuth-Metz et al. 2004; Schroeder and Vezina 2011), and contribute to 1.5%–11.6% of all paediatric CNS tumours (Stiller and Nectoux 1994; Bunin et al. 1998; Warmuth-Metz et al. 2004; Stiller 2007). Despite their benign histology, their invasive nature and location close to vital hypothalamo-pituitary structures make them the archetypal suprasellar tumour for causing neuroendocrine dysfunction, not only due to invasion and mass effects, but also from treatments targeted to this area.

There is a well-described bimodal age distribution in incidence, with peaks between 5–14 and 65–74 years, a nadir between 15 and 34 years of age (Bunin et al. 1998; Nielsen et al. 2011), and no sex difference. Thus, the incidence of craniopharyngiomas in the pae-diatric population is higher, according to a recent Danish epidemiological study estimating a WHO-standardised incidence of 2.1 cases/million/year in children <15 years versus an overall global incidence of 1.3 cases/million/year (1.4 cases/million/year in childhood by weighted meta-analysis). Although some studies suggest an increased incidence in African or Asian populations, this has not been consistently replicated and may not apply in child-hood, since it appears driven by an increased incidence in adult-onset craniopharyngioma (Bunin et al. 1998; Zacharia et al. 2012).

Aetiology

Histopathologically, childhood craniopharyngiomas are almost invariably adamantinoma-tous, referring to the presence of calcifications within the tumour (Zhang et al. 2002). Mutational screens of human tumour samples of adamantinomatous craniopharyngioma (ACP) have revealed an association with genetic aberrations in *CTNNB1*, the gene encoding the protein beta-catenin, a critical regulator of the WNT pathway (Sekine et al. 2002; Kato et al. 2004; Buslei et al. 2005; Oikonomou et al. 2005). The identified activating mutations and deletions mostly affect residues encoded by exon 3 of *CTNNB1* with important regula-tory consequences. In particular, they predict that the mutant protein may be resistant to degradation and therefore the half-life of beta-catenin would be significantly increased, leading to over-activation of the WNT pathway. This conclusion has been experimentally validated by histological findings. For instance, ACPs show clusters of cells exhibiting nucleo-cytoplasmic accumulation of beta-catenin (hereafter referred to as 'cell clusters'), which is consistent with persistence of the mutant protein. Indeed, the presence of these beta-catenin-accumulating clusters represents a histopathological hallmark of ACP of diagnostic value, as they are not present in any other pituitary tumour including the papillary form of craniopharyngioma (Hofmann et al. 2006; Buslei et al. 2007; Nguyen et al. 2012). In addition, the WNT pathway has been shown to be specifically active in the cluster cells as revealed by the expression of the transcriptional targets *AXIN2* and *LEF1* (Sekine et al. 2004; Hofmann et al. 2006). These initial human studies clearly provided enough evidence for a role of *CTNNB1* mutations and the WNT pathway in the aetiology of ACP. However, whether these mutations drive tumour formation remained to be addressed.

Further insights from genetically engineered mouse models aiming to activate the WNT pathway in the embryonic pituitary using the Cre/loxp system have shown that the expression of a mutant form of beta-catenin lacking the amino acids encoded by exon 3, and therefore functionally equivalent to the mutant beta-catenin identified in human ACP, results in the formation of mouse tumours that are histologically similar to human ACP (Gaston-Massuet et al. 2011). These similarities were based on the presence of dispersed beta-catenin-accumulating cell clusters showing a comparable co-expression of markers such as *SOX9*, *LEF1* and *AXIN2* in human and mouse tumours. These cell clusters displayed a whorl-like morphology and low to absent proliferation capacity as assessed by the lack of expression of Ki67, a marker of cycling cells. However, the mouse tumours did not show calcification or deposits of wet keratin, and so far, infiltration of the tumour into the hypothalamus has not been observed, suggesting that these characteristics may represent species-specific differences. These experiments demonstrated a causative effect of mutant beta-catenin in the initiation of ACP, thus confirming the hypotheses drawn from the human studies.

Additionally, the mouse experiments provide important insights into the cellular aetiology of these tumours; for instance, in the identification of the cell type that sustains the mutation for the tumour to develop. It has been shown that the expression of mutant beta-catenin in differentiated cells such as somatotrophs, lactotrophs, thyrotrophs, corticotrophs and gonadotrophs or even in Pit1 cell-lineage committed precursors does not result in tumorigenesis (Gaston-Massuet et al. 2011). However, tumours form when mutant beta-catenin is expressed in Rathke's pouch (RP) epithelial cells, which represent embryonic precursors of all cell lineages of the mature anterior pituitary gland (Davis et al. 2011). Therefore, these experiments demonstrate that undifferentiated precursor cells play a critical role in the genesis of this tumour variant, suggesting that human ACP is most likely a tumour of embryonic origin.

Pathogenesis

ACP is a histologically benign, slow-growing epithelial tumour of the sellar region, but prone to invade the hypothalamus and the visual pathways. Important insights have been revealed using histopathological techniques and primary tumour cell cultures of human

ACP samples. It has been proposed that beta-catenin accumulating clusters participate in the formation of finger-like protrusions at the invasion front; this is supported by data demonstrating that partial inhibition of beta-catenin reduces cell motility in vitro (Holsken et al. 2010). It has been shown that these clusters may regulate components of the extracellular matrix thus creating a specific tumour environment that facilitates invasion (Burghaus et al. 2010). Tumour cell migration could also be exacerbated as a consequence of a deregulated epidermal growth factor receptor (EGFR) cascade, as EGFR activation has been observed in cell clusters at the border between tumour and brain. Moreover, since specific inhibition of this pathway by tyrosine kinase inhibitors decreases motility in vitro, this could reflect a possible target for new medical treatment options (Holsken et al. 2011).

The combination of mouse genetics and molecular studies has revealed novel genes and pathways that are likely to play a role in the pathogenesis of ACP. This strategy has allowed us to further investigate the possible role of the beta-catenin-accumulating cell clusters in the oncogenic process. Cluster cells purified from the tumorigenic mouse model pituitaries were subjected to gene profiling analysis (Andoniadou et al. 2012). Numerous genes whose expressions were up-regulated in the mouse cell clusters were later found to be also expressed in the beta-catenin-accumulating tumour cells of human ACP. Among these genes, sonic hedgehog (*SHH*) is particularly relevant. *SHH* is a secreted factor with critical functions for the normal development of numerous organs, including the pituitary gland (Treier et al. 2001; Wang et al. 2010), and heavily involved in human tumours and cancers including medulloblastoma, gastrointestinal, lung, prostate and pancreatic cancers (Romer et al. 2004; Katoh and Katoh 2005; Rubin and de Sauvage 2006; Medina et al. 2009; Park et al. 2011; Shin et al. 2011; Theunissen and de Sauvage 2009). *SHH* expression is increased in mouse and human beta-catenin-accumulating cell clusters, and the pathway is activated in these cell groups and neighbouring areas, as demonstrated by the activation of the *SHH* direct target and receptor *PTCH1* (Andoniadou et al. 2012). Therefore, these data reveal that pathogenesis of ACP may rely on the over-activation of the *SHH* pathway. In agreement with this, Gorlin syndrome (also known as naevoid basal cell carcinoma syndrome) is a rare condition characterised by an increased risk of developing various tumours, commonly medulloblastoma, rhabdomyosarcoma and basal cell carcinoma, and is occasionally associated with ACP (Gorlin 2004). Patients normally harbour loss-of-function mutations in *PTCH1*, leading to over-activation of the SHH pathway (Theunissen and de Sauvage 2009). This finding is important because it provides an explanation for the association between Gorlin syndrome and ACP, where SHH signalling is also found to be over-activated (Musani et al. 2006) and it suggests that specific pathway inhibitors may be of therapeutic use in patients with ACP (Rudin et al. 2009; Von Hoff et al. 2009; Mas and Ruiz i Altaba 2010).

SHH is not the only molecule found to be secreted by cluster cells and a myriad of other ligands of the TGF-β, WNT and FGF families as well as numerous chemokines have been identified as possible factors influencing tumour development (Andoniadou et al. 2012). It is clear that cluster cells influence the tumour environment by secreting these factors and thereby exerting a critical non-cell autonomous role (i.e. autocrine and/or paracrine fashion). We tentatively hypothesise that counteracting some of these signals may be beneficial to patients, for instance, by using small-molecule inhibitors of critical oncogenic pathways. Further research combining mouse models and in vitro cell culture from human ACPs may provide such therapeutic targets.

Research from ACP mouse models has furthered our understanding of the pathogenesis of these tumours at a cellular level. It has been found that enlargement of the pituitary stem cell (PSC) compartment is an effect of expressing mutant beta-catenin in RP precursors (Andoniadou et al. 2012; Gaston-Massuet et al. 2011). PSCs with self-renewal and differentiating potential in vitro have been identified in the adult pituitary by several groups and are marked by expression of the transcription factor *SOX2* (Lepore et al. 2005; Fauquier et al. 2008; Gleiberman et al. 2008; Garcia-Lavandeira et al. 2009; de Almeida et al. 2010; Castinetti et al. 2011; Florio 2011). Tumorigenic pituitary glands of the ACP mouse model contain around six times more PSCs when assayed in vitro in stem cell-promoting media, suggesting a mitogenic effect of the WNT pathway on these stem cells, similar to that observed in other organs. It has been found that human ACPs express markers related to cell stemness such as SOX2 and SOX9 (amongst others), although it is not clear in which cell types (Gaston-Massuet et al. 2011; Garcia-Lavandeira et al. 2012). Enlargement of the stem cell compartment has been described in mouse models for human colorectal and breast cancer, where oncogenic stem cells are able to self-renew as well as hyperproliferate, giving rise to daughter cells that generate the bulk of the tumours. These findings have promoted the cancer stem cell paradigm to explain oncogenesis in mice and humans, a concept that is currently being thoroughly investigated (Clarke and Fuller 2006; Alison et al. 2008; Rosen and Jordan 2009; Albini et al. 2011; Nguyen et al. 2012; Visvader and Lindeman 2012). At present, it remains unknown whether higher PSC numbers in the ACP mouse model have an impact on tumour progression and whether they represent cancer stem cells. We know, however, that the beta-catenin-accumulating cluster cells derive from RP embryonic precursors and that, at least in the mouse model, some of the cluster cells are SOX2-positive and have self-renewal capacity in vitro (Gaston-Massuet et al. 2011; Andoniadou et al. 2012). It is possible that cluster cells in human ACP correspond with a more advanced stage of the disease compared with the mouse model, thus explaining the lack of SOX2 expression in human clusters. Indeed, even in the mouse, only some cells in a proportion of clusters express SOX2. Although further research is needed, the current data support a model whereby cluster cells derive from embryonic precursors and have an important function in secreting paracrine factors that control different aspects of tumour progression, from growth to vascularisation and infiltration. Whether, in addition to this non-cell autonomous role, cluster cells give rise to the tumour mass is an important question that is currently being addressed, as this will have important therapeutic implications.

Clinical features

Most studies indicate an average age at diagnosis of between 6 and 10 years (Hetelekidis et al. 1993; DeVile et al. 1996; Habrand et al. 1999; Muller et al. 2001; Merchant et al. 2002; Stripp et al. 2004; Caldarelli et al. 2005; Karavitaki et al. 2005; Puget et al. 2007; Lin et al. 2008; Schubert et al. 2009), but this ranges widely, from 17 days (pointing to its embryological origins) (Muller et al. 2001) to 18 years (Muller et al. 2001; Schubert et al. 2009). The time to diagnosis from initial symptoms is significantly delayed with median symptom durations of 8 months to 8 years (total range is between 1 day and 15 years) (Hoffman et al. 1992; Merchant et al. 2002; Van Effenterre and Boch 2002; Caldarelli et al. 2005; Karavitaki et al. 2005; Puget et al. 2007). These studies allude to the subtlety and gradual progression of symptoms in many cases, such that they remain unreported by parents and unrecognised by clinicians as being associated with possible intracranial pathology. A longitudinal study by Muller et al. (2004) showed that increases in BMI SDS (body mass index standard deviation score) and reductions in linear growth rate predate diagnosis and occur from as early as 6–7 months and 10–12 months of age, respectively, again suggesting early embryological disruption as an important step in its pathogenesis.

The most common presenting symptoms in childhood relate to raised intracranial pressure (ICP), with 51%–78% of patients experiencing headache and 31%–61% having nausea and/or vomiting (Hetelekidis et al. 1993; Merchant et al. 2002; de Vries et al. 2003; Caldarelli et al. 2005; Karavitaki et al. 2005; Lin et al. 2008) (Table 13.1). Deteriorating vision is the second commonest symptom, with either a reduction in visual acuity (23%–84%) or a restriction in visual fields (17%–57%) (Hetelekidis et al. 1993; Merchant et al. 2002; de Vries et al. 2003; Caldarelli et al. 2005; Karavitaki et al. 2005; Puget et al. 2007; Lin et al. 2008; Muller 2010), both of which may not be recognised until severe. Papilloedema is seen in 29% of patients (Hetelekidis et al. 1993; Karavitaki et al. 2005) in keeping with the frequency of raised ICP, but may also be incidentally found on visual screening in the asymptomatic patient. Neurocognitive symptoms are less common but include cranial nerve palsies (due to compression of the third and sixth cranial nerves), cognitive impairment, reduced consciousness, ataxia, hemiparesis, behavioural changes and seizures.

Symptoms related to disruption of the hypothalamo-pituitary axes are under-recognised but are the third commonest group of clinical manifestations at diagnosis. De Vile et al. (1996) demonstrated the marked discrepancy between the proportion of patients who spontaneously reported endocrine symptoms such as linear growth retardation, weight loss/gain and polyuria/polydipsia as the initial presenting complaint versus those who truly had these manifestations on direct enquiry or examination. In a cross-sectional study of 138 German children with craniopharyngioma, Muller et al. (2003) found that decelerations in height velocity occur earlier (median duration prior to diagnosis 33 months [range 12–96mo]), than increases in weight and BMI SDS (median duration 24 months [range 24–48mo]). Changes in height and weight centiles are rarely presenting features but the high proportion of patients with these protracted signs emphasises the importance of accurate interpretation of consistent auxology and a higher awareness amongst paediatricians of when to refer.

Where tested, almost all (range 40%–100%) patients have biochemical evidence of hypothalamo-pituitary insufficiency at presentation (Hetelekidis et al. 1993; DeVile et al. 1996; Caldarelli et al. 2005; Karavitaki et al. 2005; Puget et al. 2007; Muller 2013). Diabetes insipidus, in particular, is likely to go undiagnosed until the patient is water-deprived or rendered effectively adipsic by anaesthesia, coma or further hypothalamic damage sustained during surgery, with potentially fatal neurological sequelae. Non-specific symptoms such as lethargy, prolonged recovery from recurrent infections, somnolence and cold intolerance may be related to adrenocorticotropic hormone (ACTH) and/or thyroid-stimulating hormone (TSH)/thryotropin-releasing hormone (TRH) deficiencies, whilst overt hypothalamic

TABLE 13.1
**Common symptoms and signs at presentation of craniopharyngioma ranked by median
frequencies calculated from published literature**

Symptom/sign	Median frequency percentage (range %)	References
Headaches	64 (51–78)	(Hetelekidis et al. 1993; Merchant et al. 2002; de Vries et al. 2003; Caldarelli et al. 2005; Karavitaki et al. 2005; Lin et al. 2008)
Reduction in visual acuity	51 (23–73)	(Hetelekidis et al. 1993; Merchant et al. 2002; de Vries et al. 2003; Caldarelli et al. 2005; Karavitaki et al. 2005; Puget et al. 2007; Lin et al. 2008; Muller 2010)
Restriction in visual fields	46 (17–61)	(Hetelekidis et al. 1993; Merchant et al. 2002; de Vries et al. 2003; Caldarelli et al. 2005; Karavitaki et al. 2005; Puget et al. 2007; Lin et al. 2008)
Nausea/vomiting	43 (31–61)	(Hetelekidis et al. 1993; Merchant et al. 2002; de Vries et al. 2003; Caldarelli et al. 2005; Karavitaki et al. 2005; Lin et al. 2008)
Linear growth failure/ short stature	33 (14–86)	(Sorva et al. 1988; Hetelekidis et al. 1993; Sklar 1994; DeVile et al. 1996; Merchant et al. 2002; de Vries et al. 2003; Caldarelli et al. 2005; Karavitaki et al. 2005; Puget et al. 2007)
Papilloedema	29	(Hetelekidis et al. 1993)
Reduced energy/ lethargy/somnolence	21 (5–22)	(DeVile et al. 1996; Caldarelli et al. 2005; Karavitaki et al. 2005)
Cranial nerve palsies	20 (11–27)	(Hetelekidis et al. 1993; Caldarelli et al. 2005; Karavitaki et al. 2005)
Weight loss	17 (5–31)	(DeVile et al. 1996; Caldarelli et al. 2005; Karavitaki et al. 2005; Puget et al. 2007)
Polyuria/polydipsia	16 (9–28)	(Hetelekidis et al. 1993; DeVile et al. 1996; de Vries et al. 2003; Caldarelli et al. 2005; Karavitaki et al. 2005; Puget et al. 2007)
Pubertal delay/arrest	10 (5–24)	(Hetelekidis et al. 1993; DeVile et al. 1996; de Vries et al. 2003; Caldarelli et al. 2005; Karavitaki et al. 2005)
Cognitive impairment	10	(Karavitaki et al. 2005)
Ataxia	8 (7–18)	(Hetelekidis et al. 1993; Caldarelli et al. 2005; Karavitaki et al. 2005)
Hemiparesis	8 (7–12)	(Hetelekidis et al. 1993; Caldarelli et al. 2005; Karavitaki et al. 2005; Puget et al. 2007)
Decreased consciousness	8 (5–10)	(Hetelekidis et al. 1993; Karavitaki et al. 2005)
Behaviour change/ psychiatric symptoms	4 (3–10)	(Caldarelli et al. 2005; Karavitaki et al. 2005; Puget et al. 2007)

(Continued)

TABLE 13.1
(Continued)

Symptom/sign	Median frequency percentage (range %)	References
Seizures	5 (5–6)	(Hetelekidis et al. 1993; Caldarelli et al. 2005; Puget et al. 2007)
Hyperphagia/weight gain	6 (5–30)	(DeVile et al. 1996; Caldarelli et al. 2005; Karavitaki et al. 2005; Puget et al. 2007)
Optic atrophy	5	(Karavitaki et al. 2005)
Gynaecomastia/ galactorrhoea	4	(Caldarelli et al. 2005)
Precocious puberty	2 (0–3)	(DeVile et al. 1996; Hetelekidis et al. 1993; de Vries et al. 2003; Puget et al. 2007)
Blindness	9 (3–15)	(Karavitaki et al. 2005; Puget et al. 2007)
Cold intolerance	3 (0–5)	(Caldarelli et al. 2005; Karavitaki et al. 2005)
Sleep–wake cycle disturbance	2	(Caldarelli et al. 2005)

Note: Symptoms in bold indicate probable underlying endocrine or hypothalamic abnormalities which may be unrecognized.

dysfunction presenting as hyperphagia, escalating obesity, sleep–wake cycle disturbance and poor temperature control may go unrecognised or be mistaken for psychosocial dysfunction. Thus doctors must be alert to the fact that patients with growth failure, unexplained weight loss or escalating weight gain, polyuria polydipsia (without glycosuria) and early or delayed puberty may harbour a hypothalamo-pituitary lesion and necessitate urgent endocrine referral and neuroimaging. Craniopharyngiomas require differentiating from other suprasellar lesions – germinomas and Langerhans cell histiocytosis classically present with diabetes insipidus, hamartomas with central precocious puberty (Warmuth-Metz et al. 2004) and pituitary adenomas with endocrinopathies and/or specific symptoms of pituitary hormone excess. By contrast, low-grade gliomas rarely present with endocrinopathies except (often unrecognised) precocious puberty (Martinez et al. 2003; Warmuth-Metz et al. 2004).

Investigations

RADIOLOGY

The differential diagnosis of paediatric suprasellar lesions is listed in Table 13.2. Of all primary CNS tumours in children, 10% involve the sellar or suprasellar regions (Schroeder and Vezina 2011), but given their proximity to vital hypothalamo-pituitary structures, histological diagnosis is not always possible, and a radiological diagnosis is required. In this respect, the dual roles of CT and MRI in characterising the triad of solid, cystic and calcified tumour typical of an ACP (Fig 13.1) have been advocated (Spoudeas et al. 2005; Muller 2010, 2013). If MRI was the initial investigation, it is recommended that this is followed by a CT without contrast to best identify any calcification, thereby also acting as a baseline

TABLE 13.2
Differential diagnosis of paediatric suprasellar lesions

Paediatric suprasellar tumours by order of frequency

    Craniopharyngioma

    Hypothalamic/chiasmatic low-grade glioma (commonly pilocytic)

    Germinoma

    Langerhans cell histiocytosis

    Meningeal metastases

Other (rarer) tumours and malformations:

    Rathke cleft cyst (commonly asymptomatic)

    Hypothalamic hamartoma

    Pituitary adenoma (secreting e.g. PRL/ACTH or non-functioning)

    Meningioma

    Epidermoid tumour

    Aneurysms

    Arachnoid cysts

PRL, prolactin; ACTH, adrenocorticotropic hormone.

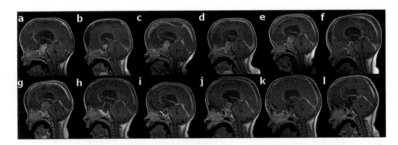

Figure 13.1. Serial TI-weighted MRI images with gadolinium contrast of a craniopharyngioma presenting in a 2-year-old boy, demonstrating solid, cystic and calcified components, as well as its tendency for multiple progressions over 7 years. (a) At diagnosis, (b) after first transcranial debulking, (c) first cystic progression, (d) after first endoscopic fenestration and cyst drainage, (e) second progression, (f) after second debulking, (g) after adjuvant radiotherapy, (h) after second cyst drainage with reservoir insertion, (i) stable appearances prior to (j) third progression, (k) after third debulking leading to radiologically apparent complete resection and (l) at last follow-up.

against which the amount of residual post-operative calcified tumour (less well-recognised macroscopically or on MRI), and thus the degree of resection, is confirmed (Warmuth-Metz et al. 2004). Between 64.7% and 93.1% of tumours are calcified (Molla et al. 2002; Zhang et al. 2002), but a combination of solid and cystic structures is highly suggestive of craniopharyngioma. The degree of T_1-weighted MRI signal varies depending on the proportion of cyst protein content, but provides better pre-operative anatomical definition. Small tumours <2cm in diameter should ideally undergo dedicated pituitary MRI scanning to provide higher resolution images of this intricate area (Spoudeas et al. 2005).

The anatomical distribution of craniopharyngiomas is relatively well-described: 5% are exclusively intrasellar, 20% exclusively suprasellar and 75% are suprasellar with an intrasellar extension (Warmuth-Metz et al. 2004; Muller 2010). Various methods of classifying these tumours have been proposed. De Vile et al. (1996) first proposed a grading system describing hypothalamic integrity and the degree of surgery-associated later morbidity in hypothalamic tumours which formed the basis of the UK risk-based consensus treatment strategy avoiding hypothalamic morbidity by limited surgery (Spoudeas et al. 2005). Since then, Puget et al. (2007) proposed a similar simplified system grading the degree of hypothalamic involvement pre-treatment (grade 0 = no hypothalamic involvement; 1 = abutting and/or displacing the hypothalamus; 2 = involving the hypothalamus, i.e. hypothalamus cannot be identified separately), accompanied by a similar system for the extent of post-operative hypothalamic damage. More recently, Flitsch et al. (2011) suggested a novel approach (Fig 13.2) to aid surgical planning, again aimed at preserving vital hypothalamic structures in the post-mamillary region by less radical resection (for stage 3b tumours).

ENDOCRINOLOGY

Accurate auxology (height, weight and BMI and SDS) is mandatory at diagnosis. Growth trajectories if available from community screening may indicate linear growth failure or rapid weight gain, and a delayed bone age provides supportive evidence especially if there is pubertal delay/arrest. Pubertal assessment for precocious, delayed or arrested puberty

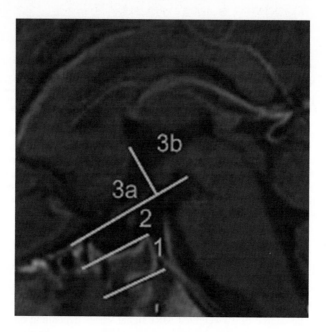

Figure 13.2. Suggested MRI classification of craniopharyngiomas. Type 1 = infrasellar, type 2 = suprasellar infrachiasmatic, type 3 = suprasellar retrochiasmatic (3a = premamillary; 3b = postmamillary) [image courtesy of Flitsch et al. 2011].

and a careful 24-hour measurement of fluid balance (particularly in the presence of nocturia or thirst) should also be documented. Higher ponderal index at birth (weight in grams/(birth length in cm)^3 × 100) and pre-treatment BMI SDS is predictive of future hypothalamic obesity, which, unlike other endocrinopathies is not treatable and negatively impacts on future morbidity (Muller et al. 2004).

Basal endocrine tests prior to any definitive treatment are important not only to determine the patient's fitness for surgery, but also to exclude the differential diagnoses of secreting germinomas α-fetoprotein [AFP], ß-human chorionic gonadotrophin [ß-hCG] or pituitary adenomas (particularly prolactin [PRL]) (Spoudeas et al. 2005), both of which may be treated medically without biopsy. Between 46% and 100% of patients have at least one endocrinopathy at diagnosis, and up to 20% have panhypopituitarism (Hetelekidis et al. 1993; Caldarelli et al. 2005). These measurements are thus also helpful in identifying which patients need prioritising for dynamic hypothalamo-pituitary assessment before treatment (Table 13.3).

In keeping with other models of hypothalamo-pituitary disruption, growth hormone deficiency (GHD) is the most common endocrinopathy at presentation (35%–100%), depending on whether dynamic tests were performed on all patients or only those with growth failure (Sorva et al. 1988; Hetelekidis et al. 1993; DeVile et al. 1996; Caldarelli et al. 2005; Karavitaki et al. 2005; Muller 2013). Serum insulin-like growth factor-1 (IGF-1 and its binding protein IGF-BP3 are useful, though less accurate, surrogate markers of GHD (Hindmarsh and Swift 1995) where formal pituitary provocation testing (with insulin-induced hypoglycaemia or glucagon stimulation) is not possible pre-treatment or may be too hazardous (Shah et al. 1992).

TABLE 13.3
Recommended pre-treatment basal endocrinology screen for craniopharyngioma

First-line	*Second-line (if first-line abnormal)*
Auxology	
Bone age	
Pubertal staging	
β-hCG, AFP, PRL*	
IGF-1/IGF-BP3	Growth hormone provocation test (e.g. insulin tolerance, glucagon stimulation)
Luteinizing hormone/FSH (if <2 and >8 years in females, >10 years in males)	GnRH test
0700, 0800, 0900 cortisol/ACTH (BEFORE commencing dexamethasone only)	Adrenal stimulation test (combined with growth hormone if insulin tolerance, or synacthen) if possible
TSH/fT$_3$/fT$_4$	
Paired plasma/urine osmolalities and electrolytes	Water deprivation test

IGF, insulin-like growth factor; FSH, follicle-stimulating hormone; ACTH, adrenocorticotropic hormone, TSH, thyroid-stimulating hormone.
*Results must be available prior to any treatment.

191

Gonadotrophin (luteinizing hormone/follicle-stimulating hormone [FSH]) deficiency is the next most prevalent endocrinopathy, with 5%–24% presenting with pubertal delay or arrest (Hetelekidis et al. 1993; DeVile et al. 1996; de Vries et al. 2003; Caldarelli et al. 2005; Karavitaki et al. 2005), and 10%–85% having hypogonadotrophic hypogonadism on biochemical testing (DeVile et al. 1996; de Vries et al. 2003; Caldarelli et al. 2005; Muller 2013). Only 3% of patients have precocious puberty at diagnosis (Hetelekidis et al. 1993; de Vries et al. 2003; Puget et al. 2007). As this axis is quiescent from 1 to 2 years of age until puberty, basal and GnRH-stimulated serum gonadotrophin measurements (luteinizing hormone/FSH) are not likely to be informative within this period and should be confined to infants below 2 years of age and peripubertal children at presentation and at intervals after treatment to identify patients at risk of early activation or deficiency.

ACTH deficiency and secondary hypoadrenalism is present in 21%–71% of patients at diagnosis, particularly where there is a history of lethargy or prolonged recovery from recurrent infections (Hetelekidis et al. 1993; Sklar 1994; DeVile et al. 1996; de Vries et al. 2003; Caldarelli et al. 2005; Karavitaki et al. 2005; Muller 2013). Importantly, early morning (0700, 0800 and/or 0900 hours) plasma cortisol and ACTH measurements should be taken *before* any dexamethasone therapy that might be administered for peri-tumoural oedema and before surgery. Morning cortisol values <200nmol/l may indicate adrenal insufficiency and will require testing by either insulin-induced hypoglycaemia (concurrently assessing growth hormone and ACTH reserve) or standard synacthen stimulation to confirm normal (peak >500nmol/l) adrenal reserve. If such a patient is not receiving dexamethasone pre-operatively, then assessment of adrenal reserve in this manner is even more crucial prior to any surgical intervention, as this can precipitate a fatal adrenal crisis if untreated. Additionally, paired early morning plasma and urine osmolalities, electrolytes and glucose are required to exclude diabetes insipidus, which can be present in up to 29% at diagnosis (Hetelekidis et al. 1993; DeVile et al. 1996; Karavitaki et al. 2005; Muller 2013), though potentially only unmasked when concurrent adrenal insufficiency is treated with glucocorticoid replacement.

Secondary and/or tertiary hypothyroidism is best assessed by measurements of serum TSH and free T_4 (± free T_3) and occurs in 13%–32% of patients (Hetelekidis et al. 1993; DeVile et al. 1996; Caldarelli et al. 2005; Karavitaki et al. 2005; Muller 2013). A normal TSH in the setting of a low free T_4 or T_3 is inappropriate and should be treated. A TRH stimulation test is often unhelpful (Mehta et al. 2003). Mild and usually clinically insignificant hyperprolactinaemia occurs in 11%–52% (DeVile et al. 1996; de Vries et al. 2003; Caldarelli et al. 2005), due to disruption of inhibitory hypothalamic dopamine by pituitary stalk compression, and is important to differentiate craniopharyngiomas from prolactinomas, where PRL secretion is usually >3000mU/l.

NEURO-OPHTHALMOLOGY AND PSYCHOLOGY

Given the prevalence of neuro-ophthalmological symptoms and signs at presentation, specialist referrals should be made for baseline neurology, visual acuity, visual fields and colour vision assessments prior to therapy. In children unable to cooperate with visual acuity testing, visual evoked potentials are useful to assess visual function. Neurocognitive testing with special assessments for the youngest and visually impaired should be performed as early as possible in the treatment pathway to provide a baseline for assessing future post-treatment brain injury.

Treatment

In the absence of high-quality level I evidence, the management of craniopharyngiomas remains controversial, with the UK paediatric endocrine and neuro-oncological societies having led the way in endorsing a consensus risk-based treatment strategy in tertiary centres of expertise (Spoudeas et al. 2005), with affiliated specialist pituitary and neuro-oncological surgical and medical services, including paediatric endocrinology, radiation oncology, neuro-oncology, neuroradiology and neuropsychology. The advantages of attempting complete tumour resection to achieve better recurrence-free survival must be balanced against the risk of causing significant hypothalamic morbidity from surgery or radiotherapy, particularly the irreversible and currently untreatable outcomes of hypothalamic obesity, adipsic diabetes insipidus and neurocognitive dysfunction.

PRE-OPERATIVE CONSIDERATIONS

If the child has presented with acute hydrocephalus and raised ICP, this may require stabilisation before transfer to a dedicated neurosurgical and neuroendocrine centre. Preoperative knowledge of early morning urine and plasma electrolytes, osmolalities and cortisol are essential with close liaison between the anaesthetist and endocrinologist; therefore samples taken prior to transfer can be useful. High-dose dexamethasone therapy is often commenced prior to transfer for peritumoral oedema. In its absence and where adrenal status has not been established pre-operatively by one of the methods in Table 13.3, then IM/IV hydrocortisone in stress doses (1–2mg/kg) should be given at induction, with repeat doses at 6–8 hourly intervals, gradually weaning to maintenance doses over 5–10 days until adrenal status can be assessed.

ACTH deficiency may mask diabetes insipidus and glucocorticoid supplementation may thus unmask it. Pre-operative diabetes insipidus warrants desmopressin administration prior to surgery (0.1–0.2μg IM/SC) with extremely careful fluid balance monitoring using an indwelling urinary catheter intra-operatively, replacing fluid losses ml for ml with an additional 300ml/m^2/day to account for insensible losses. Dangerous swings in salt and water balance may occur peri-operatively requiring close monitoring by endocrinologists and a triphasic response of temporary diabetes insipidus, syndrome of inappropriate antidiuretic hormone secretion (SIADH) and permanent diabetes insipidus may evolve over 2–3 post-operative weeks. In a patient with seizures, correction of peri-operative salt-water imbalance may obviate the need for anticonvulsants, but some such as carbamazepine and lamotrigine can potentiate the effect of desmopressin or cause an SIADH-like picture.

Supplementation of other hypothalamo-pituitary deficits must be supervised by a paediatric endocrinologist. There is no reason to delay growth hormone therapy in view of its benefits in promoting lean body mass as it has not been implicated in tumour recurrence (Moshang et al. 1996; Muller et al. 2010), but it is common practice to stop growth hormone therapy for about 2 weeks before and after surgery. It is also sensible to render a hypothyroid patient euthyroid pre-operatively. Sex hormone replacement should be timely and age-appropriate after growth hormone substitution has commenced but may be delayed until treatment is complete.

OPERATIVE TECHNIQUES

Given that craniopharygiomas are histologically benign, surgical excision or debulking remain the mainstays of treatment. A detailed review of surgical techniques is beyond the scope of this chapter and has been extensively reviewed elsewhere (Yasargil et al. 1990; Fahlbusch et al. 1999; Flitsch et al. 2011). There are essentially three means of surgical access in decreasing order of the size of operative window achieved – transcranial, trans-sphenoidal or endoscopic. The former route is most useful for suprasellar (type 2 and 3) tumours where clear views of the surrounding optic apparatus are required, whilst trans-sphenoidal access is only suitable for infrasellar and very occasionally suprasellar cystic craniopharyngiomas (Yasargil et al. 1990; Fahlbusch et al. 1999; Flitsch et al. 2011). However, the routine division of the pituitary gland to access the tumour trans-sphenoidally results in increased risk of post-operative endocrinopathy, especially diabetes insipidus. Transcranial access can be achieved via the pterional, subfrontal, transventricular or retro-sigmoid approaches. Endoscopic access routes only allow for cyst aspirations, cyst catheter insertions or tumour biopsies.

RADIOTHERAPY

The role of radiotherapy in the management of craniopharyngiomas is largely an adjuvant one, particularly where complete resection has not or cannot be achieved. Their benign histology results in reduced infiltration of surrounding tissues and a cleaner safety margin of the radiotherapy field. Conventional external beam techniques and intensity-modulated radiotherapy to a total dose of 46–50Gy are the commonest methods of administration. Fractionated stereotactic radiotherapy is advocated over conventional techniques as it reduces exposure of healthy brain tissue to high-dose irradiation (Schulz-Ertner et al. 2002; Merchant et al. 2006). There is an increasing trend to use proton beam irradiation where available in selected young patients <15 years with small tumours to further attempt to reduce radiation scatter to the surrounding normal brain. Careful planning using three-dimensional conformal techniques, and where available, fusion of CT and MRI images is recommended to improve planning target volume definition, which should encompass the entire post-operative tumour bed and any residual tumour plus an additional safety margin clearly defined in local guide-lines. However, in the absence of randomised controlled trials, there remains no consensus on the optimal dose (35–66Gy), target volume (2mm–2cm from tumour margins), degree of fractionation (1.6–3.3Gy/fraction), or modality of radiotherapy (opposing beams versus arc/rotational beams, conventional versus stereotactic/conformal, X-ray versus proton beam) that should be used (Hetelekidis et al. 1993; De Vile et al. 1996; Habrand et al. 1999; Merchant et al. 2002, 2006; Schulz-Ertner et al. 2002; Stripp et al. 2004; Caldarelli et al. 2005; Karavitaki et al. 2005; Puget et al. 2007; Lin et al. 2008; Schubert et al. 2009).

Other techniques such as single fraction 'gamma-knife' radiosurgery may also reduce exposure of surrounding healthy brain tissue to irradiation, but its applicability is limited to small tumours ($\leq$3.5cm^3) away from critical optic pathway and brainstem structures (by >3–5mm) (Chiou et al. 2001; Ulfarsson et al. 2002; Jackson et al. 2003). Brachytherapy with ^{32}P or ^{90}Y radioisotopes and intracystic sclerosant chemotherapy such as bleomycin have been anecdotally used in cystic recurrences, but carry high failure rates in large tumours, potential toxicity from leakage and no clear benefit over conservative cyst aspiration and drainage (Ulfarsson et al. 2002; Fang et al. 2012).

RISK STRATIFICATION AND OVERALL TREATMENT STRATEGY

There remains doubt as to the aetiology of long-term morbidity and what proportion of this is disease- or treatment-related. There are still those who advocate radical surgery aiming for complete resection to avoid radiation (Yasargil et al. 1990; Hoffman et al. 1992; Van Effenterre and Boch 2002; Stripp et al. 2004; Caldarelli et al. 2005) versus those who advocate more conservative surgical strategies (endoscopic/stereotactic cyst aspiration, cyst catheter and reservoir placement, shunt procedures, tumour-debulking operations) with upfront adjuvant radiotherapy for tumour remnants or as salvage treatment for relapse (De Vile et al. 1996; Fahlbusch et al. 1999; Habrand et al. 1999; Schulz-Ertner et al. 2002; Merchant et al. 2002; Lin et al. 2008; Schubert et al. 2009).

Several studies have shown that radiologically confirmed complete tumour resection increases the likelihood of progression-free survival (PFS), with 5-year and 10-year PFS ranging from 64%–100% to 73%–100%, respectively, as compared to 31%–65% to 28%–53%, respectively, for subtotal resection (De Vile et al. 1996; Fahlbusch et al. 1999; Van Effenterre and Boch 2002; Caldarelli et al. 2005; Karavitaki et al. 2005; Muller et al. 2010). Published series advocating a purely aggressive surgical strategy are often inherently specialty-biased, suffering from insufficient follow-up and non-radiologically confirmed 'complete' resections, as well as not assessing the long-term hypothalamic dysfunction associated with radical surgery found by others (Hetelekidis et al. 1993; De Vile et al. 1996; DeVile et al. 1996; Fahlbusch et al. 1999; Merchant et al. 2002; Schulz-Ertner et al. 2002; Lustig et al. 2003b; Puget et al. 2007). Radiotherapy significantly ameliorates the reduced PFS associated with incomplete resection and achieves similar cure rates to complete resection alone (5-year PFS 82% vs. 47% and 10-year PFS 77% vs. 38% for subtotal resection with and without adjuvant radiotherapy, respectively; Karavitaki et al. 2005), thereby avoiding further relapse and surgery, the two main predictors of long-term hypothalamic morbidity and premature mortality (De Vile et al. 1996; DeVile et al. 1996; Fahlbusch et al. 1999). Others have even reported better 10-year PFS after surgery and upfront radiotherapy than in those treated with surgery alone (71%–100% vs. 24%–42%) (Hetelekidis et al. 1993; Schulz-Ertner et al. 2002; Stripp et al. 2004; Lin et al. 2008; Schubert et al. 2009). Whilst PFS appears similar between those who received upfront radiotherapy as compared to those who received it only at relapse (Stripp et al. 2004; Lin et al. 2008), a randomised controlled trial looking at PFS and quality of life in relation to the timing of radiotherapy in children above 5 years of age with incompletely resected tumours is currently under way in Europe (KRANIOPHARYNGEOM 2007) (Muller 2010).

A risk-based approach to the management of paediatric craniopharyngiomas has been more recently advocated (Hetelekidis et al. 1993; De Vile et al. 1996; Fahlbusch et al. 1999;

Habrand et al. 1999; Puget et al. 2007). Several at-diagnosis predictors of poor prognosis have been identified, namely age above 5 years, tumour height >3.5–5cm in the midline, radiological or clinical evidence of hypothalamic involvement (Puget et al. grade 2; Flitsch et al. stage 3a and 3b), severe hydrocephalus (ventricular indices >55%), and tumour adherence to surrounding healthy tissue at surgery (De Vile et al. 1996; Fahlbusch et al. 1999; Habrand et al. 1999; Garre and Cama 2007; Puget et al. 2007; Flitsch et al. 2011). The risk of causing irreversible hypothalamic damage from attempted radical surgery in these subgroups outweighs any benefit in PFS from successful or attempted gross total resection (GTR), and an initial conservative surgical approach (including cyst aspirations, shunt procedures and debulking operations) with early adjuvant conformal radiotherapy for residual disease is recommended if the risk of recurrence is felt to be more neurotoxic than irradiation. At present, radiotherapy for radiologically proven completely resected tumours is not advocated in children, utilising it only in the event of recurrence during long-term follow-up (Spoudeas et al. 2005).

Experience with other CNS tumours suggests that delaying radiotherapy exposure in young patients (<5 years) may reduce the risk of long-term neurocognitive deficits (Mulhern et al. 2004). However, the reduced volumes of brain irradiated with current techniques, more focused proton beam irradiation and better neurorehabilitation may be more favourable factors in children with high-risk craniopharyngiomas where tumour progression and/ or repeated surgical interventions can also cause neurocognitive deficits in the absence of irradiation (Cavazzuti et al. 1983; Carpentieri et al. 2001). Indeed, our own historical experience at Great Ormond Street Hospital (GOSH) (De Vile et al. 1996) and the more recent St. Jude's experience (Merchant et al. 2002) indicate that surgery is the greatest risk factor for neurocognitive and endocrine sequelae in craniopharyngiomas.

POST-TREATMENT SURVEILLANCE AND FOLLOW-UP

Table 13.4 suggests a risk-stratified clinical surveillance strategy advocated in the United Kingdom (Spoudeas et al. 2005), based on the initial treatment modality(ies) employed. An immediate post-operative MRI scan is recommended within 24–72 hours of surgery, to determine the presence of residual tumour. An adjunctive CT scan is also advised to assess the possibility of residual calcified tissue not easily visualized on MRI (Muller 2010; Spoudeas et al. 2005). The presence of any residuum indicates an incomplete resection, carrying a higher risk of progression or recurrence, and thus management should ideally proceed to immediate adjuvant radiotherapy. The exception to this guidance is the situation where the child is deemed too young to undergo radiotherapy, in which case close observation and conservative surgical techniques (e.g. cyst aspiration) should be used for tumour control until the child is of appropriate age.

Transient diabetes insipidus is extremely common in the immediate post-operative period (24–48 hours), occurring in up to 100% of patients in some series (Hoffman et al. 1992; DeVile et al. 1996; Van Effenterre and Boch 2002; Poretti et al. 2004; Caldarelli et al. 2005; Karavitaki et al. 2005; Lin et al. 2008). This may be followed by a phase of SIADH, which may be missed, is rarely reported in studies but can last up to 2–3 weeks (Caldarelli et al. 2005; Spoudeas et al. 2005). Permanent diabetes insipidus can then ensue, particularly

Craniopharyngioma

Craniopharyngioma

Craniopharyngioma

TABLE 13.4
Suggested post-treatment surveillance strategy for paediatric craniopharyngiomas

Interval from treatment	Complete resection	Incomplete resection + radiotherapy	Incomplete resection + surveillance
Immediate post-operative period			
Radiology	MRI at 24–72 hours ± CT then MRI at 3 months		
Neurosurgery	For peri-operative neurosurgical complications (shunt infections, etc.)		
Endocrine	For peri-operative fluid balance management (diabetes insipidus, SIADH, salt-wasting)		
Years 1–2			
Radiology	6-monthly MRI	12-monthly MRI	4-monthly MRI
Neurosurgery	3-monthly		2-monthly
Clinical oncology	–	3-monthly	–
Endocrine		3–6 monthly	
Ophthalmology	3–6 monthly	6–12 monthly	3–4 monthly
Psychology	At 2 years		
Years 3–5			
Radiology	12-monthly MRI		6-monthly MRI
Neurosurgery	6–12 monthly		4–6 monthly
Clinical oncology	–	6–12 monthly	–
Endocrine	6-monthly		
Ophthalmology	6–12 monthly		6-monthly
Psychology	At 5 years		
After 5 years			
Radiology	At clinician's discretion		12-monthly MRI
Neurosurgery	–		At clinician's discretion
Clinical oncology	–	12-monthly	–
Endocrine	6-monthly until final adult height		
	12-monthly until transition		
	12–24-monthly thereafter		
Ophthalmology	–	12–24 monthly	–
Psychology	At 18 years (career guidance)		

SIADH, syndrome of inappropriate antidiuretic hormone.
Spoudeas et al. 2005.

if the initial diabetes insipidus or SIADH phases are prolonged or severe. The constantly changing posterior pituitary status of these patients in the post-operative period mandates extremely careful fluid balance monitoring in consultation with an endocrinologist. Diabetes insipidus is the only pituitary dysfunction that has ever been described to spontaneously resolve in this situation, and the prevalence of permanent diabetes insipidus in long-term survivors is slightly lower (42%–94%) (Hoffman et al. 1992; Hetelekidis et al. 1993; DeVile et al. 1996; Habrand et al. 1999; Merchant et al. 2002; Schulz-Ertner et al. 2002; Van Effenterre and Boch 2002; Poretti et al. 2004; Stripp et al. 2004; Caldarelli et al. 2005; Karavitaki et al. 2005; Lin et al. 2008; Crom et al. 2010; Muller et al. 2011b). However, the combination of diabetes insipidus with hypothalamic adipsia and ACTH deficiency is particularly dangerous and can prove fatal, and should be avoided where it is not evident pre-operatively. Radical surgical resection remains a consistent risk factor for diabetes insipidus if not already present pre-operatively, particularly the adipsic form (Hetelekidis et al. 1993; DeVile et al. 1996; Merchant et al. 2002; Stripp et al. 2004; Lin et al. 2008).

The risk of post-treatment endocrinopathies increases especially after radical surgery, with 97% of survivors having at least one pituitary axis affected long-term, and 31%–84% having panhypopituitarism (Hetelekidis et al. 1993; De Vile et al. 1996; DeVile et al. 1996; Habrand et al. 1999; Merchant et al. 2002; Schulz-Ertner et al. 2002; Van Effenterre and Boch 2002; Poretti et al. 2004; Stripp et al. 2004; Caldarelli et al. 2005; Lin et al. 2008; Crom et al. 2010). Our own group at GOSH have demonstrated that a conservative risk-based treatment consensus strategy significantly reduces the prevalence of life-threatening cortisol (85% to 73%) and AVP (80% to 55%) deficiencies without compromising cure rates (Ikazoboh et al. 2011). Endocrinopathies presented after 4–6 post-operative weeks are permanent and require long-term monitoring and/or supplementation, with GHD being the commonest (20%–99%), followed by secondary/tertiary hypothyroidism (39%–97%), hypogonadotrophic hypogonadism (30%–95%) and ACTH deficiency (39%–89%) (Hoffman et al. 1992; Hetelekidis et al. 1993; DeVile et al. 1996; Merchant et al. 2002; Poretti et al. 2004; Caldarelli et al. 2005; Karavitaki et al. 2005; Lin et al. 2008; Crom et al. 2010; Muller et al. 2011b). Post-operative assessment of the hypothalamopituitary-adrenal axis in patients receiving peri-operative dexamethasone is best left until 2–3 months after substitution with maintenance hydrocortisone, which allows a formal assessment of cortisol reserve off supplementation to be carried out. This should be performed with caution along with a full assessment of all other hypothalamo-pituitary axes by dynamic testing (using rescue hydrocortisone at the end of insulin-induced hypoglycaemia or glucagon stimulation) in a dedicated paediatric endocrinology centre used to managing patients with multiple coexisting endocrinopathies. Growth hormone therapy in replacement doses to the deficient child is safe and has not been shown to increase the risk of recurrence, progression or second tumours (DeVile et al. 1996; Moshang et al. 1996; Muller et al. 2010).

The hypothalamic syndrome, particularly hypothalamic obesity, remains a significant and as yet untreatable long-term problem for craniopharyngioma survivors, occurring in up to 67% by 20 years (Hoffman et al. 1992; Hetelekidis et al. 1993; De Vile et al. 1996; Fahlbusch et al. 1999; Muller et al. 2001; Schulz-Ertner et al. 2002; Poretti et al. 2004; Stripp et al. 2004; Caldarelli et al. 2005; Lin et al. 2008; Crom et al. 2010; Muller 2013), with its attendant risks of type 2 diabetes and cardiovascular mortality. Associated symptoms, apart from early (often in the first 6 months; Muller et al. 2004; Lustig 2011; Bereket et al. 2012) and often inexorable weight gain, are hyperphagia, adipsia, impaired

thermoregulation, disrupted sleep–wake cycles, memory deficits and behavioural disturbances. The aetiology and pathogenesis of this condition is poorly understood, and is currently thought to be due to disruption of energy metabolism homeostasis by the ventromedial
hypothalamic nucleus, a process controlled by a complex set of interactions between
anorexigens (leptin, pro-opiomelanocortin and α-melanocyte-stimulating hormone) and
orexigens (ghrelin, neuropeptide Y and agouti-related peptide; Horvath et al. 2001; Lustig
2002, 2011; Ramos et al. 2004; Bereket et al. 2012). More recently, the wider role of oxytocin beyond parturition and lactation has been recognised with various postulated mechanisms on its involvement in metabolism, stress and social interaction (Deblon et al. 2011;
Maejima et al. 2011; Onaka et al. 2012; Wu et al. 2012). It has been demonstrated that
hypothalamic obesity is not driven by the hyperphagia itself, but is related to disrupted
vagal tone and a dysfunctional metabolic state exacerbated by reduced physical activity
(Harz et al. 2003). It is clear that the major risk factors for the development of hypothalamic
obesity are all associated with an increased risk of hypothalamic disruption – that is hypothalamic tumour involvement (as evidenced by pre-treatment endocrinopathy and obesity),
multiple recurrences, extensive surgery and high-dose radiotherapy (>51Gy) (Habrand
et al. 1999; Muller et al. 2001; Lustig et al. 2003b). To date, there are no sustainably effective therapies for this complication, be it medical (e.g. octreotide; Lustig et al. 2003a) or
surgical (laparoscopic gastric banding; Muller et al. 2011a).

Post-operative visual acuity and field assessment should be conducted early, with the
best predictors of a good visual outcome being normal pre-treatment visual function,
tumour location away from the prechiasmatic region and less-invasive surgical techniques
(Fahlbusch et al. 1999; Merchant et al. 2002; Caldarelli et al. 2005; Muller 2013). Although
one of the major objectives of treatment is to preserve visual function, this has not been
convincingly demonstrated, with published literature contrastingly showing both reductions
(Fahlbusch et al. 1999; Schulz-Ertner et al. 2002; Van Effenterre and Boch 2002; Caldarelli
et al. 2005) and increases (Hoffman et al. 1992; Stripp et al. 2004) in the prevalence of
visual impairment post-treatment compared to at diagnosis. Neurocognitive and psychological assessments are also necessary as part of long-term follow-up, with 5%–40% of patients
requiring educational support and 3%–33% having emotional, behavioural and psychiatric
disorders (Hoffman et al. 1992; Hetelekidis et al. 1993; Carpentieri et al. 2001; Merchant
et al. 2002; Van Effenterre and Boch 2002; Poretti et al. 2004; Karavitaki et al. 2005; Crom
et al, 2010). The majority of craniopharyngioma survivors experience a reduction in all
domains of IQ, particularly in multiply relapsing tumours (Hetelekidis et al. 1993; Merchant
et al. 2002; Van Effenterre and Boch 2002; Schubert et al. 2009). Memory deficits are
particularly over-represented, affecting both language and visuospatial function, and can
importantly occur even in the absence of radiotherapy exposure (Cavazzuti et al. 1983;
Carpentieri et al. 2001; Poretti et al. 2004). These factors mandate proactive neuroendocrine
surveillance and neurorehabilitation to improve quality of life.

MANAGEMENT OF RECURRENCES
The treatment of recurrent or progressive tumours is especially difficult and remains case-
based, experimental and suboptimal. For solid recurrences, the use of external beam

conformal radiotherapy may be obviated by previous exposure, whilst systemic chemotherapy for craniopharyngiomas remains completely anecdotal and cannot be recommended at present (Bremer et al. 1984; Lippens et al. 1998; Spoudeas et al. 2005). Cystic recurrences may require repeated surgical aspirations through an indwelling catheter if it does not readily block with the proteinacious fluid, intracavitary instillation of radioisotopes (32P, 90Y) or bleomycin – none of these have been proven to be superior (De Vile et al. 1996; Merchant et al. 2002; Lin et al. 2008; Fang et al. 2012).

Prognosis

Despite these controversies, survival in paediatric craniopharyngiomas remains high, with actuarial 5-, 10-, 20- and 30-year overall survival rates in the ranges of 91%–100%, 65%–96%, 83%–96%, and 80%–92%, respectively, having improved significantly with advances in treatment strategies over time (Bunin et al. 1998; Hetelekidis et al. 1993; De Vile et al. 1996; Fahlbusch et al. 1999; Habrand et al. 1999; Schulz-Ertner et al. 2002; Van Effenterre and Boch 2002; Poretti et al. 2004; Stripp et al. 2004; Karavitaki et al. 2005; Spoudeas et al. 2005; Stiller 2007; Lin et al. 2008). This is in comparison to adult-onset craniopharyngiomas, and several studies have shown that increasing age is a predictor for mortality (Fahlbusch et al. 1999; Habrand et al. 1999; Zacharia et al. 2012). Unlike the other risk factors associated with reduced PFS, however, overall survival rate has not been consistently associated with tumour invasiveness or treatment strategy, though it is negatively associated with recurrence or disease progression (Karavitaki et al. 2005). Therefore, prognosis in paediatric craniopharyngiomas should be measured in terms of PFS rather than overall survival, accounting for the morbidities associated with tumour and/or treatment. Deaths occur not just in the immediate post-operative period from direct surgical complications such as haemorrhage and infection, but also late fluid-electrolyte imbalances secondary to endocrine dysfunction, cardiovascular events associated with hypothalamic obesity and psychology-related incidents such as drug abuse (Hetelekidis et al. 1993; DeVile et al. 1996; Fahlbusch et al. 1999; Poretti et al. 2004; Stripp et al. 2004; Caldarelli et al. 2005; Crom et al. 2010). This late mortality observed up to 30 years from diagnosis is often unaccounted for by studies that have had insufficient follow-up durations. Indeed, there have been recent calls for craniopharyngiomas to be recognised and managed as a chronic disease (Muller 2013), requiring lifelong follow-up not only for disease recurrence but predominantly for neuroendocrine, visual and cognitive morbidities.

REFERENCES

Albini A, Cesana E and Noonan DM (2011) Cancer stem cells and the tumor microenvironment: Soloists or choral singers. *Curr Pharm Biotechnol* 12: 171–181.

Alison MR, Murphy G and Leedham S (2008) Stem cells and cancer: A deadly mix. *Cell Tissue Res* 331: 109–124.

Andoniadou CL, Gaston-Massuet C, Reddy R et al. (2012) Identification of novel pathways involved in the pathogenesis of human adamantinomatous craniopharyngioma. *Acta Neuropathol* 124: 259–271.

Barkhoudarian G and Laws ER (2013) Craniopharyngioma: history. *Pituitary* 16: 1–8.

Bereket A, Kiess W, Lustig RH et al. (2012) Hypothalamic obesity in children. *Obes Rev* 13: 780–798.

Bremer AM, Nguyen TQ and Balsys R (1984) Therapeutic benefits of combination chemotherapy with vincristine, BCNU, and procarbazine on recurrent cystic craniopharyngioma. A case report. *J Neurooncol* 2: 47–51.

Bunin GR, Surawicz TS, Witman PA, Preston-Martin S, Davis F and Bruner JM (1998) The descriptive epidemiology of craniopharyngioma. *J Neurosurg* 89: 547–551.

Burghaus S, Holsken A, Buchfelder M et al. (2010) A tumor-specific cellular environment at the brain invasion border of adamantinomatous craniopharyngiomas. *Virchows Arch* 456: 287–300.

Buslei R, Holsken A, Hofmann B et al. (2007) Nuclear beta-catenin accumulation associates with epithelial morphogenesis in craniopharyngiomas. *Acta Neuropathol* 113: 585–590.

Buslei R, Nolde M, Hofmann B et al. (2005) Common mutations of beta-catenin in adamantinomatous craniopharyngiomas but not in other tumours originating from the sellar region. *Acta Neuropathol* 109: 589–597.

Caldarelli M, Massimi L, Tamburrini G, Cappa M and Di Rocco C (2005) Long-term results of the surgical treatment of craniopharyngioma: The experience at the Policlinico Gemelli, Catholic University, Rome. *Childs Nerv Syst* 21: 747–757.

Carpentieri SC, Waber DP, Scott RM et al. (2001) Memory deficits among children with craniopharyngiomas. *Neurosurgery* 49: 1053–1057; discussion 1057–1058.

Castinetti F, Davis SW, Brue T and Camper SA (2011) Pituitary stem cell update and potential implications for treating hypopituitarism. *Endocr Rev* 32: 453–471.

Cavazzuti V, Fischer EG, Welch K, Belli JA and Winston KR (1983) Neurological and psychophysiological sequelae following different treatments of craniopharyngioma in children. *J Neurosurg* 59: 409–417.

Chiou SM, Lunsford LD, Niranjan A, Kondziolka D and Flickinger JC (2001) Stereotactic radiosurgery of residual or recurrent craniopharyngioma, after surgery, with or without radiation therapy. *Neuro Oncol* 3: 159–166.

Clarke MF and Fuller M (2006) Stem cells and cancer: Two faces of eve. *Cell* 124: 1111–1115.

Crom DB, Smith D, Xiong Z et al. (2010) Health status in long-term survivors of pediatric craniopharyngiomas. *J Neurosci Nurs* 42: 323–328; quiz 329–330.

Davis SW, Mortensen AH and Camper SA (2011) Birthdating studies reshape models for pituitary gland cell specification. *Dev Biol* 352: 215–227.

De Almeida JP, Sherman JH, Salvatori R and Quinones-Hinojosa A (2010) Pituitary stem cells: Review of the literature and current understanding. *Neurosurgery* 67: 770–780.

De Vile CJ, Grant DB, Kendall BE et al. (1996) Management of childhood craniopharyngioma: Can the morbidity of radical surgery be predicted? *J Neurosurg* 85: 73–81.

De Vries L, Lazar L and Phillip M (2003) Craniopharyngioma: Presentation and endocrine sequelae in 36 children. *J Pediatr Endocrinol Metab* 16: 703–710.

Deblon N, Veyrat-Durebex C, Bourgoin L et al. (2011) Mechanisms of the anti-obesity effects of oxytocin in diet-induced obese rats. *PLoS One* 6: e25565.

Devile CJ, Grant DB, Hayward RD and Stanhope R (1996) Growth and endocrine sequelae of craniopharyngioma. *Arch Dis Child* 75: 108–114.

Fahlbusch R, Honegger J, Paulus W, Huk W and Buchfelder M (1999) Surgical treatment of craniopharyngiomas: Experience with 168 patients. *J Neurosurg* 90: 237–250.

Fang Y, Cai BW, Zhang H et al. (2012) Intracystic bleomycin for cystic craniopharyngiomas in children. *Cochrane Database Syst Rev* 4: CD008890.

Fauquier T, Rizzoti K, Dattani M, Lovell-Badge R and Robinson IC (2008) SOX2-expressing progenitor cells generate all of the major cell types in the adult mouse pituitary gland. *Proc Natl Acad Sci USA* 105: 2907–2912.

Flitsch J, Muller HL and Burkhardt T (2011) Surgical strategies in childhood craniopharyngioma. *Front Endocrinol* (Lausanne) 2: 96.

Florio T (2011) Adult pituitary stem cells: From pituitary plasticity to adenoma development. *Neuroendocrinology* 94: 265–277.

Garcia-Lavandeira M, Quereda V, Flores I et al. (2009) A GRFa2/Prop1/stem (GPS) cell niche in the pituitary. *PLoS One* 4: e4815.

Garcia-Lavandeira M, Saez C, Diaz-Rodriguez E et al. (2012) Craniopharyngiomas express embryonic stem cell markers (SOX2, OCT4, KLF4, and SOX9) as pituitary stem cells but do not coexpress RET/GFRA3 receptors. *J Clin Endocrinol Metab* 97: E80–E87.

Garre ML and Cama A (2007) Craniopharyngioma: Modern concepts in pathogenesis and treatment. *Curr Opin in Pediatr* 19: 471–479.

Gaston-Massuet C, Andoniadou CL, Signore M et al. (2011) Increased Wingless (Wnt) signaling in pituitary progenitor/stem cells gives rise to pituitary tumors in mice and humans. *Proc Natl Acad Sci USA,* 108: 11482–11487.

Gleiberman AS, Michurina T, Encinas JM et al. (2008) Genetic approaches identify adult pituitary stem cells. *Proc Natl Acad Sci USA* 105: 6332–6337.

Gorlin RJ (2004) Nevoid basal cell carcinoma (Gorlin) syndrome. *Genet Med* 6: 530–539.

Habrand JL, Ganry O, Couanet D et al. (1999) The role of radiation therapy in the management of cranio-pharyngioma: A 25-year experience and review of the literature. *Int J Radiat Oncol Biol Phys* 44: 255–263.

Harz KJ, Muller HL, Waldeck E, Pudel V and Roth C (2003) Obesity in patients with craniopharyngioma: Assessment of food intake and movement counts indicating physical activity. *J Clin Endocrinol Metab* 88: 5227–5231.

Hetelekidis S, Barnes PD, Tao ML et al. (1993) 20-year experience in childhood craniopharyngioma. *Int J Radiat Oncol Biol Phys* 27: 189–195.

Hindmarsh PC and Swift PG (1995) An assessment of growth hormone provocation tests. *Arch Dis Child* 72: 362–367; discussion 367–368.

Hoffman HJ, De Silva M, Humphreys RP, Drake JM, Smith ML and Blaser SI (1992) Aggressive surgical management of craniopharyngiomas in children. *J Neurosurg* 76: 47–52.

Hofmann BM, Kreutzer J, Saeger W et al. (2006) Nuclear beta-catenin accumulation as reliable marker for the differentiation between cystic craniopharyngiomas and rathke cleft cysts: A clinico-pathologic approach. *Am J Surg Pathol* 30: 1595–1603.

Holsken A, Buchfelder M, Fahlbusch R, Blumcke I and Buslei R (2010) Tumour cell migration in adaman-tinomatous craniopharyngiomas is promoted by activated Wnt-signalling. *Acta Neuropathol* 119: 631–639.

Holsken A, Gebhardt M, Buchfelder M, Fahlbusch R, Blumcke I and Buslei R (2011) EGFR signaling regu-lates tumor cell migration in craniopharyngiomas. *Clin Cancer Res* 17: 4367–4377.

Horvath TL, Diano S, Sotonyi P, Heiman M and Tschop M (2001) Minireview: Ghrelin and the regulation of energy balance—a hypothalamic perspective. *Endocrinology* 142: 4163–4169.

Ikazoboh E, Dattani M and Spoudeas HA (2011) Endocrine, hypothalamic and neuro-developmental out-comes after childhood craniopharyngioma. In: 43rd Congress of the International Society of Paediatric Oncology (SIOP) 2011, Auckland, New Zealand, 28th–30th October, 2011. SIOP Abstracts. *Pediatr Blood Cancer* 57: 805.

Jackson AS, St George EJ, Hayward RJ and Plowman PN (2003) Stereotactic radiosurgery. XVII: Recurrent intrasellar craniopharyngioma. *Br J Neurosurg* 17: 138–143.

Karavitaki N, Brufani C, Warner JT et al. (2005) Craniopharyngiomas in children and adults: Systematic analysis of 121 cases with long-term follow-up. *Clin Endocrinol (Oxf)* 62: 397–409.

Kato K, Nakatani Y, Kanno H et al. (2004) Possible linkage between specific histological structures and aberrant reactivation of the Wnt pathway in adamantinomatous craniopharyngioma. *J Pathol* 203: 814–821.

Katoh Y and Katoh M (2005) Hedgehog signaling pathway and gastric cancer. *Cancer Biol Ther* 4: 1050–1054.

Lepore DA, Roeszler K, Wagner J, Ross SA, Bauer K and Thomas PQ (2005) Identification and enrichment of colony-forming cells from the adult murine pituitary. *Exp Cell Res* 308: 166–176.

Lin LL, El Naqa I, Leonard JR et al. (2008) Long-term outcome in children treated for craniopharyngioma with and without radiotherapy. *J Neurosurg Pediatr* 1: 126–130.

Lippens RJ, Rotteveel JJ, Otten BJ and Merx H (1998) Chemotherapy with Adriamycin (doxorubicin) and CCNU (lomustine) in four children with recurrent craniopharyngioma. *Eur J Paediatr Neurol* 2: 263–268.

Lustig RH (2002) Hypothalamic obesity: The sixth cranial endocrinopathy. *Endocrinologist* 12: 210–217.

Lustig RH (2011) Hypothalamic obesity after craniopharyngiomas: Mechanisms, diagnosis and treatment. *Front Endocrinol* 2: 60.

Lustig RH, Hinds PS, Ringwald-Smith K et al. (2003a) Octreotide therapy of pediatric hypothalamic obesity: A double-blind, placebo-controlled trial. *J Clin Endocrinol Metab* 88: 2586–2592.

Lustig RH, Post SR, Srivannaboon K et al. (2003b) Risk factors for the development of obesity in children surviving brain tumors. *J Clin Endocrinol Metab* 88: 611–616.

Maejima Y, Iwasaki Y, Yamahara Y, Kodaira M, Sedbazar U and Yada T (2011) Peripheral oxytocin treatment ameliorates obesity by reducing food intake and visceral fat mass. *Aging* (Albany, NY), 3: 1169–1177.

Martinez R, Honegger J, Fahlbusch R and Buchfelder M (2003) Endocrine findings in patients with optico-hypothalamic gliomas. *Exp Clin Endocrinol Diabetes* 111: 162–167.

Mas C, Ruiz I and Altaba A (2010) Small molecule modulation of HH-GLI signaling: Current leads, trials and tribulations. *Biochem Pharmacol* 80: 712–723.

Medina V, Calvo MB, Diaz-Prado S and Espada J (2009) Hedgehog signalling as a target in cancer stem cells. *Clin Transl Oncol* 11: 199–207.

Mehta A, Hindmarsh PC, Stanhope RG, Brain CE, Preece MA and Dattani MT (2003) Is the thyrotropin-releasing hormone test necessary in the diagnosis of central hypothyroidism in children. *J Clin Endocrinol Metab* 88: 5696–5703.

Merchant TE, Kiehna EN, Kun LE et al. (2006) Phase II trial of conformal radiation therapy for pediatric patients with craniopharyngioma and correlation of surgical factors and radiation dosimetry with change in cognitive function. *J Neurosurg* 104: 94–102.

Merchant TE, Kiehna EN, Sanford RA et al. (2002) Craniopharyngioma: The St. Jude Children's Research Hospital experience 1984–2001. *Int J Radiat Oncol Biol Phys* 53: 533–542.

Molla E, Marti-Bonmati L, Revert A et al. (2002) Craniopharyngiomas: Identification of different semiological patterns with MRI. *Eur Radiol* 12: 1829–1836.

Moshang T Jr, Rundle AC, Graves DA, Nickas J, Johanson A and Meadows A (1996) Brain tumor recurrence in children treated with growth hormone: The National Cooperative Growth Study experience. *J Pediatr* 128 S4–S7.

Mulhern RK, Merchant TE, Gajjar A, Reddick WE and Kun LE (2004) Late neurocognitive sequelae in survivors of brain tumours in childhood. *Lancet Oncol* 5: 399–408.

Muller HL (2010) Childhood craniopharyngioma—current concepts in diagnosis, therapy and follow-up. *Nat Rev Endocrinol* 6: 609–618.

Muller HL (2013) Childhood craniopharyngioma. *Pituitary* 16: 56–67.

Muller HL, Bueb K, Bartels U et al. (2001) Obesity after childhood craniopharyngioma—German multicenter study on pre-operative risk factors and quality of life. *Klin Padiatr* 213: 244–249.

Muller HL, Emser A, Faldum A et al. (2004) Longitudinal study on growth and body mass index before and after diagnosis of childhood craniopharyngioma. *J Clin Endocrinol Metab* 89: 3298–3305.

Muller HL, Gebhardt U, Maroske J and Hanisch E (2011a) Long-term follow-up of morbidly obese patients with childhood craniopharyngioma after laparoscopic adjustable gastric banding (LAGB). *Klin Padiatr* 223: 372–373.

Muller HL, Gebhardt U, Schroder S et al. (2010) Analyses of treatment variables for patients with childhood craniopharyngioma—results of the multicenter prospective trial KRANIOPHARYNGEOM 2000 after three years of follow-up. *Horm Res Paediatr* 73: 175–180.

Muller HL, Gebhardt U, Teske C et al. (2011b) Post-operative hypothalamic lesions and obesity in childhood craniopharyngioma: Results of the multinational prospective trial KRANIOPHARYNGEOM 2000 after 3-year follow-up. *Eur J Endocrinol* 165: 17–24.

Muller HL, Kaatsch P, Warmuth-Metz M, Flentje M and Sorensen N (2003) Kraniopharyngeom im Kindes-und Jugendalter: Diagnostische und therapeutische Strategien (Childhood craniopharyngioma – diagnostic and therapeutic strategies). *Monatsschrift Kindheilkunde* 151: 1056–1063.

Musani V, Gorry P, Basta-Juzbasic A, Stipic T, Miklic P and Levanat S (2006) Mutation in exon 7 of PTCH deregulates SHH/PTCH/SMO signaling: Possible linkage to WNT. *Int J Mol Med* 17: 755–759.

Nguyen LV, Vanner R, Dirks P and Eaves CJ (2012) Cancer stem cells: An evolving concept. *Nat Rev Cancer* 12: 133–143.

Nielsen EH, Feldt-Rasmussen U, Poulsgaard L et al. (2011) Incidence of craniopharyngioma in Denmark (n = 189) and estimated world incidence of craniopharyngioma in children and adults. *J Neurooncol* 104: 755–763.

Oikonomou E, Barreto DC, Soares B, De Marco L, Buchfelder M and Adams EF (2005) Beta-catenin mutations in craniopharyngiomas and pituitary adenomas. *J Neurooncol* 73 205–209.

Onaka T, Takayanagi Y and Yoshida M (2012) Roles of oxytocin neurones in the control of stress, energy metabolism, and social behaviour. *J Neuroendocrinol* 24: 587–598.

Park KS, Martelotto LG, Peifer M et al. (2011) A crucial requirement for Hedgehog signaling in small cell lung cancer. *Nat Med* 17: 1504–1508.

Poretti A, Grotzer MA, Ribi K, Schonle E and Boltshauser E (2004) Outcome of craniopharyngioma in children: Long-term complications and quality of life. *Dev Med Child Neurol* 46: 220–229.

Puget S, Garnett M, Wray A et al. (2007) Pediatric craniopharyngiomas: Classification and treatment according to the degree of hypothalamic involvement. *J Neurosurg* 106: 3–12.

Ramos EJ, Suzuki S, Marks D, Inui A, Asakawa A and Meguid MM (2004) Cancer anorexia-cachexia syndrome: Cytokines and neuropeptides. *Curr Opin Clin Nutr Metab Care* 7: 427–434.

Romer JT, Kimura H, Magdaleno S et al. (2004) Suppression of the Shh pathway using a small molecule inhibitor eliminates medulloblastoma in Ptc1(/)p53(/) mice. *Cancer Cell* 6: 229–40.

Rosen JM and Jordan CT (2009) The increasing complexity of the cancer stem cell paradigm. *Science* 324: 1670–1673.

Rubin LL and De Sauvage FJ (2006) Targeting the Hedgehog pathway in cancer. *Nat Rev Drug Discov* 5: 1026–1033.

Rudin CM, Hann CL, Laterra J et al. (2009) Treatment of medulloblastoma with hedgehog pathway inhibitor GDC-0449. *N Engl J Med* 361: 1173–1178.

Schroeder JW and Vezina LG (2011) Pediatric sellar and suprasellar lesions. *Pediatr Radiol* 41: 287–298; quiz 404–405.

Schubert T, Trippel M, Tacke U et al. (2009) Neurosurgical treatment strategies in childhood craniopharyngiomas: Is less more? *Childs Nerv Syst* 25: 1419–1427.

Schulz-Ertner D, Frank C, Herfarth KK, Rhein B, Wannenmacher M and Debus J (2002) Fractionated stereotactic radiotherapy for craniopharyngiomas. *Int J Radiat Oncol Biol Phys* 54: 1114–1120.

Sekine S, Shibata T, Kokubu A et al. (2002) Craniopharyngiomas of adamantinomatous type harbor beta-catenin gene mutations. *Am J Pathol* 161: 1997–2001.

Sekine S, Takata T, Shibata T et al. (2004) Expression of enamel proteins and LEF1 in adamantinomatous craniopharyngioma: Evidence for its odontogenic epithelial differentiation. *Histopathology* 45: 573–579.

Shah A, Stanhope R and Matthew D (1992) Hazards of pharmacological tests of growth hormone secretion in childhood. *BMJ* 304: 173–174.

Shin K, Lee J, Guo N et al. (2011) Hedgehog/Wnt feedback supports regenerative proliferation of epithelial stem cells in bladder. *Nature* 472: 110–114.

Sklar CA (1994) Craniopharyngioma: Endocrine abnormalities at presentation. *Pediatr Neurosurg* 21(Suppl 1): 18–20.

Sorva R, Heiskanen O and Perheentupa J (1988) Craniopharyngioma surgery in children: Endocrine and visual outcome. *Childs Nerv Syst* 4: 97–99.

Spoudeas HA, Albanese A, Saran F, De Vile CJ and Mallucci C (2005) Chapter One – Craniopharyngioma. In: Spoudeas HA and Harrison B (eds.) *Paediatric Endocrine Tumours: A Multidisciplinary Consensus Statement of Best Practice from a Working Group Convened under the Auspices of the British Society for Paediatric Endocrinology & Diabetes (BSPED) and United Kingdom Children's Cancer Study Group (UKCCSG) (Rare Tumour Working Groups)*, 1st edn. Crawley, UK: Novo Nordisk Ltd.

Stiller C (2007) *Childhood Cancer in Britain: Incidence, Survival, Mortality.* Oxford: Oxford University Press.

Stiller CA and Nectoux J (1994) International incidence of childhood brain and spinal tumours. *Int J Epidemiol* 23: 458–464.

Stripp DC, Maity A, Janss AJ et al. (2004) Surgery with or without radiation therapy in the management of craniopharyngiomas in children and young adults. *Int J Radiat Oncol Biol Phys* 58: 714–720.

Theunissen JW and De Sauvage FJ, (2009) Paracrine Hedgehog signaling in cancer. *Cancer Res* 69: 6007–6010.

Treier M, O'connell S, Gleiberman A et al. (2001) Hedgehog signaling is required for pituitary gland development. *Development* 128: 377–386.

Ulfarsson E, Lindquist C, Roberts M et al. (2002) Gamma knife radiosurgery for craniopharyngiomas: Long-term results in the first Swedish patients. *J Neurosurg* 97: 613–622.

Van Effenterre R and Boch AL (2002) Craniopharyngioma in adults and children: A study of 122 surgical cases. *J Neurosurg* 97: 3–11.

Visvader JE and Lindeman GJ (2012) Cancer stem cells: Current status and evolving complexities. *Cell Stem Cell* 10: 717–728.

Von Hoff DD, Lorusso PM, Rudin CM et al. (2009) Inhibition of the hedgehog pathway in advanced basal-cell carcinoma. *N Engl J Med* 361: 1164–1172.

Wang Y, Martin JF and Bai CB (2010) Direct and indirect requirements of Shh/Gli signaling in early pituitary development. *Dev Biol* 348: 199–209.

Warmuth-Metz M, Gnekow AK, Muller H and Solymosi L (2004) Differential diagnosis of suprasellar tumors in children. *Klin Padiatr* 216: 323–330.

World Health Organization (2000) *International Classification of Diseases for Oncology (ICD-O-3)*. Geneva, Switzerland: World Health Organization.

Wu Z, Xu Y, Zhu Y et al. (2012) An obligate role of oxytocin neurons in diet induced energy expenditure. *PLoS One* 7: e45167.

Yasargil MG, Curcic M, Kis M, Siegenthaler G, Teddy PJ and Roth P (1990) Total removal of craniopharyngiomas. Approaches and long-term results in 144 patients. *J Neurosurg* 73: 3–11.

Zacharia BE, Bruce SS, Goldstein H, Malone HR, Neugut AI and Bruce JN (2012) Incidence, treatment and survival of patients with craniopharyngioma in the surveillance, epidemiology and end results program. *Neuro Oncol* 14: 1070–1078.

Zhang YQ, Wang CC and Ma ZY (2002) Pediatric craniopharyngiomas: Clinicomorphological study of 189 cases. *Pediatr Neurosurg* 36: 80–84.

14
THE HYPOTHALAMO-PITUITARY-ADRENAL AXIS AND ITS REGULATION

Elizabeth Baranowski, Tulay Guran and Nils Krone

The hypothalamic-pituitary-adrenal (HPA) axis regulates production of glucocorticoids and adrenal androgens. This regulation is essential for homeostasis and adaptation to environmental changes with appropriate metabolic, immune, behavioural and neuromodulatory responses.

The axis consists of three major levels; in the hypothalamus, corticotrophin-releasing hormone (CRH) is synthesised. CRH stimulates the production of adrenocorticotrophic hormone (ACTH) by the anterior pituitary. ACTH subsequently stimulates the adrenal cortex to produce cortisol and adrenal androgens. Cortisol plays a role in the stress response as well as exerting negative feedback on the production of CRH and ACTH (Fig 14.1).

Structure of the hypothalamic-pituitary-adrenal axis

THE HYPOTHALAMUS

The hypothalamus plays a central coordinating role in the HPA axis. Well-defined nuclei within the hypothalamus synthesise specific-releasing or inhibitory factors regulating the five anterior pituitary hormones. With regard to the HPA axis, parvocellular neuroendocrine cells originating in the paraventricular nucleus (PVN) of the hypothalamus with axons projecting to the median eminence produce CRH (Levy and Tasker 2012). CRH is a 41 amino acid peptide secreted in a pulsatile manner in response to changes in the internal or external environments (Murray and Melmed 2006). A number of inhibitory and excitatory neuronal inputs from limbic and brainstem circuits stimulate CRH production through the action of three main neurotransmitters: glutamate, gamma-amino butyric acid (GABA) and norepinephrine. Inhibitory GABAergic inputs to the PVN originate from the supraoptic nucleus, anterior perifornical region, the anterior hypothalamic area, the anterior third of the PVN itself and the bed nucleus of the striae terminalis (BNST). Excitatory glutamatergic stimuli originate from peri- and intra-PVN, and from various hypothalamic nuclei such as the paraventricular thalamic nucleus and the medial nucleus of the amygdala. Norepinephrine inputs originate in the brainstem (Levy and Tasker 2012).

CRH synthesis is stimulated by depolarisation of the cell membrane, which in turn stimulates an action potential and triggers the release of peptide from the axon terminal which is incorporated into the median eminence at the base of the brain. Here CRH is released into the hypothalamic-hypophyseal portal circulation via fenestrated portal

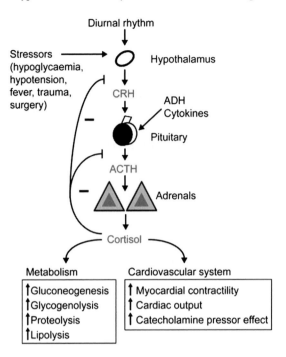

Figure 14.1. Hypothalamic-pituitary-adrenal axis. The secretion of adrenocorticotropin hormone (ACTH) from the anterior pituitary is under the influence of two principal secretagogues: corticotropin-releasing hormone (CRH) and arginine vasopressin. Other factors and stressors including cytokines also play a role. An inbuilt circadian rhythm and additional stressors regulate the hypothalamic release of CRH. The secretion of CRH and ACTH is regulated by negative feedback inhibition of cortisol.

arterioles. Subsequently, CRH stimulates the production of proopiomelanocortin (POMC) and the release of ACTH from corticotrophs in the anterior pituitary (Bonfiglio et al. 2011; Levy and Tasker 2012). Arginine vasopressin (AVP) is co-expressed and secreted by approximately half of the CRH-producing cells. In acute stress situations, CRH and AVP act synergistically to stimulate ACTH release from pituitary corticotroph cells. In addition, AVP concentrations increase while CRH secretion is suppressed in chronic stress. AVP is assumed to be important in HPA regulation during fetal and neonatal life as well as lactation periods, and there are age-dependent changes in HPA responsiveness. However, the role of AVP in chronic stress is not fully understood (Lightman 2008; Goncharova 2013).

CRH also regulates the duration of gestation and therefore the timing of birth by its various effects on myometrial contractility through progesterone and fetoplacental blood supply through nitric oxide. Furthermore, CRH influences fetal nutrition and placental corticosteroid metabolism by increasing the expression of leptin and 11β-hydroxysteroid dehydrogenase 2 (11β-HSD2) in placental trophoblasts (Fahlbusch et al. 2012).

CRH synthesis is stimulated by the cAMP-protein kinase pathway. Pituitary adenyl cyclase activating polypeptide (PACAP) is involved in the up-regulation of CRH synthesis.

PACAP and its receptor, the PAC1 receptor, are highly expressed in the hypothalamus and specifically in the PVN. PACAP stimulates adenylate cyclase, resulting in increased intracellular cAMP. Cyclic AMP in turn induces CRH and AVP gene transcription through the PKA pathway mediated by the cAMP-response element (CRE) in hypothalamic cells. Activation of the PKA pathway leads to CRE-binding protein binding to the CRE on the CRH promoter in the hypothalamus. Protein kinase C and p38 mitogen-activating protein (MAP) are also involved in the regulation of gene expression (Kageyama and Suda 2009). Furthermore epigenetic chromatin modification processes such as inhibition of histone deacetylases are involved in the differential tissue expressions of CRH in hypothalamus and placenta (Abou-Seif et al. 2012).

CRH acts through binding to G-protein coupled receptors (GPCRs) – the CRH receptors (CRHR). These receptors belong to the class B or secretin-like receptor family. There are two types, CRHR1 and CRHR2, located in different brain areas and with different ligand-binding preferences. CRH has a high affinity for CRHR1 but not for CRHR2. Other CRH-related neuropeptides like Urocortins I, II and III can also bind to the CRHRs. Urocortin II and III bind with high affinity to CRHR2, while Urocortin I can bind to both receptors. Urocortins have been implicated in the regulation of the stress response (Bonfiglio et al. 2011).

THE PITUITARY

In the pituitary, corticotrophs constitute approximately 20% of the cells of the anterior pituitary around the central median pituitary wedge. Abnormalities of the commitment, differentiation and function of the corticotrophs account for HPA dysfunction. In the development of the pituitary, corticotrophs are seen from around 6 weeks of gestation (Murray and Melmed 2006). Pluripotent stem cells in the primitive anterior pituitary begin to differentiate into corticotroph lineage precursors, relying on transcription factors such as HESX1, LHX3, LHX4, PROP1 and SOX3. Mutations in any of these transcription factors lead to combined pituitary hormone deficiency including ACTH deficiency. Function of the corticotrophs is regulated by the various other transcription factors such as NeuroD1, TPIT and PITX1 through the regulation of POMC gene expression.

TPIT is a T-box transcription factor only found in POMC-expressing cells in the pituitary. It is important for final cell fate decision between late POMC lineage differentiation and late events of gonadotroph differentiation. It is also essential for POMC gene transcription. TPIT forms a functional heterodimer with PITX1, a pan-pituitary transcription factor involved in binding to the regulatory sequences of the coding genes for all of the pituitary hormones. This heterodimer binds to the PITX1/TPIT response element leading to the activation of POMC expression and antagonises SF1 to prevent gonadotroph differentiation. The TPIT-dependent differentiation of the two alternate POMC lineages is influenced by PAX7. PAX7 is crucial for the activation of melanotrope-specific genes and a critical positive regulator of the melanotrope fate, whereas it acts as repressor of corticotrope-specific genes. Thus, PAX7 is regarded as pioneer factor and selector gene for differentiation following TPIT recruitment and action (Budry et al. 2012).

Hypothalamic CRH binds to CRHR1 in the pituitary and activates adenyl cyclase to generate cAMP. Subsequently, this activates the MAPK signalling pathway, resulting in

ERK1/2 activation via a series of phosphorylation steps from the B-Raf kinase. The end product, phosphorylated ERK1/2, recruits transcription factor (Nurr1 and Nurr77) binding to the Nurr response element of the POMC gene promoter inducing POMC transcription.

POMC is a 31 kDa prohormone precursor protein synthesised not just in the pituitary but also in the hypothalamus, medulla, skin and several peripheral tissues (Wardlaw 2011). POMC is processed in a tissue-specific manner depending on the prohormone convertases (PCs). Within the corticotrophs of the anterior pituitary, POMC undergoes proteolysis by prohormone convertase 1 (PC1) into ACTH, lipotropin and a 16 kDa N-terminal fragment. Within other structures, such as the hypothalamus, prohormone convertase 2 (PC2) is present, further processing POMC to other products including α, β, γ-MSH (Bonfiglio et al. 2011). ACTH is a 39 amino acid peptide released in a circadian rhythm with pulsatile secretion. After cleavage from POMC in the corticotroph cells, ACTH is secreted and released into the cavernous sinus and thus enters the systemic circulation to reach its final target organ – the adrenal cortex (Murray and Melmed 2006).

THE ADRENAL GLANDS

The adrenal cortex arises from the urogenital ridge. The early differentiation of the adreno-gonadal primordium requires the signalling cascade involving transcription factors such as GLI3, SALL1, FOXD2, WT1, PBX1, WNT4, and the regulator of telomerase activity, ACD at, around 4 weeks of gestation. The adrenal primordium derives from the adrenogonadal primordium under the influence of transcription factors SF1, DAX1, WNT4 and CITED2 at around 8 weeks of gestation. The adrenal primordium contains two distinctive zones – the inner fetal zone and the outer definitive zone. These two distinct zones persist up to 12 months of postnatal age. The inner fetal zone increases in size during the second trimester of pregnancy as it secretes large amounts of dehydroepiandrostene (DHEA) and dehydroepiandrosten sulphate (DHEAS). The fetal zone reduces in size after birth while the definitive zone proliferates. The definitive zone develops into the zona glomerulosa and fasciculata. The islets of the innermost zona reticularis can be seen after two years of age (Stewart and Krone 2011).

ACTH acts to maintain the adrenal gland structure and function and controls the production of glucocorticoids from the zona fasciculata. It also stimulates to a lesser extent the production of adrenal androgens. The main circulating adrenal androgen is DHEA. The adrenal gland cortex has three zones involved in hormone production. Mineralocorticoid production occurs in the zona glomerulosa, glucocorticoids are synthesised in the zona fasciculata and androgens derive from the zona reticularis. This zone-specific production is a result of the localised expression of specific enzymes involved in important steps in steroidogenesis. For example, for the steroidogenic pathway to be directed from mineralocorticoid production to glucocorticoid production, the enzyme 17α-hydroxylase is required. This is expressed in the zona fasciculata but not the zona glomerulosa, confining glucocorticoid generation to the former (Stewart and Krone 2011).

The adrenal cortex does not store hormone ready for release like some other chemical messenger systems in the body, so it is required to have the ability to rapidly synthesise hormones in response to ACTH. ACTH binds to the G-protein coupled melanocortin-

2-receptor (MC2R) within the adrenal cortex and acts in three ways, over three time frames. First, it acts over weeks to months to stimulate adrenal growth through hyperplasia and hypertrophy of adrenal cells. Second, it acts over days to facilitate gene transcription of steroidogenic enzymes and co-factors. Third, over only a matter of minutes, it causes steroidogenic acute regulatory protein (*StAR*) gene transcription which leads to recruitment and transport of cholesterol to the inner mitochondrial membrane, and acceleration of the initial catalytic reaction by P450 side chain cleavage enzymes (CYP11A1; Miller and Auchus 2011).

NEGATIVE FEEDBACK OF GLUCOCORTICOIDS ON THE HPA AXIS

Controlled termination of the stress response is an important function of the HPA axis to protect systems against the catabolic and immunosuppressive effects of glucocorticoid overexposure. This important function is accomplished through the glucocorticoids and their receptors. Glucocorticoids predominantly bind to a hepatic-derived cortisol-binding globulin with approximately 5% as the biologically active free hormone in the circulation. Glucocorticoids have a direct inhibitory action on the HPA axis. Glucocorticoid negative feedback occurs at the level of the hypothalamus, the pituitary, at upstream limbic structures such as the hippocampus, paraventricular thalamus and prefrontal cortex, and also downstream at the adrenal cortex (Grossman 2010). Cortisol exerts its negative effect via the glucocorticoid and mineralocorticoid receptors. After glucocorticoid binding, the glucocorticoid receptor (GR) translocates to the nucleus where it binds to glucocorticoid response elements (GREs) and activates gene transcription (Chesnokova and Melmed 2002). Rapid negative feedback action develops in only minutes at the membrane level whereas delayed negative feedback signalling occurs over minutes to hours and occurs at the level of gene expression (Evanson et al. 2010).

Within the hypothalamus, glucocorticoids interact with GR located on the extracellular membrane of CRH neurosecretory cells within the PVN. This interaction results in a rapid decrease in the secretion of excitatory glutamate and suppression of CRH release. In addition, CRH and AVP mRNA transcription is down-regulated in neurons over a period of hours. Recently it has been demonstrated that neurotrophic factors, such as brain-derived neurotrophic factor (BDNF) and its receptor, TrkB, are both expressed in the PVN and are involved in the maintenance of CRH expression and glucocorticoid bioavailability. BDNF and glucocorticoids regulate CRH homeostasis in opposite directions through the action on cAMP response-element binding protein cofactor CRTC2 (Jeanneteau et al. 2012).

Activation of the GR in the pituitary corticotrophs leads to inhibition of ACTH release and repression of POMC transcription. Nuclear proteins BRG1 and HDAC2 scaffold a repression complex with GR and NGFI-B at the *POMC* gene to inhibit its transcription (Bonfiglio et al. 2011).

The GR is highly expressed in the prefrontal cortex and hippocampus. These limbic structures transmit glutaminergic excitatory outputs to the BNST that are reversed via inhibitory relays inhibiting the PVN activity. Glucocorticoid action on these structures is excitatory and therefore exhibits an inhibitory effect on the CRH neurons in the PVN and subsequently on the HPA axis. The negative feedback control of the HPA axis via the limbic system appears to be specific to psychological stressors rather than physiological stressors. This mechanism plays a role in the termination of stress response and is mediated by genomic actions of glucocorticoids with a delayed response (Hill and Tasker 2012).

The mineralocorticoid receptor is mainly located in the limbic structures of the brain, specifically the hippocampus. The mineralocorticoid receptor is involved in maintaining basal HPA activity. This is facilitated via its higher affinity for glucocorticoids than mineralocorticoids at the low glucocorticoid concentrations, thereby preventing the occupation of the glucocorticoid receptor at the trough states of circadian rhythm, rendering the HPA axis at a pro-active state. The mineralocorticoid conveys tonic inhibitory signals to the PVN through GABAergic neurons. The mineralocorticoid receptor agonist fludrocortisone can inhibit the HPA axis in a dose-dependent fashion (Karamouzis et al. 2013).

Sex hormones have a role in regulating the HPA axis and CRH expression, particularly in enhancing the stress response. Oestrogens enhance stress-induced CRH activation through the oestrogen receptor β pathway which is co-localised within CRH neurons in the PVN. Increased oestrogen concentrations during the mid-luteal phase of the menstrual cycle may directly enhance ACTH and cortisol response by stimulating CRH production (Kageyama and Suda 2009). The crosstalk between the reproductive and HPA axes has also been evidenced by immunohistochemical studies in rats showing co-localisation of the CRH receptor and GR in kisspeptin neurons in the hypothalamus of female rats. This may explain stress-induced amenorrhea through the inhibition of gonadotrophins by CRH and glucocorticoids via the kisspeptin pathway (Takumi et al. 2012).

Modulation of the hypothalamic-pituitary-adrenal axis and glucocorticoid synthesis

THE CIRCADIAN RHYTHM

The entire HPA axis is a conserved circadian clock system. This circadian clock has three major components: First, peripheral inputs from all organs and tissues; second, a self-oscillating pacemaker; and third, output rhythms. Glucocorticoids are secreted in a circadian and pulsatile fashion with plasma cortisol concentrations reaching a peak around 07.00h and a nadir between 23.00h and 03.00h. The suprachiasmatic nucleus (SCN), a small paired nucleus in the anterior hypothalamus, acts as a central master clock driving the circadian rhythm. The SCN controls the HPA axis, leading to circadian oscillation of circulating CRH, ACTH and cortisol. The HPA axis coordinates the central clock signals with circadian rhythmicity of the peripheral clocks against various external stressors through the GR. Changes in the external environment affect the circadian rhythmicity by modulating the function of the SCN. The SCN receives light input from the eyes via the retinohypothalamic tract. Retinal ganglion cells expressing melanopsin project directly into the SCN. This light input triggers a signalling cascade, changing gene expression and the neuronal firing rate at the SCN. The SCN has output projections towards various brain regions including the PVN, subparaventricular zone and dorsomedial nucleus.

The main components at the molecular level are self-oscillating molecular pacemakers consisting of the Clock-Bmal1 heterodimer and other transcription factors. The bHLH transcription factors CLOCK and BMAL1 dimerise and bind to the E-box regulatory sequence to activate transcription of period (*PER*) and cryptochrome (*CRY*) genes. Over several hours, *PER* and *CRY* accumulate and localise to the nucleus. *CRY* and *PER* then act to inhibit their own transcription by inhibiting the action of the CLOCK-BMAL1 heterodimer. Clock-Bmal1 regulates the response to glucocorticoids in peripheral tissues through acetylation of the GR. Many cell types and tissues express peripheral clock genes in a circadian fashion. Central drivers of circadian rhythm coordinate peripheral tissues that oscillate autonomously. For example, AVP acts to stimulate ACTH secretion, but also inhibits SCN control of the PVN by blocking the glucocorticoid peaks. An autonomic neural SCN-adrenal gland connection, consisting of a multisynaptic pathway from the SCN to the adrenal gland, passes via autonomic nervous system neurons. It is independent of the HPA axis targeted pathways from SCN to PVN. Light can directly affect the adrenal gland circadian rhythm via this pathway. This pathway is also responsible for regulating the adrenal sensitivity to ACTH, possibly by affecting the adrenal glands' own clock mechanism. The adrenal also expresses clock genes and is partly capable of regulating autonomously its own internal circadian rhythm. The adrenal clock regulates the sensitivity of the adrenal to ACTH and the cyclic expression of rate-limiting StAR through the CLOCK:BMAL1 heterodimer.

Outside the SCN, a food-related oscillator clock exists. This influences the rhythmicity of glucocorticoid secretion according to feed-fasting cycles. The clock genes BMAL1 and PER1 have been implicated in this regulatory action. Overall, the circadian pattern of the HPA axis regulates the balance between circulating cortisol and tissue sensitivity. Disturbed rhythmicity has been implicated in the pathophysiology of various health problems including obesity, metabolic syndrome and cardiovascular diseases (Chung et al. 2011).

ENDOCANNABINOID SIGNALLING

The endocannabinoid system is involved in the maturation and central regulation of the HPA axis under basal conditions and in the stress response. The endocannabinoid system is a lipid-signalling system found throughout the brain and body. It consists of two types of G-protein-coupled receptor – CB1 and CB2 receptors. CB1 receptors are expressed mainly in the brain and in some peripheral systems including all major endocrine glands. CB2 receptors are mainly found in organs involved in the immune response and are also present in the brain.

The endocannabinoid system is widely distributed around the corticolimbic and hypothalamic circuitry, which is involved in regulating the HPA axis. The predominant effect is the inhibition of the HPA axis. However, a role in activation has also been suggested. Under steady-state conditions, the endocannabinoid system suppresses the amplitude of ACTH peaks. Inhibition of endocannabinoid system by knocking out the CB1 receptor leads to increased basal HPA activity by increased CRH mRNA synthesis within the PVN with an increase in ACTH and corticosteroid synthesis. Endocannabinoids are involved in the rapid glucocorticoid-mediated negative feedback of the HPA axis at the level of the PVN via binding to membrane-associated GR. Glucocorticoids act to mobilise endocannabinoids within the PVN, resulting in reduced excitatory input to CRH neurons. Glucocorticoids increase endocannabinoid levels in the amygdala, and specifically the basolateral nucleus of the amygdala (BLA), which in turn suppresses the HPA axis. This mechanism may also play a role in the termination of the stress response.

In addition, the endocannabinoid system contributes to delayed feedback loops of glu-cocorticoids via the prefrontal cortex and the hippocampus where the GR is abundantly expressed. In the prefrontal cortex, glucocorticoids can induce endocannabinoid signalling, increasing the activity of the prefrontal cortical outputs by a reduction of local inhibitory tone on these neurons. Consequently, this results in the augmentation of negative feedback response by triggering inhibitory relays in the BNST suppressing neuronal activity in the PVN. This has been elicited in the prefrontal cortex but less is known about the mechanism of action in the hippocampus (Crosby and Bains 2012; Hill and Tasker 2012; Lee and Gorzalka 2012).

NEUROENDOCRINE EFFECT OF INFLAMMATION AND CYTOKINES

Cytokines can affect pituitary development and function. Exposure to endotoxins and inflammation in utero or at birth can have long-term endocrine effects, such as decreased GR binding, decreased negative feedback by steroids during the stress response and an increased predisposition to inflammatory disease. (Brunton 2010; Lee and Gorzalka 2012).

The HPA axis is activated by pro-inflammatory cytokine production. Interleukin (IL)-6 production stimulates the HPA axis and results in increased glucocorticoid production. Glucocorticoids can suppress IL-6 production via a negative feedback mechanism. IL-6 is co-expressed with CRH and AVP in PVN neurons positively regulating their expression in the hypothalamus. PACAP stimulates endogenous IL-6 mRNA expression, and IL-6 acts as an autocrine stimulus sustaining gene transcription of CRH and AVP.

Stimulation of the HPA axis is not confined to IL-6. The entire gp130 family of cyto-kines including IL-6, leucocyte inhibitory factor (LIF), IL-11, ciliary neurotrophic factor (CNTF) and oncostatin M (OSM) as well as other cytokines such as IL-1 and TNF can affect the HPA axis. These factors mediate the HPA response to stress and inflammation by stimulating CRH production, stimulating POMC expression, inducing ACTH secretion or inducing the release of corticosteroids from the adrenal cortex. LIF, similar to IL-6, has a role in sustaining the HPA axis stress response and also has a protective role for neurons and peripheral tissues during injury. CRH and cytokines can act synergistically to induce POMC production through different pathways. CRH acts via cAMP signalling via PKA pathways, whereas cytokines act via the JAK/STAT/SOCS pathways. The crosstalk between these systems allows the HPA axis to respond rapidly to acute inflammatory processes. The activation of JAK2 leads to the transcriptional activation of StAR, representing a novel mechanism regulating steroidogenesis (Lefrancois-Martinez et al. 2011).

Glucocorticoids negatively affect pro-inflammatory cytokines through activation of the glucocorticoid. Once bound, the GR antagonises nuclear factor κB (NF-κB), which is required by TNF and IL-1 to initiate an inflammatory signal cascade to result in transcrip-tion of pro-inflammatory genes. Negative regulation of cytokine-induced HPA axis activa-tion involves SOCS proteins, which inhibit the JAK-STAT signalling pathway. *SOCS-3* gene expression is induced by the activation of the JAK-STAT pathway by LIF and IL-1, leading to the resistance of the cell to further stimulation by gp130 cytokines. Prolonged exposure to inflammatory cytokines, such as in chronic inflammation, increases the steady-state proportion of the βGR isoform. This blocks the activation of αGR-promoting glucocorticoid resistance and hence desensitisation of the HPA axis (Chesnokova and Melmed 2002; Priftis et al. 2009).

Clinical conditions affecting the hypothalamic-pituitary-adrenal axis
ISOLATED ACTH DEFICIENCY
Isolated ACTH deficiency (IAD) is characterised by low plasma concentrations of ACTH, leading to secondary adrenal insufficiency with lack of cortisol synthesis, whilst mineralocorticoid production is preserved. In clinical practice, isolated ACTH deficiency commonly results from chronic excess glucocorticoid administration for various inflammatory conditions. Congenital isolated ACTH deficiency is extremely rare. It can be a result of mutations in transcription factors such as T-box pituitary-restricted transcription factor (TPIT) or in the gene encoding POMC.

TPIT (also known as *TBX19*) deficiency results in the development of very few POMC expressing cells, very low plasma ACTH concentrations and adrenal hypoplasia with very low or undetectable cortisol concentrations. Commonly, patients present in the neonatal period with severe hypoglycaemia often associated with seizures. In addition, patients often have prolonged cholestatic jaundice as a sign of glucocorticoid deficiency. A high rate of neonatal death has been suggested for this condition. Low maternal plasma oestriol concentrations during pregnancy are detectable during maternal pregnancy tests.

Psychomotor development is normal if glucocorticoid replacement therapy is started early. *TPIT* mutations account for about two-thirds of neonatal onset complete IAD. However, *TPIT* mutations cause severe neonatal onset IAD rather than partial or juvenile onset forms. Mutations are located throughout the entire *TPIT* gene but mainly affect the T-box domain of the protein, and follow an autosomal recessive inheritance (Couture et al. 2012).

Defects in POMC synthesis or processing lead to impaired production of POMC-derived peptides including ACTH and MSH. MSH is also involved with hair pigmentation and food-intake regulation. Mutations in the gene encoding POMC leads to a stereotypical phenotype of early-onset severe obesity, red pigmented hair and ACTH insufficiency leading to hypocortisolism, and usually presents in early childhood. However, there have been some reports of *POMC* mutations that have not been associated with the typical red hair and pale skin features. Mutations in proconvertase-1 (PC-1) result in a typical phenotype of abnormal glucose homeostasis, ACTH deficiency, elevated POMC concentrations, childhood obesity and hypogonadism (Andrioli et al. 2006; Mendiratta et al. 2011). Coexistence of obesity is an important clue for the differential diagnosis of POMC and PC-1 gene defects in cases of IAD.

Deficit in anterior pituitary function and variable immune deficiency (DAVID) syndrome has been recently described in three unrelated families. The underlying aetiology remains elusive. This syndrome is characterised by the association of ACTH deficiency and combined variable immune deficiency. Patients present with severe hypoglycaemia, ACTH deficiency and variable degrees of other anterior pituitary hormone deficiencies, recurrent respiratory tract infections, low IgG concentrations and abnormal lymphocytes (Quentien et al. 2012).

ACTH DEFICIENCY AS PART OF MULTIPLE PITUITARY HORMONE DEFICIENCY

Combined pituitary deficiency is much more common than isolated ACTH deficiency. It can be acquired secondary to pituitary trauma, inflammation, tumours or surgery. Defects in transcription factors involved with early pituitary cell differentiation result in congenital combined pituitary deficiencies of which ACTH is variably associated. For example, *HESX1* and *LHX4* deficiencies are associated with corticotroph deficiency in 50% of cases, whereas *PROP1* mutations are associated in 40% and *LHX3* defects are associated in 33%. These are described in detail in Chapter 2.

MENTAL HEALTH DISORDERS

Mental health disorders such as depression and anxiety have been linked with HPA axis dysregulation. Children and young people with depression tend to have a dysregulated response to the dexamethasone suppression test and moderately higher plasma cortisol concentrations throughout the day. The effects of suppression of the HPA axis appear to be age-dependent. Depressed preschool children showed reduced reactivity but a higher peak plasma cortisol concentration whereas depressed adolescents showed higher reactivity and delayed recovery. The higher baseline cortisol does not correlate with sex or age, nor is it specific to any particular time of day. However, the cortisol response to CRH infusion is normal in depressed patients, suggesting a normal sensitivity of the hypothalamus to CRH and a normal adrenal sensitivity to ACTH (Lopez-Duran et al. 2009).

ASTHMA

Prospective studies in children have shown a positive association between psychosocial factors and future atopic disease. In asthmatics, there is a link between low socio-economic status and higher inflammatory markers, cytokines and eosinophil count. Lower socio-economic groups also demonstrated marginally lower morning plasma cortisol concentrations possibly indicating HPA axis suppression. It is thought that this is secondary to chronic emotional stress and threat perception. Children with asthma who experienced acute or chronic stressors show reduced expression of GR mRNA. Early psychological and physical stress aggravates asthma later in life by inducing hyporesponsiveness of the HPA axis by causing dysregulation of the immune system function. Lower cortisol responses to stress as a marker of reduced HPA axis activity are seen in children with chronic allergic conditions. Production of pro-inflammatory cytokines may be involved in the pathogenesis of this. Some children with severe disease were found to have relative adrenal insufficiency compared to those with milder conditions. The circadian rhythm is disrupted in asthmatic children, and they show a reduced response to ACTH stimulation testing. Treatment with lower and appropriate doses of inhaled corticosteroids does not suppress the HPA axis, but with higher doses, some changes in adrenal function have been noted. This suppressive effect seems to be dose-dependent (Priftis et al. 2009).

Testing the hypothalamic-pituitary-adrenal axis

Accurate testing of the HPA axis remains challenging. It is important to consider that reported cortisol concentrations are assay-dependent. Liquid chromatography tandem mass spectrometry commonly measures lower cortisol concentrations than immune-based assays due to reduced cross-reactivity with other steroid hormones. There are also differences between different immune-based assays. Thus, absolute cut-offs published in the literature have to be potentially adjusted to local settings.

Early morning cortisol concentrations of <150nmol/L are highly suggestive of adrenal insufficiency, whereas concentrations of >525nmol/L make the diagnosis unlikely. Random cortisol measurements can be problematic unless concentrations are >600nmol/L, demonstrating a clear capacity for a stress response. Dynamic testing represents a more reliable way to assess the intact HPA axis and its response to stress. The insulin tolerance test (ITT) remains the criterion standard and defines the integrity of the entire HPA axis but it is not without risk.

The short synacthen test (SST) using a pharmacological dose of synthetic $ACTH_{1-24}$ represents a safe alternative to the ITT. The SST only stimulates the adrenal cortex, but a sufficient response indicates an intact HPA axis. The 30-minute cortisol response to $ACTH_{1-24}$ correlates well with the cortisol response observed to ITT. Plasma cortisol concentrations >550nmol/L are generally considered as a normal response. It is, however, important to realised that the different local cut-offs are also depending on the employed cortisol assay. An ongoing debate continues as to whether a low-dose synacthen test ($500ng/1.73m^2$) would be more sensitive to diagnose mild cases of adrenal deficiency, particularly for secondary adrenal insufficiency and for patients on chronic steroid treatment (Chrousos et al. 2009).

The glucagon test represents a safe alternative to the ITT checking the entire axis. The glucagon test leads to an increase of both cortisol and growth hormone, although the cortisol response is less consistent. The measurement of ACTH concentrations and CRH stimulation tests can be useful to differentiate between secondary and primary adrenal deficiency.

REFERENCES

Abou-Seif C, Shipman KL, Allars M et al. (2012) Tissue specific epigenetic differences in CRH gene expression. *Front Biosci* (Landmark Ed) 17: 713–725.

Andrioli M, Pecori Giraldi F and Cavagnini F (2006) Isolated corticotrophin deficiency. *Pituitary* 9: 289–295.

Bonfiglio JJ, Inda C, Refojo D, Holsboer F, Arzt E and Silberstein S (2011) The corticotropin-releasing hormone network and the hypothalamic-pituitary-adrenal axis: Molecular and cellular mechanisms involved. *Neuroendocrinology* 94: 12–20.

Brunton PJ (2010) Resetting the dynamic range of hypothalamic-pituitary-adrenal axis stress responses through pregnancy. *J Neuroendocrinol* 22: 1198–1213.

Budry L, Balsalobre A, Gauthier Y et al. (2012) The selector gene Pax7 dictates alternate pituitary cell fates through its pioneer action on chromatin remodeling. *Genes Dev* 26: 2299–2310.

Chesnokova V and Melmed S (2002) Minireview: Neuro-immuno-endocrine modulation of the hypothalamic-pituitary-adrenal (HPA) axis by gp130 signaling molecules. *Endocrinology* 143: 1571–1574.

Chrousos GP, Kino T and Charmandari E (2009) Evaluation of the hypothalamic-pituitary-adrenal axis function in childhood and adolescence. *Neuroimmunomodulation* 16: 272–283.

Chung S, Son GH and Kim K (2011) Circadian rhythm of adrenal glucocorticoid: Its regulation and clinical implications. *Biochim Biophys Acta* 1812: 581–591.

Couture C, Saveanu A, Barlier A et al. (2012) Phenotypic homogeneity and genotypic variability in a large series of congenital isolated ACTH-deficiency patients with TPIT gene mutations. *J Clin Endocrinol Metab* 97: E486–E495.

Crosby KM and Bains JS (2012) The intricate link between glucocorticoids and endocannabinoids at stress-relevant synapses in the hypothalamus. *Neuroscience* 204: 31–37.

Evanson NK, Tasker JG, Hill MN, Hillard CJ and Herman JP (2010) Fast feedback inhibition of the HPA axis by glucocorticoids is mediated by endocannabinoid signaling. *Endocrinology* 151: 4811–4819.

Fahlbusch FB, Ruebner M, Volkert G et al. (2012) Corticotropin-releasing hormone stimulates expression of leptin, 11beta-HSD2 and syncytin-1 in primary human trophoblasts. *Reprod Biol Endocrinol* 10: 80.

Goncharova ND (2013) Stress responsiveness of the hypothalamic-pituitary-adrenal axis: Age-related features of the vasopressinergic regulation. *Front Endocrinol* (Lausanne) 4: 26.

Grossman AB (2010) Clinical Review#: The diagnosis and management of central hypoadrenalism. *J Clin Endocrinol Metab* 95: 4855–4863.

Hill MN and Tasker JG (2012) Endocannabinoid signaling, glucocorticoid-mediated negative feedback, and regulation of the hypothalamic-pituitary-adrenal axis. *Neuroscience* 204: 5–16.

Jeanneteau FD, Lambert WM, Ismaili N et al. (2012) BDNF and glucocorticoids regulate corticotrophin-releasing hormone (CRH) homeostasis in the hypothalamus. *Proc Natl Acad Sci USA* 109: 1305–1310.

Kageyama K and Suda T (2009) Regulatory mechanisms underlying corticotropin-releasing factor gene expression in the hypothalamus. *Endocr J* 56: 335–344.

Karamouzis I, Berardelli R, Marinazzo E et al. (2013) The acute effect of fludrocortisone on basal and hCRH-stimulated hypothalamic–pituitary–adrenal (HPA) axis in humans. *Pituitary* 16: 378–385.

Lee TT and Gorzalka BB (2012) Timing is everything: Evidence for a role of corticolimbic endocannabinoids in modulating hypothalamic-pituitary-adrenal axis activity across developmental periods. *Neuroscience* 204: 17–30.

Lefrancois-Martinez AM, Blondet-Trichard A, Binart N et al. (2011) Transcriptional control of adrenal steroidogenesis: Novel connection between Janus kinase (JAK) 2 protein and protein kinase A (PKA) through stabilization of cAMP response element-binding protein (CREB) transcription factor. *J Biol Chem* 286: 32976–32985.

Levy BH and Tasker JG (2012) Synaptic regulation of the hypothalamic-pituitary-adrenal axis and its modulation by glucocorticoids and stress. *Front Cell Neurosci* 6: 24.

Lightman SL (2008) The neuroendocrinology of stress: A never ending story. *J Neuroendocrinol* 20: 880–884.

Lopez-Duran NL, Kovacs M and George CJ (2009) Hypothalamic-pituitary-adrenal axis dysregulation in depressed children and adolescents: A meta-analysis. *Psychoneuroendocrinology* 34: 1272–1283.

Mendiratta MS, Yang Y, Balazs AE et al. (2011) Early onset obesity and adrenal insufficiency associated with a homozygous POMC mutation. *Int J Pediatr Endocrinol* 2011: 5.

Miller WL and Auchus RJ (2011) The molecular biology, biochemistry, and physiology of human steroidogenesis and its disorders. *Endocr Rev* 32: 81–151.

Murray RD and Melmed S (2006) The Pituitary. *Encyclopedia of Life Sciences*. doi: 10.1038/npg.els.0000065.

Priftis KN, Papadimitriou A, Nicolaidou P and Chrousos GP (2009) Dysregulation of the stress response in asthmatic children. *Allergy* 64: 18–31.

Quentien MH, Delemer B, Papadimitriou DT et al. (2012) Deficit in anterior pituitary function and variable immune deficiency (DAVID) in children presenting with adrenocorticotropin deficiency and severe infections. *J Clin Endocrinol Metab* 97: E121–E128.

Stewart PM and Krone N (2011) The adrenal cortex. In: Melmed S, Polonsky KS, Larsen PR Kronenberg HM (eds) *Williams Textbook of Endocrinology*. Vol 1. 12th ed. Philadelphia, PA: Saunders Elsevier, 479–544.

Takumi K, Iijima N, Higo S and Ozawa H (2012) Immunohistochemical analysis of the colocalization of corticotropin-releasing hormone receptor and glucocorticoid receptor in kisspeptin neurons in the hypothalamus of female rats. *Neurosci Lett* 531: 40–45.

Wardlaw SL (2011) Hypothalamic proopiomelanocortin processing and the regulation of energy balance. *Eur J Pharmacol* 660: 213–219.

15
THE EFFECT OF STRESS ON THE HYPOTHALAMIC-PITUITARY-ADRENAL AXIS: AN UPDATE

Evangelia Charmandari and George P. Chrousos

Introduction

Life exists through maintenance of a complex dynamic equilibrium, termed 'homeostasis' or 'eustasis', which is constantly challenged by intrinsic or extrinsic, real or perceived, adverse forces, the 'stressors'. 'Stress' is defined as a state of threatened, or perceived as threatened, homeostasis. The human body and mind react to stress by activating a complex repertoire of physiologic and behavioural central nervous system (CNS) and peripheral adaptive responses, which, if inadequate, excessive or prolonged, may affect development and behaviour, and may have adverse consequences on physiologic functions, such as growth, metabolism, circulation, reproduction and the inflammatory/immune response. This chronic dynamic state in which the adaptive response fails to fully reestablish homeostasis during stress is called 'dyshomeostasis' or 'cacostasis', and may have detrimental effects on the organism, including dysphoria of various forms, development of chronic disease and curtailment of life expectancy (Fig 15.1a). Of course, stress is not always bad (distress); it might actually be beneficial, resulting in an improved steady state called 'hyperstasis' characterised by a better quality of life and prolonged life expectancy (Chrousos and Gold 1992; Chrousos 1995, 2002, 2009, 2012; Charmandari et al. 2003, 2005, 2012).

The pre-Socratic philosophers Pythagoras and Alcmaeon, respectively, used the terms 'harmony' and 'isonomia' to express the dynamic balance or homeostasis of life, while the Hippocratics equated this harmony with health and disharmony with disease. The Stoics, the Skeptics and the Epicurians, philosophic schools that concentrated on the study of stress and its management, considered the attainment of 'ataraxia', or imperturbability of the mind to stressors, as the ultimate goal of life, while Epicurus himself spoke of 'eustatheia' or 'eustasis', which refers to the serene and satisfactory emotional state of a harmonious balance in a human being. Based on these ancient seminal ideas, appropriate responsiveness of the human stress system to stressors is a crucial prerequisite for a sense of well-being, adequate performance of tasks and positive social interactions, and hence for the survival of the self and the species. By contrast, inappropriate, over- or under- responsiveness of the stress system through its hormonal and inflammatory

218

(a)

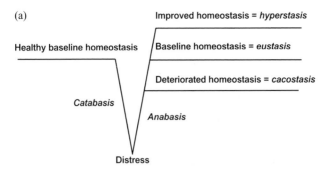

(b)

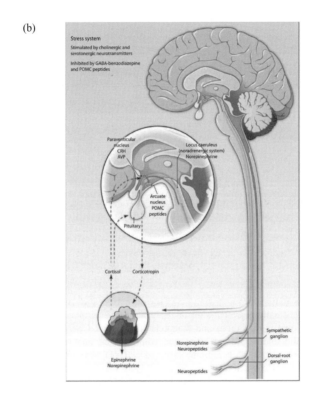

Figure 15.1. (a) After exposure to a stressor and descent (catabasis) into disturbed homeostasis (stress or distress), a healthy organism's adaptive response brings homeostasis back (anabasis), with one of three possible outcomes: first, the adaptive response succeeds and returns the organism to its previous healthy homeostasis (eustasis); second, the adaptive response succeeds partly, either because it is inadequate or because it is excessive and/or prolonged, and the organism returns to an unhealthy form of homeostasis (cacostasis) that is damaging the host, producing frailty and curtailing life expectancy; and, third, the adaptive response succeeds and the organism gains from the experience returning to an improved homeostasis, a superior state that is to the benefit of the host, improving its resilience and chances to survive (hyperstasis). (Adapted from Chrousos 2012.) (b) Schematic representation of the central and peripheral components of the stress system involved in the stress response. GABA, ?-aminobutyric acid; POMC, proopiomelanocortin. (Adapted from Chrousos 1995.)

(c)

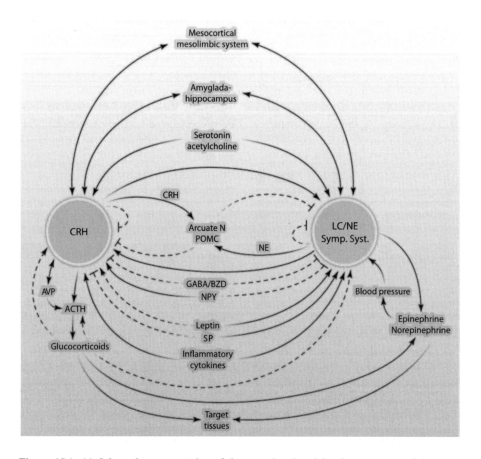

Figure 15.1. (c) Schematic representation of the central and peripheral components of the stress system, their functional interrelations and their relation to other CNS components involved in the stress response. Solid lines represent activation, while dashed lines represent inhibition. ACTH: Adrenocorticotropic hormone; AVP, arginine vasopressin; BZD, benzodiazepine; CRH, corticotropin-releasing hormone; GABA, γ-aminobutyric acid; LC, locus ceruleus; NE. noradrenergic; NPY, neuropeptide Y; SP, substance P. (Adapted from Chrousos and Gold 1992.)

mediators may impair growth and development, and may account for the many chronic behavioural, endocrine, metabolic and allergic/autoimmune disorders that plague contemporary humanity. The development and severity of these conditions primarily depend on the genetic vulnerability of the individual, the exposure to adverse environmental factors, including psychosocial and economic ones, and the timing and duration of the stressful event(s) (Chrousos and Gold 1992; Chrousos 1995, 2002, 2009, 2012; Charmandari et al. 2003, 2005, 2012).

Endocrinology of the stress response

NEUROENDOCRINE EFFECTORS OF THE STRESS RESPONSE

The stress response is subserved by the stress system, which has both CNS and peripheral components. The central components of the stress system are located in the hypothalamus and the brainstem, and include (i) the parvocellular neurons of corticotropin-releasing hormone (CRH); (ii) the arginine vasopressin (AVP) neurons of the paraventricular nuclei (PVN) of the hypothalamus; (iii) the CRH neurons of the paragigantocellular and para-branchial nuclei of the medulla and the locus ceruleus; and (iv) other mostly noradren-ergic cell groups in the medulla and pons (locus ceruleus/noradrenergic system). The peripheral components of the stress system include (i) the hypothalamic-pituitary-adrenal (HPA) axis; (ii) the efferent systemic sympathetic-adrenomedullary systems (SNS); and (iii) components of the parasympathetic system (Chrousos and Gold 1992; Chrousos 1995, 2002, 2009, 2012; Charmandari et al. 2003, 2005, 2012) (Fig 15.1b). The central neurochemical circuitry responsible for activation of the stress system and the multiple sites of interaction among the various components of the stress system are illustrated in Figure 15.1c.

CORTICOTROPIN-RELEASING HORMONE, ARGININE VASOPRESSIN

AND CATECHOLAMINERGIC NEURONS

CRH is a 41-amino acid peptide that represents the principal hypothalamic regulator of the pituitary-adrenal axis. CRH and CRH receptors have been detected in many extrahypotha-lamic sites of the brain, including parts of the limbic system, the basal forebrain and the locus ceruleus–noradrenergic sympathetic system in the brainstem and spinal cord. Intra-cerebroventricular administration of CRH results in a series of behavioural and peripheral responses, as well as activation of the pituitary-adrenal axis and the sympathetic nervous system (SNS), indicating that CRH has a much broader role in coordinating the stress response than initially recognised (Chrousos and Gold 1992; Bale and Vale 2004; Chrousos 1995, 2002, 2009, 2012; Charmandari et al. 2003, 2005, 2012) (Table 15.1).

In addition to its primary role in the regulation of adrenocorticotropic hormone (ACTH) release from the anterior pituitary, and the subsequent release of glucocorticoids from the adrenal gland, CRH plays the role of a bona fide neurotransmitter in the CNS and offers a novel approach for the discovery of potential therapeutics to treat a variety of stress-related psychiatric disorders. The primary target for hypothalamic CRH is a G-protein coupled receptor that was also elucidated and cloned by Vale and colleagues from a human ACTH-secreting adenoma almost a decade after the discovery of CRH itself. The cloning of the CRH receptor brought forth a new opportunity for the understanding of the interactions of small molecules that could block the actions of CRH. The first published clinical study of a small molecule CRF1 receptor antagonist, NBI-30775/R121919, demonstrated a pharma-cological improvement in patients with severe depression (Grigoriadis 2002).

A subset of PVN parvocellular neurons synthesise and secrete both CRH and AVP, while another subset secretes AVP only. During stress, the relative proportion of the subset of neurons that secrete both CRH and AVP increases significantly. The terminals of the parvocellular PVN CRH and AVP neurons project to different sites, including the

TABLE 15.1
Behavioural and physical adaptation during acute stress

Behavioural adaptation: adaptive redirection of behaviour	Physical adaptation: adaptive redirection of energy
Increased arousal and alertness	Oxygen and nutrients directed to the central nervous system and stressed body site(s)
Increased cognition, vigilance and focused attention	Altered cardiovascular tone, increased blood pressure and heart rate
Euphoria (or dysphoria)	Increased respiratory rate
Heightened analgesia	Increased gluconeogenesis and lipolysis
Increased temperature	Detoxification from toxic products
Suppression of appetite and feeding behaviour	Inhibition of growth and reproduction
Suppression of reproductive axis	Inhibition of digestion-stimulation of colonic motility
Containment of the stress response	Containment of the inflammatory/immune response
	Containment of the stress response

Adapted from Chrousos and Gold (1992).

noradrenergic neurons of the brainstem and the hypophyseal portal system in the median eminence. PVN CRH and AVP neurons also send projections to and activate proopi-omelanocortin (POMC)-containing neurons in the arcuate nucleus of the hypothalamus, which in turn project to the PVN CRH and AVP neurons, innervate locus ceruleus-noradrenergic sympathetic neurons of the central stress system in the brainstem, and terminate on pain control neurons of the hind brain and spinal cord. Thus, activation of the stress system via CRH and catecholamines stimulates the secretion of hypothalamic β-endorphin and other POMC-derived peptides, which reciprocally inhibit the activity of the stress system and also result in 'stress-induced' analgesia (Chrousos and Gold 1992; Chrousos 1995, 2002, 2009, 2012; Charmandari et al. 2003, 2005, 2012; Bale and Vale 2004).

THE HYPOTHALAMIC-PITUITARY-ADRENAL AXIS
CRH is the principal hypothalamic regulator of the pituitary-adrenal axis, which stimulates the secretion of ACTH from the anterior pituitary gland. AVP, although a potent synergistic factor of CRH on ACTH secretion, has very little ACTH secretagogue activity on its own (Gillies et al. 1982). In non-stressful situations, both CRH and AVP are secreted in the portal system in a circadian, pulsatile and highly concordant fashion (Iranmanesh et al. 1990). The amplitude of the CRH and AVP pulses increases early in the morning, resulting in increases primarily in the amplitude of the pulsatile ACTH and cortisol secretion. During acute stress, there is an increase in the amplitude and synchronisation of the PVN CRH and AVP pulsatile release into the hypophyseal portal system. In addition, depending on

the stressor, other factors, such as angiotensin II, various cytokines, and lipid mediators of inflammation, are secreted and act on the hypothalamic, pituitary and/or adrenal components of the HPA axis and potentiate its activity.

The adrenal cortex is the main target of ACTH, which regulates glucocorticoid and adrenal androgen secretion by the zonae fasciculata and reticularis, respectively, and participates in the control of aldosterone secretion by the zona glomerulosa. Other hormones, cytokines and neuronal information from the autonomic nerves of the adrenal cortex may also participate in the regulation of cortisol secretion (Bornstein and Chrousos 1999).

Glucocorticoids are the final effectors of the HPA axis. Named for their effects on glucose metabolism, glucocorticoids are involved in almost every cellular, molecular and physiologic network of the organism and regulate a broad spectrum of physiologic functions essential for life, including growth, reproduction, cognition, behaviour, cell proliferation and survival, as well as immune, CNS and cardiovascular functions. Glucocorticoids regulate both the basal activity of the HPA axis and the termination of the stress response by acting at extrahypothalamic regulatory centres, the hypothalamus and the pituitary gland. The negative feedback of glucocorticoids on the secretion of CRH and ACTH serves to limit the duration of the total tissue exposure of the organism to glucocorticoids, thus minimising the catabolic, lipogenic, anti-reproductive and immunosuppressive effects of these hormones (Chrousos and Kino 2009).

The actions of glucocorticoids at the cellular level are mediated by an intracellular protein, the glucocorticoid receptor (NR3C1). The human glucocorticoid receptor (hGR) belongs to the steroid/thyroid/retinoic acid nuclear receptor superfamily of transcription factor proteins and functions as a ligand-dependent transcription factor (Nicolaides et al. 2010). Consistent with the pleiotropic effects of glucocorticoids, the hGR is ubiquitously expressed in almost all human tissues and cells. The unliganded hGRα resides mostly in the cytoplasm of cells as part of a large multiprotein complex, which contains chaperone heat shock proteins 90 and 70, as well as other proteins. Ligand-induced activation of the receptor leads to conformational changes that result in dissociation from this multiprotein complex and translocation into the nucleus. Within the nucleus of cells, the hGRα binds as a homodimer to glucocorticoid-response elements (GREs) in the promoter regions of target genes and regulates their expression positively or negatively. When bound to the GREs, conformational changes ensue in the receptor that lead to coordinated recruitment of coregulators and chromatin-remodelling complexes that influence the activity of RNA polymerase II and modulate gene transcription. The ligand-activated hGRα can also modulate gene expression independently of DNA-binding, by interacting, possibly as a monomer, with other transcription factors, such as nuclear factor-κB (NF-κB), activator protein-1 (AP-1), p53 and signal transducers and activators of transcription. The interaction of hGR with the pro-inflammatory transcription factors NF-κB and AP-1 inhibits their activity and accounts for the major anti-inflammatory and immunosuppressive effects of glucocorticoids (Nicolaides et al. 2010).

Multiple mechanisms, such as pre-receptor ligand metabolism, receptor isoform expression and receptor-, tissue- and cell type-specific factors, exist to generate diversity, as well as specificity in the response to glucocorticoids. Indeed, the cellular response to glucocorticoids displays profound variability both in magnitude and in specificity of action. Tissue sensitivity to glucocorticoids differs among individuals, within tissues of the same individual and even the same cell at different states. Furthermore, tissue-specific glucocorticoid resistance often develops in patients receiving chronic glucocorticoid therapy (Gross et al. 2009; Oakley and Cidlowski 2011).

In addition to the above mechanisms, transcription factors important for the circadian rhythmicity of glucocorticoids, such as CLOCK/BMAL1, also play an important role in determining tissue sensitivity to glucocorticoids. Recent studies have demonstrated that CLOCK/BMAL1 is a reverse-phase negative regulator of glucocorticoid action in target tissues, antagonising the biological actions of diurnally fluctuating circulating glucocorticoids and providing a local target tissue counter-regulatory feedback loop of the central CLOCK on the HPA axis. Therefore, the elevated cortisol concentrations in the morning coincide with reduced tissue sensitivity to glucocorticoids, while the very low cortisol concentrations at night coincide with increased tissue sensitivity to these hormones (Nader et al. 2009, 2010) (Fig 15.2).

The circadian clock system and the HPA axis regulate the activity of one another through multilevel interactions to ultimately coordinate homeostasis against the day/night change and various unforeseen random internal and external stressors. Uncoupling of or dysfunction in either system alters internal homeostasis and causes pathologic changes virtually in all organs and tissues, including those responsible for intermediary metabolism and immunity. Disrupted coupling of cortisol secretion and target tissue sensitivity to glucocorticoids may explain the development of central obesity and the metabolic syndrome in chronically stressed individuals, whose HPA axis circadian rhythm is characterised by blunting of the evening decreases of circulating glucocorticoids. Similarly, disrupted coupling of cortisol secretion and target tissue sensitivity to glucocorticoids may explain the increased cardiometabolic risk of individuals exposed to frequent jet lag because of travelling across time zones and of people performing night shift work over long periods of time (Chrousos 2000). Furthermore, administration of glucocorticoids at a specific period of the circadian cycle might increase their pharmacological efficacy or enhance the incidence of unwanted side effects (Nader et al. 2009, 2010).

THE LOCUS CERULEUS–NORADRENERGIC, SYSTEMIC SYMPATHETIC, ADRENOMEDULLARY AND PARASYMPATHETIC SYSTEMS

The autonomic nervous system (ANS) responds rapidly to stressors and controls a wide range of functions. Cardiovascular, respiratory, gastrointestinal, renal, endocrine and other systems are regulated by the SNS and/or the parasympathetic system. In general, the parasympathetic system can both assist and antagonise sympathetic functions by withdrawing or by increasing its activity, respectively (Chrousos and Gold 1992; Chrousos 1995, 2002, 2009, 2012; Charmandari et al. 2003, 2005, 2012).

Sympathetic innervation of peripheral organs is derived from the efferent preganglionic fibers, whose cell bodies lie in the intermediolateral column of the spinal cord. These nerves synapse in the bilateral chain of sympathetic ganglia with postganglionic sympathetic

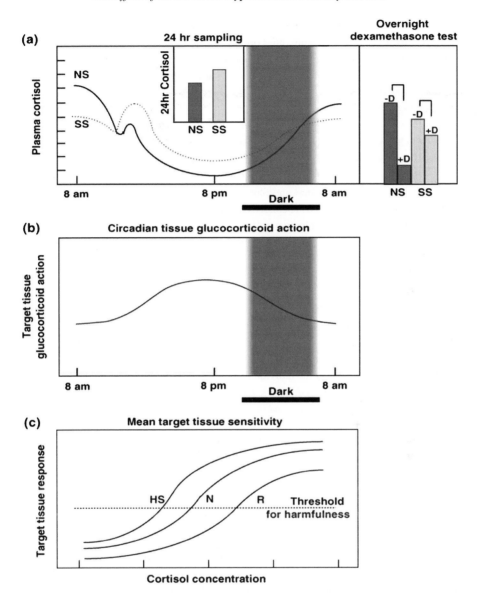

Figure 15.2. A heuristic scheme of (a) circadian secretion of cortisol in non-stressed and chronically stressed humans (left panel) and their responses to midnight dexamethasone administration (right panel), (b) the corresponding circadian changes of target tissue sensitivity to glucocorticoids and (c) mean target tissue sensitivity to glucocorticoids in the human population. Even mild evening cortisol elevations, as those seen in chronically stressed individuals, will exert disproportionately increased glucocorticoid effects because of the natural circadian target tissue sensitivity increase at this time of the day. CS, chronically stressed individuals; D, midnight dexamethasone administration; HS, hypersensitivity; N, normal sensitivity; NS, non-stressed individuals; R, resistance. (Adapted from Chrousos 2000; Nader 2010.)

neurons, which innervate widely the smooth muscle of the vasculature, the heart, skeletal muscles, kidney, gut, fat and many other organs. The pre-ganglionic neurons are primarily cholinergic, while the post-ganglionic neurons are mostly noradrenergic. The sympathetic system of the adrenal medulla also provides all of circulating epinephrine and some of the norepinephrine (Chrousos and Gold 1992; Chrousos 1995, 2002, 2009, 2012; Charmandari et al. 2003, 2005, 2012).

Effects of chronic hyperactivation of the stress system

The stress system receives and integrates a diversity of cognitive, emotional, neurosensory and peripheral somatic signals, which arrive through distinct pathways. Activation of the stress system leads to behavioural and physical changes that are remarkably consistent in their qualitative presentation and are collectively defined as the stress syndrome (Table 15.1). These changes are normally adaptive and time-limited, and improve the chances of the individual for survival (Chrousos and Gold 1992; Chrousos 1995, 2002, 2009, 2012; Charmandari et al. 2003, 2005, 2012).

In general, the stress response is meant to be of short or limited duration. The time-limited nature of this process renders its accompanying anti-growth, anti-reproductive, catabolic and immunosuppressive effects temporarily beneficial and/or of no adverse consequences to the individual. However, chronic activation of the stress system may lead to a number of disorders, which are due to increased and/or prolonged secretion of CRH and/or glucocorticoids and catecholamines (Table 15.2).

The adaptive response of an individual to stress is determined by multiple genetic, environmental and developmental factors. Excessive and/or prolonged in duration stressors may affect personality development and behaviour, and may have adverse consequences on physiologic functions, such as growth, metabolism, reproduction and the inflammatory/immune response (Chrousos and Gold 1992; Chrousos 1995, 2002, 2009, 2012; Charmandari et al. 2003, 2005, 2012).

EFFECTS OF CHRONIC HYPERACTIVATION OF THE STRESS SYSTEM ON GROWTH HORMONE/IGF-I AXIS

The growth axis is inhibited at many levels during stress. Prolonged activation of the HPA axis leads to suppression of growth hormone secretion (GHS) and glucocorticoid-induced inhibition of the effects of insulin-like growth factor-I (IGF-I) and other growth factors on target tissues (Chrousos and Gold 1992; Magiakou et al. 1994b; Chrousos 1995, 2002, 2009, 2012; Charmandari et al. 2003, 2005, 2012). Children with Cushing syndrome have delayed or arrested growth and achieve a final adult height, which is on average 7.5–8.0cm below their predicted height (Magiakou et al. 1994a). In addition, CRH-induced increases in somatostatin secretion, and therefore inhibition of GHS, have been implicated as a potential mechanism of chronic stress-related suppression of GHS. It is worth noting, however, that acute elevations of serum growth hormone concentrations may occur at the onset of the stress response or following acute administration of glucocorticoids, most likely due to stimulation of the growth hormone gene by glucocorticoids through GREs in its promoter region (Raza et al. 1998) (Fig 15.3a).

TABLE 15.2
States associated with altered hypothalamic-pituitary-adrenal (HPA) axis activity and altered regulation or dysregulation of behavioural and/or peripheral adaptation

Increased HPA axis activity	*Decreased HPA axis activity*
Chronic stress	Adrenal insufficiency
Melancholic depression	Atypical/seasonal depression
Anorexia nervosa	Chronic fatigue syndrome
Malnutrition	Fibromyalgia
Obsessive-compulsive disorder	Hypothyroidism
Panic disorder	Nicotine withdrawal
Excessive exercise (obligate athleticism)	Discontinuation of glucocorticoid therapy
Chronic active alcoholism	After Cushing syndrome cure
Alcohol and narcotic withdrawal	Premenstrual tension syndrome
Diabetes mellitus	Postpartum period
Truncal obesity (metabolic syndrome X)	After chronic stress
Childhood sexual abuse	Rheumatoid arthritis
Psychosocial short stature	Menopause
Attachment disorder of infancy	
'Functional' gastrointestinal disease	
Hyperthyroidism	
Cushing syndrome	
Pregnancy (last trimester)	

Adapted from Chrousos and Gold (1992).

EFFECTS OF CHRONIC HYPERACTIVATION OF THE STRESS SYSTEM ON THYROID FUNCTION

Activation of the HPA axis is associated with decreased production of thyroid-stimulating hormone (TSH) and inhibition of peripheral conversion of the relatively inactive thyroxine to the biologically active triiodothyronine. These alterations are likely to be caused by the increased concentrations of CRH-induced somatostatin and glucocorticoids and may help to conserve energy during stress (the 'euthyroid sick' syndrome). Somatostatin suppresses both TRH and TSH, while glucocorticoids inhibit the activity of the enzyme 5-deiodinase, which converts thyroxine to triiodothyronine.

Furthermore, the increased secretion of inflammatory cytokines during stress activates CRH secretion and inhibits 5-deiodinase activity (Chrousos and Gold 1992; Chrousos 1995, 2002, 2009, 2012; Charmandari et al. 2003, 2005, 2012) (Fig 15.3b).

EFFECTS OF CHRONIC HYPERACTIVATION OF THE STRESS SYSTEM ON REPRODUCTION

The reproductive axis is inhibited at all levels by various components of the HPA axis. CRH suppresses the secretion of gonadotropin-releasing hormone (GnRH) either directly or

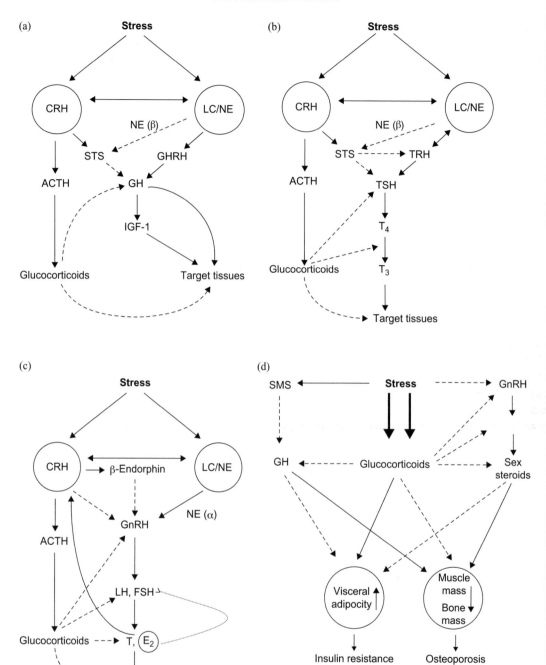

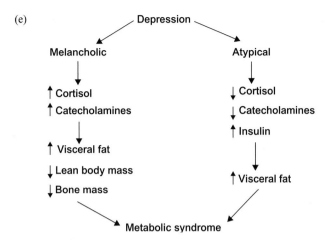

Figure 15.3. Schematic representation of the interactions between the stress system and (a) the growth hormone/IGF-I axis, (b) the thyroid axis, (c) the hypothalamic-pituitary-gonadal axis and (d) metabolic functions. (Adapted from Chrousos and Gold 1992.) (e) Melancholic and atypical depression, representing, respectively, a stress system-hyperactive/hyperreactive or hypoactive/hyporeactive state, which are both associated with development of the metabolic syndrome and its cardiovascular and other sequelae through two opposed but metabolically converging pathways. The central stress system and the peripheral sympathetic system, which normally restrain appetite and insulin secretion, respectively, when hypoactive, allow increased food intake and excessive insulin secretion, both of which promote obesity, including accumulation of visceral fat. (Adapted from Peeke and Chrousos 1995.)

indirectly, via stimulation of arcuate POMC peptide-secreting neurons. Glucocorticoids, on the other hand, exert an inhibitory effect on the GnRH neuron, the pituitary gonadotroph and the gonads, and render target tissues of gonadal steroids resistant to these hormones. The inflammatory cytokines, which are elevated during inflammatory stress, also suppress the reproductive function by inhibiting both the pulsatile secretion of GnRH from the hypothalamus and ovarian/testicular steroidogenesis. The interaction between CRH and the gonadal axis appears to be bidirectional. Estrogen-responsive elements are present in the promoter region of the CRH gene and estrogen stimulates CRH gene expression. These findings implicate the *CRH* gene as an important target of gonadal steroids and a potential mediator of sex-related differences in the stress response and the activity of the HPA axis (Chrousos and Gold 1992; Chrousos 1995, 2002, 2009, 2012; Charmandari et al. 2003, 2005, 2012) (Fig 15.3c).

EFFECTS OF CHRONIC HYPERACTIVATION OF THE STRESS SYSTEM ON METABOLISM

In addition to their direct catabolic effects, glucocorticoids also antagonise the actions of growth hormone and sex steroids on fat tissue catabolism (lipolysis) and muscle and bone anabolism. Chronic activation of the stress system is associated with increased visceral adiposity, decreased lean body (bone and muscle) mass and suppressed osteoblastic activity. This phenotype is observed in patients with Cushing syndrome, some patients with melancholic depression and patients with the metabolic syndrome (visceral obesity, insulin resistance, dyslipidemia, hypertension, hypercoagulation, atherosclerotic cardiovascular disease, sleep apnoea) (Chrousos and Gold 1992; Chrousos 1995, 2002, 2009, 2012; Charmandari et al. 2003, 2005, 2012) (Fig 15.3d).

Activation of the HPA axis during stress may also contribute to the poor control of diabetic patients with emotional stress or concurrent inflammatory or other diseases. Over time, progressive glucocorticoid-induced visceral adiposity causes further insulin resistance and deterioration of glycaemic control. Therefore, chronic activation of the stress system in patients with diabetes mellitus may result in a vicious cycle of hyperglycemia, hyperlipidemia and progressively increasing insulin resistance and insulin requirements.

Osteoporosis is almost invariably seen in association with hypercortisolism and growth hormone deficiency (GHD), and represents another example of the adverse effects of elevated cortisol concentrations and decreased growth hormone/IGF-I concentrations on osteoblastic activity. The chronic elevations of catecholamines and interleukin-6, the stress-induced hypogonadism and the reduced concentrations of sex steroids may further contribute to the development of osteoporosis (Chrousos and Gold 1992; Chrousos 1995, 2002, 2009, 2012; Charmandari et al. 2003, 2005, 2012) (Fig 15.3d).

PSYCHIATRIC DISORDERS
Depression
Stress precipitates major depression and influences its incidence, severity and course. The stress response and major depression share many common features because of using similar brain circuitries and mediators. Each is associated with a diminution of cognitive and affective flexibility, alterations in arousal and perturbations in neuroendocrine and autonomic function. Major depression is a heterogeneous disorder with two main subtypes, the melancholic and atypical depression. In melancholic depression, there is hyperactivity of the stress system, which is associated with anxiety, low self-esteem, guilt, fear for the future, insomnia, loss of appetite and HPA axis activation. Patients suffering from the condition have hypersecretion of hypothalamic CRH, as evidenced by the elevated 24h urinary cortisol excretion, the decreased ACTH responses to exogenous CRH administration, and the elevated concentrations of CRH in the cerebrospinal fluid (CSF) throughout the 24h period. These patients also have continuously elevated concentrations of norepinephrine in the CSF, which remain elevated even during sleep and a marked increase in the number of PVN CRH neurons on autopsy. Atypical depression, on the other hand, seems to be the reverse of melancholia: it is characterised by lethargy, fatigue, hypersomnia and hyperphagia, which are associated with down-regulation of the HPA axis of central origin (Chrousos and Gold 1992; Chrousos 1995, 2002, 2009, 2012; Gold et al. 2002; Charmandari et al. 2003, 2005, 2012).

The enhanced susceptibility of patients with major depression to the premature onset of chronic complex non-communicable diseases that are frequently seen as we age suggests that the pathophysiologic changes of major depression, especially the form that includes melancholic features, leads to a premature ageing. Melancholic patients have an increased incidence of coronary artery disease, osteoporosis and sleep disturbances, as well as premature progressive decrements in growth hormone and DHEA secretion. Patients with atypical depression develop obesity, metabolic syndrome and their chronic cardiovascular consequences, including cardiovascular disease (Chrousos and Gold 1992; Chrousos 1995, 2002, 2009, 2012; Charmandari et al. 2003, 2005, 2012). Figure 15.3e compares the pathopsysiologic pathways of the two forms of depression.

POSTTRAUMATIC STRESS DISORDER

Posttraumatic stress disorder (PTSD) develops following exposure to traumatic life experiences and is characterised by dysregulation of both the HPA axis and the locus ceruleus/noradrenergic–SNS. Adults with this disorder display a unique neuroendocrine profile, with centrally elevated CRH and catecholamines, and low peripheral cortisol concentrations (Pervanidou and Chrousos 2010). Traumatic experiences early in life predispose strongly to PTSD development later in life. In studies that included children and adolescents involved in motor vehicle accidents, elevated evening salivary cortisol and morning serum interleukin-6 concentrations were predictive of persistent PTSD development 6 months later. Longitudinal analysis showed a progressive divergence of the two main axes of the stress system that may be part of the pathophysiologic mechanism responsible for PTSD maintenance. An initial elevation of cortisol in the aftermath of the trauma, followed by a gradual normalisation and finally low cortisol secretion together with a gradual elevation of catecholamines over time, may represent the natural history of neuroendocrine changes in pediatric PTSD. Thus, low cortisol concentrations found in adult studies may reflect prior trauma and might represent a biologic vulnerability factor for later PTSD development (Pervanidou and Chrousos 2010).

Conclusion

The stress system coordinates the adaptive response of the organism to stressors and plays an important role in maintenance of basal and stress-related homeostasis. Activation of the stress system leads to behavioural and peripheral changes that improve the ability of the organism to adapt and increase its chances for survival. Inadequate and/or prolonged response to stressors may impair growth and development, and may result in a variety of endocrine, metabolic, autoimmune and psychiatric disorders. The development and severity of these conditions primarily depend on genetic, developmental and environmental factors.

The prenatal life, infancy, childhood and adolescence are periods of increased plasticity for the stress system and, therefore, are particularly sensitive to stressors. Excessive or sustained activation of the stress system during these critical periods may have profound effects on its function. These environmental triggers or stressors may have not a transient, but rather a permanent, effect on the organism, reminiscent of the 'organisational' effects of several hormones exerted on certain target tissues, which last long after cessation of the exposure to these hormones.

Today, the presence of stress and 'cacostasis' in an individual can be evaluated and graded. There are rational and proven methods to prevent and ameliorate distress that starts from changes in lifestyle (healthy diet, exercise, stable daily timing of food uptake and sleep onset, adequate sleep), to cognitive and behavioural therapies, to the use of appropriate medications. Indeed, the currently available medications control risk factors and prolong life function primarily by blocking the stress system and inflammatory mediators. The key issue is that nature provides flexibility and well-being and hyperstasis are attainable.

Granted that chronic stress in early life augments the risk of developing chronic behavioural and non-communicable disorders, preventing distress in pregnancy and the first 5 years of life or interrupting the vicious cycle of distress during this period is imperative and, in the long run, the most cost-effective approach. Interventions beyond the age of 5 may be quite useful, but one should note that major stress-related brain organisational and epigenetic damage has already occurred. L. Tolstoy had intuitively said, 'from the child of five to myself is but a step. But from the newborn baby to the child of five is an appalling distance'. This is based on robust evidence and calls for early interventions, starting with the education of prospective parents (Carneiro and Heckman 2003).

Therefore, to interrupt the vicious effects of stress in a society and its members, one should, first, eliminate or at least moderate the stressors, and second, one should improve the coping of individuals with such stressors – aka improving their resilience to stress. Political actions can influence both strategies. Granted that stress in today's industrialised world is mostly anthropogenic, a well-run country itself in homeostasis, in which people feel enfranchised, dignified and dealt with fairness and justice, is bound to have happier and healthier citizens. On the other hand, preventing early life stressors and their effects on the very young will eliminate development of risks for the later behavioural and chronic non-communicable disorders that plague our societies today. Finally, like many human endeavours, coping with stress is a learnable process and the basis of the most effective psychological therapy employed today, cognitive behavioural therapy. It is the duty of a society to ensure the well-being and happiness of its people with political strategies that prevent stress and enhance the ability of its citizens to cope.

REFERENCES

Bale TL and Vale WW (2004) CRF and CRF receptors: role in stress responsivity and other behaviors. *Annu Rev Pharmacol Toxicol* 44: 525–557.

Bornstein SR and Chrousos GP (1999) Clinical review 104: Adrenocorticotropin (ACTH) and non-ACTH-mediated regulation of the adrenal cortex: Neural and immune inputs. *J Clin Endocrinol Metab* 84(5): 1729–1736.

Carneiro P and Heckman JJ (2003) Human capital policy. Discussion Paper No821. IZA Discussion Papers, IZA, Bonn, Germany. http://ssrn.com/abstract434544.

Charmandari E, Achermann JC, Carel JC, Soder O and Chrousos GP (2012) Stress response and child health. *Sci Signal* 5(248): mr1.

Charmandari E, Kino T, Souvatzoglou E and Chrousos GP (2003) Pediatric stress: Hormonal mediators and human development. *Horm Res* 59(4): 161–179.

Charmandari E, Tsigos C and Chrousos G (2005) Endocrinology of the stress response. *Annu Rev Physiol* 67: 259–284.

Chrousos GP (1995) The hypothalamic-pituitary-adrenal axis and immune-mediated inflammation. *N Engl J Med* 332(20): 1351–1362.

Chrousos GP (2000) The role of stress and the hypothalamic-pituitary-adrenal axis in the pathogenesis of the metabolic syndrome: neuro-endocrine and target tissue-related causes. *Int J Obes Relat Metab Disord.* 24; Suppl 2: S50–5.

Chrousos GP (2002) Organization and integration of the endocrine system. In: Sperling M (ed) *Pediatric Endocrinology.* Philadelphia, PA: WB Saunders, 1–14.

Chrousos GP (2009) Stress and disorders of the stress system. *Nat Rev Endocrinol* 5(7): 374–381.

Chrousos GP (2012) Stress in early life: A developmental and evolutionary perspective. In: Hochberg Z (ed) *Evo-Devo of Child Growth*. Hoboken, NJ: Wiley-Blackwell Co, 29–40.

Chrousos GP and Gold PW (1992) The concepts of stress and stress system disorders. Overview of physical and behavioral homeostasis. *JAMA* 267(9): 1244–1252.

Chrousos GP and Kino T (2009) Glucocorticoid signaling in the cell: Expanding clinical implications to complex human behavioral and somatic disorders. In: Glucocorticoids and mood: Clinical manifestations, risk factors, and molecular mechanisms. *Proc. NY Acad Sci* 1179: 153–166.

Gillies GE, Linton EA and Lowry PJ (1982) Corticotropin releasing activity of the new CRF is potentiated several times by vasopressin. *Nature* 299(5881): 355–357.

Gold PW, Gabry KE, Yasuda MR and Chrousos GP (2002) Divergent endocrine abnormalities in melancholic and atypical depression: Clinical and pathophysiologic implications. *Endocrinol Metab Clin North Am* 31(1): 37–62.

Grigoriadis DE (2002) The corticotropin releasing factor receptor: A novel target for the treatment of depression and anxiety-related disorders. *Expert Opin. Ther. Targets* 9(4): 651–684.

Gross KL, Lu NZ and Cidlowski JA (2009) Molecular mechanisms regulating glucocorticoid sensitivity and resistance. *Mol Cell Endocrinol* 300(1–2): 7–16.

Iranmanesh A, Lizarralde G, Short D and Veldhuis JD (1990) Intensive venous sampling paradigms disclose high frequency adrenocorticotropin release episodes in normal men. *J Clin Endocrinol Metab* 71(5): 1276–1283.

Magiakou MA, Mastorakos G and Chrousos GP (1994a) Final stature in patients with endogenous Cushing's syndrome. *J Clin Endocrinol Metab* 79(4): 1082–1085.

Magiakou MA, Mastorakos G, Gomez MT, Rose SR and Chrousos GP (1994b) Suppressed spontaneous and stimulated growth hormone secretion in patients with Cushing's disease before and after surgical cure. *J Clin Endocrinol Metab* 78(1): 131–137.

Nader N, Chrousos GP and Kino T (2009) Circadian rhythm transcription factor CLOCK regulates the transcriptional activity of the glucocorticoid receptor by acetylating its hinge region lysine cluster: Potential physiological implications. *FASEB J* 23(5): 1572–1583.

Nader N, Chrousos GP and Kino T (2010) Interactions of the circadian CLOCK system and the HPA axis. *Trends Endocrinol Metab* 21(5): 277–286.

Nicolaides NC, Galata Z, Kino T, Chrousos GP and Charmandari E (2010) The human glucocorticoid receptor: Molecular basis of biologic function. *Steroids* 75(1): 1–12.

Oakley RH and Cidlowski JA (2011) Cellular processing of the glucocorticoid receptor gene and protein: New mechanisms for generating tissue-specific actions of glucocorticoids. *J Biol Chem* 286(5): 3177–3184.

Peeke PM and Chrousos GP (1995) Hypercortisolism and obesity. *Ann N Y Acad Sci* 771: 665–676.

Pervanidou P and Chrousos GP (2010) Neuroendocrinology of posttraumatic stress disorder. *Prog. Brain Res* 182: 149–160.

Raza J, Massoud AF, Hindmarsh PC, Robinson IC and Brook CG (1998) Direct effects of corticotrophin-releasing hormone on stimulated growth hormone secretion. *Clin Endocrinol (Oxf)* 48(2): 217–222.

16
ADRENOLEUKODYSTROPHY: NEUROLOGICAL ASPECTS

Patrick Aubourg

Introduction

X-linked adrenoleukodystrophy (X-ALD; OMIM, phenotype MIM number #300100) is the most common inherited peroxisomal disorder. The combined incidence of hemizygotes (all phenotypes) plus heterozygous female carriers is 1:16 800 newborn infants (Bezman and Moser 1998).

Adrenomyeloneuropathy

Adrenomyeloneuropathy (AMN) is the most frequent clinical phenotype of X-ALD and affects both males and heterozygous women in adulthood (Engelen et al. 2012). The initial symptoms are restricted exercise, stiffness in the lower limbs, gait imbalance with impaired vibration sense in the lower limbs, bladder problems and often scarce scalp hair (alopecia) in males (Powers et al. 2000, 2001; Engelen et al. 2012). AMN progresses to a severe spastic paraplegia within one or two decades. AMN is not a demyelinating disease and results from a slowly progressive axonopathy affecting sensory-ascending and motor-descending tracts in the spinal cord with 100% penetrance in men and 65% in heterozygous women by the age of 60 years (Powers et al. 2000; Engelen et al. 2012). AMN is one of the most common causes of hereditary spastic paraplegia. About 66% of male AMN patients (Blevins et al. 1994) but less than 5% of female patients (El-Deiry et al. 1997) have adrenal insufficiency. In AMN males, the diagnosis of Addison disease is often made years or decades before the onset of neurological symptoms (Engelen et al. 2012). Magnetic resonance imaging (MRI) studies reveal abnormal signals within the pyramidal tracts in the brainstem and internal capsule. While many patients with AMN show subtle involvement of white matter in the centrum ovale, there is no overt MRI sign of cerebral demyelination (Van der Voorn et al. 2011; Engelen et al. 2012).

Cerebral X-linked adrenoleukodystrophy

Approximately 60%–65% of males with X-ALD are at risk of developing inflammatory cerebral demyelination (cerebral X-ALD, CALD) (Engelen et al. 2012). It may occur in childhood (35%), usually between 5 and 12 years of age, or in adulthood (30%) when X-ALD males have already developed neurologic symptoms of AMN (Van Geel et al. 2001; Engelen et al. 2012). The cerebral demyelination starts most often in the corpus callosum (splenium or genu) and extends relentlessly outwards as symmetric, confluent lesions either in the parieto-occipital or in the frontal white matter. Clinically, this coincides with a devastating decline in cognitive and neurologic functions, leading to a vegetative state or death within 3 to 5 years. Occasionally, a spontaneous arrest of cerebral disease can be observed, particularly into adulthood. In females, cerebral disease is exceedingly rare and has only been verified in a case where both X chromosomes were affected (Hershkovitz et al. 2002).

Clinical signs of Addison disease are present in 92% of boys with CALD with an onset of symptoms before 6 years of age, and 63% with onset of symptoms before 15 years of age (Korenke et al. 1997).

Treatment options

There is no treatment for AMN but allogeneic hematopoietic stem cell transplantation (HSCT) or autologous transplantation of hematopoietic stem cell corrected with lentiviral vector can arrest the cerebral demyelination when the procedure is performed at an early stage of cerebral disease (Shapiro et al. 2000; Peters et al. 2004; Cartier et al. 2009). In practice, transplantation should be undertaken when boys have started to develop cerebral demyelination on brain MRI but there are no significant cognitive or neurologic symptoms.

A 2011 survey showed that at least 40% of X-ALD boys who were considered as candidates for HSCT had Addison disease as the presenting feature of X-ALD before the onset of CALD (Polgreen et al. 2011). Among 90 X-ALD patients consecutively evaluated at the University of Minnesota for treatment of CALD with HSCT, the first indicator of X-ALD was Addison disease in 17 (19%), brain MRI and/or neurologic changes in 52 (58%) and a family history in 21 (23%). The frequency of X-ALD phenotypes was 2% Addison disease only, 12% cerebral disease only and 86% Addison disease and cerebral disease. Of the boys with cerebral disease, adrenal insufficiency was the presenting sign in 40%.

Importantly, boys diagnosed with unexplained adrenal insufficiency who had a delay in the diagnosis of X-ALD greater than 12 months and then developed CALD had more advanced cerebral disease at the time of evaluation for HSCT than boys diagnosed with X-ALD at the time of the diagnosis of adrenal insufficiency.

Screening family members

It is likely that X-ALD is under-diagnosed in boys with Addison disease (Bezman et al. 2001; Dubey et al. 2005). Screening of at-risk family members has demonstrated a high prevalence of unrecognised adrenocortical insufficiency in asymptomatic boys with X-ALD at an early age of 4–5 years. At baseline, 80% had impaired adrenal function. Serum adrenocorticotropic hormone (ACTH) was elevated in 69% patients and the ACTH stimulation test was abnormal in 43% of patients. By the end of the follow-up 2 to 3 years later, 86% patients had borderline or clear adrenal insufficiency (age at onset: 4.8 ± 3.7 years). A key finding was that 70% of the patients studied by 2 years of age already showed increased serum ACTH levels. Another study showed that 83% of boys with unexplained adrenal insufficiency did indeed have X-ALD (Ronghe et al. 2002).

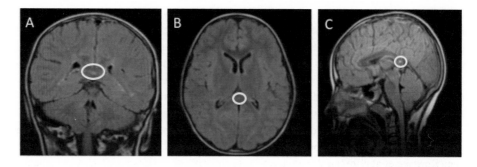

Figure 16.1. Brain MRI of a 6-year-old boy with Addison disease due to X-linked adrenoleukodys-trophy. Melanodermia appeared at 3 years and this boy had several episodes of unexplained abdominal pain and vomiting from the age of 5 years before he developed acute adrenal crisis at 6 years. Following the diagnosis of Addison disease, very-long-chain fatty acid assay in plasma demonstrated he had X-ALD. Brain MRI was rapidly performed and showed on coronal (a), axial (b) and sagittal (c) FLAIR sequences abnormal hyperintense signal of the splenium of corpus callosum indicating that he was already developing cerebral X-ALD.

It is therefore essential to screen all boys with Addison disease without another identified etiology even if neurological signs or symptoms are absent (Fig. 16.1). The diagnosis of X-ALD is reliably established by characteristic abnormalities in fasting saturated very-long-chain fatty acids (VLCFAs) profile in a serum or plasma sample (Moser et al. 1981).

Genetic and biochemical aspects of X-linked adrenoleukodystrophy
All X-ALD patients have mutations in the adenosine triphosphate (ATP)-binding cassette (ABC) transporter subfamily D member 1 (*ABCD1*) gene (Mosser et al. 1993). More than 693 different *ABCD1* gene mutations have been identified (see http://www.x-ald.nl). There is no genotype–phenotype correlation. The same *ABCD1* gene mutation can lead to CALD or AMN within the same kindred and a complete loss of ABCD1 protein (due to frameshift, nonsense or large deletion mutation) or an *ABCD1* gene mutation leading to a stable but non-functional ABCD1 protein in peroxisomes can also result in either CALD or AMN (Berger et al. 1994; Smith et al. 1999). There remains the possibility that mutations, in particular missense mutations, may play a role in the phenotypic variation of AMN in terms of age at onset and severity.

The ABCD1 protein is a half transporter that forms homodimers (Liu et al. 1999). The ATP-binding domain of ABCD1 is facing the cytosol, and substrates are transported from the cytosol into the peroxisome with ATP consumption. Saturated VLCFAs accumulate in tissues (including adrenal glands, brain, spinal cord and peripheral nerves) and plasma of X-ALD patients. In fact, VLCFAs accumulate not as free fatty acids but as coenzyme A (CoA) esters acylated to various lipids and proteins. The ABCD1 protein imports VLCFA-CoA (as well as other fatty acid-CoA) into peroxisomes where they are degraded by sequential reactions of oxidation (Van Roermund et al. 2008). Failure to import

VLCFA-CoA into peroxisomes results in the accumulation of these fatty acid-CoAs in the cytosol where they are redirected towards different pathways and deficient peroxisomal β-oxidation of VLCFA in vitro. The majority of VLCFAs are derived from endogenous synthesis and the VLCFA burden observed in X-ALD is not only due to a defect of degradation in peroxisomes but also due to an increased synthesis involving mostly the activity of the elongase ELOVL1 (Ofman et al. 2010). There is no correlation between X-ALD clinical phenotypes and the accumulation of VLCFAs in plasma or fibroblasts from X-ALD patients. Nevertheless, the amount of VLCFA is higher in the normal appearing white matter of patients with CALD compared with patients with AMN (Asheuer et al. 2005). Oligodendrocytes derived from induced pluripotent stem cells of patients with CALD accumulate more VLCFAs than those derived from patients with AMN (Jang et al. 2011).

Pathophysiology of adrenomyeloneuropathy and cerebral X-linked adrenoleukodystrophy

With the availability of an ABCD1-deficient mouse model that develops an 'AMN-like' phenotype (Pujol et al. 2002), significant progress has been made in the pathophysiology of AMN which is fully penetrant in X-ALD male patients. The die-back axonopathy of AMN seems to be the consequence of oligodendrocyte failure to maintain normal axonal function independent of myelination. Loss of ABCD1 protein function and accumulation of VLCFA-CoA esters result in abnormal oxidative stress; mitochondrial dysfunction (OXPHOS disruption and mitochondrial depletion) and malfunctioning of the ubiquitin-proteasome system lead to axonal degeneration in the spinal cord (Fourcade et al. 2014).

The CALD phenotype is not fully penetrant and its physiopathogenesis remains an enigma (reviewed in Berger et al. 2013). There is no mouse model of CALD. Different mechanisms are likely involved in the initial cerebral demyelination, and then the severe neuro-inflammation process that induces rapidly progressive demyelination. The initial phase of spontaneous demyelination might be related to the level of VLCFAs in myelin sheaths. However, even with the same loss of ABCD1 protein function, concentrations of VLCFAs can be modulated by the ability of oligodendrocytes to synthesise more or less VLCFA (linked to ELOVL1 activity) as well as to degrade VLCFA-CoA by alternative pathways, in particular omega-oxidation. The amount of VLCFA-CoA in different lipids or proteins together with environmental and epigenetic factors may determine whether or not and when spontaneous myelin breakdown occurs.

The molecular mechanisms responsible for the conversion into full-blown inflammation are poorly understood. The neuro-inflammation process is associated with an opening of the blood–brain barrier. Impairment of the neuro-vascular unit as well as the contribution of blood volume and vascular density may contribute to the pathogenesis of inflammatory CALD, as in multiple sclerosis. The therapeutic benefit of *HSCT* and *HSC* gene therapy indicates that correction of brain myeloid cells, including microglia, is an important factor to arrest the progression of CALD. It is important to mention that in contrast to HSCT performed for lysosomal central nervous system diseases, there is no cross-correction of other cell types after HSCT in X-ALD because ABCD1, as a peroxisomal membrane protein, cannot be released from normal or corrected cells. Dysfunction of X-ALD microglia might therefore contribute to demyelination and/or neuroinflammation and possibly alters the neurovascular unit. Another important factor might be that lysophosphatidylcholine with excess of VLCFA-CoA can lead to microglial activation and apoptosis (Eichler et al. 2008). Yet, the accumulation of T and B cells in the active cerebral demyelinating lesions is strongly suggestive of an immune attack. Which antigens elicit autoimmunity within the brain remains unknown.

Physiopathogenesis of Addison disease

Pathologic changes of adrenal glands are already detectable at 20 weeks of gestation (Powers et al. 1982). After birth, the adrenal glands show a marked atrophy of the cortex which is progressive and can be imaged using ultrasound, CT scan or MRI (Shaumburg et al. 1972; Powers and Shaumburg 1973). The atrophy is more marked in the zona fasciculata and reticularis than in the glomerulosa. Ballooned cells with the presence of lamellar lipid striations and fine clefts are visible by light microscopy. There is no accumulation of inflammatory cells and the medulla is preserved. ABCD1 protein is expressed in the adrenal cortex but not in the adrenal medulla (Troffer-Charlier et al. 1998; Hoftberger et al. 2007, 2010) in good agreement with the pathological findings.

VLCFAs are extremely hydrophobic and their rate of desorption from biological membranes is about 10 000 times slower than that of long-chain fatty acids causing disruptive effects on the structure, stability and function of cell membranes (Ho et al. 1995). Excess of VLCFAs in cultured cells decreases the ACTH-stimulated cortisol release by human adrenocortical cells (Whitcomb et al. 1988). VLCFAs are proposed to be toxic to the adrenal cortex, resulting in apoptotic cell death (Powers et al. 1982). The mechanism leading to the activation of apoptotic pathway is however unknown. Not all patients with X-ALD develop biological or clinical adrenal insufficiency, indicating that factors other than the accumulation of VLCFA-CoA play a role in the progressive loss of adrenocortical cells. There is no evidence for a reversal of adrenal failure after hematopoietic cell transplantation in X-ALD (Petryk et al. 2012). Treatment of Addison disease has no impact on CALD or AMN (onset, severity and disease course).

Adrenal insufficiency due to X-ALD affects first the glucocorticoid function, but the mineralocorticoid function is ultimately deficient in approximately half of ALD patients (Sadeghi-Nejad and Senior 1990; Aubourg and Chaussain 1991; Laureti et al. 1998). In boys, melanodermia appear frequently around 2–3 years of age and several years may pass before severe impairment of adrenal function results in adrenal crisis with abdominal pain, vomiting, drowsiness, hypoglycemia, salt wasting and sometimes blood pressure collapse. Moderate adrenal crisis with only abdominal pain and vomiting are frequent before the onset of severe adrenal crisis and the diagnosis of Addison disease is often not made because salt wasting in the urine is not checked. There are many other causes of Addison disease than X-ALD in boys aged from 3 to 12 years (Hsieh and White 2011). X-ALD patients with Addison disease do not develop antibodies against 21-hydroxylase (P450c21) (Falorni et al. 1995; Laureti et al. 1996b). Yet, we recommend not to wait for a 21-hydroxylase antibody result, and to urgently perform VLCFA screening in plasma from boys with Addison disease.

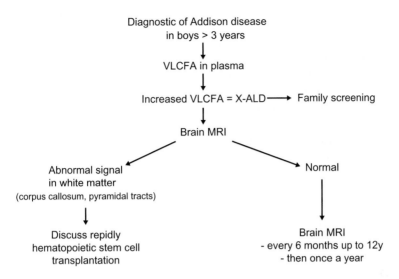

Figure 16.2. Flowchart describing the management of boys with Addison disease and X-linked adrenoleukodystrophy.

Long-term monitoring

Once the aetiology of Addison disease has been linked to X-ALD and the patient's brain MRI is normal, regular monitoring is required. In the absence of biomarkers predicting CALD or AMN, the only strategy is to perform brain MRI every 6 months from the age of 4 to 12 years and then once a year up to at least 50 years of age (Fig. 16.2). After the age of 12 years, the risk of CALD decreases sharply but is not null.

X-ALD is also a frequent cause of Addison disease in adult males (Laureti et al. 1996a; Horn et al. 2013). Adults with X-ALD have a 30% chance of developing CALD usually between 25 and 40 years.

Conclusion

Making an early diagnosis of X-ALD diagnosis is important to attenuate progression to CALD by early instigation of HSCT. Less than 10% of *ABCD1* gene mutations are de novo mutations. It is not unusual, therefore, to identify an adult with X-ALD and Addison disease who has other affected family members. Family studies are essential in terms of screening with VLCFA measurement in all males. Early and frequent MRI brain imaging is essential for early detection of cerebral complications.

REFERENCES

Asheuer M, Bieche I, Laurendeau I et al. (2005) Decreased expression of ABCD4 and BG1 genes early in the pathogenesis of X-linked adrenoleukodystrophy. *Hum Mol Genet* 14: 1293–1303.
Aubourg P and Chaussain JL (1991) Adrenoleukodystrophy presenting as Addison's disease in children and adults. *Trends Endocrinol Metab* 2: 49–52.

Berger J, Forss-Petter S and Eichler FS (2013) Pathophysiology of X-linked adrenoleukodystrophy. *Biochem Biophys Acta*, in press.

Berger J, Molzer B, Fae I and Bernheimer H (1994) X-linked adrenoleukodystrophy (ALD): A novel mutation of the ALD gene in 6 members of a family presenting with 5 different phenotypes. *Biochem Biophys Res Commun* 205: 1638–1643.

Bezman L, Moser AB, Raymond GV et al. (2001) Adrenoleukodystrophy: Incidence, new mutation rate, and results of extended family screening. *Ann Neurol* 49: 512–517.

Bezman L and Moser HW (1998) Incidence of X-linked adrenoleukodystrophy and the relative frequency of its phenotypes. *American J Med Genet* 76: 415–419.

Blevins LS Jr, Shankroff J, Moser HW and Ladenson PW (1994) Elevated plasma adrenocorticotropin concentration as evidence of limited adrenocortical reserve in patients with adrenomyeloneuropathy. *J Clin Endocrinol Metab* 78: 261–265.

Cartier N, Hacein-Bey-Abina S, Bartholomae CC et al. (2009) Hematopoietic stem cell gene therapy with a lentiviral vector in X-linked adrenoleukodystrophy. *Science* 326: 818–823.

Dubey P, Raymond GV, Moser AB, Kharkar S, Bezman L and Moser HW (2005) Adrenal insufficiency in asymptomatic adrenoleukodystrophy patients identified by very long-chain fatty acid screening. *J Pediatr* 146: 528–532.

Eichler FS, Ren JQ, Cossoy M et al. (2008) Is microglial apoptosis an early pathogenic change in cerebral X-linked adrenoleukodystrophy? *Ann Neurol* 63: 729–742.

El-Deiry SS, Naidu S, Blevins LS and Ladenson PW (1997) Assessment of adrenal function in women heterozygous for adrenoleukodystrophy. *J Clin Endocrinol Metab* 82: 856–860.

Engelen M, Kemp S, De Visser M et al. (2012) X-linked adrenoleukodystrophy (X-ALD): Clinical presentation and guidelines for diagnosis, follow-up and management. *Orphanet J Rare* 7: 51.

Falorni A, Nikoshkov A, Laureti S et al. (1995) High diagnostic accuracy for idiopathic Addison's disease with a sensitive radiobinding assay for autoantibodies against recombinant human 21-hydroxylase. *J Clin Endocrinol Metab* 80: 2752–2755.

Fourcade S, López-Erauskin J, Ruiz M, Ferrer I and Pujol A (2014) Mitochondrial dysfunction and oxidative damage cooperatively fuel axonal degeneration in X-linked adrenoleukodystrophy. *Biochimie* 98: 143–149.

Hershkovitz E, Narkis G, Shorer Z et al. (2002) Cerebral X-linked adrenoleukodystrophy in a girl with Xq 27-Ter deletion. *Ann Neurol* 52: 234–237.

Ho JK, Moser H, Kishimoto Y and Hamilton JA (1995) Interactions of a very long chain fatty acid with model membranes and serum albumin. Implications for the pathogenesis of adrenoleukodystrophy. *J Clin Invest* 96: 1455–1463.

Hoftberger R, Kunze M, Voigtlander T et al. (2010) Peroxisomal localization of the proopiomelanocortin-derived peptides beta-lipotropin and beta-endorphin. *Endocrinology* 151: 4801–4810.

Hoftberger R, Kunze M, Weinhofer I et al. (2007) Distribution and cellular localization of adrenoleukodystrophy protein in human tissues: Implications for X-linked adrenoleukodystrophy. *Neurobiol Dis* 28: 165–174.

Horn MA, Erichsen MM, Wolff AS et al. (2013) Screening for X-linked adrenoleukodystrophy among adult men with Addison's disease. *Clin Endocrinol* 79: 316–320.

Hsieh S and White PC (2011) Presentation of primary adrenal insufficiency in childhood. *J Clin Endocrinol Metab* 96: E925–E928.

Jang J, Kang HC, Kim HS et al. (2011) Induced pluripotent stem cell models from X-linked adrenoleukodystrophy patients. *Ann Neurol* 70: 402–409.

Korenke GC, Roth C, Krasemann E, Hüfner M, Hunneman DH and Hanefeld F (1997) Variability of endocrinological dysfunction in 55 patients with X-linked adrenoleucodystrophy: Clinical, laboratory and genetic findings. *Eur J Endocrinol* 137: 40–47.

Laureti S, Aubourg P, Calcinaro F et al. (1998) Etiological diagnosis of primary adrenal insufficiency using an original flowchart of immune and biochemical markers. *J Clin Endocrinol Metab* 83: 3163–3168.

Laureti S, Casucci G, Santeusanio F, Angeletti G, Aubourg P and Brunetti P (1996a) X-linked adrenoleukodystrophy is a frequent cause of idiopathic Addison's disease in young adult male patients. *J Clin Endocrinol Metab* 81: 470–474.

Laureti S, Falorni A, Volpato M et al. (1996b) Absence of circulating adrenal autoantibodies in adult-onset X-linked adrenoleukodystrophy. *Horm Metab* 28: 319–343.

Liu LX, Janvier K, Berteaux-Lecellier V, Cartier N, Benarous R and Aubourg P (1999) Homo- and heterodimerization of peroxisomal ATP-binding cassette half-transporters. *J Biol Chem* 274: 32738–32743.

Moser HW, Moser AB, Frayer KK et al. (1981) Adrenoleukodystrophy: Increased plasma content of saturated very long chain fatty acids. *Neurology* 31: 1241–1249.

Mosser J, Douar AM, Sarde CO et al. (1993) Putative X-linked adrenoleukodystrophy gene shares unexpected homology with ABC transporters. *Nature* 361: 726–730.

Ofman R, Dijkstra IM, van Roermund CW et al. (2010) The role of ELOVL1 in very long-chain fatty acid homeostasis and X-linked adrenoleukodystrophy. *EMBO Ol Med* 2: 90–97.

Peters C, Charnas LR, Tan Y et al. (2004) Cerebral X-linked adrenoleukodystrophy: The international hematopoietic cell transplantation experience from 1982 to 1999. *Blood* 104: 881–888.

Petryk A, Polgreen LE, Chahla S, Miller W and Orchard PJ (2012) No evidence for the reversal of adrenal failure after hematopoietic cell transplantation in X-linked adrenoleukodystrophy. *Bone Marrow Transplant* 47: 1377–1378.

Polgreen LE, Chahla S, Miller W et al. (2011) Early diagnosis of cerebral X-linked adrenoleukodystrophy in boys with Addison's disease improves survival and neurological outcomes. *Eur J Pediatr* 170: 1049–1054.

Powers JM, DeCiero DP, Cox C et al. (2001) The dorsal root ganglia in adrenomyeloneuropathy: Neuronal atrophy and abnormal mitochondria. *J Neuropathol Exp Neurol* 60: 493–501.

Powers JM, DeCiero DP, Ito M, Moser AB and Moser HW (2000) Adrenomyeloneuropathy: Aneuropathologic review featuring its noninflammatory myelopathy. *J Neuropathol Exp Neurol* 59: 89–102.

Powers JM, Moser HW, Moser AB and Shaumburg HH (1982) Fetal adrenoleukodystrophy: The significance of pathologic lesions in adrenal gland and testis. *Hum Pathol* 13: 1013–1019.

Powers JM and Shaumburg HH (1973) The adrenal cortex in adrenoleukodystrophy. *Arch Pathol* 96: 305–310.

Pujol A, Hindelang C, Callizot N, Bartsch U, Schachner M and Mandel JL (2002) Late onset neurological phenotype of the X-ALD gene inactivation in mice: A mouse model for adrenomyeloneuropathy. *Hum Mol Genet* 11: 499–505.

Ronghe MD, Barton J, Jardine PE et al. (2002) The importance of testing for adrenoleucodystrophy in males with idiopathic Addison's disease. *Arch Dis Child* 86: 185–189.

Sadeghi-Nejad and A Senior B (1990) Adrenomyeloneuropathy presenting as Addison's disease in childhood. *N Engl J Med* 322: 13–16.

Shapiro E, Krivit W, Lockman L et al. (2000) Long-term effect of bone-marrow transplantation for childhood-onset cerebral X-linked adrenoleukodystrophy. *Lancet* 356: 713–718.

Shaumburg HH, Richardson EP and Johnson PC (1972) Schilder's disease: Sex-linked recessive transmission with specific adrenal changes. *Arch Neurol* 27: 458–460.

Smith KD, Kemp S, Braiterman LT et al. (1999) X-linked adrenoleukodystrophy: Genes, mutations and phenotypes. *Neurochem Res* 24: 521–535.

Troffer-Charlier N, Doerflinger N, Metzger E, Fouquet F, Mandel JL and Aubourg P (1998) Mirror expression of adrenoleukodystrophy and adrenoleukodystrophy related genes in mouse tissues and human cell lines. *Eur J Cell Biol* 75: 254–264.

Van der Voorn JP, Pouwels PJ, Powers JM et al. (2011) Correlating quantitative MR imaging with histopathology in X-linked adrenoleukodystrophy. *AJNR Am J Neuroradiol* 32: 481–489.

Van Geel BM, Bezman L, Loes DJ, Moser HW and Raymond GV (2001) of phenotypes in adult male patients with X-linked adrenoleukodystrophy. *Ann Neurol* 49: 186–194.

Van Roermund CW, Visser WF, Ijlst L et al. (2008) The human peroxisomal ABC half transporter ALDP functions as a homodimer and accepts acyl-CoA esters. *FASEB J* 22: 4201–4208.

Whitcomb RW, Linehan WM and Knazek RA (1988) Effects of long-chain, saturated fatty acids on membrane microviscosity and adrenocorticotropin responsiveness of human adrenocortical cells in vitro. *J Clin Invest* 81: 185–188.

17
CUSHING DISEASE: DIAGNOSIS AND MANAGEMENT

Helen L Storr and Martin O Savage

Incidence of paediatric Cushing syndrome

Cushing syndrome is a clinical syndrome, which comprises many symptoms and signs reflecting excessive circulating glucocorticoid concentrations. It is very rare in childhood and adolescence. The incidence of paediatric-onset Cushing syndrome is estimated as 10% of the adult Cushing syndrome prevalence, i.e. ~0.5 new cases/million/year (Newell-Price et al. 2006). Cushing syndrome within the paediatric age range can be classified into two groups: adrenocorticotrophic hormone (ACTH)-independent and ACTH-dependent causes (Table 17.1). Iatrogenic exogenous glucocorticoid administration remains the most common cause in paediatric as well as adult patients with Cushing syndrome. These patients are rarely referred for endocrine review and therefore this chapter will not discuss iatrogenic Cushing syndrome further.

Aetiology of paediatric Cushing disease

Cushing syndrome can occur throughout childhood and adolescence; however, different aetiologies are more commonly associated with particular age groups (Fig 17.1). Cushing disease is the commonest cause in children after the pre-school years, reaching a peak incidence at 14 years (Magiakou et al. 1994c). The commonest cause of Cushing disease is an ACTH-secreting pituitary corticotroph adenoma (Magiakou et al. 1994c; Savage and Besser 1996; Magiakou and Chrousos 2002). Cushing disease accounts for 75%–80% of paediatric patients with Cushing syndrome compared to 49%–71% of adult cases (Weber et al. 1995; Magiakou and Chrousos 2002).

Paediatric Cushing disease is almost always caused by a pituitary microadenoma (diameter <5mm) (Fahlbusch et al. 1995). Children with macroadenomas are only rarely reported in the literature (Khadilkar et al. 2004; Storr et al. 2005) but can be aggressive with invasion of the cavernous sinus (Damiani et al. 1998). Pituitary macroadenomas have been described as an early manifestation of multiple endocrine neoplasia type 1 (MEN1 syndrome) (Stratakis et al. 2000) and therefore should alert the clinician to the possibility of this diagnosis in children.

In adults, Cushing disease has a female preponderance (Besser and Trainer 2002) whereas in our series of 50 patients with Cushing disease aged 6 to 30 years, there was a significant predominance of males in the pre-pubertal patients (Storr et al. 2004).

Cushing Disease: Diagnosis and Management

TABLE 17.1
Classification of paediatric Cushing syndrome

ACTH-independent

1. Exogenous glucocorticoid administration (tablets, nose drops, inhalers, nasal spray, skin cream)

2. Adrenocortical tumour (adenoma or carcinoma)

3. Primary adrenocortical hyperplasia

   a. Primary pigmented nodular adrenocortical disease

   b. Macronodular adrenal hyperplasia

   c. McCune–Albright syndrome

ACTH-dependent

1. Cushing disease (ACTH-secreting pituitary adenoma)

2. Ectopic ACTH syndrome

ACTH, adrenocorticotrophic hormone.

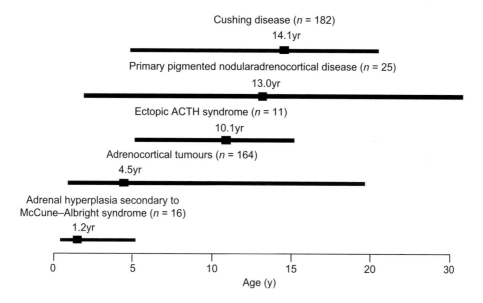

Figure 17.1. Different aetiologies of paediatric patients with Cushing syndrome from the literature (*n* = 398 cases) shown at ages of peak incidence (boxes).

The incidence in males and females during puberty was similar, with an increasing predominance of females in post-pubertal patients. A similar distribution was observed in the National Institutes of Health (NIH) series (Magiakou et al. 1994c). No clear explanation for this exists. It might simply reflect small sample sizes or an effect of increasing estrogen concentrations in females through puberty.

Clinical features in paediatric Cushing disease

Most paediatric endocrinologists have limited experience in the diagnosis and treatment of children with Cushing disease, and therefore evaluation should be undertaken in centres with a high throughput and adult endocrine liaison. Some aspects of paediatric Cushing disease do differ from those in adults (Storr et al. 2011) such as the sex ratio, the frequent absence of radiological evidence of a corticotroph adenoma on pituitary scanning and the higher incidence of lateralisation of ACTH secretion demonstrated by inferior petrosal sinus sampling. Children also have a more exuberant cortisol response to an intravenous bolus of corticotrophin-releasing factor (CRF) and a more rapid response to external beam pituitary radiotherapy. Clinically children can present differently from adults, most notably with reduced height velocity associated with rapid weight gain.

GENERAL CLINICAL FEATURES

The early recognition of the salient features of Cushing disease is crucial to allow prompt diagnosis and effective treatment. Key presenting features include reduced height velocity, weight gain and a change in facial appearance. Most children and adolescents have a typical Cushingoid appearance. A subtle or subclinical presentation or even cyclical features are uncommon. Changes evolve slowly over time, which leads to a delay in diagnosis. For example, the mean length of symptoms prior to diagnosis in our 43 paediatric patients with Cushing disease was 2.5 ± 1.7 years (range 0.3–6.6 years). Table 17.2 lists the clinical appearances, with striae present in 49% of patients (more frequently in the older patients; mean age 14.2 ± 2.6yrs). Additional features commonly noted in some children included emotional lability (60%), fatigue (60%) and hypertension (49%). Muscle weakness and easy bruising are rare symptoms. Figure 17.2 illustrates the clinical features.

TABLE 17.2
Clinical features at diagnosis of paediatric Cushing disease ($N = 43$)

Major symptoms	Patients (*n*)	Percentage of total
Facial changes	43	100
Weight gain	42	98
Weight loss	1	2
Pre-pubertal virilisation	17/22	77
Fatigue	26	60
Emotional lability/depression	26	60
Hirsutism	25	58
Headaches	21	49
Striae	21	49
Hypertension	21	49
Acne	19	44

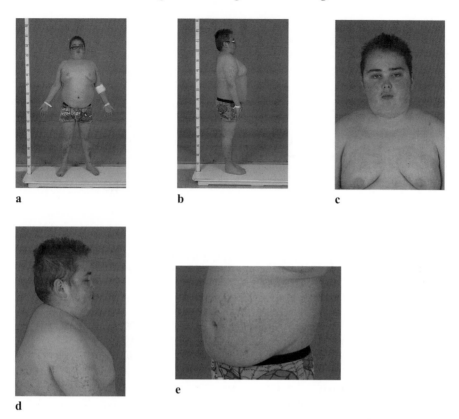

Figure 17.2. Clinical features of Cushing syndrome: (a) full body, (b) profile full body, (c) frontal view showing facial features, (d) profile of face and (e) abdominal striae.

CHARACTERISTICS OF GROWTH AND AUXOLOGICAL PARAMETERS

Short stature (height less than −2.0 SD) was present in 40% of the study patients and height velocity when available was subnormal. Growth failure has been attributed to growth hormone deficiency (GHD), resistance to insulin-like growth factor 1 (Magiakou et al. 1994b) and prolonged exposure to supraphysiological free-circulating glucocorticoids (Magiakou et al. 1994a, 1994c). One of the most striking features is that height SD score (SDS) is nearly always below the mean whereas body mass index (BMI) SDS is consistently above the mean (Fig 17.3; Magiakou and Chrousos 2002). One of the principal features of Cushing disease, obesity, is now extremely common in the general population so this alone is non-specific. However, there is an important difference in the growth pattern between obesity due to Cushing disease and simple obesity: Cushing disease is almost always associated with a reduction in height velocity and growth failure while simple obesity is usually accompanied by normal height velocity and often bone age advance. Greening et al. (2006) compared height and BMI SDS in 29 patients with Cushing disease and 44 age-matched patients with simple obesity. There was a significant difference in the ratio of these two

245

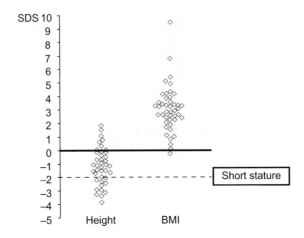

Figure 17.3. Height and body mass index (BMI) standard deviation score (SDS) values in 43 paediatric patients with Cushing disease. The dotted line indicates the SDS value below which patients are significantly shorter than average.

variables between the two groups: height increased in simple obesity and decreased in Cushing disease. Bone age at diagnosis of Cushing disease was delayed in 15 of 17 patients (mean delay, 2.0yrs; range, −0.5 to 4.1yrs) and correlated negatively with height SDS ($r = 0.70$; $p < 0.01$), duration of symptoms ($r = 0.48$; $p = 0.05$) and age at diagnosis ($r = 0.48$; $p = 0.05$) (Peters et al. 2007).

PUBERTAL DEVELOPMENT

True precocious puberty in Cushing disease is unusual with very few cases reported in the literature. However, virilisation with pseudo-precocious puberty is recognised as an important presenting feature (Magiakou et al. 1994c; Magiakou and Chrousos 2002). This was also demonstrated in our cohort. Abnormal virilisation, defined as unusual advance of Tanner pubic hair stage compared to testicular volume or breast development, was identified in 12 of 27 patients (Dupuis et al. 2007). In these patients, the values of serum androstenedione, DHEAS (as previously reported by Hauffa et al. 1984), and testosterone SDS were higher ($p = 0.03$, 0.008, 0.03, respectively) than in patients without abnormal virilisation, and sex hormone binding globulin SDS values were lower ($p = 0.006$). Gonadotrophin concentrations were subnormal in patients, suggesting a suppressive effect of chronic hypercortisolaemia and/or the effect of the elevated adrenal androgens.

Investigation of paediatric Cushing disease

The investigation of patients with suspected Cushing disease has been extensively reviewed (Newell-Price et al. 1998; Arnaldi et al. 2003) and guidelines for the diagnosis of paediatric patients with Cushing disease have also been published (Magiakou and Chrousos 2002). A recent consensus statement advised that only those obese children who have demonstrated slowing of their height velocity should be investigated, as a combined reduction in height

TABLE 17.3
Scheme for the investigation of patients with suspected Cushing syndrome

Confirmation or exclusion of Cushing syndrome

1. Urinary-free cortisol excretion (24h urine collection) daily for 3 days
2. Serum cortisol circadian rhythm study (09.00h, 18.00h, midnight [sleeping])
3. Low-dose dexamethasone suppression test
   a. Dose 0.5mg 6 hourly (09.00, 15.00, 21.00, 03.00h) for 48h
   b. Dose for patients weighing < 40kg: 30µg/kg/day
   c. Serum cortisol measured at 0h (day 0) and 48h at 08.00h

Definition of aetiology of Cushing syndrome

1. Plasma adrenocorticotrophic hormone (09.00h)
2. Corticotropin-releasing hormone test (1.0 = g/kg IV)
3. Analysis of change in serum cortisol during low-dose dexamethasone suppression test
4. Adrenal or pituitary MRI scan
5. Bilateral inferior petrosal sinus sampling for adrenocorticotrophic hormone (with corticotropin-releasing hormone)

velocity with increased weight was felt to have a high sensitivity and specificity for Cushing disease (Nieman et al. 2009).

The algorithm for testing in children should be based on that performed in adults (Newell-Price et al. 1998), and should consist initially of confirmation or exclusion of the diagnosis of Cushing syndrome followed by investigations to determine the aetiology. This scheme is listed in Table 17.3. The initial screening investigations shown have a high sensitivity (particularly urinary free cortisol); if the initial test results are normal, the patient is very unlikely to have Cushing syndrome. We have highlighted some aspects, which we found helpful during the management of 43 patients with Cushing disease over the past 30 years. Prior to embarking on biochemical evaluation, it is important to investigate the possible forms of glucocorticoid use detailed in Table 17.1, as exogenous Cushing syndrome is much more common than the endogenous form.

CONFIRMATION OR EXCLUSION OF CUSHING SYNDROME

Consistent with current recommendations (Nieman et al. 2009), our initial screening test includes three consecutive 24-hour urine collections for urinary-free cortisol. This provides an integrated assessment of cortisol secretion over a 24-hour period and measures only free, unbound hormone. If there is doubt about the interpretation of these values, we proceed to admit the child for measurement of serum cortisol at three time-points (09.00h, 18.00h and midnight [sleeping]) to assess circadian rhythm. Determination of midnight cortisol in the sleeping child gives the highest sensitivity for the diagnosis of Cushing syndrome (Batista et al. 2007). The value in normal childen is <50nmol/L (<1.8µg/dl), although some young children may reach their cortisol nadir earlier than midnight. Midnight serum cortisol was measurable in all the patients with Cushing syndrome whom we have managed. Late-night salivary cortisol has also been evaluated as a screening test in the paediatric obese population to differentiate children with Cushing syndrome. A high sensitivity and specificity have been reported (Martinelli et al. 1999); however, the influence of age has not been fully characterised. It can also be technically difficult to obtain a salivary sample in younger children; hence our protocol uses midnight serum cortisol.

Following assessment of midnight cortisol we perform a low-dose dexamethasone suppression test (LDDST), using the adult dose regimen of 0.5mg every 6h (at 09.00h, 15.00h, 21.00h and 03.00h) for 48h, unless the child weighs <40kg when we use the NIH-recommended dose of 30micrograms/kg/day (Magiakou et al. 1994c). In the LDDST, blood is taken for serum cortisol at 0h and at 48h at 08.00h. The serum cortisol should be undetectable (<50nmol/L, <1.8μg/dl) in normal children. These tests performed individually and particularly in combination have a high sensitivity for Cushing syndrome and an even higher specificity for the exclusion of this diagnosis. The 1mg overnight dexamethasone test has been used as a screening test in children but there are no available data on its interpretation or reliability (Nieman et al. 2009).

CONFIRMATION OF CUSHING DISEASE
Following confirmation of Cushing syndrome, the priority is to determine the cause of the hypercortisolism. Cushing disease is most easily confirmed by determination of basal plasma ACTH. In all of our patients with Cushing disease, ACTH was detectable, ranging from 13ng/L to 125ng/L (normal 10–50ng/L) (Fig 17.4). In ACTH-independent Cushing syndrome, plasma ACTH is always low and usually undetectable.

We routinely perform a CRF test using human sequence CRH (1 microgram/kg IV), and in 37 of 40 (93%) patients with Cushing disease serum cortisol increased by >20% (range of cortisol increase from baseline 2%–454%). Ectopic ACTH syndrome is so rare in children that the need for a CRF test is questionable; however, we find an increased cortisol response contributes to the diagnosis of Cushing disease.

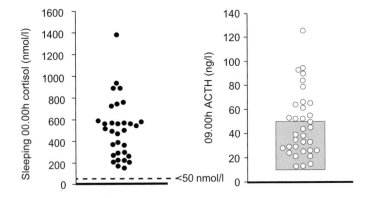

Figure 17.4. Midnight serum cortisol was >50nmol/l with detectable plasma adrenocorticotrophic hormone (ACTH), ranging from 13ng/L to 125ng/L, in all paediatric patients with Cushing disease. Shaded box indicates normal plasma ACTH range (10–50ng/L).

It may no longer be necessary to perform a high-dose dexamethasone suppression test (HDDST). This recent decision follows an analysis of serum cortisol suppression during LDDST and HDDST in our paediatric patients with Cushing disease (Dias et al. 2006). In 24 patients, mean baseline serum cortisol values of 590.7 ± 168.8nmol/L (21.4 ± 4.7μg/dl) decreased to 337.4 ± 104.0nmol/L (12.2 ± 3.8μg/dl) at 48h during LDDST (P <0.05; mean decrease, 45.1%) with 66% decreasing by >30%. Cortisol suppression during LDDST correlated with that during HDDST ($r = +0.45$, $p < 0.05$). Consequently, decrease of cortisol during the LDDST strongly supports the diagnosis of Cushing disease and negates the need for a HDDST. These results have also been demonstrated in adult patients with Cushing disease (Dias et al. 2006), as the change in cortisol during LDDST has been shown to distinguish between pituitary and ectopic ACTH secretion, again questioning the value of the HDDST.

IMAGING STUDIES

Most ACTH-secreting pituitary tumours occurring in the paediatric age range are microadenomas. The majority of these have a hypointense signal on MRI, which fails to enhance with gadolinium (Newell-Price et al. 1998). Approximately 50% of microadenomas are visible on pituitary MRI (Magiakou et al. 1994c) with only 33% concordance with surgical finding in terms of lateralisation (Storr et al. 2005). Therefore, although pituitary imaging using MRI is an important step towards the successful treatment of Cushing disease by trans-sphenoidal surgery (TSS), results should be interpreted together with bilateral inferior petrosal sinus sampling (BIPSS) for ACTH (see below). In some cases, the distinction between Cushing disease and ectopic ACTH syndrome may be in doubt. A CT scan of the chest using 0.5cm cuts will usually exclude a bronchial carcinoid tumour.

BILATERAL INFERIOR PETROSAL SINUS SAMPLING FOR ACTH

BIPSS was initially piloted in adults at the NIH (Oldfield et al. 1991) to enable distinction between Cushing disease and ectopic ACTH syndrome and also to provide a method of identifying a lateral versus central source of pituitary ACTH secretion (Newell-Price et al. 1998). It has now become routine in adult practice unless the MRI unequivocally shows a pituitary adenoma.

In children, ectopic ACTH secretion is extremely rare and so the primary aim of BIPSS is to contribute to the localisation of the microadenoma by demonstrating lateral or midline ACTH secretion. The first paediatric data were reported in the NIH series where a predictive value of lateralisation was 75%–80% (Magiakou et al. 1994c; Magiakou and Chrousos 2002). Similar values have been reported in smaller series with surgical concordance of 87% (Storr et al. 2005).

A more recent study from the NIH described their further experience of BIPSS in 94 paediatric patients and reported that localisation of ACTH secretion concurred with the site of the adenoma at surgery in 58% of cases, concluding that the technique was not an essential part of a paediatric investigation protocol (Batista et al. 2006). The percentage of predictive lateralisation, however, increased to 70% (51/73) after exclusion of 18 centrally located and 4 bilateral lesions. One of the difficulties is that false localisation can occur due to altered pituitary blood flow, so in theory an additional stimulus to other pituitary cells should be given to determine if the localisation is specific to ACTH or simply a reflection of altered blood flow.

Treatment of paediatric Cushing disease

Cushing disease in childhood requires urgent evaluation, diagnosis and prompt treatment to minimise the associated morbidity and maximise potential improvements in growth and body composition post-cure. It is clear that curative treatment in patients with moderate to severe Cushing syndrome reduces morbidity and mortality. Furthermore, as there is a finite time available for normal growth, it could be argued that rapid diagnosis and treatment are even more important in children and may reduce the risk of residual morbidity post-cure.

Treatment options have advanced significantly over the past 50 years. Initially bilateral adrenalectomy was practised widely and, although effective in lowering hypercortisolaemia, had considerable consequences. The pituitary adenoma remained in situ and there was an appreciable risk of post-adrenalectomy Nelson syndrome (Hopwood and Kenny 1977; McArthur et al. 1979). In addition, patients required lifelong glucocorticoid and mineralocorticoid replacement. Adrenalectomy has been considered where there was uncontrollable cortisol secretion, but with the use of agents such as etomidate, adrenalectomy as an option has almost disappeared from the repertoire (Greening et al. 2005; Chan et al. 2011). Medical therapy to lower cortisol using metyrapone or ketoconazole is a useful short-term option prior to surgery or radiotherapy but cannot be recommended as a long-term definitive therapy for Cushing disease.

TRANS-SPHENOIDAL SURGERY

Definitive cure of Cushing disease can be achieved by TSS or radiotherapy. Transsphenoidal pituitary surgery is a safe and effective procedure in children (Knappe and Ludecke 1996; Massoud et al. 1997; Joshi et al. 2005; Kanter et al. 2005) and is now considered first-line therapy as it involves selective removal of the adenoma, maximising the potential for normal pituitary tissue to remain in situ. Low rates of post-operative hypopituitarism have been reported in several large studies (Knappe and Ludecke 1996; Linglart and Visot 2002). However, selective microadenomectomy can be technically very difficult in children.

We recently analysed our experience over the past 25 years and considered the factors which contributed to successful surgical therapy (Storr et al. 2005). The variable surgical success rates reported depend on which definition of cure is adopted in that unit. Storr et al. (2005) use the definition used in adult endocrine practice (Trainer et al. 1993) as an undetectable post-operative serum cortisol <50nmol/L (<1.8μg/dl) and reported an overall cure rate using TSS of 68% for patients with microadenomas rising to 75% in those who had routine BIPSS pre-operatively (Magiakou et al. 1994b). Other paediatric case series report cure rates varying from 45% to 78% (Styne et al. 1984; Leinung et al. 1995; Devoe et al. 1997; Linglart and Visot 2002), but very few report rates of over 90% (Magiakou et al. 1994c).

PITUITARY RADIOTHERAPY

Pituitary radiotherapy has been considered a therapeutic option for paediatric patients with Cushing disease for many years. External beam radiotherapy is often used as second-line therapy, following unsuccessful TSS. The time to introducing radiotherapy varies with some groups proceeding to radiotherapy within 2–4 weeks of TSS, when it is clear from circulating cortisol levels that complete cure has not been achieved (Storr et al. 2003). The radiotherapy protocol we follow consists of delivering 45Gy in 25 fractions over 35 days (PN 1997), reflecting evidence demonstrating that children with Cushing disease respond more rapidly than adults (Thoren et al. 1986; Jennings et al. 1977). We have treated 14 patients during the past 26 years with a successful cure rate of 93%, which occurred at a mean interval of 0.8yrs (range 0.3–2.9) following completion of therapy.

POST-CURE GROWTH AND DEVELOPMENT AND PITUITARY FUNCTION

Growth failure and resultant short stature are almost always seen at diagnosis in paediatric patients with Cushing disease (Lebrethon et al. 2000; Magiakou and Chrousos 2002). Virilisation may lead to acceleration of bone age and a further compromise in height potential (Hayles et al. 1966). A key article from the NIH described the abnormalities of height and growth hormone secretion (Magiakou et al. 1994b) together with a poor outcome for post-treatment catch-up growth and adult height (Magiakou et al. 1994a). This finding has been confirmed in other studies and radiotherapy will also add to the problem (Lebrethon et al. 2000). The challenge is to reverse these problems and maximise growth potential so as to achieve acceptable adult height and body composition.

One approach is to test for GHD 3 months after TSS or completion of radiotherapy. If growth hormone therapy is required, conventional GHD doses can be used (0.025mg/kg/day). Gonadotropin-releasing hormone analogue therapy may be added to delay puberty and epiphyseal closure. Results demonstrate that this regimen usually enables adequate catch-up growth and adult height within the range of target height for the majority of patients (Davies et al. 2005). Combined treatment with growth hormone and aromatase inhibitors may also be a therapeutic alternative in male patients (Boronat et al. 2012). Normal body composition is more difficult to achieve. Many patients remain obese and BMI SDS remained elevated at a mean interval of 3.9 years after cure (Davies et al. 2005). A long-term follow-up study of childhood and adolescent patients with Cushing disease showed that total body fat and the ratio of visceral to subcutaneous fat was abnormally high in the majority of patients studied 7 years after cure (Leong et al. 2007). The implications of chronic excess visceral fat in terms of risk for adult metabolic syndrome deserve future study. Bone mineral density was closer to normal (Scommegna et al. 2005).

Although GHD is frequent initially, some recovery may occur in adult life (Chan et al. 2007). Gonadotrophin secretion is generally preserved with normal or early puberty, the latter a well-recognised complication of cranial radiotherapy. TSH and ACTH deficiency are minimal (Chan et al. 2007). It is important to note that the risk of hypopituitarism may continue to increase in the years after radiation.

Studies of adult patients with Cushing syndrome have reported brain atrophy, cognitive impairment and psychopathology, most commonly depression, associated with excess

251

endogenous circulating glucocorticoids (Dorn et al. 1997). A study from the NIH (Merke et al. 2005) also found significant cerebral atrophy in children with Cushing disease at diagnosis; however, there were no differences in IQ scores between patients and controls. Interestingly, NIH found an almost complete reversal of the cerebral atrophy but a significant decline in cognitive function 1 year after cure with TSS. This was also observed in one of our cases who presented with severe psychosis (Chan et al. 2011). This is in contrast to adult studies, which report reversible cognitive impairment and reversible loss of brain volume associated with eucortisolaemia (McEwen 2002; Merke et al. 2005). In a more recent article, the NIH group reported that children with Cushing disease have impaired health-related quality of life, which has not fully resolved 1 year post-treatment (Keil et al. 2009).

Conclusion

Paediatric patients with Cushing disease manifest a number of characteristic features distinct from adult patients with Cushing disease, most notably the significant impact on linear growth. Once Cushing disease is suspected, the patient requires investigation using a formal protocol and the choice and interpretation of tests are most productively discussed with an adult specialist with experience of Cushing disease. Referral should be considered to a centre combining paediatric and adult endocrinology, BIPSS, TSS and pituitary radiotherapy. In addition, choosing a neurosurgeon experienced in TSS in children is likely to significantly improve the chance of effective and curative therapy. The prognosis for cure is good in the majority of children and adolescents and full recovery of the hypothalamic-pituitary-adrenal axis is possible. However post-treatment management frequently presents challenges for the optimisation of growth, puberty and body composition.

REFERENCES

Arnaldi G, Angeli A, Atkinson AB et al. (2003) Diagnosis and complications of Cushing's syndrome: A consensus statement. *J Clin Endocrinol Metab* 88: 5593–5602.

Batista D, Gennari M, Riar J et al. (2006) An assessment of petrosal sinus sampling for localization of pituitary microadenomas in children with Cushing disease. *J Clin Endocrinol Metab* 91: 221–224.

Batista DL, Riar J, Keil M and Stratakis CA (2007) Diagnostic tests for children who are referred for the investigation of Cushing syndrome. *Pediatrics* 120: e575–e586.

Besser GM and Trainer PJ (2002) Cushing's syndrome; In Besser GM and Thorner MO (eds) *Comprehensive Clinical Endocrinology* 3rd edn. Edinburgh: Mosby.

Boronat M, Marrero D, Lopez-Plasencia Y, Novoa Y, Garciadelgado Y and Novoa FJ (2012) Combined treatment with GH and anastrozole in a pubertal boy with Cushing's disease and postsurgical GH deficiency. *Eur J Endocrinol* 166: 1101–1105.

Chan LF, Storr HL, Plowman PN et al. (2007) Long-term anterior pituitary function in patients with paediatric Cushing's disease treated with pituitary radiotherapy. *Eur J Endocrinol* 156: 477–482.

Chan LF, Vaidya M, Westphal B et al. (2011) Use of intravenous etomidate to control acute psychosis induced by the hypercortisolaemia in severe paediatric Cushing's disease. *Horm Res Paediatr* 75: 441–446.

Damiani D, Aguiar CH, Crivellaro CE, Galvao JA, Dichtchekenian V and Setian N (1998) Pituitary macroadenoma and Cushing's disease in pediatric patients: Patient report and review of the literature. *J Pediatr Endocrinol Metab* 11: 665–669.

Davies JH, Storr HL, Davies K et al. (2005) Final adult height and body mass index after cure of paediatric Cushing's disease. *Clin Endocrinol (Oxf)* 62: 466–472.

Devoe DJ, Miller WL, Conte FA et al. (1997) Long-term outcome in children and adolescents after transs-phenoidal surgery for Cushing's disease. *J Clin Endocrinol Metab* 82: 3196–3202.

Dias R, Storr HL, Perry LA, Isidori AM, Grossman AB and Savage MO (2006) The discriminatory value of the low-dose dexamethasone suppression test in the investigation of paediatric Cushing's syndrome. *Horm Res* 65: 159–162.

Dorn LD, Burgess ES, Friedman TC, Dubbert B, Gold PW and Chrousos GP (1997) The longitudinal course of psychopathology in Cushing's syndrome after correction of hypercortisolism. *J Clin Endocrinol Metab* 82: 912–919.

Dupuis CC, Storr HL, Perry LA et al. (2007) Abnormal puberty in paediatric Cushing's disease: Relationship with adrenal androgen, sex hormone binding globulin and gonadotrophin concentrations. *Clin Endocrinol (Oxf)* 66: 838–843.

Fahlbusch R, Honegger J and Buchfelder M (1995) Neurosurgical management of Cushing's disease in children. In: Savage MO, Bourguignon JP and Grossman AB (eds) *Frontiers of Paediatric Neuroendocrinolog.* Oxford: Blackwell Scientific, 68–72.

Greening JE, Brain CE, Perry LA et al. (2005) Efficient short-term control of hypercortisolaemia by low-dose etomidate in severe paediatric Cushing's disease. *Horm Res* 64: 140–143.

Greening JE, Storr HL, Mckenzie SA et al. (2006) Linear growth and body mass index in pediatric patients with Cushing's disease or simple obesity. *J Endocrinol Invest* 29: 885–887.

Hauffa BP, Kaplan SL and Grumbach MM (1984) Dissociation between plasma adrenal androgens and cortisol in Cushing's disease and ectopic ACTH-producing tumour: Relation to adrenarche. *Lancet* 1: 1373–1376.

Hayles AB, Hahn HB, Sprague RG, Bahn RC and Priestley JT (1966) Hormone-secreting tumors of the adrenal cortex in children. *Pediatrics* 37: 19–25.

Hopwood NJ and Kenny FM (1977) Incidence of Nelson's syndrome after adrenalectomy for Cushing's disease in children: Results of a nationwide survey. *Am J Dis Child* 131: 1353–1356.

Jennings AS, Liddle GW and Orth DN (1977) Results of treating childhood Cushing's disease with pituitary irradiation. *N Engl J Med* 297: 957–962.

Joshi SM, Hewitt RJ, Storr HL et al. (2005) Cushing's disease in children and adolescents: 20 years of experience in a single neurosurgical center. *Neurosurgery* 57: 281–285; discussion 281–285.

Kanter AS, Diallo AO, Jane JA et al. (2005) Single-center experience with pediatric Cushing's disease. *J Neurosurg* 103: 413–420.

Keil MF, Merke DP, Gandhi R, Wiggs EA, Obunse K and Stratakis CA (2009) Quality of life in children and adolescents 1-year after cure of Cushing syndrome: A prospective study. *Clin Endocrinol (Oxf)* 71: 326–333.

Khadilkar VV, Khadilkar AV and Navrange JR (2004) Cushing's disease in an 11-month-old child. *Indian Pediatr* 41: 274–276.

Knappe UJ and Ludecke DK (1996) Transnasal microsurgery in children and adolescents with Cushing's disease. *Neurosurgery* 39: 484–493.

Lebrethon MC, Grossman AB, Afshar F, Plowman PN, Besser GM and Savage MO (2000) Linear growth and final height after treatment for Cushing's disease in childhood. *J Clin Endocrinol Metab* 85: 3262–3265.

Leinung MC, Kane LA, Scheithauer BW, Carpenter PC, Laws ER and Zimmerman D (1995) Long term follow-up of transsphenoidal surgery for the treatment of Cushing's disease in childhood. *J Clin Endocrinol Metab* 80: 2475–2479.

Leong GM, Abad V, Charmandari E et al. (2007) Effects of child- and adolescent-onset endogenous Cushing syndrome on bone mass, body composition, and growth: A 7-year prospective study into young adulthood. *J Bone Miner Res* 22: 110–118.

Linglart A and Visot A (2002) Cushing's disease in children and adolescents. *Neurochirurgie* 48: 271–280.

Magiakou MA and Chrousos GP (2002) Cushing's syndrome in children and adolescents: Current diagnostic and therapeutic strategies. *J Endocrinol Invest* 25: 181–194.

Magiakou MA, Mastorakos G and Chrousos GP (1994a) Final stature in patients with endogenous Cushing's syndrome. *J Clin Endocrinol Metab* 79: 1082–1085.

Magiakou MA, Mastorakos G, Gomez MT, Rose SR and Chrousos GP (1994b) Suppressed spontaneous and stimulated growth hormonesecretion in patients with Cushing's disease before and after surgical cure. *J Clin Endocrinol Metab* 78: 131–137.

Magiakou MA, Mastorakos G, Oldfield EH et al. (1994c) Cushing's syndrome in children and adolescents. Presentation, diagnosis, and therapy. *N Engl J Med* 331: 629–636.

Martinelli CE, Sader SL, Oliveira EB, Daneluzzi JC and Moreira AC (1999) Salivary cortisol for screening of Cushing's syndrome in children. *Clin Endocrinol (Oxf)* 51: 67–71.

Massoud AF, Powell M, Williams RA, Hindmarsh PC and Brook CGD (1997) Transsphenoidal surgery for pituitary tumours. *Arch Dis Child* 76: 398–404.

Mcarthur RG, Hayles AB and Salassa RM (1979) Childhood Cushing disease: Results of bilateral adrenalectomy. *J Pediatr* 95: 214–219.

McEwen BS (2002) Cortisol, Cushing's syndrome, and a shrinking brain-new evidence for reversibility. *J Clin Endocrinol Metab* 87: 1947–1948.

Merke DP, Giedd JN, Keil MF et al. (2005) Children experience cognitive decline despite reversal of brain atrophy one year after resolution of Cushing syndrome. *J Clin Endocrinol Metab* 90: 2531–2536.

Newell-Price J, Bertagna X, Grossman AB and Nieman LK (2006) Cushing's syndrome. *Lancet* 367: 1605–1617.

Newell-Price J, Trainer P, Besser GM and Grossman AB (1998) The diagnosis and differential diagnosis of Cushing's syndrome and pseudo-Cushing's states. *Endocr Rev* 19: 647–672.

Nieman L, Biller B, Findling J et al. (2009) The diagnosis of Cushing's syndrome: An Endocrine Society clinical practice guideline. *Eur J Endocrinol.*

Oldfield EH, Doppman JL, Nieman LK et al. (1991) Petrosal sinus sampling with and without corticotropin-releasing hormone for the differential diagnosis of Cushing's syndrome. *N Engl J Med* 325: 897–905.

Peters CJ, Ahmed ML, Storr HL et al. (2007) Factors influencing skeletal maturation at diagnosis of paediatric Cushing's disease. *Horm Res* 68: 231–235.

Pn P (1997) Pituitary radiotherapy: Techniques and potential complications. In: Jenkins PJ, Wass JAH and Sheaves R (eds) *Clinical Endocrine Oncology*, Oxford: Blackwell Science Publications, 185–188.

Savage MO and Besser GM (1996) Cushing's disease in childhood. *Trends in Endocrinology and Metabolism* 7: 213–216.

Scommegna S, Greening JP, Storr HL et al. (2005) Bone mineral density at diagnosis and following successful treatment of pediatric Cushing's disease. *J Endocrinol Invest* 28: 231–235.

Storr HL, Afshar F, Matson M et al. (2005) Factors influencing cure by transsphenoidal selective adenomectomy in paediatric Cushing's disease. *Eur J Endocrinol* 152: 825–833.

Storr HL, Alexandraki KI, Martin L et al. (2011) Comparisons in the epidemiology, diagnostic features and cure rate by transsphenoidal surgery between paediatric and adult-onset Cushing's disease. *Eur J Endocrinol* 164: 667–674.

Storr HL, Isidori AM, Monson JP, Besser GM, Grossman AB and Savage MO. (2004) Prepubertal Cushing's disease is more common in males, but there is no increase in severity at diagnosis. *J Clin Endocrinol Metab* 89: 3818–3820.

Storr HL, Plowman PN, Carroll PV et al. (2003) Clinical and endocrine responses to pituitary radiotherapy in pediatric Cushing's disease: An effective second-line treatment. *J Clin Endocrinol Metab* 88: 34–37.

Stratakis CA, Schussheim DH, Freedman SM et al. (2000) Pituitary macroadenoma in a 5- year-old: An early expression of multiple endocrine neoplasia type 1. *J Clin Endocrinol Metab* 85: 4776–4780.

Styne DM, Grumbach MM, Kaplan SL, Wilson CB and Conte FA (1984) Treatment of Cushing's disease in childhood and adolescence by transsphenoidal microadenomectomy. *N Engl J Med* 310: 889–893.

Thoren M, Rahn T, Hallengren B et al. (1986) Treatment of Cushing's disease in childhood and adolescence by stereotactic pituitary irradiation. *Acta Paediatr Scand* 75: 388–395.

Trainer PJ, Lawrie HS, Verhelst J et al. (1993) Transsphenoidal resection in Cushing's disease: Undetectable serum cortisol as the definition of successful treatment. *Clin Endocrinol (Oxf)* 38: 73–78.

Weber A, Trainer PJ, Grossman AB et al. (1995) Investigation, management and therapeutic outcome in 12 cases of childhood and adolescent Cushing's syndrome. *Clin Endocrinol (Oxf)* 43: 19–28.

18
THE HYPOTHALAMIC-PITUITARY-GONADAL AXIS

Pierre-Marc G Bouloux

Introduction

Mammalian reproduction is under the tightly controlled regulation of a three-tiered body axis comprising gonadotrophin-releasing hormone (GnRH) neurons, located in the hypothalamus, the gonadotropin-secreting cells of the adenohypophysis and their respective target organs, the ovaries or testes, making up the hypothalamo-pituitary-gonadal (HPG) axis. In the male, the axis is under classic negative feedback control from testicular steroids and inhibin, whereas in the female, both negative and positive feedback loops operate.

ANATOMY AND REGULATION OF GONADOTROPHIN-RELEASING HORMONE NEURONAL ACTIVITY

GnRH neurons, the most upstream regulatory component of this axis, form the final common output pathway from the hypothalamus in the neuroendocrine control of reproduction, comprising approximately 1 000–2 000 neurons dispersed in the anterior hypothalamus; in rodents their axons project to the external zone of the median eminence from where the decapeptide GnRH is neurosecreted in a coordinated pulsatile pattern into the median eminence capillaries, reaching the adenohypophysis via the long portal veins. These 'quanta' of neurosecreted GnRH bind to cell membrane GnRHR1 receptors on gonadotrophs in a periodic manner, entraining pulsatile release of luteinizing hormone and follicle-stimulating hormone (FSH).

In the human, the post-infundibular eminence of the hypothalamus contains both superficial and deep capillary plexuses, both draining into the hypophyseal portal system and, partly, also to the general circulation (Duvernoy et al. 1971). These capillary networks are surrounded by GnRH-immunoreactive axons (Anthony et al. 1984), suggesting releasing sites for the hypophysiotropic GnRH axon terminals. Some GnRH projections enter the infundibular stalk and also travel down to the neurohypophysis (King and Anthony 1984), implying that GnRH may also reach gonadotrophs via short portal veins.

Phasic occupancy of gonadotroph GnRHR1 receptors by pulsatile GnRH secretion thus leads to the synthesis and secretion of the glycoprotein gonadotrophins, luteinizing hormone and FSH, which, when released into the systemic circulation, stimulate steroidogenesis and gametogenesis in the gonads. The axis is regulated by classic predominantly negative feedback inhibitory effects of steroidal and non-steroidal gonadal products, acting at pituitary and suprapituitary levels (Fig 18.1).

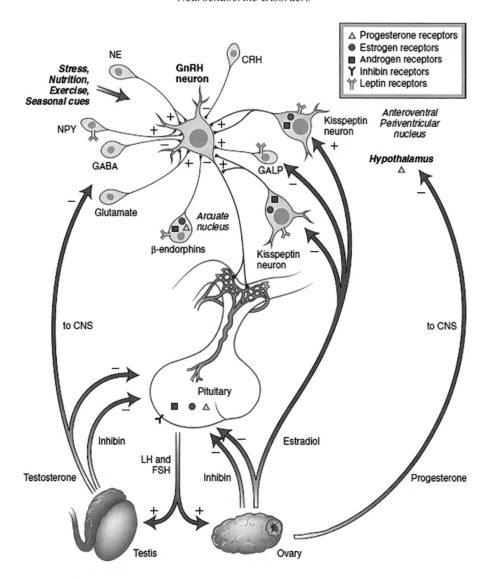

Figure 18.1. The hypothalamo-pituitary-gonadal axis and feedback regulation of gonadotrophin secretion. (Adapted from Low MJ. Neuroendocrinology. In: Melmed S, Polonsky KS, Reed Larsen P and Kronenberg (eds) *Williams Textbook of Endocrinology 13th Edition*. Canada: Elsevier, 110–175, 2016. With permission.)

THE GNRH PULSE GENERATOR

The afferent pathways to GnRH neurons convey physiological signals to the reproductive axis, including metabolic, nutritional (leptin, Ghrelin), stress, sex steroid, lactational and circadian rhythm signals. Post-puberty, the pulse frequency of GnRH and therefore luteinizing hormone and FSH release is about 60–90 minutes in men and, depending on the phase of the menstrual cycle, 60–240 minutes in women. The mechanism of pulsatile GnRH release is not fully established, but requires the coordinated activity of GnRH neurons which are dispersed in the anterior hypothalamus. GnRH-secreting cell lines (GT1-7) demonstrate intrinsic pulsatility, which may involve voltage-gated calcium channels and interconnectivity via gap junctions (Martínez de la Escalera et al. 1992). Classic axo-somatic and axo-dendritic synapses interconnecting GnRH neurons are found in rats and humans, and synchronisation of the GnRH network is likely to be mediated at the axo-dendritic level, dendrites representing the primary sites of action potential generation in the mouse GnRH neuron (Roberts et al. 2008).

ORIGINS OF THE PULSE GENERATOR: EFFECTS OF KISSPEPTIN-GPR54 REGULATION ON GnRH PULSE GENERATION

Explants of mediobasal hypothalamus from fetal and adult human brains release GnRH in a pulsatile manner. In many species, hypothalamic arcuate and infundibular neurons (ARC/Inf) which co-synthesise kisspeptin, neurokinin B (NKB) and dynorphins ('KNDy neurons') appear to represent an important component of the pulse generator (Fig 18.2). These kisspeptin-expressing neurons represent an important constituent of this hypothalamic pulse generator (*vide infra*). Kisspeptins exist in different lengths—Kp-54 (metastin), Kp-14, Kp-13 and Kp-10—all generated by cleavage of a common 145 amino acid precursor. They all share a 10 amino acid carboxyterminal sequence, sufficient to fully activate their specific receptor (GPR54), and contain the distinctive Arg–Phe–NH_2 motif, characteristic of the large RF-amide peptide superfamily (Kotani et al. 2001).

Recent animal models (Smith et al. 2009; Cheng et al. 2010; Lehman et al. 2010) have strongly supported kisspeptin as the major output signal toward GnRH neuron secretion, and have complemented observations made by two independent clinical studies reported in 2003 and documenting the connection between the kisspeptin system and reproductive function (de Roux et al. 2003; Seminara et al. 2003). Patients bearing loss-of-function mutations in the kisspeptin receptor *GPR54* present with isolated hypogonadotropic hypogonadism, with absence of puberty and infertility, a phenotype reproduced in mice lacking functional *GPR54* or *KISS1* genes (Colledge 2009).

Kisspeptin stimulates GnRH release from median eminence fragments of wild type, but not *KISS1R* mutant mice (d'Anglemont et al. 2008), an effect independent of action potential generation. Moreover, in vivo release of kisspeptin into the monkey median eminence is pulsatile, with kisspeptin peaks coinciding with luteinizing hormone secretory pulses (Keen et al. 2008); in the human, peripheral injection of kisspeptin, which does not cross the blood–brain barrier, results in a rapid increase of luteinizing hormone release (Dhillo et al. 2007), consistent with kisspeptin action on GnRH projections in circumventricular organs or the median eminence (both outside the blood–brain barrier).

Kisspeptins are now regarded as the most potent naturally occurring stimulators of GnRH and, therefore, gonadotropin secretion (Roa et al. 2008; Oakley et al. 2009).

The hypothalamus is the likely primary site for activation of the HPG axis by Kisspeptins, with direct kisspeptin activation of GnRH neurons. Thus, GnRH neurons express GPR54 and kisspeptins induce *Fos* expression (a sign of early activation) in GnRH neurons

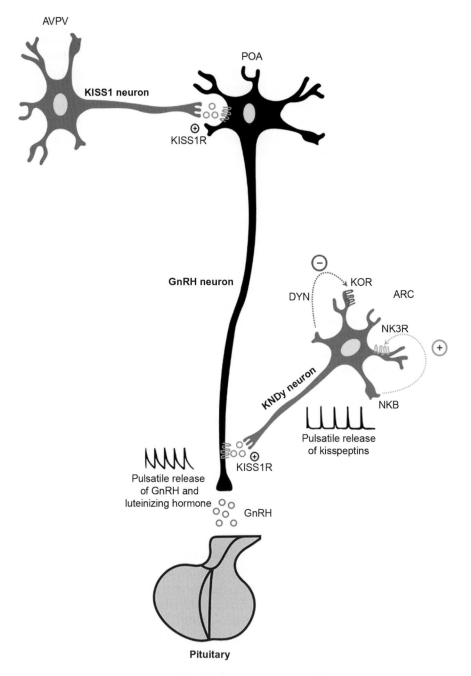

Figure 18.2. Kisspeptin neurons in the infundibular (humans)/arcuate (rodents) nucleus co-express neurokinin B and dynorphin (KNDy neurons), which via neurokinin B receptor and kappa opioid peptide receptor autosynaptically regulate pulsatile kisspeptin (and therefore GnRH) secretion, with neurokinin B being stimulatory and dynorphin inhibitory. GnRH, gonadotrophin-releasing hormone.

(Irwig et al. 2004). Kisspeptins exert potent depolarising effects on GnRH neurons, as measured by voltage recordings in hypothalamic slice preparations (Pielecka-Fortuna et al. 2008) and kisspeptins stimulate GnRH release from hypothalamic explants ex vivo and into the cerebrospinal fluid in vivo (Messager et al. 2005). By contrast, GnRH antagonists abrogate the release of gonadotropins evoked by kisspeptins (Navarro et al. 2005), and blockade of kisspeptin signalling by a specific antagonist decreases GnRH neuronal firing and the pulsatile release of GnRH (Roseweir et al. 2009). Additional indirect stimulation of GnRH via excitatory afferents to GnRH neurons cannot be discounted however, nor can the possibility of additional direct actions at the pituitary level to stimulate secretion of gonadotropes.

ROLE OF KISSPEPTIN IN SEX-STEROID FEEDBACK IN FEMALES

Independently of the species, kisspeptin neurons of the ARC/Inf are also implicated in the negative feedback effects of gonadal steroids on GnRH neurons; in the rat, its neurotoxic ablation prevents the rise in serum luteinizing hormone and attenuates the rise in serum FSH following ovariectomy (Mittelman-Smith et al. 2012a). In sheep and possibly in primates, kisspeptin neurons of the ARC may also play a role in positive oestrogen feedback to GnRH neurons. Both ovariectomy and a surge-inducing E2 (oestradiol) treatment induce Fos expression in kisspeptin neurons of the sheep ARC (Hoffman et al. 2011).

Oestrogens that originate from the ovary or that are locally produced after aromatisation of testosterone play essential parts in positive and negative feedback loops, mainly via signalling by oestrogen receptor α (Wintermantel et al. 2006). GnRH neurons seem, however, to lack functional estrogen receptor α, implicating interneuronal pathways in the transmission of sex-steroid feedback actions to GnRH neurons. KISS1 neuronal populations appear to participate in these phenomena through nucleus-specific specialisation: arcuate nucleus KISS1 neurons participate in negative feedback events, whereas those in the antero-ventral periventricular (AVPV) nucleus, at least in rodents, seem to have a dominant role in conveying positive feedback effects of oestradiol and, therefore, essential for the generation of the preovulatory surge of gonadotropins (Oakley et al. 2009).

In rodents, evidence links arcuate nucleus KISS1 neurons in negative feedback also. Thus, elimination of sex steroids by gonadectomy increases *KISS1* mRNA levels in the arcuate nucleus while sex-steroid replacement abrogates the rise of *KISS1* expression in this nucleus after gonadectomy. Absence of oestrogen receptor α or the androgen receptor prevents the rise of *KISS1* mRNA levels at this site after gonadectomy (Smith et al. 2005a, 2005b). KISS1 neurons in the arcuate nucleus express oestrogen receptor α and androgen receptor, and a mouse model of estrogen-receptor-α ablation in KISS1-expressing cells has shown the importance of signalling via this receptor in arcuate nucleus KISS1 neurons in mediation of the negative feedback on GnRH and gonadotropin secretion. The functional relevance of this pathway is further reinforced by the observation that *GPR54* knockout mice fail to display the usual rise in circulating gonadotropin concentrations after gonadectomy (Dungan et al. 2007). Similarly, increases in luteinizing hormone secretion after gonadectomy are attenuated in rodents pretreated with a selective kisspeptin antagonist (Roseweir et al. 2009).

OTHER PEPTIDERGIC AND MONOAMINERGIC NEURONS AND INTERACTIONS WITH GnRH NEURONS

In humans, monoaminergic and peptidergic nerves also input onto GnRH neurons, particularly at the infundibular and preoptic areas (Fig 18.1). About 50% of GnRH-IR neurons receive histaminergic appositions (Fekete et al. 1999) with kisspeptin immunoreactive (KPIR) appositions observed on over half of GnRH neurons in the infundibulum (Molnar et al. 2012). Axo-axonal appositions occur in the human postinfundibular eminence, wherein KPIR axons establish axo-axonal contacts on GnRH-IR fibres within the human postinfundibular eminence (Hrabovszky et al. 2010). The most abundant afferent inputs are given off by γ-aminobutyric acid (GABA)ergic and glutamatergic (VGLUT1 and VGLUT2) neurons. Amino-acidergic contacts (glutaminergic > GABAergic) are also encountered frequently on GnRH neuron dendrites (Hrabovszky et al. 2012).

NEUROPEPTIDE Y

The 36 amino acid peptide NPY acts at the hypophyseal level, to potentiate luteinizing hormone secretion in response to GnRH by modulating GnRH binding to anterior pituitary GnRH receptors (Parker et al. 1991), but at the level of the median eminence, it stimulates GnRH secretion from GnRH axon terminals (Crowley and Kalra 1987) via the Y5 receptor isoform (Campbell et al. 2001). NPY plays an important role in the metabolic regulation of fertility (Evans and Anderson 2012). Although a chronic increase in NPY tone inhibits luteinizing hormone and FSH (Raposinho et al. 2001) and delays sexual maturation (Pierroz et al. 1995), suppressing oestrous cyclicity (Catzeflis et al. 1993), the direction of acute NPY effects depends upon the sex steroid milieu. Thus in castrated animals, intracerebroventricular (ICV) NPY decreases gonadotropin secretion (Kerkerian et al. 1985), whereas in intact rodents or gonadectomised and steroid-primed rodents, it increases gonadotropin levels (Kaynard et al. 1990).

SUBSTANCE P AND THE TACHYKININS

Substance P, which exhibits the highest affinity to the G-protein-coupled NK1 receptor, can influence reproduction at the hypothalamic, pituitary and gonadal levels of the reproductive axis (Lasaga and Debeljuk 2011). In primates, substance P immunoreactive neurons densely innervate the neurovascular zone of the infundibulum (Hokfelt et al. 1978), and substance P inhibits GnRH-stimulated luteinizing hormone secretion from cultured human pituitary cells (Wormald et al. 1989).

Substance P neurons appear to form a network within the infundibulum similar to the networking among the NKB (neurokinin B) neurons (Burke et al. 2006), and NKB-signalling through these NKB/NKB contacts employs NK3 autoreceptors; this communication could also be implicated in the mechanism of pulsatile GnRH/luteinizing hormone secretion (Rance and Young 1991).

NEUROKININ B

The majority of human kisspeptin neurons in the infundibulum contain NKB immunoreactivity (NKB-IR) and similarly to kisspeptin, NKB appears to play a crucial role in the regulation of puberty and reproduction in the human. Thus inactivating mutations of the genes encoding for NKB (*TAC3*) or the NKB receptor NK3 (*TACR3*) cause hypogonado-tropic hypogonadism in humans (Guran et al. 2009; Topaloglu et al. 2009). Kisspeptin neurons of the ARC in various mammalian species also contain the NK3 autoreceptor, and NKB-signalling via the NK3 autoreceptor can significantly modulate the frequency of the GnRH neurosecretory pulses. For example, central administration of NKB increases the frequencies of multiunit activity volleys and luteinizing hormone secretory pulses in ovari-ectomised goats, likely via acting on this NK3 autoreceptor.

Similarly to kisspeptin neurons, NKB neurons in the human hypothalamus form afferent contacts with the somatic, dendritic and axonal compartments of GnRH neurons. Interest-ingly, the incidence of NKB immunoreactive contacts onto GnRH neurons is significantly higher than that of kisspeptin immunoreactive (KP-IR) inputs, and depending on the human model, only 10%–30% of the kisspeptin-IR and NKB-IR inputs to GnRH neurons are found to be double-labelled for the other peptide (Hrabovszky et al. 2009).

GALANIN

Galanin, a 29 amino acid peptide, is synthesised both locally in the anterior pituitary and in the hypothalamus in the ARC and the paraventricular nucleus, reaching gonadotroph cells via the hypophyseal portal circulation; it is secreted into the portal blood in a pulsatile manner and enhances GnRH receptor binding on gonadotroph cells (Lopez et al. 1991; Sahu et al. 1994). Galaninergic neurons also regulate reproduction at the level of the hypo-thalamus in rodents, partly via providing direct innervation to GnRH neurons.

Dual-label immunohistochemical studies have localised the majority of galaninergic neurons posteriorly to the lamina terminalis in humans; high numbers are present in the infundibulum around the portal capillary vessels.

CORTICOTROPIN-RELEASING HORMONE

Central corticotropin-releasing hormone (CRH) signalling has long been known to play an important role in the stress-induced suppression of the GnRH pulse generator in rodents. Juxtaposition of CRH immunoreactive fibres to GnRH neurons has been observed in the human hypothalamus in the infundibular region (Dudas and Merchenthaler 2002). ICV administration of CRH decreases luteinizing hormone pulse frequency in rats whereas stress-induced suppression of luteinizing hormone pulses by insulin-induced hypoglycae-mia is blocked by ICV administration of a CRH antagonist (Cates et al. 2004).

ENDORPHINS

Endogenous opioid peptides are important central inhibitors of the reproductive axis. Microinjection of β-endorphin into the mediobasal hypothalamus and the medial preoptic area significantly suppresses luteinizing hormone secretion in rats whereas administration of β-endorphin antiserum into these areas elevated luteinizing hormone (Schulz et al. 1981).

Light microscopic contacts have also been observed between β-endorphin-IR axons and GnRH-IR neurons in humans; the contacts were most abundant in the infundibular region (Dudas and Merchenthaler 2004). Administration of the opioid antagonist naloxone in humans stimulates luteinizing hormone release (Tenhola et al. 2012) whereas opiates and opioid administration suppress gonadotrophin secretion (Pfeiffer and Herz 1984)

ENKEPHALINS AND DYNORPHIN

In humans, dual-label immunohistochemical studies have established that Leu-enkephalin-IR cell bodies are concentrated in the periventricular area of the tuberal region, in the infundibulum in the close proximity to the portal vessels and in the medial preoptic area periventricularly (Dudas and Merchenthaler 2003). The infundibulum of the human hypothalamus also contains prodynorphin mRNA expressing neurons and GnRH neurons in the human hypothalamus have close contacts with dynorphin fibres.

RF-AMIDE-RELATED PEPTIDES/GONADOTROPIN-INHIBITING HORMONE

Gonadotropin-inhibiting hormone (GnIH) plays a crucial role in the inhibitory regulation of the reproductive axis of several subhuman species (Kriegsfeld et al. 2006). In a study using affinity column purified rabbit anti-white-crowned sparrow GnIH antibodies for the immunohistochemical detection of GnIH-IR structures, IR cell bodies in the rhesus macaque monkey were found to be located in the dorsomedial nucleus, sending axonal projections to GnRH neurons in the preoptic area as well as to the median eminence (Ubuka et al. 2009). There are currently no data pertaining to the role of these peptides in human physiology.

LEPTIN AND THE GONADOTROPIN-GONADAL AXIS

Leptin, the 167 amino acid protein product of the *ob* gene, belongs to the cytokine family and is expressed primarily in adipose tissue, as well as stomach, placenta and the mammary gland. It is secreted from adipose tissue in a pulsatile fashion with a significant circadian rhythm (Licinio et al. 1997, 1998) and influences gonadotropin secretion from the hypothalamus and pituitary as well as gonadal steroid output from the gonads. Leptin conveys a signal of the amount of peripheral energy stores to the brain, and may represent the key link between energy reserves and neural networks controlling reproduction (Cunningham et al. 1999). States of leptin deficiency and excess demonstrate the key role of leptin in the regulation of the reproductive system. The latter is highly sensitive to states of energy deficit, providing an efficient mechanism in preventing the energy demands of pregnancy and lactation under unfavourable conditions (Mantzoros 1999). Paradoxically, the excessive energy storage of obesity also interferes with proper regulation of the reproductive system (Yura et al. 2000).

The pulsatile release of leptin showed a significant pattern synchrony with serum luteinizing hormone and oestradiol levels, especially at night when leptin levels peak, suggesting that leptin may regulate the physiological levels and rhythmicity of reproductive hormones. Studies in patients with Kallmann syndrome following 7 days of GnRH administration show that while converting the baseline apulsatile release pattern of luteinizing hormone into a pulsatile pattern, GnRH fails to modify serum leptin concentrations and their pulsatile patterns, demonstrating the independence of episodic leptin release from luteinizing hormone secretion (Sir-Petermann et al. 1999). Taken together, this suggests that either leptin regulates luteinizing hormone release or that another factor regulates both leptin and luteinizing hormone secretion in a synchronous manner.

LEPTIN AND THE HYPOTHALAMUS

A number of studies have provided evidence that leptin may influence gonadotropin release at the level of the hypothalamus. Leptin administered peripherally to adult ovariectomised oestrogen-treated rats during a 48-hour fast prevents the suppression of luteinizing hormone pulse frequency that occurs during fasting, providing evidence that leptin may regulate GnRH since changes of luteinizing hormone pulse frequency reflect timing of GnRH release (Sir-Petermann et al. 1999). The fact that leptin had the same effect in the presence or absence of estrogen suggested that there was no modulation of negative feedback. Leptin given through ICV to 3-day starved rats restores luteinizing hormone surges, and leptin 116–130 (an active fragment of the native molecule) administered ICV to fasted adult male rats has been shown to increase luteinizing hormone pulse frequency, amplitude, mean concentrations and net secretion (Gonzalez et al. 1999) whereas sc leptin administered to fasted adult male sheep prevents the marked decline in luteinizing hormone pulse frequency (Nagatani et al. 2000). The stimulatory effect of leptin on luteinizing hormone secretion can be blocked by GnRH antiserum, further supporting a hypothalamic site of action of leptin (Dearth et al. 2000).

MONOAMINES INVOLVED IN GnRH SECRETION: CATECHOLAMINES AND HISTAMINE

Catecholamines of hypothalamic and extrahypothalamic origins partly modulate gonadal functions via direct interactions with hypothalamic GnRH neurons. Tyrosine hydroxylase immunoreactive (TH-IR) dopaminergic perikarya have been located in the periventricular, paraventricular and supraoptic hypothalamic nuclei and also in the median eminence (Dudas and Merchenthaler 2001). The TH-IR fibres are numerous in septal, infundibular, periventricular and lateral hypothalamic regions, and GnRH neurons in the infundibular and medial preoptic areas receive TH-immunopositive axon contacts. About half of GnRH neurons receive histamine-immunoreactive axonal appositions and there is evidence in rodents that positive feedback effect of oestradiol on the preovulatory luteinizing hormone surge may involve oestrogen-receptive histamine-containing neurons within the tuberomamillary regions which communicate with GnRH neurons via H1 receptors (Panula et al. 1989).

GHRELIN AND GnRH SECRETION

Ghrelin, a 28 amino acid peptide, represents the endogenous ligand for the growth hormone secretagogue receptor (Kojima et al. 1999) and is produced primarily in gastric mucosa and a variety of other tissues. Ghrelin circulates in the blood and stimulates the secretion of growth hormone, prolactin and adrenocorticotrophic hormone from the pituitary (Takaya et al. 2000) as well as stimulating appetite and promoting food intake via an action at the hypothalamus (Nonogaki 2008). Animal studies demonstrate that either centrally or peripherally administered ghrelin reduces luteinizing hormone pulse frequency in ovariectomised rats and rhesus monkeys (Furuta et al. 2001) and decreases basal luteinizing hormone levels in intact rats and sheep (Iqbal et al. 2006). Intravenous administration of four consecutive ghrelin boluses (Kluge et al. 2007) effects a delay and suppresses the amplitude of luteinizing hormone pulses; a ghrelin infusion also suppresses luteinizing hormone pulsatility in response to the opiate antagonist naloxone without affecting the response of luteinizing hormone to GnRH (Lanfranco et al. 2008).

AMINO ACID NEUROTRANSMITTERS AND GnRH RELEASE

The most abundant inhibitory and excitatory neurotransmitters in the hypothalamus are GABA and glutamate, respectively (Leranth et al. 1985; Decavel and Van den Pol 1990), and there is good evidence that that GABA and glutamate modulate GnRH neuron excitability (DeFazio et al. 2002; Herbison and Moenter 2011). Dual-labelling investigations have shown that GnRH neurons express receptor subunits required for α-amino-3-hydroxy-5-methyl-4-isoxazolepropionic acid (AMPA), N-Methyl-D-aspartate (NMDA) and kainate signalling, and electrophysiological and calcium imaging studies have confirmed that while the majority of adult GnRH neurons express AMPA/kainate receptors, only small subpopulations have functional NMDA or metabotropic glutamate receptors. Direct glutamate signalling at GnRH neurons occurs during the activation of puberty, and peripubertal changes in AMPA receptor expression may be dominant in the mouse. Glutamatergic inputs to the GnRH neurons include those originating from the anteroventral periventricular nucleus (Iremonger et al. 2010).

GnRH AND ITS ACTIONS

The decapeptide GnRH, encoded from a single gene on the short arm of chromosome 8, is derived from the post-translational processing of the large 92 amino acid precursor pre-pro-GnRH which has a tripartite structure (23 amino acid signal peptide followed by a Gly-Lys-Arg sequence, essential for proteolytic processing and carboxy terminal amidation of GnRH molecules) with the last 56 amino acid residues designated as GnRH-associated peptide. GnRH has a very short half-life in the blood (approximately 2 to 5 minutes), and is neurosecreted in episodic bursts at the median eminence into hypophyseal-portal blood, thereby exposing the pituitary gonadotrophs to phasic high concentrations of GnRH. Pulsatile GnRH release is essential for its stimulatory effects on luteinizing hormone and FSH release; by contrast, constant exposure to GnRH results in paradoxical inhibitory effects on luteinizing hormone and FSH release (Belchetz et al. 1978) after an initial period of stimulation. The response of the pituitary to GnRH is influenced by the gonadal steroid milieu. For example, testosterone and oestradiol deficiency in patients with primary hypogonadal disorders results in an exaggerated gonadotrophin response to exogenous GnRH administration.

MECHANISM OF GnRH ACTION

The GnRH receptor belongs to a family of G-coupled receptors linked by the typical seven-transmembrane domain structure (Fan et al. 1995). At 328 amino acids, it is the smallest known G-protein-coupled receptor, with a short extracellular and an absent intracellular domains. Signal transduction occurs via the unusually long third intracellular loop. Following GnRH-receptor complex formation, an interaction with the Gq protein occurs, leading to phosphoinositide hydrolysis generating diacylglycerol and inositol triphosphate, calcium mobilisation from intracellular stores and influx of extracellular calcium into the cell. Diacylglycerol and calcium activate protein kinase C, inducing protein phosphorylation and further activation of calcium channels. (Shacham et al. 2001) Increased intracellular calcium evokes prompt gonadotrophin release by exocytosis and, with time, more sustained gonado-trophin synthesis and secretion. GnRH modulates the number and activity of its own recep-tors (*vide supra*), the effect depending on the secretory pattern of GnRH and the dose of the neurohormone. Receptor expression is higher when exposure to pulsatile GnRH occurs, this 'self priming' effect leading to an increase in GnRH binding sites before the next pulse.

GONADOTROPHINS

Luteinizing hormone and FSH are heterodimeric glycopeptides consisting of two peptide chains (alpha and beta) synthesised and released from the same gonadotroph cell, whose function is to control development, maturation and function of the gonads. Structurally, they share a common alpha peptide subunit with thyroid-stimulating hormone (TSH) and human chorionic gonadotropin (hCG) and differ from each other by the presence of a specific beta chain, the latter providing specificity of biological action. These two hormones have a different terminal glycosylation; luteinizing hormone is rich in N-acetylglucosamine sulphate and, following an interaction with specific liver receptors that recognise sulphate terminals, is quickly cleared from the circulation. By contrast, FSH is sialylated and pro-tected from immediate capture and metabolism in the liver, hence its longer half-life. The half-life of luteinizing hormone is about 60–90 minutes and FSH is 180–200 minutes (Ludwig et al. 2003).

Luteinizing hormone and FSH are stored in different granules, ready for release by exocytosis. A proportion of molecules are not stored in granules however, and do not enter the regulated pathway of secretion; rather, they are constitutively secreted. FSH in particular follows this route. Low GnRH pulse frequency causes preferential release of FSH, faster pulse frequency favouring luteinizing hormone release (Kaiser 1998). Luteinizing hormone and FSH are measurable in the human pituitary by the tenth week of gestation, and by the twelfth week in peripheral blood. In fetal life and infancy, FSH is predominant over lutein-izing hormone, the FSH/luteinizing hormone ratio being higher in females. Testosterone is produced by the developing testes by the tenth week, its early production dependent on maternal hCG, rather than luteinizing hormone.

GONADOTROPHIN RECEPTORS

The pattern of circulating gonadotrophins reflects the pattern of GnRH release from the hypo-thalamus. In the testis, luteinizing hormone and FSH bind to their specific receptors on Leydig cells and Sertoli cells, respectively, stimulating testosterone secretion (luteinizing hormone) while FSH is important in the initiation and maintenance of spermatogenesis. In the ovary, FSH (acting on granulosa cells to induce aromatase activity) and luteinizing hormone (acting on theca cells to produce androgens) act sequentially and in concert to produce ovarian follicu-lar maturation, ovulation and secretion of oestradiol and progesterone.

Both luteinizing hormone receptors and FSH receptors (LHR/FSHR) contain an N-terminal extracellular domain that binds the respective ligands with high affinity and specificity, and seven transmembrane domains responsible for signal transduction. The extracellular domains of LHR and FSHR contain a number of irregular leucine-rich repeats thought to contain successive β-strands and α-helices that organise into a cusp-shaped structure. The β-strands form a parallel β-sheet along the concave surface of this structure, a common feature of all three glycoprotein hormone receptors (LHR, FSHR and TSH). Based on sequence similarity, the structure of the hormone-binding domain appears to be conserved across the glycoprotein hormone receptors. There is evidence for dimerisation of FSH-FSHR ectodomain complex in solution by chemical cross-linking, analytical centrifugation and light scattering (Kreuchwig et al. 2013).

LHR is thought to remain in an inactive state via an extensive intra-helical hydrogen bonding network. Upon binding of the ligand on the extracellular domain, the receptor is activated by disrupting some of these hydrogen bonding interactions.

Mutations of both luteinizing hormone and FSH receptors have been identified and are classified as both inactivating (loss of function) and activating (gain of function) mutations. Activating mutations of the first and third transmembrane helices of the luteinizing hormone receptor in the male result in precocious puberty (Muller et al. 1998) whereas inactivating mutations involving the seventh and first transmembrane helices are associated with testicular resistance (Simoni et al. 1998).

HYPOTHALAMO-PITUITARY-GONADAL AXIS IN THE MALE

Actions of luteinizing hormone on leydig cells

Upon receptor occupancy, luteinizing hormone activates the cAMP pathway through a guanosine triphosphate–binding protein, leading to a number of events resulting in the provision of cholesterol substrate and stimulation of the side chain cleavage enzyme to convert cholesterol to pregnenolone, with subsequent biosynthesis of testosterone, a process which takes 30–60 minutes after exposure to luteinizing hormone. This pathway is operational in both Leydig cells and theca cells of the ovary. A longer response can be seen after repeated luteinizing hormone stimulation or after a single injection of hCG, when the initial rise in testosterone peaks within 12h with the concentration subsequently declining to an elevated plateau at 24h, again rising to a peak 48–72h after the initial injection. This reflects the long half-life of hCG, and a likely down-regulation/loss of luteinizing hormone receptors after initial exposure followed by recovery of receptor numbers after several days, when there is sufficient hCG remaining to stimulate steroidogenesis (Sharpe 1976). Conversion of testosterone to oestradiol and the suppressive effect of the latter on 17,20-lyase activity may also contribute to this biphasic response. Testosterone is the main secretory product of the testes, together with dihydrotestosterone (DHT), androsterone, androstenedione, 17-alphahydroxyprogesterone, progesterone and pregnenolone.

TESTOSTERONE SYNTHESIS, SECRETION AND TRANSPORT

Testosterone and DHT are transported in plasma mainly bound to the liver derived βglobulin sex hormone–binding globulin (SHBG), which has a single androgen binding site per molecule, and in total binds about 44% of circulating testosterone. Albumin binds 55% testosterone, with only 2% testosterone being free. SHBG also binds oestradiol but with weaker

TABLE 18.1
Factors regulating plasma SHBG concentrations

Stimulation of SHBG synthesis	Inhibition of SHBG synthesis
Thyroxine	Hypothyroidism
Pregnancy	Androgens/anabolic steroids
PCOS	Polycystic ovarian syndrome
Liver disease/cirrhosis	Diabetes mellitus
Phenytoin therapy	Obesity
Anorexia nervosa	Cushing syndrome

affinity. The half-life of testosterone is about 12 minutes, and it is estimated that the adult testes produce about 5mg to 7mg daily (Wang et al. 2004). The binding affinity of testosterone for albumin is 100 times lower than for SHBG, but since the albumin concentration is much higher than SHBG, the binding capacity of both proteins is about the same. SHBG concentration in blood is regulated by a number of hormones (see Table 18.1).

METABOLISM OF TESTOSTERONE

Testosterone can be 5α-reduced by the endoplasmic reticulum enzyme 5α reductase to generate the highly biologically active DHT, which is 10 times more active than testosterone. Testosterone is also a substrate for aromatisation to oestradiol. There are two 5α reductases, type 1 (localised to skin, liver and brain, whose optimal pH is alkaline) and type 2 (active in the penis, scrotum, epididymis and prostate, whose optimal pH is acidic) (Thigpen et al. 1993). DHT, whose generation from testosterone is organ dependent, sustains differentiation and growth, and the type 2 enzyme is particularly important for normal sexual development and virilisation in men (phallic development, scrotum, prostate), as evidenced by the phenotypic changes induced by its loss of function in patients with 5α reductase deficiency.

DETERMINANTS OF SENSITIVITY TO ANDROGENS: ANDROGEN RECEPTOR POLYMORPHISMS

The androgen receptor gene, located on the X chromosome, is more than 90kb long and 8 exons encode a protein with three major functional domains: the N-terminal domain (exon 1), a two zinc finger DNA-binding domains (exon 2 and 3) and an androgen-binding domain (exon 4–8) (Quigley et al. 1995). The protein functions as a steroid-hormone activated transcription factor. Upon binding the hormone ligand, the receptor dissociates from accessory proteins (HSP90) and becomes phosphorylated, translocates into the nucleus, dimerises and then stimulates transcription of androgen responsive genes. This gene contains two polymorphic trinucleotide repeat segments that encode polyglutamine and polyglycine tracts in the N-terminal transactivation domain of its protein. Expansion of the polyglutamine tract (CAG repeats) leads to increasing degrees of androgen insensitivity, such as that associated with spinal bulbar muscular atrophy (Kennedy disease). Loss-of-function mutations in this gene are also associated with complete androgen insensitivity (CAIS). Shorter lengths of the CAG trinucleotide repeat are associated with increased sensitivity to testosterone action (Giovannucci et al. 1997).

LOCAL INTRATESTICULAR ACTIONS OF TESTOSTERONE

The secreted testosterone and its 5α-reduced derivative DHT act on numerous target end organs causing the development of male secondary sexual characteristics and inhibiting the pituitary secretion of luteinizing hormone and FSH. Within the testes, testosterone is the best documented local regulator of spermatogenesis, acting locally in the seminiferous tubules. A good example of this effect is seen in testosterone-producing Leydig cell tumours which are surrounded by seminiferous tubules which maintain spermatogenesis, whereas long-loop negative feedback inhibition of gonadotrophins by tumorous sex steroids impairs spermatogenesis in the tumour free areas. The actions of testosterone on spermatogenesis are enhanced by FSH, which acts on FSHR located on Sertoli cells. Peritubular cells express androgen receptors, and testosterone acts on these cells to stimulate production of peritubular modifying substance (PmodS), which mediates stromal/epithelial cell interactions (Verhoeven et al. 2000).

Sertoli cells themselves express the androgen receptor. The main locally produced growth factors participating in the local regulation of spermatogenesis are transforming growth factor (TGF)-alpha/beta, inhibin (inhibitor of spermatogonial proliferation) and activin (stimulators of spermatogonial proliferation), nerve growth factor, insulin-like growth factor-1 and epidermal growth factor.

FEEDBACK REGULATION OF GNRH AND GONADOTROPHIN RELEASE IN THE MALE

Negative-feedback of GnRH release is exerted by testosterone through androgen and oestrogen receptors present in the hypothalamic neurons and in the pituitary. This is easily demonstrated by the rise in serum luteinizing hormone and serum FSH that occurs after orchiectomy. Luteinizing hormone and FSH blood levels continue to rise for a long period after castration, reaching maximum levels as late as 25 to 50 days after surgery. Although it was previously thought that testosterone, the major secretory product of the testis, was the primary inhibitor of luteinizing hormone secretion in men, a number of testicular secretory products, including oestrogens and other androgens, have the ability to inhibit luteinizing hormone secretion. Oestradiol (E2), a potent oestrogen, is produced both from the testis and from peripheral conversion of androgens and androgen precursors by aromatase enzyme and is the predominant regulator of luteinizing hormone secretion in the male. Although the concentration of oestradiol in the blood of men is relatively low compared with testosterone, it is a much more potent inhibitor of luteinizing hormone and FSH secretion (approximately 1 000-fold) than testosterone. In the human male, oestrogen has dual sites of negative feedback, acting at the hypothalamus to decrease GnRH pulse frequency and at the pituitary to decrease responsiveness to GnRH (Hayes et al. 2000). Thus E2 and testosterone act primarily to feedback inhibit gonadotrophins at the level of the hypothalamus, whereas estrogens provide feedback to the pituitary also to modulate the gonadotropin secretion response to each GnRH surge. Testosterone exerts both direct and indirect feedback on luteinizing hormone secretion, whereas its effects on FSH appear to be mediated largely by aromatisation to oestradiol (E2). Thus in terms of sex steroid feedback, E2 is the predominant regulator of FSH secretion in the human male. DHT does not appear to play a significant role in feedback regulation of gonadotrophins (Canovatchel et al. 1994).

INHIBINS

Inhibin B, a peptide growth factor produced by Sertoli cells, is also important in the negative feedback regulation of FSH (Hayes et al. 2001), acting predominantly at the pituitary level, binding to a coreceptor composed of type III TGF-beta receptor and the type IIB activin receptor.

    Two forms of inhibin have been isolated. They have the same alpha subunit, but their beta subunits are different. Inhibin B (alpha subunit and B variant of the beta subunit) is the form secreted by the Sertoli cells, which selectively suppresses FSH secretion by gonadotropes by inhibiting transcription of the FSH beta subunit gene. Men who have selective injury to the germinal epithelium (seminiferous tubules) have elevated serum FSH, but normal luteinizing hormone and testosterone concentrations. Selective damage to the germinal epithelium occurs following testis irradiation, anti-spermatogenic agents, pesticides, chemotherapy and early cryptorchidism. In addition to inhibin B, a number of other gonadal peptide growth factors, such as follistatin and transforming growth factors, are also modulators of FSH secretion. In humans, inhibin B rises progressively at the time of puberty correlating with FSH concentrations and FSH-stimulated Sertoli cell proliferation, adult concentrations being reached by mid-puberty.

CLINICAL UTILITY OF INHIBIN B MEASUREMENTS IN MALES

The potential regulation of inhibin B concentrations by the interaction between Sertoli and spermatogenic cells suggests its use as a marker of spermatogenesis. Inhibin B concentrations correlate with total sperm count (von Eckardstein et al. 1999) and testicular volume. In men treated with chemotherapy for haematologic malignancy, inhibin B decreased as expected based on known evidence for seminiferous tubule damage in these patients. The inverse correlation between inhibin B and testicular biopsy score suggests that decreasing inhibin B concentrations reflect progressive testicular damage. In addition, the potential to discriminate between spermatidic arrest in which inhibin B concentrations are normal and Sertoli cell-only syndrome in which concentrations are generally low point to a potential use in the evaluation of male infertility.

ACTIVINS AND FOLLISTATIN

The activins (closely related to inhibins) are also secreted in the testis, primarily by the Sertoli cells. They are also composed of heterodimers and homodimers of beta subunits. They stimulate transcription of the FSH beta subunit and are in turn negatively regulated by the binding protein follistatin. Inhibin, activin and follistatin were first identified as gonadal hormones that could exert selective effects on FSH secretion without affecting luteinizing hormone. Although the primary source of inhibin remains the gonad, both activin and follistatin are produced in extragonadal tissues (e.g. the pituitary) and can exert effects on FSH through an autocrine-paracrine mechanism. These proteins can affect the regulation of the gonadotropins at many levels. First, activin can directly stimulate FSH biosynthesis and release from the gonadotrope cells of the pituitary gland. Second, activin up-regulates GnRH receptor (*GnRHR*) gene expression, leading to alterations in the synthesis and release of both gonadotropins in response to GnRH. Third, activin can stimulate GnRH release from GnRH neurons in the hypothalamus and thereby affect FSH and luteinizing hormone secretion. Follistatins are glycoproteins produced by the gonadotrophs and by folliculostellate cells of the pituitary gland that bind and antagonise the actions of activins. Both inhibin and follistatin can negatively regulate the effects of activin by preventing activin binding to the activin receptor at the cell membrane and blocking activation of downstream signal transduction pathways (de Kretser et al. 2004; Gregory and Kaiser 2004). The overall organisation of the hypothalamo-pituitary testicular axis is depicted diagrammatically in Figure 18.1.

GERM CELL DEVELOPMENT IN THE MALE

The development of the male germ cells in the seminiferous tubule essentially consists of three phases: spermatogonal clonal expansion, meiosis and spermatogenesis. Spermatogenesis is a 60- to 73-day process by which a primitive stem cell, the type A spermatogonium, passes through a series of transformations to give rise to spermatozoa (Misell et al. 2006).

In the seminiferous epithelium, cells in these developmental phases are arranged in defined stages. Along the seminiferous tubules, these stages follow one another in a regular fashion, giving rise to the wave of the seminiferous epithelium. Spermatogenesis is dependent on pituitary FSH and on intratesticular testosterone. FSH and androgens seem to have different preferential sites of action during spermatogenesis. Stages VII and VIII appear to be androgen-dependent, whereas maximal binding of FSH and activation of FSH-dependent enzymes occurs in stages XIII to XV of the spermatogenic cycle.

Luteinizing hormone affects spermatogenesis by increasing intratesticular testosterone concentrations. The concentrations of FSH required to initiate spermatogenesis in patients with hypogonadotrophic hypogonadism are, in general, low (Bouloux et al. 2003). Thus, both FSH and luteinizing hormone are apparently required for the initiation and completion of spermatogenesis. However, in patients with gonadotropin deficiency acquired after puberty, sperm production can be stimulated with only hCG, suggesting that the reinitiation and maintenance of spermatogenesis in adults can be achieved by luteinizing hormone alone. Studies of selective gonadotropin replacement in normal men, in whom hypogonadotropic hypogonadism was induced with exogenous testosterone administration, show that qualitatively normal sperm production can be achieved by replacement of either FSH or luteinizing hormone alone. Both FSH and luteinizing hormone are necessary to maintain quantitatively normal spermatogenesis in man.

THE HYPOTHALAMO-PITUITARY OVARIAN AXIS

The menstrual cycle: feedback control of gonadotropins in the female

In the human menstrual cycle, serum concentrations of both luteinizing hormone and FSH begin to increase a few days prior to the menses. FSH concentrations initially increase more rapidly than those of luteinizing hormone and attain maximal concentrations during the first few days of the follicular phase, and then decline in the latter half of the follicular phase, and with the exception of a brief peak at mid-cycle, continue to fall until the lowest concentrations in the cycle are reached during the second half of the luteal phase. The preovulatory decline in FSH is a consequence of the rising concentration of oestradiol in this period. Luteinizing hormone concentrations rise gradually throughout the follicular phase. At mid-cycle, there is a large peak in the concentration of luteinizing hormone, lasting 1–3 days, and subsequently luteinizing hormone concentrations gradually decline reaching their lowest concentration late in the luteal phase (Fig 18.3). During the follicular phase, luteinizing hormone pulses occur hourly, but in the luteal phase, luteinizing hormone pulses occur every 4–8h, then decrease in frequency, secondary to the feedback effects of rising concentrations of progesterone, which slow down the hypothalamic GnRH pulse generator.

In females, feedback mechanisms are more complex in that, while oestradiol and progesterone evoke negative feedback, oestradiol also has a positive feedback role responsible for generating the pre-ovulatory GnRH and luteinizing hormone surge. Inhibin B is produced and secreted by ovarian granulosa cells during the follicular phase (under FSH control) and inhibin A by the corpus luteum under the control of luteinizing hormone. Inhibins act synergistically with oestradiol to inhibit FSH production.

Activin and follistatin are produced in the ovary and in the pituitary, and appear to act on FSH in the pituitary by autocrine or paracrine but not endocrine pathways, activin stimulating FSH production, whereas follistatin suppresses this action of activin.

Oestrogen receptors and GnRH neurons

The classic 'α' form of oestrogen receptor (ERα) is absent in GnRH neurons (Simonian et al. 1999). Feedback inhibition of oestrogen on GnRH secretion is thought to be mediated via an interneuron or by oestrogen-sensitive glial elements. Oestrogen modulates the activity of neuronal networks by both slow genomic and rapid (non-genomic) actions. In the case of oestrogen positive feedback, classic genomic mechanisms underlie the oestrogen activation of GnRH neurons occurring only after several hours of oestrogen exposure. After oestrogen exposure for a sufficient period, oestrogen can be removed without having any negative effect upon subsequent GnRH neuron activation. Thus, rapid and immediate actions of oestrogen are unlikely to be crucial for GnRH neuron activation, whereas positive feedback relies upon a classic genomic mechanism. The finding of ERβ mRNA and protein in GnRH neurons in mouse, rat and the sheep raises the possibility that oestrogen might act directly upon GnRH neurons via this isoform to generate the GnRH/luteinizing hormone surge. However, in terms of both luteinizing hormone secretion and immediate early gene expression in GnRH neurons, oestrogen positive feedback is normal in the global ERβ mutant mouse, strongly suggesting that ERβ-regulated signalling within GnRH neurons is not critical for oestrogen's positive feedback effects upon these cells.

ERβ immunoreactivity is present in 11%–28% of GnRH neurons in adult human males. In mouse GnRH neurons, ERβ causes rapid phosphorylation of cAMP-response element-binding (CREB) protein and stimulates intracellular calcium oscillations via non-genomic

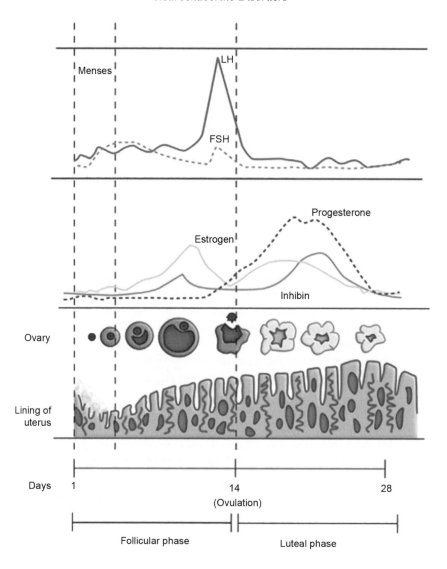

Figure 18.3. Hormonal changes during the human menstrual cycle. Inhibin B is predominantly secreted in the follicular phase, and inhibin A in the luteal phase.

effects, as well as in vitro, mediating ligand-independent transcriptional activation and a ligand-dependent transcriptional repression of the mouse GnRH promoter. ERβ-selective agonists induce galanin mRNA expression in GnRH cells of ovariectomised rats in vivo, possibly via an ERβ-mediated direct action.

ERα containing interneurons however dominate in the regulation of reproduction over the ERβ-mediated direct effects and both negative and positive oestrogen feedback mechanisms are disrupted in the ERα-knockout mice. Accidents of nature in humans show that

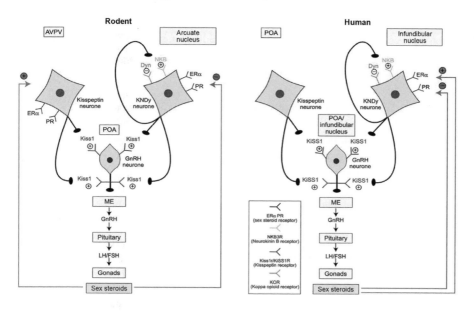

Figure 18.4. Organization of the kisspeptin–GnRH pathway and KNDy/GnRH neurons in rodents and humans. Kisspeptin signals directly to kisspeptin receptor-expressing GnRH neurons. The location of kisspeptin neuron populations within the hypothalamus is species-specific, residing within the anteroventral periventricular nucleus (AVPV) and the arcuate nucleus in rodents, and within the pre-optic area (POA) and the infundibular nucleus in humans. Kisspeptin neurons in the infundibular (humans)/arcuate (rodents) nucleus co-express neurokinin B and dynorphin (KNDy neurons), which via neurokinin B receptor and kappa opioid peptide receptor autosynaptically regulate pulsatile kis-speptin secretion, with neurokinin B being stimulatory and dynorphin inhibitory. Negative (red) and positive (green) sex steroid feedback is mediated via distinct kisspeptin populations in rodents, via the AVPV and the arcuate nucleus, respectively. In humans, KNDy neurons in the infundibular nucleus relay both negative (red) and positive (green) feedback. The role of the POA kisspeptin population in mediating sex steroid feedback in humans is incompletely explored. ME, median eminence; +, stimulatory; −, inhibitory; ERα, estrogen receptor alpha; PR, progesterone receptor; KISS1/KiSS1, kisspeptin; NKB, neurokinin B; Dyn, dynorphin. (A colour version of this figure can be seen in the plate section at the end of the book)

disruption of ERα signalling causes profound oestrogen resistance in women, with delayed puberty and the absence of menstrual cyclicity (Quaynor et al. 2013).

Oestrogen-sensitive interneurons of the infundibular region

The absence of negative oestrogen feedback in post-menopausal women causes profound anatomical changes in the human infundibulum, with significant hypertrophy of ERα, substance P, NKB, kisspeptin and prodynorphin (Rometo and Rance 2008) expressing cells. The high levels of kisspeptin and NKB immunoreactivities detectable in the infundibulum of postmenopausal women support the notion that inhibitory control of kisspeptin and NKB synthesis in these cells is diminished in the absence of oestradiol. This is supported by recent experimental evidence from animal studies confirming that DYN/kisspeptin/NKB neurons are critical in gonadal steroid feedback to GnRH neurons (Figs 18.1 and 18.2). When these cells are ablated in the rat by locally applied microinjection of the NK3-saporin neurotoxin, serum luteinizing hormone and FSH increments are attenuated following ovariectomy (Mittelman-Smith et al. 2012b).

ROLE OF THE KISS1 SYSTEM IN THE PREOVULATORY GONADOTROPIN SURGE

KISS1 neurons in anteroventral periventricular nucleus (AVPV)/preoptic periventricular nucleus (PeN) are implicated in the positive feedback effects of oestrogen in female rodents. Thus, oestrogen stimulates the expression of *KISS1* selectively in the AVPV/PeN and KISS1 neurons in these nuclei become activated during the preovulatory period and following sex-steroid induction of luteinizing hormone surges; moreover, immunoneutralisation of endogenous kisspeptins in the preoptic area abrogates the preovulatory luteinizing hormone surge (Roa et al. 2009). Since almost all AVPV/PeN KISS1 neurons express oestrogen receptor α, essential for luteinizing hormone surge generation, given their projections to GnRH neurons, this KISS1 neuron population is thought to play an important role in the preovulatory gonadotropin surge generation. This theory is supported by initial observations of the anovulatory state of *GPR54* and *KISS1* knockout mice (Clarkson et al. 2008) and is supported by the prevention of the preovulatory surge after antagonisation of GPR54 (Pineda et al. 2010). Further evidence comes from the disruption to ovulation in mice after selective ablation of oestrogen receptor α from *KISS1*-expressing cells. This effect is probably due to impairment of development, function, or both, of KISS1 neurons in the AVPV/PeN.

Besides their roles as transcriptional regulators of *KISS1*, sex steroids are also important modulators of GnRH/gonadotropin responses to kisspeptins. For instance, activation of oestrogen receptor α in female rats increases the responsiveness of luteinizing hormone to Kp-10, especially in the presence of activated progesterone receptors. This effect probably contributes to the generation of full preovulatory gonadotropin surges (Roa et al. 2008).

NEUROKININ B

ARC KISS1 neurons coexpress NKB and dynorphin A and are therefore termed KNDy. NKB and dynorphin A are thought to operate in a reciprocal manner (stimulatory and inhibitory, respectively) as autosynaptic regulators of the kisspeptin output to GnRH neurons (see later section). Thus, they play crucial parts in the control of the pulsatile secretion of GnRH.

ENDOCRINE DISORDERS OF THE HYPOTHALAMO-PITUITARY-GONADAL AXIS

Assessment of hypogonadal patients

Hypogonadotrophic hypogonadism This describes the association of low circulating sex steroids with inappropriately low gonadotrophin levels. It may occur as a consequence of a primarily hypothalamic pathology, or a pituitary disorder, and may be congenital or acquired. Congenital disorders of the hypothalamo-pituitary axis causing hypergonadotropic hypogonadism are discussed more fully below and in Chapter 19.

Hypergonadotropic hypogonadism Males with primary testicular disease (hypergonadotropic hypogonadism) with Leydig and Sertoli cell damage exhibit diminished feedback inhibition of gonadotropin secretion, resulting in high-serum luteinizing hormone and FSH concentrations. In hypergonadotropic hypogonadism, patients have a diminished Leydig cell reserve and a blunted testosterone response to administered luteinizing hormone or to the luteinizing hormone–like effects of hCG.

PATHOLOGIES AFFECTING GNRH NEUROSECRETION CAUSING
HYPOGONADOTROPHIC HYPOGONADISM

Insufficient pulsatile secretion of GnRH with resulting deficiency of luteinizing hormone and FSH leads to sexual infantilism and delayed sexual maturation, depending on the severity in qualitative or quantitative defects in amplitude or frequency of GnRH pulses (Spratt et al. 1987); thus at one end of the spectrum, patients may present with sexual infantilism, while at the other extreme, separation from constitutional pubertal delay may be challenging. GnRH deficiency may be secondary to genetic or developmental defects present in the neonate but undetected until the age of expected puberty, or secondary to pathologies such as tumours, inflammatory processes, vascular lesions, radiation damage or trauma. Lesions which affect growth hormone secretion also will result in decreased growth velocity especially at the time of the expected pubertal growth spurt. Isolated luteinizing hormone and FSH deficiency usually results in normal height for age in early and middle adolescent age, whereas those with constitutional growth and pubertal delay have a normal growth rate for bone age, but are short for chronological age.

TUMOURS

It is unusual for these to solely cause hypogonadotrophic hypogonadism, but rather they are associated with multiple pituitary hormonal deficiencies.

Craniopharyngioma

These represent the commonest non-glial brain tumours of childhood causing disturbed hypothalamo-pituitary malfunction and sexual infantilism. This is more fully discussed in Chapter 13. They originate from Rathke's pouch from epithelial rests along the pituitary stalk extending superiorly to the hypothalamus, and more rarely remain solely intrasellar, and very occasionally in the nasopharynx or third ventricle (Fig 18.5). The peak incidence is between 6 and 14 years (Fahlbusch et al. 1999). Presentation is with headache, visual disturbance, short stature, diabetes insipidus, optic atrophy and signs of growth hormone deficiency, delayed puberty and hypothyroidism. Surgical correction is often attempted but the recurrence rate is high.

Germinoma

These are the second most common extrasellar tumours associated with hypogonadotrophic hypogonadism. The diagnosis is often made in the second decade of life, symptoms of diabetes insipidus being most frequent (Mootha et al. 1997) followed by visual difficulties

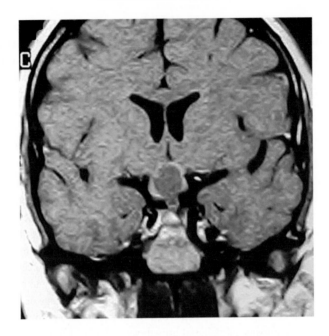

Figure 18.5. Contrast enhanced MRI scan of suprasellar craniopharyngioma presenting with panhypopituitarism.

and abnormalities of growth and puberty. Other endocrine abnormalities include hyperprolactinaemia, due to a stalk effect. The elevated concentrations of hCG in spinal fluid and serum are important markers of this disease. In boys, hCG secretion from these tumours may cause isosexual precocious puberty. As these lesions are generally suprasellar, untreated, subependymal spread in the lining of the third ventricle and seeding into the lower spinal cord and cauda equine may occur. Pure germinomas are radiosensitive, and surgery is rarely required except for making a diagnosis (Wara et al. 1977). Mixed germ cell tumours require both radiation and chemotherapy.

Hypothalamic and optic gliomas/astrocytoma
These can occur as part of von Reckinghausen disease, or sporadically, and may lead to hypogonadotrophic hypogonadism.

PITUITARY DISEASE
Pituitary function may be impaired in cases of pituitary surgery, infarction, tumours, radiation or infectious diseases. Patients with prepubertal onset of pituitary disease are usually diagnosed prior to a fertility evaluation as a result of growth retardation or adrenal or thyroid deficiency. Infertility, impotence, visual field abnormalities and severe headaches may be presenting symptoms in the adult male with pituitary dysfunction. Normal male secondary sexual characteristics are usually present unless adrenal insufficiency exists. Small, soft

testes may be demonstrated on physical examination. This is in contrast to cases of primary testicular failure with tubular and peritubular sclerosis, in which case the testes are small and firm to palpation. Plasma testosterone concentrations are low and gonadotropin concentrations are low or normal. Thus, a normal luteinizing hormone value associated with a low-serum testosterone value is abnormal and further evaluation of the pituitary is mandated. Evaluation of other pituitary hormones and endocrine functions should be performed in appropriate cases.

Pituitary tumours are rare in childhood, but include both functioning (prolactinoma 50%, growth hormone secretion 20%) and non-functioning lesions (30%), and may lead to pubertal delay because of hypogonadotrophic hypogonadism (De Menis 2001). Prolactin-producing tumours tend to be larger in boys, whereas microadenomas are commoner in girls.

HAEMOCHROMATOSIS

Hereditary haemochromatosis is a genetically transmitted disease characterised by excessive absorption of dietary iron, which may result in parenchymal iron overload and subsequent tissue damage. Early reports recognised the frequent involvement of the endocrine system; iron deposition in pituitary gonadotrophs causes hypogonadotropic hypogonadism, which is the most frequently encountered nondiabetic endocrinopathy in hereditary haemochromatosis, reported to occur in 10%–100% of cases (McNeil et al. 1983). Biochemical evidence of iron overload is necessary to make a diagnosis, with elevated serum ferritin values and abnormally high transferrin saturation. Other possible causes for iron overload (e.g. porphyria cutanea tarda, disorders of erythropoiesis and transfusional iron overload) should be excluded. Transfusion haemosiderosis, for example in patients with haemoglobinopathies, can cause similar endocrine damage.

Mutations in the *HAMP*, *HFE*, *HFE2*, *SLC40A1* and *TFR2* genes cause haemochromatosis (Kanwar and Kowdley 2014). The *HAMP*, *HFE*, *HFE2*, *SLC40A1* and *TFR2* genes play an important role in regulating the absorption, transport and storage of iron. Mutations in these genes impair the control of iron absorption during digestion and alter the distribution of iron to other parts of the body. As a result, iron accumulates in tissues and organs, which can disrupt their normal functions. Each type of hemochromatosis is caused by mutations in a specific gene. Type 1 haemochromatosis is caused by mutations in the *HFE* gene, and type 2 haemochromatosis is caused by mutations in either the *HFE2* or *HAMP* gene. Mutations in the *TFR2* gene cause type 3 haemochromatosis, and mutations in the *SLC40A1* gene cause type 4 haemochromatosis.

LANGERHANS' CELL HISTIOCYTOSIS

Clinical symptoms are related to the site of disease. Commonly affected organs include the lungs, skin and bone; however, virtually any tissue may be involved, including the stomach, central nervous system, thyroid and liver. Patterns of involvement are classified as single system, single system multifocal and multisystem (disseminated). In general, better outcomes are observed in older patients and patients with single system disease; worse outcomes are observed in multisystem disease, in patients with organ dysfunction,

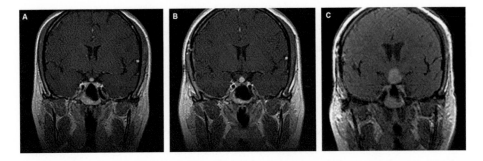

Figure 18.6. Example of Langerhans' cell histiocytosis on MRI in patient presenting with diabetes insipidus and anterior pituitary insufficiency, including hypogonadotrophic hypogonadism.

in isolated pulmonary disease and in younger patients (Arico et al. 2003). Multisystem disease can be further classified as low risk or high risk (hematopoietic system, lungs, liver and spleen) based on involvement of specific organs (Stockschlaeder and Sucker 2006).

Endocrine abnormalities are relatively common in Langerhans' cell histiocytosis (LCH) multisystem disease (Figure 18.6). In one study, 81 of 188 (43.1%) adult patients with multisystem disease developed diabetes insipidus. In the same study, no patient with single system disease developed diabetes insipidus. Hypothyroidism was also noted in 18 (9.6%) patients with multisystem disease and in no patients with single system disease. It is unclear whether these abnormalities in this series were attributable to pituitary and/ or hypothalamic lesions or to compression of the pituitary stalk by nearby osseous lesions. Several pathologies may present with thickening of the pituitary stalk (Table 18.2). The 'criterion standard' for histopathological diagnosis is the presence of characteristic Birbeck granules on electron microscopy of the biopsied lesion. Other histological features seen in LCH lesions include detection of CD1a, CD207, S100 protein, adenosine triphosphate (ATP)ase or alpha-D-mannosidase on the cell surface (Arico et al. 2003). In practice, the presence of CD1a and S100 on histiocytes is thought to be highly specific for LCH (Gangwani et al. 2007).

LCH involvement of the pituitary stalk and hypothalamus frequently leads to central diabetes insipidus, affecting 12%–30% of patients with the condition (Nanduri et al. 2000; Makras et al. 2007). The presence of LCH in either the pituitary stalk or hypothalamus is likely in multisystem disease and craniofacial LCH involvement. Radiological abnormalities can be demonstrated by MRI in the large majority of patients with central diabetes insipidus and LCH and may include enhancing stalk or hypothalamic lesions and loss of the posterior bright spot, thought to represent depletion of vasopressin-containing secretory granules in the posterior pituitary (Figure 18.6).

Anterior pituitary hormone deficits usually occur in patients with central diabetes insipidus and sellar abnormalities detected on MRI scans. Growth hormone deficiency is the most common, followed by gonadotropin deficiency, whereas TSH or corticotropin

TABLE 18.2
Causes of an abnormal pituitary stalk

Congenital

Stalk hypoplasia or aplasia

Stalk duplication

Traumatic

Traumatic brain injury

Surgery

Inflammatory

Lymphocytic infundibuloneurohypophysitis

Sarcoidosis

Wegener granulomatosis

Idiopathic granulomatous infundibuloneurohypophysitis

Infectious

Tuberculosis

Whipple disease

Neoplastic

Langerhans cell histiocytosis

Germ cell tumours

Craniopharyngiomas

Metastases (including breast or lung primary)

Leukaemias and lymphomas

Other primary brain tumours (astrocytomas, ependymomas, meningiomas, pituicytomas, tanycytomas)

deficiencies occur less frequently. Patients with hypothalamic LCH lesions may also experience disturbances of thirst (adipsia), appetite (morbid obesity), thermoregulation (hypothermia), sleep and short-term memory (Kaltsas et al. 2000).

High-dose glucocorticoid therapy has been used in an attempt to decrease the size of inflammatory lesions in patients with a thickened pituitary stalk suspected of having lymphocytic hypophysitis or infundibuloneurohypophysitis, and has been combined with antineoplastic chemotherapy in some patients with LCH.

Endocrine deficiencies require treatment with standard replacement therapies, including desmopressin for diabetes insipidus and regular neuroendocrine evaluation is necessary to detect development of pituitary hormone deficiencies. Growth hormone replacement does not seem to influence the natural history of LCH (Donadieu et al. 2004).

Annual brain MRI scans and periodic skeletal surveys will detect progression. Radiation therapy may be used to treat patients with expanding sellar lesions that might impinge on the optic chiasm and threaten vision, but this incurs the additional long-term risk of hypopituitarism, so lifelong surveillance with periodic assessment of their pituitary function is advisable.

Patients with systemic LCH involvement may be treated with antineoplastic chemo-therapy, including vinblastine and glucocorticoids in pharmacological doses. Etoposide administration is generally avoided because of an increased risk of leukaemia associated with its use. Surgery may be used in selected cases to resect symptomatic or expanding mass lesions. 2-CDA (2-chlorodeoxyadenosine) demonstrates significant effectiveness in patients with LCH and CNS involvement with enhancing space-occupying lesions, as evidenced by a response in all 12 patients in one series herein reported achieving a sustained complete or partial radiographic response (Dhall et al. 2008).

HYPOTHALAMIC SYNDROMES ASSOCIATED WITH GNRH DEFICIENCY

Prader–Willi syndrome (PWS) is a rare imprinted genetic disorder with an incidence of between 1 in 25 000 and 1 in 10 000 live births, in which seven genes (or some subset thereof) on chromosome 15 (q 11–13) are deleted or unexpressed (chromosome 15q partial deletion) on the paternal chromosome (Cassidy and Driscoll 2009). PWS is characterised by low muscle tone, short stature, incomplete sexual development, cognitive disabilities, problem behaviours and a chronic feeling of hunger that can lead to excessive eating and life-threatening obesity.

For the genes affected in PWS, it is the maternal copy of these genes that are silenced, while the mutated paternal copy is not functional. If the maternally derived genetic material from the same region is affected instead, the sister syndrome Angelman syndrome ensues.

Patients demonstrate luteinizing hormone and FSH deficiencies because of a lack of GnRH. This is manifested as undescended testes in males. Benign premature adrenarche may occur in females. Testes may descend with time or can be managed with surgery or testosterone replacement. Treatment is identical to that for Kallmann syndrome. A similar picture is found in Laurence–Moon Bardet–Biedl syndrome, which consists of obesity, hypogonadotropic hypogonadism, retinitis pigmentosa and polydactyly. Hypogonadotrophic hypogonadism is also observed with Gordon-Holmes syndrome and CHARGE syndrome, when it is associated with coloboma of the eye, heart defects, choanal atresia, growth retardation, ear abnormalities with hearing loss and learning difficulties (see Chapter 19).

HYPERGONADOTROPHIC HYPOGONADISM

Primary testicular disorders

Approximately 6% of infertile men are found to have chromosomal abnormalities, with the incidence increasing as the sperm count decreases. The highest incidence is found in azoospermic patients, with up to 21% of cases demonstrating abnormalities of the karyotype. The majority of these cases are associated with Klinefelter syndrome. One gene locus localised to the long arm of the Y chromosome is a region referred to as AZF (azoospermia factor) (Navarro-Costa et al. 2010).

This locus is subdivided into a, b and c, of which AZFc contains the gene *DAZ* (deleted in azoospermia). Men with complete deletions of the entire AZFa region uniformly show a Sertoli cell-only pattern (see below). The AZFa region contains a gene *DBY*, a transcriptional regulator. The AZFb region appears to be critical for completion of sper-matogenesis. No patients with AZFb deletion have shown completely developed sperma-tozoa present on testicular biopsy.

KLINEFELTER SYNDROME

The presence of an extra X chromosome is the genetic hallmark of Klinefelter syndrome. This is due to non-dysjunction of the meiotic chromosomes of the gametes from either parent. Hypogonadism, with the classic triad of small, firm testes, gynecomastia and elevated plasma and urinary gonadotropins, has an incidence of 1 of every 600 male births, but clinically may not be identifiable until puberty (Kamischke et al. 2003). Although secondary sexual characteristics begin developing at the appropriate time, the completion of puberty is usually delayed with features of eunuchoidism, gynaecomastia and impotence.

Virilisation may be complete in some patients and the diagnosis for them may be delayed until adulthood, at which point the patient may present with infertility (azoospermia) with associated gynaecomastia and small, firm testes. Intellectual disability and various psychi-atric disturbances may also occur (Simm and Zacharin 2006). Testicular biopsy reveals seminiferous tubular sclerosis and an occasional Sertoli cell or spermatozoa.

Owing to the absence of normal seminiferous tubules, Leydig cells may appear hyper-plastic. Plasma FSH concentrations are usually markedly elevated as a result of the severe seminiferous tubular injury, whereas luteinizing hormone concentrations may be elevated or normal. Total plasma testosterone concentrations are decreased in 60% of patients and normal in 40%. The physiologically active free testosterone concentrations are usually decreased. In addition, plasma oestradiol levels are usually increased, stimulating increased levels of testosterone-binding globulin and resulting in a decreased testosterone to oestrogen ratio leading to gynecomastia.

The diagnosis may be made with a chromatin-positive buccal smear, indicating the presence of an extra X chromosome. Karyotypes usually demonstrate 47 XXY or, less commonly, a mosaic pattern, 46 XY/47 XXY. Less severe abnormalities are present in patients with the mosaic form of Klinefelter syndrome, and occasional patients are fertile, either spontaneously or more usually using TESE (testicular sperm extraction) retrieval techniques (Fullerton et al. 2010). Patients with Klinefelter syndrome have increased mor-tality (Bojesen et al. 2004). There is growing evidence that the length of the (CAG)n repeat sequence within the androgen receptor may in part explain the variability in the severity of the phenotype (Zinn et al. 2005).

XYY SYNDROME

The XYY karyotype occurs in 0.1% to 0.4% of newborn infants. This karyotype has been linked to aggressive and criminal behaviour. Not all investigators agree that this behaviour is secondary to the karyotype, but feel that it may be secondary to tall stature, which may predispose individuals to this behaviour. Patients are characteristically tall, whereas semen analyses typically reveal severe oligospermia or azoospermia (Aksglaede et al. 2008). Testicular biopsy specimens reveal patterns of maturation arrest to complete germinal aplasia as well as occasional cases demonstrating seminiferous tubular sclerosis. Plasma gonadotropins and testosterone concentrations are most often within the normal range in these patients. However, elevations of plasma FSH concentrations may be found in association with more severe patterns of testicular dysfunction.

NOONAN SYNDROME

The appearance of these patients is similar to that of Turner syndrome (XO). They have short stature, hypertelorism, webbed neck, low-set ears, cubitus valgus, ptosis and cardio-vascular abnormalities. Chromosomal analysis reveals a 46 XY karyotype. Despite identi-fication of several causative genes, the diagnosis of Noonan syndrome is still based on clinical features.

The following genes are known to cause Noonan syndrome with the percentage of cases in brackets: *PTPN11* (50%), *RAF1* (3–17%), *SOS1* (10%), *KRAS* (1%), *NRAS* (unknown) or *BRAF* (unknown) (Van Der Burgt and Brunner 2000; Tartaglia et al. 2001; Bentires-Alj et al. 2006; Schubbert et al. 2006; Razzaque et al. 2007; Roberts et al. 2007; Shchelochkov et al. 2008).

Cryptorchidism and testicular atrophy with elevation of gonadotropins may be present in some patients. Androgens may be given to complete virilisation, but these patients remain infertile.

SERTOLI CELL-ONLY SYNDROME

Although the etiology of Sertoli cell-only syndrome is unknown, patients usually present with bilaterally small testes and azoospermia. Phenotypically, these patients have normal secondary characteristics. Seminiferous tubules are lined by Sertoli cells with a complete absence of germ cells. The testes of patients with Sertoli cell-only syndrome are reasonably normal in consistency. Plasma FSH concentrations are often but not invariably elevated. Plasma testosterone and luteinizing hormone concentrations are normal. Micro-deletions in the AZFb/b+c region are responsible for this condition (Yang et al. 2008).

MYOTONIC DYSTROPHY

Patients who have myotonic dystrophy have myotonia, a condition of delayed muscle relax-ation after contraction. In addition, patients demonstrate premature frontal baldness, pos-terior subcapsular cataracts and cardiac conduction defects.

Testicular atrophy may develop in up to 80% of patients. Testicular damage usually occurs in adulthood; Leydig cells typically are not involved, with biopsy specimens dem-onstrating severe tubular sclerosis (Harper et al. 1972). Serum FSH is elevated with severe tubular atrophy. The disease, classified as DM1 and DM2, is transmitted as an autosomal dominant trait with variable penetrance. DM1 results from an expansion of a CTG trinucleo-tide repeat in the 3'-untranslated region of the dystrophia myotonica protein kinase gene (*DMPK* gene) on chromosome 19q 13.3 (Mahadevan et al. 1992). Wild-type individuals have 5 to 34 CTG repeats at this locus, whereas individuals with DM1 have repeats in the hundreds to thousands. In DM1, a new mutation, which is the expansion of a normal allele (<35 repeats) into the abnormal range, is rare.

DM2 is caused by an expanded CCTG tetranucleotide repeat expansion located in intron 1 of the zinc finger protein 9 gene (*ZNF9* gene, also known as the *CNBP* gene) on chromosome 3q 21.3 (Liquori et al. 2001). On normal alleles, there are 11 to 26 tetranucleotide repeats; on pathogenic alleles, the number of repeats ranges from 75 to more than 11 000, with a mean of 5 000 repeats. There is no therapy for the testicular dysfunction in these patients.

OTHER FORMS OF TESTICULAR FAILURE

Radiation to the gonads may cause testicular failure usually resulting in azoospermia, although normal testosterone secretion can be maintained in the presence of elevated luteinizing hormone and FSH values. Doses of 0.35Gy to the testes may cause temporary aspermia, >2Gy permanent azoospermia while doses over 15Gy impair testosterone production and Leydig cell function (Barrett et al. 1987).

TESTICULAR BIOSYNTHETIC DEFECTS

Mutations in *CYP17* affecting 17α-hydroxylase/17,20 lyase in males is associated with a female phenotype, because androgen biosynthesis is impaired at all stages of development. Gonadotrophins are raised, and there is associated cortisol deficiency and increased mineralocorticoid synthesis with hypokalaemic alkalosis and hypertension.

HYPOGONADISM IN FEMALES

Although amenorrhea may result from a number of different conditions, a systematic evaluation including a detailed history, physical examination and laboratory assessment of selected serum hormone concentrations can usually identify the underlying cause. Initial workup of primary and secondary amenorrhoea includes a pregnancy test and serum concentrations of luteinizing hormone, FSH, oestradiol, prolactin and TSH.

Primary amenorrhoea, defined as failure to reach menarche, is often the result of chromosomal abnormalities leading to primary ovarian insufficiency (e.g. Turner syndrome XO) or anatomical abnormalities (e.g. Müllerian agenesis). Secondary amenorrhoea, defined as the cessation of regular menses for 3 months or the cessation of irregular menses for 6 months, is most commonly caused by polycystic ovary syndrome, hypothalamic amenorrhoea, hyperprolactinaemia or primary ovarian insufficiency – having excluded pregnancy in all cases. Women presenting with primary ovarian insufficiency (raised FSH/luteinizing hormone, low oestradiol and anti-Müllerian hormone concentrations) can retain unpredictable ovarian function and are not always infertile. Those with secondary hypogonadism will typically have low oestradiol concentrations associated with inappropriately normal or low gonadotrophin concentrations (see also Chapter 19).

HYPOGONADOTROPIC HYPOGONADISM IN THE FEMALE

Congenital and acquired causes of hypogonadotrophic hypogonadism are listed in Table 18.3.

TABLE 18.3

Causes of hypergonadotrophic hypogonadism in the female

Ovarian dysgenesis

  Turner syndrome (XO)

Gonadal toxins (chemotherapy/radiation)

  Cytotoxic drugs (e.g. chemotherapy)

Enzyme defects

  17α-hydroxylase deficiency

Miscellaneous

Mumps

Pelvic radiation

  Gonadal failure (in adults)

Menopause

Premature ovarian failure

HYPOTHALAMIC AMENORRHOEA

Patients with hypothalamic amenorrhoea should be evaluated for eating disorders and are at risk for decreased bone density. The condition can also arise in the context of women who perform considerable amounts of exercise on a regular basis or lose a significant amount of weight, who are at risk of developing hypothalamic (or 'athletic') amenorrhoea. Functional hypothalamic amenorrhoea (FHA) can result from stress, weight loss and/or excessive exercise. Women who eat a persistently hypocaloric diet or who exercise to high intensity without consuming enough calories to compensate for their exercise are particularly prone to hypothalamic amenorrhoea. The threshold of developing amenorrhoea appears to be dependent on low energy availability rather than absolute weight because a critical minimum amount of stored, easily mobilised energy is necessary to maintain regular menstrual cycles.

Energy imbalance and weight loss can disrupt menstrual cycles through several hormonal mechanisms. Weight loss can cause elevations in the hormone ghrelin which inhibits the hypothalamic-pituitary-ovarian axis (Cummings et al. 2013; Rak-Mardyla 2013).

Elevated concentrations of ghrelin alter the frequency and amplitude of GnRH pulses, which cause diminished pituitary release of luteinizing hormone and FSH. Patients with hypothalamic amenorrhoea frequently have a low luteinizing hormone and a higher FSH, the consequence of reduced GnRH pulse frequency. The altered interaction between ghrelin and the hypothalamic-pituitary-ovarian axis is also responsible for the prolongation of amenorrhea in patients who have regained normal weight. Low concentration of the hormone leptin in females with low body weight is another hormonal factor that can contribute to secondary amenorrhea. A critical leptin concentration is necessary to maintain regular menstrual cycles and circulating leptin concentrations are low in underweight females caused by excessive exercise or eating disorders such as anorexia nervosa. Like ghrelin, leptin acts as an indicator of energy balance and fat stores to the reproductive axis. Decreased concentrations of leptin are closely related to low levels of body fat, and correlate with a slowing of GnRH pulsing (Andrico et al. 2002).

Thus, women who suffer from FHA but maintain a normal weight experience less severe menstrual irregularities than underweight amenorrhoeic patients.

HYPERGONADOTROPHIC HYPOGONADISM IN THE FEMALE

The pathogenesis of spontaneous Primary Ovarian Insufficiency (POI)/Primary Ovarian Failure (POF) in most cases is caused by follicle dysfunction or follicle depletion, the latter being the major mechanism (Goswami and Conway 2005).

FOLLICLE DEPLETION

At the beginning of puberty in the female, some 300 000–400 000 primordial follicles are present in the ovaries. Full maturation of one dominant follicle is dependent on the simultaneous development of a support cohort of nondominant follicles. These, although destined to undergo atresia, play an important role in the fine-tuning of the hypothalamic-pituitary-ovarian axis by secreting regulatory hormones such as oestradiol, inhibins, activins and androgens (*vide supra*).

Depletion or a reduction of the follicle number thus disrupts the highly coordinated process of follicular growth and ovulation with reduced circulating oestradiol and inhibin concentrations and elevated serum FSH and luteinizing hormone. Occasionally, a 'lonely' follicle may develop, stimulated by the high levels of FSH; however, instead of progressing to a normal ovulation, it is inappropriately luteinised (by the high luteinizing hormone concentrations) presenting as a cystic structure on ovarian ultrasound.

The ovarian follicle reserve can be depleted prematurely because of a low initial number or an accelerated rate of follicle atresia.

A low initial ovarian follicle reserve may be caused by a defect in step of germ cell formation, migration, oogonia proliferation and meiosis resulting in a deficient initial follicle number. The final outcome could be a formation of streak gonads and primary amenorrhea, as in familial 46,XX gonadal dysgenesis, an autosomal-dominant disease with sex-linked inheritance.

In milder cases, the initial follicle number can support pubertal development, initiation of menstrual cycles and occasionally fertility, but premature follicle depletion then results in ovarian failure.

Accelerated follicle atresia or destruction can result from X chromosome monosomy/aneuploidy or mosaicism (as observed in Turner syndrome or some cases with 47,XXX karyotype), X chromosome abnormalities (X chromosome rearrangement, X isochromosome and ring chromosome, translocations of X chromosome material to an autosome [t(X;A)], fragile X permutation), as well as in galactosaemia. It more commonly occurs as an acquired lesion following cytotoxic therapy, ovarian radiation or inflammatory/infective processes (e.g. mumps oophoritis).

Multiple X chromosome genes are involved in regulating female fertility and reproductive lifespan and deletions or disruptions of critical regions of the short arm of the X chromosome (*Xp11, Xp22.1-21.3*) as well as several genes on the long arm of the X chromosome (*Xq13-21*, *Xq22-25* and *Xq26-28*) are associated with gonadal dysgenesis and primary or secondary amenorrhea. These include the *FMR1* gene (Conway 2010), the XIST locus (X inactivation site) and the *DIA* gene (diaphanous gene).

Autosomal abnormalities including Trisomies 13 and 18 are associated with ovarian dysgenesis and failure. Mutations in *FOXL2* and *BMP15* have also been incriminated (Harris et al. 2002; Di Pasquale et al. 2004).

Approximately two-thirds of cases with gonadal dysgenesis in XX individuals are genetic. The inheritance is autosomal recessive, with variable penetrance. 46,XX gonadal dysgenesis is sometimes part of a genetic syndrome, such as gonadal dysgenesis and sensorineural deafness (Perrault syndrome); gonadal dysgenesis and cerebellar ataxia; gonadal dysgenesis, arachnodactyly and microcephaly; and gonadal dysgenesis, short stature and metabolic acidosis. Autosomal recessive disorders associated with POI/POF include Cockayne syndrome, Nijmegen breakage syndrome, Werner syndrome and Bloom syndrome. The *ATM* gene (ataxia-telangiectasia intellectual disability gene) encodes a protein kinase involved in DNA metabolism and cell cycle control, which when mutated is associated with ovarian atrophy and amenorrhea despite normal female sexual differentiation (Persani et al. 2010).

TURNER SYNDROME (XO)

Occurring in 1 in 2000–5000 phenotypic females the syndrome characteristically presents with short stature, limb swelling, broad chest, low hairline, low-set ears and webbed necks. Girls with Turner syndrome typically experience gonadal dysfunction, which results in amenorrhoea and sterility. Non-gonadal-associated anomalies include congenital heart disease, hypothyroidism, diabetes, visual problems, hearing loss and several autoimmune diseases. Finally, a specific pattern of cognitive deficits is often observed, with particular difficulties in visuospatial, mathematical and memory areas.

17α-HYDROXYLASE DEFICIENCY

Genetic 46XX females affected by 17α-hydroxylase deficiency are born with normal female internal and external anatomy. At the expected time of puberty, neither the adrenals nor the ovaries can synthesise sex steroids, so neither breast development nor pubic hair appears. Investigation of delayed puberty yields elevated gonadotropins and normal karyotype but absent oestradiol levels, while imaging confirms the presence of ovaries and an infantile uterus. Discovery of hypertension and hypokalemic alkalosis usually suggests the presence of one of the proximal forms of CAH, and the characteristic mineralocorticoid elevations confirm the specific diagnosis (Kater and Biglieri 1994).

A few milder forms of this deficiency in genetic females have allowed relatively normal breast development and irregular menstruation. Evidence suggests that only 5% of normal enzyme activity may be sufficient to allow at least the physical changes of female puberty, if not ovulation and fertility. In these girls, the elevated blood pressure was the primary clinical problem.

Conclusion

Significant inroads have been made in our understanding of the biology of gonadotrophin secretion in recent years. The identification of molecules such as kisspeptin, leptin and neurokinin B and their receptors have generated excitement in the field. However, basic questions with respect to the onset of puberty and the factors required still remain to be answered. Molecular advances will reveal new players in the field over the next few years, and these will eventually lead to the elucidation of the mechanisms underlying normal and abnormal gonadal development and puberty.

REFERENCES

Aksglaede L, Skakkebaek NE and Juul A (January 2008). Abnormal sex chromosome constitution and longitudinal growth: Serum levels of insulin-like growth factor (IGF)-I, IGF binding protein-3, luteinizing hormone, and testosterone in 109 males with 47,XXY, 47,XYY, or sex-determining region of the Y chromosome (SRY)-positive 46,XX karyotypes. *J Clin Endocrinol Metab* 93(1): 169–176.

Andrico S, Gambera A, Specchia C, Pellegrini C, Falsetti L and Sartori E (2002) Leptin in functional hypothalamic amenorrhoea. *Hum Reprod* 17(8): 2043–2048.

Anthony EL, King JC and Stopa EG (1984) Immunocytochemical localization of LHRH in the median eminence, infundibular stalk, and neurohypophysis. Evidence for multiple sites of releasing hormone secretion in humans and other mammals. *Cell Tissue Res* 236(1): 5–14.

Arico M, Girschikofsky M, Genereau T et al. (2003) Langerhans cell histiocytosis in adults. Report from the International Registry of the Histiocyte Society. *Eur J Cancer* 39(16): 2341–2348.

Barrett A, Nicholls J and Gibson B (1987) Late effects of total body irradiation. *Radiother Oncol* 9: 131–135.

Belchetz PE, Plant TM, Nakai Y, Keogh EJ and Knobil E (1978) Hypophysial responses to continuous and intermittent delivery of hypopthalamic gonadotropin-releasing hormone. *Science* 202(4368): 631–633.

Bentires-Alj M, Kontaridis MI and Neel BG (2006) Stops along the RAS pathway in human genetic disease. *Nat Med* 12(3): 283–285.

Bojesen A, Juul S, Birkebaek N and Gravholt CH (August 2004) Increased mortality in Klinefelter syndrome. *J Clin Endocrinol Metab* 89(8): 3830–3834.

Bouloux PM, Nieschlag E, Burger HG et al. (2003) Induction of spermatogenesis by recombinant follicle-stimulating hormone (puregon) in hypogonadotropic azoospermic men who failed to respond to human chorionic gonadotropin alone. *J Androl* 24(4): 604–611.

Burke MC, Letts PA, Krajewski SJ and Rance NE (2006) Co-expression of dynorphin and neurokinin B immunoreactivity in the rat hypothalamus: Morphologic evidence of interrelated function within the arcuate nucleus. *J Comp Neurol* 498(5): 712–726.

Campbell RE, French-Mullen JM, Cowley MA, Smith MS and Grove KL (2001) Hypothalamic circuitr of neuropeptide Y regulation of neuroendocrine function and food intake via the Y5 receptor subtype. *Neuroendocrinology* 74(2): 106–119.

Canovatchel WJ, Volquez D, Huang S et al. (1994) Luteinizing hormone pulsatility in subjects with 5-alpha-reductase deficiency and decreased dihydrotestosterone production. *J Clin Endo Metab* 78: 916–921.

Cassidy SB and Driscoll DJ (2009) Prader-Willi syndrome. *Eur J Hum Genet* 17: 3–13.

Cates PS, Li XF and O'Byrne KT (2004) The influence of 17 beta-oestradiol on corticotrophin-releasing hormone induced suppression of luteinising hormone pulses and the role of CRH in hypoglycaemic stress-induced suppression of pulsatile LH secretion in the female rat. *Stress* 7(2): 113–118.

Catzeflis C, Pierroz DD, Rohner-Jeanrenaud F, Rivier JE, Sizonenko PC and Aubert ML (1993) Neuropeptide Y administered chronically into the lateral ventricle profoundly inhibits both the gonadotropic and the somatotropic axis in intact adult female rats. *Endocrinology* 132(1): 224–234.

Cheng G, Coolen LM, Padmanabhan V, Goodman RL and Lehman MN (2010) The kisspeptin/neurokinin B/dynorphin (KNDy) cell population of the arcuate nucleus: Sex differences and effects of prenatal testosterone in sheep. *Endocrinology* 151(1): 301–311.

Clarkson J, d'Anglemont de Tassigny X, Moreno AS, Colledge WH and Herbison AE (2008) Kisspeptin-GPR54 signaling is essential for preovulatory gonadotropin-releasing hormone neuron activation and the luteinizing hormone surge. *J Neurosci* 28: 8691–8697.

Colledge WH (2009) Transgenic mouse models to study Gpr54/kisspeptin physiology. *Peptides* 30: 34–41.

Conway GS (2010) Premature ovarian failure and *FMR1* gene mutations: An update. *Ann Endocrinol* 71(3): 215–217.

Crowley WR and Kalra SP (1987) Neuropeptide Y stimulates the release of luteinizing hormone-releasing hormone from medial basal hypothalamus in vitro: Modulation by ovarian hormones. *Neuroendocrinology* 46(2): 97–103.

Cummings DE, Weigle DS, Frayo RS et al. (2002) Plasma ghrelin levels after diet-induced weight loss or gastric bypass surgery. *N Engl J Med* 346(21): 1623–1630.

Cunningham MJ, Clifton DK and Steiner RA (1999) Leptin's actions on the reproductive axis: Perspectives and mechanisms. *Biol Reprod* 60: 216–222.

d'Anglemont de Tassigny X, Fagg LA, Carlton MB and Colledge WH (2008) Kisspeptin can stimulate gonadotropin-releasing hormone (GnRH) release by a direct action at GnRH nerve terminals. *Endocrinology* 149(8): 3926–3932.

de Kretser DM, Buzzard JJ, Okuma Y et al. (2004) The role of activin, follistatin and inhibin in testicular physiology. *Mol Cell Endocrinol* 225: 57–64.

De Menis S, Visentin A, Billeci D et al. (2001) Pituitary adenomas in childhood and adolescence. Clinical analysis of 10 cases. *J Endocrinol Invest* 24: 92–97.

de Roux N, Genin E, Carel JC, Matsuda F, Chaussain JL and Milgrom E (2003) Hypogonadotropic hypogonadism due to loss of function of the KiSS1-derived peptide receptor GPR54. *Proc Natl Acad Sci USA* 100: 10972–10976.

Dearth RK, Hiney JK and Dees WL (2000) Leptin acts centrally to induce the prepubertal secretion of luteinizing hormone in the female rat. *Peptides* 21: 387–392.

Decavel C and Van den Pol AN (1990) GABA: A dominant neurotransmitter in the hypothalamus. *J Comp Neurology* 302(4): 1019–1037.

DeFazio RA, Heger S, Ojeda SR and Moenter SM (2002) Activation of A-type gamma-aminobutyric acid receptors excites gonadotropin-releasing hormone neurons. *Mol Endocrinol* 16(12): 2872–2891.

Dhall G, Finlay JL, Dunkel IJ et al. (2008) Analysis of outcome for patients with mass lesions of the central nervous system due to Langerhans cell histiocytosis treated with 2-chlorodeoxyadenosine. *Pediatr Blood Cancer* 50: 72–79.

Dhillo WS, Chaudhri OB, Thompson EL et al. (2007) Kisspeptin-54 stimulates gonadotropin release most potently during the preovulatory phase of the menstrual cycle in women. *J Clin Endocrinol Metab* 92(10): 3958–3966.

Di Pasquale E, Beck-Peccoz P and Persani L (2004) Hypergonadotropic ovarian failure associated with an inherited mutation of human bone morphogenetic protein-15 (BMP15) gene. *Am J Hum Genet* 75: 106–111.

Donadieu J, Rolon MA, Pion I et al. (2004) Incidence of growth hormone deficiency in pediatric-onset Langerhans cell histiocytosis: Efficacy and safety of growth hormone treatment. *J Clin Endocrinol Metab* 89: 604–609.

Dudas B and Merchenthaler I (2001) Catecholaminergic axons innervate LH-releasing hormone immunoreactive neurons of the human diencephalon. *J Clin Endocrinol Metab* 86(11): 5620–5626.

Dudas B and Merchenthaler I (2002) Close juxtapositions between LHRH immunoreactive neurons and substance P immunoreactive axons in the human diencephalon. *J Clin Endocrinol Metab* 87(6): 2946–2953.

Dudas B and Merchenthaler I (2003) Topography and associations of leu-enkephalin and luteinizing hormone-releasing hormone neuronal systems in the human diencephalon. *J Clin Endocrinol Metab* 88(4): 1842–1848.

Dudas B and Merchenthaler I (2004) Close anatomical associations between beta-endorphin and luteinizing hormone-releasing hormone neuronal systems in the human diencephalon. *Neuroscience* 124(1): 221–229.

Dungan HM, Gottsch ML, Zeng H et al. (2007) The role of kisspeptin-GPR54 signaling in the tonic regulation and surge release of gonadotropin-releasing hormone / luteinizing hormone. *J Neurosci* 27: 12088–12095.

Duvernoy H, Koritke JG and Monnier G (1970) Vascularization of the posterior tuber in man and its relation to the tuber-hypophyseal vasculature. *J Neurovisc Relat* 32(2): 112–142.

Evans JJ and Anderson GM (2012) Balancing ovulation and anovulation: Integration of the reproductive and energy balance axes by neuropeptides. *Hum Reprod Update* 18(3): 313–332.

Fahlbusch R, Honneger J, Paulus W et al. (1999) Surgical treatment of craniopharyngiomas: Experience with 168 patients. *J Neurosurg* 90: 237–250.

Fan NC, Peng C, Krisinger J and Leung PCK (1995) The human gonadotrophin receptor gene: Complete structure including multiple promoters, transcription initiation sites and polyadenylation signals. *Mol Cell Endocrinol* 107: R1–R8.

Fekete CS, Strutton PH, Cagampang FR et al. (1999) Estrogen receptor immunoreactivity is present in the majority of central histaminergic neurons: Evidence for a new neuroendocrine pathway associated with luteinizing hormone-releasing hormone-synthesizing neurons in rats and humans. *Endocrinology* 140(9): 4335–4341.

Fullerton G, Hamilton M and Maheshwari A (2010) Should non-mosaic Klinefelter syndrome men be labelled as infertile in 2009. *Hum Reprod* 25(3): 588–597.

Furuta M, Funabashi T and Kimura F (2001) Intracerebroventricular administration of ghrelin rapidly suppresses pulsatile luteinizing hormone secretion in ovariectomized rats. *Biochem Biophys Res Commun* 288: 780–785.

Gangwani V, Walker M, El-Defrawy H, Nicoll JA, Reck A and Pathmanathan T (2007) Langerhans cell histiocytosis of the optic chiasm. *Clin Experiment Ophthalmol* 35(1): 66–68.

Giovannucci E, Stampfer MJ, Krithivas K et al. (1997) The CAG repeat within the androgen receptor gene and its relationship to prostate cancer. *Proc Natl Acad Sci USA* 94(7): 3320–3323.

Gonzalez LC, Pinilla L, Tena-Sempere M and Aguilar E (1999) Leptin$_{116-130}$ stimulates prolactin and luteinizing hormone secretion in fasted adult male rats. *Neuroendocrinology* 70: 213–220.

Goswami D and Conway GS (2005) Premature ovarian failure. *Hum Reprod Update* 11: 391–410.

Gregory SJ and Kaiser UB (2004) Regulation of gonadotropins by inhibin and activin. *Semin Reprod Med* 22(3): 253–267.

Guran T, Tolhurst G, Bereket A et al. (2009) Hypogonadotropic hypogonadism due to a novel missense mutation in the first extracellular loop of the neurokinin B receptor. *J Clin Endocrinol Metab* 94(10): 3633–3639.

Harper P, Penny R, Foley TP Jr, Migeon CJ and Blizzard RM (1972) Gonadal function in males with myotonic dystrophy. *J Clin Endocrinol Metab* 35(6): 852.

Harris SE, Chand AL, Winship IM, Gersak K, Aittomaki K and Shelling AN (2002) Identification of novel mutations in FOXL2 associated with premature ovarian failure. *Mol Hum Reprod* 8: 729–733.

Hayes FJ, Pitteloud N, DeCruz S, Crowley WF Jr and Boepple PA (2001) Importance of inhibin B in the regulation of FSH secretion in the human male. *J Clin Endocrinol Metab* 86(11): 5541–5546.

Hayes FJ, Seminara SB, Decruz S, Boepple PA and Crowley WF Jr (2000) Aromatase inhibition in the human male reveals a hypothalamic site of estrogen feedback. *J Clin Endocrinol Metab* 85(9): 3027–3035.

Herbison AE and Moenter SM (2011) Depolarising and hyperpolarising actions of GABA(A) receptor activation on gonadotrophin-releasing hormone neurones: Towards an emerging consensus. *J Neuroendocrinol* 23(7): 557–569.

Hoffman GE, Le WW, Franceschini I, Caraty A and Advis JP (2011) Expression of fos and *in vivo* median eminence release of LHRH identifies an active role for preoptic area kisspeptin neurons in synchronized surges of LH and LHRH in the ewe. *Endocrinology* 152(1): 214–222.

Hokfelt T, Pernow B, Nilsson G, Wetterberg L, Goldstein M and Jeffcoate SL (1978) Dense plexus of substance P immunoreactive nerve terminals in eminentia medialis of the primate hypothalamus. *Proc Natl Acad Sci USA* 75(2): 1013–1015.

Hrabovszky E, Ciofi P, Vida B et al. (2010) The kisspeptin system of the human hypothalamus: Sexual dimorphism and relationship with gonadotropin-releasing hormone and neurokinin B neurons. *Eur J Neurosci* 31(11): 1984–1998.

Hrabovszky E, Molnar CS, Nagy R et al. (2012) Glutamatergic and GABAergic innervation of human gonadotropin-releasing hormone- I neurons. *Endocrinology* 153(6): 2766–2776.

Hrabovszky E, Molnar CS, Sipos MT et al. (2011) Sexual dimorphism of kisspeptin and neurokinin B immunoreactive neurons in the infundibular nucleus of aged men and women. *Front Endocrinol (Lausanne)* 2: 80.

Iqbal J, Kurose Y, Canny B and Clarke IJ (2006) Effects of central infusion of ghrelin on food intake and plasma levels of growth hormone, luteinizing hormone, prolactin, and cortisol secretion in sheep. *Endocrinology* 147: 510–519.

Irwig MS, Fraley GS, Smith JT et al. (2004) Kisspeptin activation of gonadotropin releasing hormone neurons and regulation of KiSS-1 mRNA in the male rat. *Neuroendocrinology* 80: 264–272.

Kaiser UB (1998) Molecular mechanism of the regulation of gonadotrophin gene expression by gonadotrophin-releasing hormone. *Mol Cells* 8: 647–656.

Kaltsas GA, Powles TB, Evanson J et al. (2000) Hypothalamo-pituitary abnormalities in adult patients with langerhans cell histiocytosis: Clinical, endocrinological, and radiological features and response to treatment. *J Clin Endocrinol Metab* 85: 1370–1376.

Kamischke A, Baumgardt A, Horst J and Nieschlag E (2003) Clinical and diagnostic features of patients with suspected Klinefelter syndrome. *J Androl* 24(1): 41–48.

Kater CE and Biglieri EG (1994) Disorders of steroid 17 alpha-hydroxylase deficiency. *Endocrinol Metab Clin North Am* 23(2): 341–357.

Kanwar P and Kowdley KV (2014) Metal storage disorders: Wilson disease and hemochromatosis. *Med Clin North Am* 98(1): 87–102.

Kaynard AH, Pau KY, Hess DL and Spies HG (1990) Third-ventricular infusion of neuropeptide Y 132. suppresses luteinizing hormonesecretion in ovariectomized rhesus macaques. *Endocrinology* 127(5): 2437–2444.

Keen KL, Wegner FH, Bloom SR, Ghatei MA and Terasawa E (2008) An increase in kisspeptin-54 release occurs with the pubertal increase in luteinizing hormone-releasing hormone-1 release in the stalk-median eminence of female rhesus monkeys in vivo. *Endocrinology* 149(8): 4151–4157.

Kerkerian L, Guy J, Lefevre G and Pelletier G (1985) Effects of neuropeptide Y (NPY) on the release of anterior pituitary hormones in the rat. *Peptides* 6(6): 1201–1204.

King JC and Anthony EL (1984) LHRH neurons and their projections in humans and other mammals: species comparisons. *Peptides* 5(Suppl 1): 195–207.

Kluge M, Schüssler P, Uhr M, Yassouridis A and Steiger A (2007) Ghrelin suppresses secretion of luteinizing hormone in humans. *J Clin Endocrinol Metab* 92: 3202–3205.

Kojima M, Hosoda H, Date Y, Nakazato M, Matsuo H and Kangawa K (1999) Ghrelin is a growth-hormone-releasing acylated peptide from stomach. *Nature* 402: 656–650.

Kotani M, Detheux M, Vandenbogaerde A et al. (2001) The metastasis suppressor gene KiSS-1 encodes kisspeptins, the natural ligands of the orphan, G. protein-coupled receptor GPR54. *J Biol Chem* 276: 34631–34636.

Kreuchwig A, Kleinau G and Krause G (2013) Research resource: Novel structural insights bridge gaps in glycoprotein hormone receptor analyses. *Mol Endocrinol* 27(8): 1357–1363.

Kriegsfeld LJ, Mei DF, Bentley GE et al. (2006) Identification and characterization of a gonadotropin-inhibitory system in the brains of mammals. *Proc Natl Acad Sci USA* 103(7): 2410–2415.

Lanfranco F, Bonelli L, Baldi M, Me E, Broglio F and Ghigo E (2008) Acylated ghrelin inhibits spontaneous LH pulsatility and responsiveness to naloxone, but not that to GnRH in young men: Evidence for a central inhibitory action of ghrelin on the gonadal axis. *J Clin Endocrinol Metab* 93: 3633–3639.

Lasaga M and Debeljuk L (2011) Tachykinins and the hypothalamo-pituitary-gonadal axis: An update. *Peptides* 32(9): 1972–1978.

Lehman MN, Coolen LM and Goodman RL (2010) Minireview: Kisspeptin/neurokinin B/dynorphin (KNDy) cells of the arcuate nucleus: A central node in the control of gonadotropin-releasing hormone secretion. *Endocrinology* 151(8): 3479–3489.

Leranth C, MacLusky NJ, Sakamoto H, Shanabrough M and Naftolin F (1985) Glutamic acid decarboxylase-containing axons synapse on LHRH neurons in the rat medial preoptic area. *Neuroendocrinology* 40(6): 536–539.

Licinio J, Mantzoros C, Negrao AB et al. (1997) Human leptin levels are pulsatile and inversely related to pituitary-adrenal function. *Nat Med* 3: 575–579.

Licinio J, Negrao AB, Mantzoros C et al. (1998) Synchronicity of frequently sampled, 24-h concentrations of circulating leptin, luteinizing hormone, and estradiol in healthy women. *Proc Natl Acad Sci USA* 95: 2541–2546.

Liquori CL, Ricker K, Moseley ML et al. (2001) Myotonic dystrophy type 2 caused by a CCTG expansion in intron 1 of ZNF9. *Science* 293(5531): 864.

Lopez FJ, Merchenthaler I, Ching M, Wisniewski MG and Negro-Vilar A (1991) Galanin: A hypothalamic-hypophysiotropic hormone modulating reproductive functions. *Proc Natl Acad Sci USA* 88(10): 4508–4512.

Low MJ (2016) Neuroendocrinology. In: Melmed S, Polonsky KS, Reed Larsen P and Kronenberg (eds) *Williams Textbook of Endocrinology 13th Edition*. Canada: Elsevier, 110–175.

Ludwig M, Westergaard LG, Diedrich K and Andersen CY (2003) Developments in drugs for ovarian stimulation. *Best Pract Res Clin Obstet Gynaecol* 17(2): 231–247.

Mahadevan M, Tsilfidis C, Sabourin L et al. (1992) Myotonic dystrophy mutation: An unstable CTG repeat in the 3' untranslated region of the gene. *Science* 255(5049): 1253–1255.

Makras P, Alexandraki KI, Chrousos GP, Grossman AB and Kaltsas GA (2007) Endocrine manifestations in Langerhans cell histiocytosis. *Trends Endocrinol Metab* 18: 252–257.

Mantzoros CS (1999) The role of leptin in human obesity and disease: A review of current evidence. *Ann Intern Med* 130: 671–680.

Martínez de la Escalera G, Choi AL and Weiner RI (1992) Generation and synchronization of gonadotropin-releasing hormone (GnRH) pulses: Intrinsic properties of the GT1-1 GnRH neuronal cell line. *Proc Natl Acad Sci USA* 89(5): 1852–1855.

McNeil LW, McKee LC, Lorber D and Rabin D (1983) The endocrine manifestations of hemochromatosis. *Am J Med Sci* 285: 7–13.

Messager S, Chatzidaki EE, Ma D et al. (2005) Kisspeptin directly stimulates gonadotropin-releasing hormone release via G. protein-coupled receptor 54. *Proc Natl Acad Sci USA* 102: 1761–1766.

Misell LM, Holochwost D, Boban D et al. (2006) A stable isotope-mass spectrometric method for measuring human spermatogenesis kinetics in vivo. *J Urol* 175(1): 242–246.

Mittelman-Smith MA, Williams H, Krajewski-Hall SJ et al. (2012a) Arcuate kisspeptin/neurokinin B/dynorphin (KNDy) neurons mediate the estrogen suppression of gonadotropin secretion and body weight. *Endocrinology* 153(6): 2800–2812.

Mittelman-Smith MA, Williams H, Krajewski-Hall SJ et al. (2012b) Role for kisspeptin/neurokinin B/dynorphin (KNDy) neurons in cutaneous vasodilatation and the estrogen modulation of body temperature. *Proc Natl Acad Sci USA* 109(48): 19846–19851.

Molnar CS, Vida B, Sipos MT et al. (2012) Morphological evidence for enhanced kisspeptin and neurokinin B signaling in the infundibular nucleus of the aging man. *Endocrinology* 153(11): 5428–5439.

Mootha SL, Barkovic AJ, Grumbach MM et al. (1997) Idiopathic hypothalamic diabetes insipidus, pituitary stalk thickening and the occult intracranial germinoma in children and adolescents. *J Clin Endocrinol Metab* 82: 1362–1367.

Muller J, Gondos B and Kosugi S (1998) Severe testotoxicosis phenotype associated with Asp578: Tyr mutation of the lutrophin/choriogonadotrophin receptor gene. *J Med Genet* 35: 340–341.

Nagatani S, Zeng Y, Keisler DH, Foster DL and Jaffe CA (2000) Leptin regulates pulsatile luteinizing hormone and growth hormone secretion in the sheep. *Endocrinology* 141: 3965–3975.

Nanduri VR, Bareille P, Pritchard J and Stanhope R (2000) Growth and endocrine disorders in multisystem Langerhans' cell histiocytosis. *Clin Endocrinol (Oxf)* 53: 509–515.

Navarro VM, Castellano JM, Fernández-Fernández R et al. (2005) Characterization of the potent luteinizing hormone-releasing activity of KiSS-1 peptide, the natural ligand of GPR54. *Endocrinology* 146: 156–163.

Navarro-Costa P, Gonçalves J and Plancha CE (2010) The AZFc region of the Y chromosome: At the crossroads between genetic diversity and male infertility. *Hum Reprod Update* 16(5): 525–542.

Nonogaki K (2008) Ghrelin and feedback systems. *Vitam Horm* 77: 149–170.

Oakley AE, Clifton DK and Steiner RA (2009) Kisspeptin signaling in the brain. *Endocr Rev* 30: 713–743.

Panula P, Pirvola U, Auvinen S and Airaksinen MS (1989) Histamine-immunoreactive nerve fibers in the rat brain. *Neuroscience* 28(3): 585–610.

Parker SL, Kalra SP and Crowley WR (1991) Neuropeptide Y modulates the binding of a gonadotropin-releasing hormone (GnRH) analog to anterior pituitary GnRH receptor sites. *Endocrinology* 128(5): 2309–2316.

Pfeiffer A and Herz A (1984) Endocrine actions of opioids. *Horm Metab Res* 16(8): 386–397.

Pielecka-Fortuna J, Chu Z and Moenter SM (2008) Kisspeptin acts directly and indirectly to increase gonadotropin-releasing hormone neuron activity and its effects are modulated by estradiol. *Endocrinology* 149: 1979–1986.

Pierroz DD, Gruaz NM, d'Alieves V and Aubert ML (1995) Chronic administration of neuropeptide Y into the lateral ventricle starting at 30 days of life delays sexual maturation in the female rat. *Neuroendocrinology* 61(3): 293–300.

Pineda R, Garcia-Galiano D, Roseweir A et al. (2010) Critical roles of kisspeptins in female puberty and preovulatory gonadotropin surges as revealed by a novel antagonist. *Endocrinology* 151: 722–730.

Quaynor SD, Stradtman EW Jr, Kim HG et al. (2013) Delayed puberty and estrogen resistance in a woman with estrogen receptor alpha variant. *N Engl J Med* 369(2): 164–171.

Quigley CA, De Bellis A, Marschke KB, el-Awady MK, Wilson EM and French FS (June 1995). Androgen receptor defects: Historical, clinical, and molecular perspectives. *Endocr Rev* 16(3): 271–321.

Rak-Mardyla A (2013) Ghrelin role in hypothalamus-pituitary-ovarian axis. *J Physiol Pharmacol* 64(6): 695–704.

Rance NE and Young WS III (1991) Hypertrophy and increased gene expression of neurons containing neurokinin-B and substance-P messenger ribonucleic acids in the hypothalami of post-menopausal women. *Endocrinology* 128(5): 2239–2247.

Raposinho PD, Pierroz DD, Broqua P, White RB, Pedrazzini T and Aubert ML (2001) Chronic administration of neuropeptide Y into the lateral ventricle of C57BL/6J male mice produces an obesity syndrome including hyperphagia, hyperleptinemia, insulin resistance, and hypogonadism. *Mol Cell Endocrinol* 185(1–2): 195–204.

Razzaque MA, Nishizawa T, Komoike Y et al. (2007) Germline gain-of-function mutations in *RAF1* cause Noonan syndrome. *Nat Genet* 39(8): 1013–1017.

Roa J, Aguilar E, Dieguez C, Pinilla and L Tena-Sempere M (2008) New frontiers in kisspeptin/GPR54 physiology as fundamental gatekeepers of reproductive function. *Front Neuroendocrinol* 29: 48–69.

Roa J, Castellano JM, Navarro VM, Handelsman DJ, Pinilla L and Tena-Sempere M (2009) Kisspeptins and the control of gonadotropin secretion in male and female rodents. *Peptides* 30: 57–66.

Roa J, Vigo E, Castellano JM et al. (2008) Follicle-stimulating hormone responses to kisspeptin in the female rat at the preovulatory period: Modulation by estrogen and progesterone receptors. *Endocrinology* 149: 5783–5790.

Roberts AE, Araki T, Swanson KD et al. (2007). Germline gain-of-function mutations in SOS1 cause Noonan syndrome. *Nat Genet* 39(1): 70–74.

Roberts CB, Campbell RE, Herbison AE and Suter KJ (2008) Dendritic action potential initiation in hypothalamic gonadotropin-releasing hormone neurons. *Endocrinology* 149(7): 3355–3360.

Rometo AM and Rance NE (2008) Changes in prodynorphin gene expression and neuronal morphology in the hypothalamus of postmenopausal women. *J Neuroendocrinol* 20(12): 1376–1381.

Roseweir AK, Kauffman AS, Smith JT et al. (2009) Discovery of potent kisspeptin antagonists delineate physiological mechanisms of gonadotropin regulation. *J Neurosci* 29: 3920–3929.

Sahu A, Xu B and Kalra SP (1994) Role of galanin in stimulation of pituitary luteinizing hormone secretion as revealed by a specific receptor antagonist, galantide. *Endocrinology* 134(2): 529–536.

Schubbert S, Zenker M, Rowe SL et al. (2006). Germline KRAS mutations cause Noonan syndrome. *Nat Genet* 38(3): 331–336.

Schulz R, Wilhelm A, Pirke KM, Gramsch C and Herz A (1981) Beta-endorphin and dynorphin control serum luteinizing hormone level in immature female rats. *Nature* 294(5843): 757–759.

Seminara SB, Messager S, Chatzidaki EE et al. (2003) The GPR54 gene as a regulator of puberty. *N Engl J Med* 349: 1614–1627.

Shacham S, Harris D, Ben-Shlomo H et al. (2001) Mechanism of GnRH receptor signaling on gonadotropin release and gene expression in pituitary gonadotrophs. *Vitam Horm* 63: 63–90.

Sharpe RH (1976) hCG induced decrease in availability of rat testes receptors. *Nature* 264: 644–646.

Shchelochkov OA, Patel A and Weissenberger GM et al. (2008) Duplication of chromosome band 12q24.11q24.23 results in apparent Noonan syndrome. *Am J Med Genet* 146A(8): 1042–1048.

Simm PJ and Zacharin MR (April 2006). The psychosocial impact of Klinefelter syndrome – A 10 year review. *J Pediatr Endocrinol Metab* 19(4): 499–505.

Simoni M, Gromoll J and Nieschlag E (1998) Molecular pathophysiology and clinical manifestations of gonadotrophin receptor defects. *Steroids* 63: 288–293.

Simonian SX, Spratt DP and Herbison AE (1999) Identification and characterization of estrogen receptor alpha-containing neurons projecting to the vicinity of the gonadotropin-releasing hormone perikarya in the rostral preoptic area of the rat. *J Comp Neurol* 411(2): 346–358.

Sir-Petermann T, Maliqueo M, Palomino A, Vantman D, Recabarren SE and Wildt L (1999) Episodic leptin release is independent of luteinizing hormone secretion. *Hum Reprod* 14: 2695–2699.

Smith JT, Li Q, Pereira A and Clarke IJ (2009) Kisspeptin neurons in the ovine arcuate nucleus and preoptic area are involved in the preovulatory luteinizing hormone surge. *Endocrinology* 150(12): 5530–5538.

Smith JT, Dungan HM, Stoll EA et al. (2005a) Differential regulation of KiSS-1 mRNA expression by sex steroids in the brain of the male mouse. *Endocrinology* 146: 2976–2984.

Smith JT, Cunningham MJ, Rissman EF, Clifton DK and Steiner RA (2005b) Regulation of Kiss1 gene expression in the brain of the female mouse. *Endocrinology* 146: 3686–3692.

Spratt DI, Carr DH, Merriam GR et al. (1987) The spectrum of abnormal patterns of gonadotrophin-releasing hormone secretion in men with idiopathic hypogonadotrophic hypogonadism: Clinical and laboratory correlations. *J Clin Endoc* 64: 283–291.

Stockschlaeder M and Sucker C (2006) Adult Langerhans cell histiocytosis. *Eur J Haematol* 76(5): 363–368.

Takaya K, Ariyasu H, Kanamoto N et al. (2000) Ghrelin strongly stimulates growth hormone release in humans. *J Clin Endocrinol Metab* 85: 4908–4911.

Tartaglia M, Mehler EL, Goldberg R et al. (2001). Mutations in PTPN11, encoding the protein tyrosine phosphatase SHP-2, cause Noonan syndrome. *Nat Genet* 29(4): 465–468.

Tenhola H, Sinclair D, Alho H and Lahti T (2012) Effect of opioid antagonists on sex hormone secretion. *J Endocrinol Invest* 35(2): 227–230.

Thigpen AE, Silver RI, Guileyardo JM, Casey ML, McConnell JD and Russell DW (1993) Tissue distribution and ontogeny of steroid 5 alpha-reductase isozyme expression. *J Clin Invest* 92(2): 903–910.

Topaloglu AK, Reimann F, Guclu M et al. (2009) TAC3 and TACR3 mutations in familial hypogonadotropic hypogonadism reveal a key role for Neurokinin B in the central control of reproduction. *Nat Genet* 41(3): 354–358.

Ubuka T, Lai H, Kitani M et al. (2009) Gonadotropin-inhibitory hormone identification, cDNA cloning, and distribution in rhesus macaque brain. *J Comp Neurology* 517(6): 841–855.

Van Der Burgt I and Brunner H (2000) Genetic heterogeneity in Noonan syndrome: Evidence for an autosomal recessive form. *American Journal of Medical Genetics* 94(1): 46–51.

Verhoeven G, Hoeben E and De Gendt K (2000) Peritubular cell-Sertoli cell interactions: Factors involved in PmodS activity. *Andrologia* 32(1): 42–45.

von Eckardstein S, Simoni M, Bergmann M et al. (1999) Serum inhibin-B in combination with serum follicle-stimulating hormone (FSH) is a more sensitive marker than serum FSH alone for impaired spermatogenesis in men, but cannot predict the presence of sperm in testicular tissue samples. *J Clin Endocrinol Metab* 84: 2496–2501.

Wang C, Catlin DH, Starcevic B et al. (2004) Testosterone metabolic clearance and production rates determined by stable isotope dilution/tandem mass spectrometry in normal men: Influence of ethnicity and age. *J Clin Endocrinol Metab* 89(6): 2936–2941.

Wara WM, Fellows FC and Sheline GE (1977) Radiation therapy for pineal tumours and suprasellar germinomas. *Radiology* 124: 221–223.

Wintermantel TM, Campbell RE, Porteous R et al. (2006) Definition of estrogen receptor pathway critical for estrogen positive feedback to gonadotropin-releasing hormone neurons and fertility. *Neuron* 52: 271–280.

Wormald PJ, Millar RP and Kerdelhue B (1989) Substance P receptors in human pituitary: A potential inhibitor of luteinizing hormone secretion. *J Clin Endocrinol Metab* 69(3): 612–615.

Yang Y, Ma MY, Xiao CY, Li L, Li SW and Zhang SZ (2008) Massive deletion in AZFb/b+c and azoospermia with Sertoli cell only and/or maturation arrest. *Int J Androl* 31(6): 573–578.

Yura A, Ogawa Y, Sagawa N et al. (2000) Accelerated puberty and late-onset hypothalamic hypogonadism in female transgenic skinny mice overexpressing leptin. *J Clin Invest* 105: 749–755.

Zinn AR, Ramos P, Elder FF, Kowal K, Samango-Sprouse C and Ross JL (2005) Androgen receptor CAGn repeat length influences phenotype of 47, XXY (Klinefelter) syndrome. *J Clin Endocrinol Metabol* 90(9): 5041–5046.

19
THE INHERITED BASIS OF HYPOGONADOTROPIC HYPOGONADISM

Pierre-Marc G Bouloux

Introduction

Congenital isolated hypogonadotropic hypogonadism (CIHH) is a well-known cause of absent pubertal development in both sexes and results directly from inadequate secretion of the gonadotrophins, luteinizing hormone (LH) and follicle-stimulating hormone (FSH), most commonly secondary to subnormal secretion of hypothalamic gonadotrophin-releasing hormone (GnRH), with consequent impairment of normal testicular or ovarian function. With a prevalence estimation, based on a civilian and military hospital series, of 1/4000 to 1/10 000 in males (Fromantin et al. 1973), CIHH is reported to be between two and five times more common in boys than in girls (Seminara et al. 1998). CIHH patients usually come to clinical attention during adolescence or adulthood because of incomplete or absent pubertal development; owing to progress in molecular genetics and clinical practice, the diagnosis can be made earlier in cases where the diagnosis is specifically sought.

Congenital hypogonadotropic hypogonadism is a component of several syndromes, usually managed in the paediatric setting (Table 19.1), when it may occur together with non-gonadal features such as short stature due to growth hormone deficiency and other anterior pituitary hormone deficiencies (Netchine et al. 2000; Reynaud et al. 2005), primary adrenal failure (Lin et al. 2006), (early onset) childhood obesity (Clement et al. 1998; Strobel et al. 1998) or in association with several neurological disorders (Quinton et al. 1999a; Dollfus et al. 2005; Goldstone et al. 2008), when early onset of the extragonadal features may predominate.

Current understanding of the pathophysiology and origins of CIHH can be gleaned from the ontogeny of the GnRH neuronal system and the rapid progress made in the molecular genetics that have unravelled this condition.

Ontogeny of the gonadotrophin-releasing hormone system

Embryological studies conducted in mammals (Schwanzel-Fukuda and Pfaff 1989; Wray et al. 1989; Schwanzel-Fukuda 1999; Wray 2001), birds (Murakami et al. 2002), amphibians (Muske and Moore 1990) and fish (Parhar 2002) have established that neuroendocrine GnRH cells originate, proliferate and then migrate from the medial part of the olfactory pit

TABLE 19.1
Genetic syndromes associated with hypogonadotropic hypogonadism

Symptoms	Phenotype	Genetic defect
Prader–Willi	Intellectual disability, morbid obesity, hypotonia	Deletions within paternally imprinted 15q 11.2-12 region
	Carbohydrate intolerance	
	Cryptorchidism	
Laurence–Moon–Bardet–Biedl	Intellectual disability, obesity, retinitis pigmentosa, autosomal recessive post-axial polydactyly	BBS-1-11 (multiple loci)
		20p12
		16q21, 15q22.3-23, 14q32.1
Biemond	Iris coloboma, polydactyly, developmental delay	
Congenital adrenal hypoplasia	Adrenal hypoplasia	
	Primary adrenal deficiency, hypogonadotrophic hypogonadism	DAX-1
CHARGE syndrome	Coloboma, heart anomaly, Choanal atresia, growth retardation, genital anomalies, ear anomalies	CHD7
Septo-optic dysplasia	Small, dysplastic pale optic discs	HESX1
	Pendular nystagmus, midline Hypothalamic defect with DI, GH, ACTH, TSH and LH/FSH deficiency, absent seotum pellucidum	
Solitary median maxillary incisor syndrome	Prominent midpalatal ridge	SHH 7q3
	Hypopituitarism	
	GH, TSH, LH/FSH deficiency	PROP1 5q
	LH, FSH + multiple hormone deficiencies	LHX3
	Severe restriction of head rotation due to rigid cervical spine	
	Anterior pituitary hypoplasia	SOX2
	Anophthalmia, microphthalmia	
	Coloboma	
Borjeson–Forssman–Lehmann syndrome	Intellectual disability	X-linked ataxia
Gorden Holmes	HH, ataxia, dementia	Inactivating mutations in RNF216/OTUD4

into the brain in an axonophilic manner along the olfactory–vomeronasal nerve pathway. The stem cell population giving rise to GnRH neurons is as yet unknown because cells are only identifiable once they express GnRH. In humans, GnRH neuronal migration begins during the sixth embryonic week, at a time when axon terminals of the olfactory sensory neurons first come into contact with the rostral pole of the forebrain just before the emergence of the olfactory bulbs. On reaching the base of the telencephalon, GnRH neurons penetrate into the brain, just caudal to the olfactory bulb anlage, before making their way superficially along the medial wall of the cerebral hemisphere to their final resting location in the septopreoptic hypothalamic region (Muller and O'Rahilly 1989).

The fully developed GnRH system consists between 1500 and 2000 neurons scattered in the anterior septopreoptic area of the hypothalamus, whose axons converge and abut the basement membrane of the median eminence portal capillaries where GnRH neurosecretion occurs. This full developmental sequence, completed by the eighth to ninth week of embryonic development, can therefore be compartmentalised into several discrete but well-coordinated events, starting with (1) fate specification of GnRH neurons; (2) expansion of cell numbers (mitosis and apoptosis); (3) cell migration (a mixture of chemorepulsive and chemorepellent events); (4) coalescence of individual GnRH neurons into a responsive, secreting and coordinating network functioning in an integrated manner; and (5) the development of a capacity to incorporate and integrate internal and external feedback signals into the final feedback control mechanisms that modulate GnRH release. Mutations in the genes whose actions determine any one or more of these pathways could theoretically underpin congenital forms of hypogonadotropic hypogonadism. Postnatally, a further tier of regulation of these neurosecretory events involves the reversible detachment of these nerve endings onto the capillary loops of the median eminence (Prevot et al. 2010).

Over the past 22 years, steady progress has been made towards unravelling the molecular genetic abnormalities that can underpin the inherited forms of hypogonadotropic hypogonadism. What has emerged is a complex group of genes and patterns of inheritance spanning from classic monogenic to what seems to be increasingly recognised as an oligogenic disorder involving potentially interacting genes underpinning the phenotype.

Development of reproductive activity

In humans, the fetal GnRH pulse generator and its downstream gonadotrope and gonadal axis activation are functional in both sexes by the end of the first trimester of gestation but then become quiescent in utero such that by the time of parturition, cord blood serum luteinizing hormone and FSH are fully suppressed, the consequence of negative feedback inhibition from placentally derived sex steroids. Shortly after birth, male infants demonstrate a brief surge of luteinizing hormone and testosterone that persists for about 12h, followed by, about 1–2 weeks later (with the gradual elimination of placentally derived inhibitory hormonal influences), what is tantamount to a minipuberty, differing in its duration between the two sexes (Massa et al. 1992). Thus, in males, luteinizing hormone, FSH and testosterone peak between 4 and 10 weeks. The hypothalamo–pituitary axis then gradually becomes less active until around 6 months, after which GnRH quiescence becomes complete (Andersson et al. 1998), only to be reawakened with the onset of puberty. At the onset of puberty, Sertoli cells undergo a radical change in their morphology and function, switching from an immature proliferative state to a mature, nonproliferative state. FSH induces proliferation of immature Sertoli cells, and the number of Sertoli cells is directly associated with sperm-producing capability. In females, there is a greater persistence of GnRH secretory activation for up to 3 years, with a greater preponderance of FSH secretion throughout. The male minipuberty serves to expand the pool of Sertoli cells, with a concomitant increase in germ cells available for future fertility (Sharpe et al. 2003). In macaque monkeys, exposure to superactive GnRH analogues at this critical phase leads to the suppression of future fertility potential (Mann et al. 1985). A further effect of the minipuberty is the exposure of the developing male brain to testosterone concentrations not far short of adult values, as well as those of hormone-sensitive tissues such as the penis and for completion of testicular descent. Absence of in utero and early postnatal sex steroid exposure may explain in part the frequency of micropenis seen in males with idiopathic hypogonadotropic hypogonadism (IHH).

Gonadotrophin secretion then becomes effectively silenced by an ill-understood restraint mechanism until the onset of puberty.

Clinical presentation of hypogonadotropic hypogonadism

Hypogonadotropic hypogonadism is suspected when onset of pubertal development is incomplete or absent after the age of 13 years in girls and 14 years in boys, particularly if pubertal delay is associated with cryptorchidism or micropenis or is persistent after the age of 18 years. In females, it is likely to present as failure of breast and secondary sexual hair development in association with primary amenorrhoea, associated with low concentrations of FSH, luteinizing hormone and oestradiol.

Prepubertal diagnosis in boys with CIHH is rarely made before puberty, although the presence of neonatal unilateral or bilateral cryptorchidism or micropenis or hyposmia/ anosmia may suggest the diagnosis; the finding of low gonadotrophins and testosterone during the expected minipuberty (within the first 6 months of postnatal life) can establish an early diagnosis if cryptorchidism, micropenis or both are present (Grumbach et al. 2005).

Constitutional short stature and pubertal delay (CSSPD) can cause diagnostic confusion: in complete forms, CIHH can be usually distinguished from CSSPD by virtue of the growth pattern, with CIHH having normal height for chronological age and CSSPD tending to be short. (Uriarte et al. 1992) In mild or partial forms, additional associated physical signs (e.g. cryptorchidism or micropenis) suggestive of a syndromic form can be helpful. CIHH has a normal growth pattern during childhood but lacks the usual pubertal growth spurt. The absence of long-bone epiphyseal closure results in eunuchoid proportions and relative tall stature, and an arm span exceeding height. Lack of exposure to testosterone not only leads to relative stunting of upper-segment growth, and general retardation of bone maturation, but also predisposes to osteopenia, and osteoporosis in later life (Finkelstein et al. 1987).

Gynaecomastia is occasionally seen in patients with untreated CIHH, although more usually after human chorionic gonadotropin (hCG) or supraphysiological testosterone exposure, the latter being due to aromatisation into oestradiol. Partial congenital gonadotropin deficiency affects only a minority of male patients and is characterised by incomplete virilisation, gynaecomastia and a testicular volume >4mL or even close to normal and with only moderate clinical and endocrine abnormalities.

Congenital isolated hypogonadotropic hypogonadism in women

In >90% of women, CIHH is characterised by primary amenorrhoea, with variable breast development ranging from absent to almost normal. Pubic hair may be absent, sparse or even normal. Partial forms may lead to an underestimation of the true prevalence of this condition in females. The mildest form, present in a minority of women, is associated with isolated chronic anovulation, with oestradiol secretion adequate for endometrial development as evidenced by progestogen-induced endometrial stripping; oligomenorrhoea may be present in these women. These attenuated forms have also been described in women having conceived spontaneously.

Diagnostic difficulty may arise in women with primary amenorrhoea, normal olfaction and no identified mutation where the differential diagnosis lies between CIHH and functional hypothalamic amenorrhoea. In such cases, it is important to exclude other causes of hypogonadotropic hypogonadism such as those due to low body mass, eating disorders, excessive physical activity and chronic underlying conditions. Sometimes, only after a period of observation with later reassessment of the hypothalamo–pituitary ovarian axis can the diagnosis be established. It has recently become recognised that a genetic lesion responsible for CIHH may be present in a significant number of women presenting with hypothalamic amenorrhoea (Caronia et al. 2011).

Clinical evaluation of suspected congenital isolated hypogonadotropic hypogonadism

The first step in the evaluation is a thorough anamnesis and family history followed by physical examination. Certain physical signs will increase suspicion of underlying CIHH, such as hyposmia/anosmia, cleft lip/palate, bimanual synkinesia (Conrad et al. 1978; Schwankhaus et al. 1989) and features suggesting the CHARGE syndrome (Pinto et al. 2005) as well as skeletal abnormalities (Fig 19.1). Pubertal status according to Tanner staging should be established. Family history should focus on the reproductive histories of male and female family members.

The many non-reproductive phenotypes associated with CIHH therefore include the following: mirror movements of the upper limbs (bimanual synkinesis) (Quinton et al. 1996, 2001; Mayston et al. 1997; Krams et al. 1999), eye movement abnormalities (Schwankhaus et al. 1989), congenital ptosis and abnormal visual spatial attention (Kertzman et al. 1990), hearing impairment (Santen and Paulsen 1972), renal agenesis (Wegenke et al. 1975), cleft lip or palate (Murray and Schutte 2004), agenesis of one or several teeth (hypodontia) (Molsted et al. 1997), obesity and digital abnormalities (Lieblich et al. 1982).[40]

Kallmann syndrome

Kallmann syndrome is diagnosed when low serum gonadotropins and gonadal steroids are coupled with a compromised sense of smell (hyposmia or anosmia), with the latter being

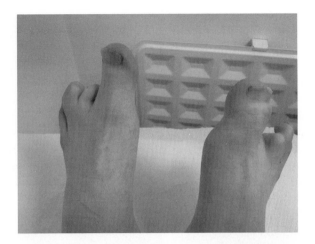

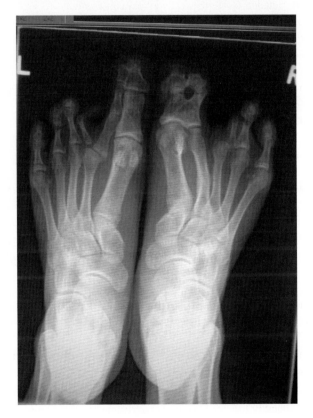

Figure 19.1. Digital abnormality of the toes with corresponding radiograph, with broad great toe in a male with a de novo mutation of fibroblast growth factor receptor 1 (*FGFR1*), anosmia and hypogonadotropic hypogonadism. The hands were normal.

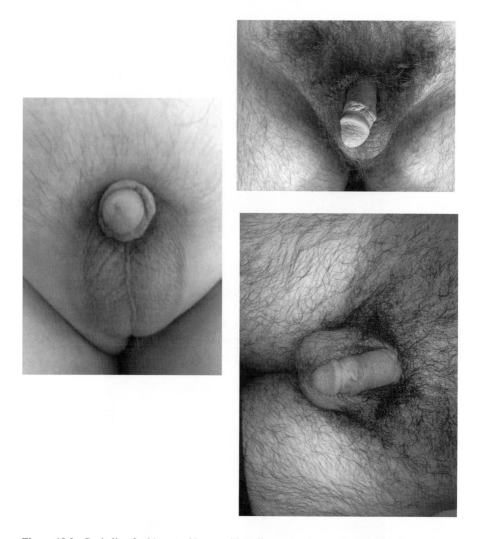

Figure 19.2. Genitalia of a 21-year-old man with Kallmann syndrome. Sparse pubic hair represents the effects of adrenarche, and the penile shaft is short and the scrotum hypoplastic. Luteinizing hormone <0.1 IU/L, follicle-stimulating hormone <0.1 IU/L, testosterone <0.5nmol/L and testes are <4ml. The responses to human chorionic gonadotropin (hCG) alone (1 500U twice weekly for 6 months and after 6 months of combined hCG and cofollitrophin treatment) are shown.

ascertainable on the anamnesis (subjective) or by means of detailed questioning or objectively by formal olfactory test, such as the Pennsylvania smell test.

Even severe CIHH in men is not associated with ambiguous external genitalia, and the penis can range from normal to micropenis proportions (Fig 19.2). Although luteinizing hormone and FSH will have been deficient in these cases, testosterone secretion secondary to fetal Leydig cell stimulation by placental hCG will have occurred during early development.

INVESTIGATIONS

In males, the diagnosis of hypogonadotropic hypogonadism is based on low plasma total testosterone concentrations, usually associated with an inappropriately low or 'normal' luteinizing hormone and FSH. Although it was thought that the use of ultrasensitive gonadotrophin assays might also give an insight into the central control of gonadotrophin secretion in affected individuals, with some patients showing no discernible pulsatile luteinizing hormone secretion, others demonstrating reduced luteinizing hormone pulse frequency or amplitude and still others an exclusively luteinizing hormone nocturnal secretion, it has become evident that there is no genotype–phenotype relationship between the luteinizing hormone secretion profile and underlying genetic abnormality (see Fig 19.3).

Patients with complete gonadotropin deficiency pose no diagnostic difficulties with prepubertal range testosterone concentrations and low inhibin B concentrations, a marker of FSH deficiency. Difficulties arise in partial forms of CIHH when gonadotrophin and inhibin B concentrations can be in the reference range. Other studies have shown that patients with CIHH retain prepubertal circulating anti-Müllerian hormone concentrations indicative of absent pubertal FSH-dependent testicular maturation, induced by intratesticular testosterone (Young et al. 1999). Its use for diagnostic purposes is still under evaluation.

Short and long gonadotropin-releasing hormone test
It is doubtful whether the GnRH test provides any additional information to that gleaned from ultrasensitive baseline gonadotrophin assays. The conventional 100μg GnRH test does

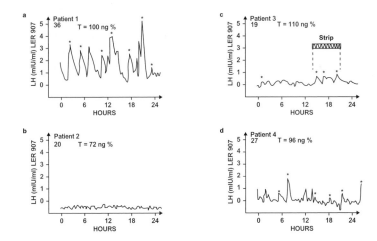

Figure 19.3. Heterogeneity in the profiles of luteinizing hormone (LH) and follicle-stimulating hormone secretion in patients with isolated hypogonadotropic hypogonadism (IHH). The pulsatile LH secretion in a healthy young man (a) is contrasted with a complete absence of LH pulses in a man with IHH (b). The patient in (c) has a few low-amplitude, night-time LH pulses, reminiscent of early puberty, while the patient in (d) has a normal frequency of LH pulses, all of which have low amplitude. It now seems likely that this clinical heterogeneity in LH pulsatile secretion is due to different degrees of gonadotropin-releasing hormone deficiency and reflects genetic heterogeneity in the pathophysiology of this syndrome. (Adapted from Crowley WF Jr et al. *Recent Prog Horm Res*, 41, 473–531, 1985.)

not usually discriminate between gonadotrophin deficiency of hypothalamic or pituitary origin, and a partial response is usually present in partial pituitary deficiency, both in patients with CIHH and in those with acquired postpubertal hypogonadotropic hypogonadism. In congenital gonadotropin deficiencies, the response to GnRH test is highly variable; absent responses are seen when the testes are very small in men and breast development is absent in women. In complete forms with testicular volumes <2mL, a slight or totally absent gonadotrophin response is observed. In partial forms with testicular volume >6mL, the response can be positive, or even supranormal in the case of luteinizing hormone.

Plasma oestradiol concentrations are often near the detection limit in CIHH, paralleling the degree of breast development, whereas oestradiol can range from just detectable when a little breast development is present to the concentrations seen in the mid-follicular phase in patients with Tanner 3–4 breast development.

Finally, before making a firm diagnosis of isolated congenital gonadotropin deficiency, all anterior pituitary functions must be investigated to exclude hyperprolactinaemia or other anterior pituitary deficiencies or an associated endocrine disorder that may be a part of syndromic forms of CHH. In all cases of CIHH, the diagnostic work-up should include serum iron-binding capacity and ferritin concentrations to rule out haemochromatosis, and the anamnesis should rule out other underlying chronic illness and opioid use.

Ultrasound examination

Renal ultrasound examination can reveal malformation or unilateral agenesis in patients with X-linked *KAL1* but is invariably normal in other causes of CIHH (euosmic and hyposmic) (Kirk et al. 1994). Ultrasound examination of the scrotum and testes is helpful in situations where there is difficulty palpating the testes, and to give objective evidence of maldescent and its level.

In women, transabdominal ultrasound can help size the uterus, an indicator of estrogenic exposure, and transvaginal ultrasound, where possible, can enable direct visualisation of endometrial thickness, ovary volume and the number of developing follicles and their size, which reflects the severity of gonadotrophin deficiency.

Hypothalamo-pituitary imaging

Magnetic resonance imaging (MRI) of the brain and olfactory bulbs is useful in CIHH and can demonstrate absent or hypoplastic olfactory bulbs and sulci in cases of Kallmann syndrome (Klingmüller et al. 1987; Quinton et al. 1996) (Fig 19.4). MRI is also useful to exclude hypothalamic or pituitary lesions as the cause of hypogonadotropic hypogonadism. MRI is invariably normal in IHH but can occasionally show structural abnormalities such as absent corpus callosum and abnormal cerebellum, in specific cases.

Classification of genetic causes of hypogonadotropic hypogonadism

Rapid progress has been made in unravelling the genetic basis of CIHH. Targeted clinical investigation, together with the catalyst provided by mapping of the human genome, has enabled the identification of several genes involved in GnRH ontogeny and whose loss of function, singly or in combination, results in the phenotype of hypogonadotropic

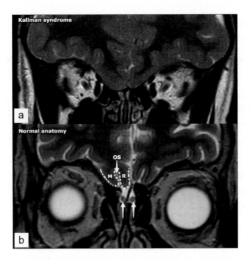

Figure 19.4. Coronal MRI showing absent bullbs and sulci in (a) a patient with Kallmann syndrome and normal olfactory sulci and bulbls in (b) a typical individual The arrows point to the anatomy of normal olfactory bulbs on the cribriform plate.

hypogonadism. The genes whose loss of function results in hypogonadotropic hypogonadism can broadly be classified into four groups (Fig 19.5).

1. Genes that appear to represent purely neurodevelopmental genes whose loss of function affects the development and migration of GnRH neurons into the hypothalamus (*KAL1, NELF*, fibroblast growth factor receptor 1 [*FGFR1*], fibroblast growth factor 8 *[FGF8]* and its synexpression group, *PROKR2, PROK2, CHD7, SEM3A, SEM3E, HS6ST1, WDR11*)
2. Genes that appear to be involved in GnRH synthesis and release (*GnRH1, KISS 1, KISS1R (GPR54), TAC3, TACR3*, Leptin and its receptor, *SF1, DAX1*)
3. Genes involved in GnRH action (*GnRHR*)
4. Genes involved in gonadotrophin synthesis (*LH*β, *FSH*β)

Genes mutated in hypogonadotropic hypogonadism

Multiple genetic defects can cause Kallmann syndrome (Table 19.2), and multiple inheritance patterns have been reported, including X-linked recessive, autosomal dominant and autosomal recessive. Frequently, however, the condition is sporadic. For each genetic form of Kallmann syndrome identified so far, the clinical heterogeneity of the disease within affected families clearly indicates that the manifestation of Kallmann syndrome phenotypes is dependent on factors other than the mutated gene itself. These factors may include epigenetic factors and modifier genes. More recently, it has become evident that CIHH is not infrequently a digenic or oligogenic condition, a further explanation for the variable penetrance of the disease within pedigrees (Pitteloud et al. 2007).

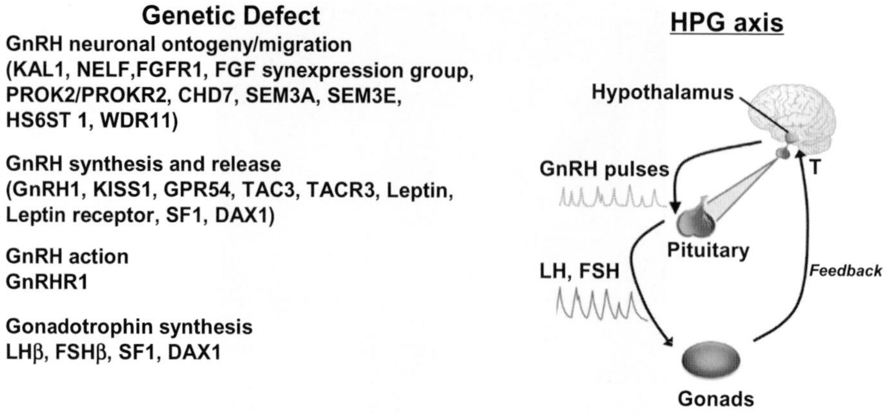

Genetic Defect

GnRH neuronal ontogeny/migration
(KAL1, NELF,FGFR1, FGF synexpression group,
PROK2/PROKR2, CHD7, SEM3A, SEM3E,
HS6ST 1, WDR11)

GnRH synthesis and release
(GnRH1, KISS1, GPR54, TAC3, TACR3, Leptin,
Leptin receptor, SF1, DAX1)

GnRH action
GnRHR1

Gonadotrophin synthesis
LHβ, FSHβ, SF1, DAX1

HPG axis

Figure 19.5. Genetic defects causing hypogonadotropic hypogonadism. GnRH, gonadotropin-releasing hormone; LH, luteinizing hormone; FSH, follicle-stimulating hormone.

A greater variability in the degree of hypogonadism has been observed in patients carrying mutations in *FGFR1*, *FGF8*, *PROKR2* or *PROK2* than in *KAL1* patients, in which the phenotype is invariably severe (Hardelin and Dodé 2008; Salenave et al. 2008). Spontaneously fertile individuals carrying mutations in many of the autosomal Kallmann syndrome genes account for the transmission of the disease over several generations, whereas the X-linked form of Kallmann syndrome is usually transmitted by the female carriers of *KAL1* mutations, who are clinically unaffected. Among the variety of non-reproductive and non-olfactory disorders that affect a fraction of patients with Kallmann syndrome, some clinical features have been reported for specific genetic forms of the disease.

Unilateral renal agenesis occurs in approximately 30% of *KAL1* patients (Kirk et al. 1994) but has so far not been reported in patients with *FGFR1*, *FGF8*, *PROKR2* or *PROK2* mutations. The loss of nasal cartilage, external ear hypoplasia and skeletal anomalies of the hands or feet have only been reported in *KAL2* (*FGFR1*) patients. In contrast, hearing impairment is common to several genetic forms of Kallmann syndrome, although it should be noted that the underlying defect (conductive, perceptive or mixed) is likely to vary between different genetic forms. Palate defects should also be considered as one of these shared traits, even though the severity differs between *KAL1* (high-arched palate) and *KAL2* (cleft palate). The cleft lip, palate or both may occur in as many as 25%–30% of the *KAL2* cases. Finally, bimanual synkinesis is highly prevalent in *KAL1* (maybe >75% of the cases), but it seems to be much less common in *KAL2*.

KAL1 (Anosmin 1)

The *KAL1* gene, located on the X chromosome at the Xp22.3 locus, was the first gene identified to be mutated in X-linked Kallmann syndrome (Legouis et al. 1991). It encodes an extracellular cell membrane associated glycoprotein (anosmin 1) involved in cellular adhesion, cell migration and neurite outgrowth and is bound extracellularly to heparan (Hu et al. 2004).

TABLE 19.2
Genetic loci incriminated in inherited forms of hypogonadotropic hypogonadism

Gene	Gene product	Function	Inheritance	Clinical phenotype
IL17RD	Interleukin 17 receptor D	FGF8 synexpression member, inhibits FGF signaling by acting both at the level of the FGF receptors (FGFR1 and FGFR2) and on downstream components of the Ras–extracellular-signal-regulated kinase (ERL)1/2 pathway by capturing active mitogen-activated protein kinase (MEK) and ERK complexes at the Golgi apparatus and inhibiting their dissociation	One allelic defect is most likely not sufficient	KS individuals and strongly linked to hearing loss
DUSP6	Dual-specificity phosphatase 6	FGF8 synexpression member, inhibits MAPK pathway by dephosphorylating and thereby inactivating MAP kinases	One allelic defect is most likely not sufficient	Congenital hypogonadotropic hypogonadism
SPRY4	Sprouty homolog 4	FGF8 synexpression member, inhibits MAPK pathway	One allelic defect is most likely not sufficient	Congenital hypogonadotropic hypogonadism
FLRT3	Fibronectin leucine-rich transmembrane protein 3	FGF8 synexpression member, stimulates FGFR by increasing ERK phosphorylation via intracellular domain interaction with FGFR	One allelic defect is most likely not sufficient	Congenital hypogonadotropic hypogonadism
NELF	Nasal embryonic LHRH factor	GnRH neuronal migration	Heterozygous mutation, mutation of one NELF allele may not be sufficient to result in disease	Normosmic IHH and KS
CHD7 (KAL5)	Chromodomain helicase DNA-binding protein-7	Hydrolyze ATP to alter nucleosome structure (DNA wrapped in histones), two N-terminal chromodomains that function to bind histones, whereas SNF2/helicase domains are important in chromatin remodeling; CHD7 may function in DNA binding, transcription regulation, cell cycle regulation, apoptosis, and embryonic stem cell pluripotency	Predominantly inherited in an autosomal dominant manner	nIHH, KS + hearing loss, CHARGE syndrome: eye coloboma, heart malformations, atresia of the choanae, retardation of growth/development, genital anomalies, and ear abnormalities

(Continued)

TABLE 19.2
(Continued)

Gene	Gene product	Function	Inheritance	Clinical phenotype
PROK2	Ligand for G protein-coupled prokineticin receptor-2	Effects on neuronal survival, gastrointestinal smooth muscle contraction, circadian locomotor rhythm, survival and migration of adrenal cortical capillary endothelial cells; in appetite regulation its anorectic effect is mediated partly by the melanocortin system; *PROK2* deficiency in mice leads to a loss of normal olfactory bulb architecture and accumulation of neuronal progenitors in the rostral migratory stream; PROK2 is a clock-controlled gene; PROK2-null mice show accelerated acquisition of food anticipatory activity during a daytime food restriction, exhibit reduced total sleep time predominantly during the light period, and also have an impaired response to sleep disturbance	Heterozygous mutations in most cases and homozygous in minority (or compound heterozygous) indicating a digenic or oligogenic mode of inheritance in heterozygous patients	IHH, KS, but not associated with hypopituitarism and septo-optic dysplasia
PROKR2	G protein-coupled prokineticin receptor-2	*Prokr2-/-* knockout mice exhibit early hypoplasia of the olfactory bulbs and severe atrophy of the reproductive organs in both sexes	Heterozygous mutations in most cases and homozygous in minority (or compound heterozygous), indicating digenic or oligogenic mode of inheritance in heterozygous patients	IHH, KS, hypopituitarism and septo-optic dysplasia
WRD11	WD repeat-containing protein 11 and also known as bromodomain and WD repeat containing protein 2 (BRWD2)	Expressed in the developing olfactory and GnRH migratory pathway, as well as in the hypothalamus in adults; in addition, WDR11 protein was found to colocalize with EMX1 *in vivo* and *in vitro*, and three of the human mutations failed to bind EMX1	Heterozygous missense mutations	nIHH, KS

Gene	Protein	Function	Mutation	Phenotype
GPR54	KISS1-derived peptide receptor/kisspeptin receptor	G protein-coupled receptor for kisspeptin to stimulate GnRh release	Recessive mutation in affected patients	nIHH
KISS1	Metastin or kisspeptin	Ligand for GPR54 to stimulate gonadotropin release in several species by inducing GnRH secretion from hypothalamic GnRH neurons expressing GPR54	Recessive mutation in all affected family members as an autosomal recessive trait	nIHH
TACR3	Neurokinin B receptor/NK3R	Coordinated activity with kisspeptin to regulate GnRH secretion	Most affected individuals are homozygous for loss-of-function mutations	nIHH
TAC3	Neurokinin B	Substance P-related tachykinin family, coordinated activity with kisspeptin to regulated GnRH secretion	Most affected individuals are homozygous for loss-of-function mutations	nIHH
LEP	Leptin	Regulation of kisspeptin expression and involved in coordinating metabolic status with the reproductive axis	Recessive mutations	Severe early-onset obesity with major hyperphagia associated with HH
LEPR	Leptin receptor	Regulation of kisspeptin expression and involved in coordinating metabolic status with the reproductive axis	Recessive mutations	Severe early-onset obesity with major hyperphagia associated with HH
GnRH	Gonadotropin-releasing hormone	Ligand for GnRH receptor to induce signal transduction; GnRH is released from the hypothalamus and stimulates cells in the anterior pituitary to release LH and FSH	Recessive frameshift mutation and heterozygous variants	nIHH

(Continued)

TABLE 19.2
(Continued)

Gene	Gene product	Function	Inheritance	Clinical phenotype
GnRHR	Gonadotropin-releasing hormone receptor	Secretion of LH and FSH in anterior pituitary	As the first gene involved in autosomal recessive normosmic IHH	nIHH
LHβ	Luteinizing hormone β	Triggers ovulation and development of the corpus luteum and stimulates production of testosterone	Compound heterozygous state	HH
FSHβ	Follicle-stimulating hormone β	Regulates the development, growth, pubertal maturation, and reproductive processes of the body	homozygous mutations	HH
SEMA3A	Semaphorin-3A	A secreted guidance protein acting on neuropilin-1 with repulsive effects on primary olfactory axons and GnRH neurons	Autosomal dominant	KS
SOX10	SOX10	Transcription factor, maintenance of progenitor cell multipotency, lineage specification, cell differentiation, OEC development	*SOX10* mutations in the heterozygous state in both KS and WS individuals	KS individuals and strongly linked to hearing loss, pigmentation defects, intellectual disability, psychomotor delay
NR0B1	DAX-1	Act on both the hypothalamus and pituitary	X-linked	X-linked adrenal hypoplasia congenita and HH
KAL1	Anosmin 1	Promotes neurite outgrowth, axon branching and targeting, chemoattractive on GnRH neuronal migration, cell adhesion	X-KS	KS (anosmia + HH), bimanual synkinesis, renal agenesis, cryptorchidism, neurosensorial deafness

Gene	Gene name	Function	Inheritance	Phenotype
FGFR1 (KAL2)	FGF receptor 1	FGF signaling for cell proliferation, differentiation and GnRH neuronal migration	Autosomal dominant	Normosmic IHH, KS, primary amenorrhoea, craniofacial defects, abnormal limb development, cleft palate, dental agenesis, digital bony abnormalities
FGF8 (KAL3)	Fibroblast growth factor 8	Ligand of FGFR for the genesis of the GnRH neuronal system and olfactory bulb development, *Fgf8*-conditional-knockout mice exhibit increased levels of apoptosis in the developing olfactory epithelium	Predominantly inherited in an autosomal dominant manner	Normosmic IHH, KS, primary amenorrhoea, sesorineural cleft lip and palate, neurosensorial deafness, digital bony abnormalities, dental agenesis, recessive holoprosencephaly, craniofacial defects, and hypothalamo-pituitary dysfunction
FGF17	Fibroblast growth factor 17	FGF8 synexpression member, mice lacking FGF17 have cerebellar defects and selective reduction in the size of the dorsal frontal cortex, but normal OB	One allelic defect is most likely not sufficient	Congenital hypogonadotropic hypogonadism
HS6ST1	Heparan-sulfate 6-0-sulfotransferase 1	An enzyme involved in 60 sulfation on glycosaminoglycan heparan sulfate, regulates neural branching *in vivo* in concert with other IHH-associated genes, including *kal-1*, the *FGF receptor*, and *FGF*	Heterozygous/homozygous mutations; complex inheritance patterns not readily conforming to Mendelian definitions of autosomal dominant or recessive transmission	IHH, KS, microphallus, unilateral cryptorchidism

FGF, fibroblast growth factor; FGFR, fibroblast growth factor receptor; ERK, extracellular signal regulated kinase; MAPK, Mitogen-activated protein kinase; GnRH, gonadotrophin-releasing hormone; KH, Kallman syndrome; HH, hypogonadotropic hypogonadism; IHH, idiopathic hypogonadotropic hypogonadism.hypogonadism; IHH, idiopathic hypogonadotropic hypogonadism.

Structurally, *KAL1* is a modular protein comprising a large cysteine-rich N-terminal domain, a whey acidic protein (WAP)–like domain, four contiguous fibronectin-like type III (FnIII) repeats and a small C-terminal domain rich in basic residues (Soussi-Yanicostas et al. 1996). The WAP domain is structurally similar to those of many serine protease inhibitors, whereas the FnIII repeats are structurally related to some cell adhesion molecules. Early indicators, gleaned from a human fetus carrying a chromosomal deletion at Xp22.3 that included *KAL1*, showed that GnRH cellular migration was abnormal, with GnRH neurons accumulating in the upper nasal region (Schwanzel-Fukuda et al. 1989); the olfactory bulbs were also absent. It was inferred that *KAL1* gene mutations have led to the failure of the later phases of GnRH neuronal migration (GnRH neuronal arrest in the subcribriform plate area) coupled with failed olfactory bulb development.

Mutations in *KAL1* are mainly nonsense or frameshift mutations, or large gene deletions. They tend to be associated with a more severe Kallmann syndrome phenotype, with anosmia and hypogonadotropic hypogonadism, a high frequency of cryptorchidism, microphallus and small testes in males. All reported families with *KAL1* mutations and hypogonadotropic hypogonadism have exclusively anosmic hypogonadotropic hypogonadism. Indeed, in a patient with Kallmann syndrome, a family history of normosmic hypogonadotropic hypogonadism makes an underlying *KAL1* mutation unlikely.

In the embryo, anosmin 1 is expressed in the interstitial matrix of the presumptive olfactory bulbs during the sixth embryonic week (Hardelin et al. 1999), although it is also present in the olfactory pit epithelium. Such a distribution is consistent with a role of anosmin 1 in the initial stage of olfactory bulb morphogenesis, which occurs at the end of the sixth embryonic week. Evidence has accrued that anosmin 1 is a modulator of *FGFR1* signalling (Gonzalez-Martinez et al. 2004), with *FGFR1* having an important role in the evagination of the olfactory bulbs from the neuroepithelial wall (Hébert et al. 2003).

FGFR1 (*KAL2*) mutations

FGFR1, a member of the receptor tyrosine kinase superfamily located on chromosome 8, is also implicated in cell migration and has an obligatory requirement for heparin sulfate (as does anosmin 1) for its signalling. In the presence of heparan sulfate proteoglycans, FGF binds with high affinity to FGFR and induces receptor dimerisation, thereby triggering transautophosphorylation of tyrosine residues in the intracellular domain. FGF signalling also controls cell proliferation, differentiation and survival and thus plays essential roles in various processes of embryonic development. Several signalling proteins are phosphorylated in response to FGF stimulation (Shc, phospholipase Cγ, STAT1, Gab1, FRS2α), leading to activation of downstream signalling pathways that include Ras/mitogen-activated protein kinase and phosphatidylinositol-3 kinase/Akt pathways. *FGF8* can activate the FGFR1c splice form of *FGFR1* (Zhang et al. 2006).

Both *FGFR1* and anosmin 1 represent separate though interacting genes involved in GnRH neuronal migration to the hypothalamus. Although loss-of-function mutations in *FGFR1* and *KAL1* can present with very similar phenotypes, FGFR1-related phenotypes are highly variable, with patients having both normosmic or anosmic forms of hypogonadotropic hypogonadism; indeed females with anosmia and normal reproductive function have

TABLE 19.3
Non-reproductive phenotypic abnormalities reported in patients with *FGFR1* mutations

Cleft lip/palate
Dental agenesis
Absent nasal cartilage
External ear hypoplasia
Mandibular hypoplasia
Thoracic dystrophia
Asymmetry of limbs
Cubitus valgus
Syndactyly
Clinodactyly
Osteoporosis
Miscellaneous phenotypes
Synkinesia
Agenesis of corpus callosum
Frontal bossing
Hypertelorism
Iris coloboma
Hearing loss
Epilepsy
Sleep disorder
Obesity

been described with *FGFR1* mutations (Pitteloud et al. 2006; Trarbach et al. 2006). Moreover, reversal of GnRH deficiency has even been reported in some male patients with *FGFR1* mutations after therapy with testosterone.

FGF8 mutations

FGF8 is one of the ligands for *FGFR1*. Mutations in *FGF8* have been associated with Kallmann syndrome in humans; in mice, homozygous mutation in *FGF8* leads to absent hypothalamic GnRH neurons, whereas heterozygous mice had markedly fewer hypothalamic GnRH neurons (Chung et al. 2008). As with *FGFR1* mutations, humans with *FGF8* mutations have a range of phenotypes, including adult-onset hypogonadotropic hypogonadism (Falardeau et al. 2008). In common with patients with *FGFR1* mutations, patients with *FGF8* mutations have a cleft palate in 30% of cases and may also display ear, cartilage and digital abnormalities (Table 19.3). The presence of these abnormalities in a patient with hypogonadotropic hypogonadism should raise suspicion for *FGFR1/FGF8* mutation.

PROKR2/PROK2

The clinical phenotypes of *PROKR2/PROK2* mutations, encoding prokineticin receptor-2 and prokineticin-2, respectively, range from both classic Kallmann syndrome to normosmic hypogonadotropic hypogonadism (Pitteloud et al. 2007). Non-reproductive phenotypes include fibrous dysplasia, bimanual synkinesia and epilepsy. Patients with more severe reproductive dysfunction tend to have biallelic mutations in *PROK2/PROKR2* and fewer associated non-reproductive abnormalities. Patients with monoallelic mutations have less severe reproductive dysfunction and more non-reproductive abnormalities. PROKR2 is a G protein–coupled receptor that binds to the ligand PROK2. Mouse *PROK2* knockout models have small, abnormally shaped olfactory bulbs with an accumulation of neurons in the rostral migratory stream between the subventricular zone and the olfactory bulb (Matsumoto et al. 2006).

Putative loss-of-function mutations in *PROKR2* or *PROK2* have been detected in approximately 9% of the patients with Kallmann syndrome (Cole et al. 2008; Leroy et al. 2008; Monnier et al. 2008). Most of these mutations are missense (loss-of-function) mutations, and many have also been found in apparently unaffected individuals, challenging their pathogenic role in the disease. Although the *PROK2/ PROKR2* system regulates various biological processes, including intestinal contraction, circadian rhythms and vascular function, its role in GnRH neuronal migration remains unclear. It is not expressed in GnRH neurons.

CHARGE syndrome

CHARGE stands for coloboma, heart malformations, atresia of the choanae, retardation of growth and development, genital anomalies and ear anomalies (auditory and vestibular). In addition, hypogonadotropic hypogonadism may be present, and most if not all patients with CHARGE syndrome have both olfactory bulb aplasia and hypoplasia, two Kallmann syndrome-defining features (Topaloglu and Kotan 2010). CHARGE syndrome has an estimated birth incidence of 1 in 8 500–12 000. Other infrequently occurring features include characteristic face and hand dysmorphia, hypotonia, arhinencephaly, semicircular canal agenesis or hypoplasia, hearing impairment, urinary tract anomalies, orofacial clefting, dysphagia and tracheoesophageal anomalies. Multiple sets of diagnostic criteria for CHARGE syndrome have been proposed (Kim and Layman 2011).

The causative *CHD7* gene encodes a chromodomain (chromatin organisation modifier domain) helicase DNA–binding protein expressed in the olfactory placode, which gives rise to GnRH neurons, spinal cord, nasopharynx and eye. This protein may explain some of the organ involvement. Most patients are heterozygous for loss-of-function mutations in *CHD7*.

Kallmann syndrome occurring in association with congenital heart disease or choanal atresia may represent unrecognised mild CHARGE syndrome. Additional traits shared between CHARGE syndrome and the *KAL2* (FGFR1) genetic form of Kallmann syndrome include cleft lip or palate (present in 20%–35% of patients with *KAL2* and CHARGE syndrome), external ear malformation (present in virtually all patients with CHARGE syndrome and a few patients with *KAL2*), agenesis of the corpus callosum and coloboma. Because of the similarity between CHARGE and *KAL2* phenotypes, it is tempting to speculate that there are functional interactions between CHD7 and FGFR1 signalling. Thus, IHH/ Kallmann syndrome may be a mild allelic form of the CHARGE syndrome; indeed, CHD7 has been designated as KAL5.

Kisspeptin and *GPR54*

Kisspeptin, a peptide encoded by the gene *KISS1*, was originally described as a metastasis suppressor in melanoma and breast cancer (Ohtaki et al. 2001). It binds to *GPR54*, encoded by the gene *KISSR1*. The kisspeptin–*KISS1R* system is established as an important positive regulator of GnRH secretion, and in humans, intravenous kisspeptin acutely releases gonad-otrophins (Roa et al. 2008). Loss-of-function mutations in *GPR54/KISSR1* in patients can cause both familial and sporadic forms of normosmic CIHH (de Roux et al. 2003; Seminara et al. 2003), although they represent a rare cause of hypogonadotropic hypogonadism. Further studies in affected humans and in knockout mice have revealed that mutations in *GPR54* resulted in normosmic (n) IHH with an autosomal recessive mode of inheritance. Although animal models have not conclusively demonstrated hypogonadotropic hypogo-nadism with loss of function in kisspeptin, a loss-of-function mutation leading to normos-mic isolated hypogonadotrphic hypogonadism (nIHH) has been recently described in the kisspeptin gene *KISS1* in humans (Topaloglu et al. 2012).

Clinical and endocrinological evaluation of individuals with CIHH affected by muta-tions in *GPR54* reveals low sex steroid levels and low gonadotrophin levels. In males, micropenis and cryptorchidism are frequently noted, and in females primary amenorrhoea and partial breast development are evident. Exogenous gonadotrophin therapy leads to testicular maturation, with the appearance of sperm in the ejaculate and subsequent fertility ruling out primary testicular dysfunction. Pulsatile GnRH therapy in affected females leads to ovulation and conception. These findings indicate that loss-of-function mutations in *GPR54/KISSR1* do not diminish the sensitivity of gonadotropic cells to GnRH nor the sensitivity of the gonads to gonadotropins. Thus, in humans as in mice, *GPR54/KISSR1* loss of function mainly appears to affect hypothalamic GnRH secretion, with no discernible direct effect on the pituitary or gonads. Patients with *GPR54* defects demonstrate a mark-edly higher sensitivity to exogenous pulsatile GnRH than a cohort of CIHH patients receiv-ing similar therapy; indeed, some patients retain a persistent pulsatile luteinizing hormone secretion with a normal frequency but a very low amplitude, suggesting that *GPR54* inac-tivation impaired but did not prevent the neuroendocrine onset of puberty.

GnRH1 mutations as a cause of congenital isolated hypogonadotropic hypogonadism in humans

GnRH is crucial for regulating reproduction in mammals. It is synthesised by hypothalamic neurons and released from nerve endings into the portal circulation; it binds to the membrane *GnRHR* type 1 receptor, stimulating the gonadotropic cells of the anterior pituitary to synthe-sise and release luteinizing hormone and FSH, which in turn, stimulate synthesis and secretion of sex steroid hormones and gametogenesis. Proof that *GnRH* mutations are involved in CIHH pathogenesis appeared in two reports in 2009 (Bouligand et al. 2009; Chan et al. 2009).

As would be anticipated, pulsatile GnRH administration restored the patient's ovarian function, as indicated by increased circulating oestradiol and inhibin B concentrations and the appearance of a single dominant follicle seen on ultrasonography. Both index patients were homozygous for the mutation, whereas their unaffected parents and sisters were het-erozygous and had a normal reproductive phenotype.

Leptin and leptin receptor mutations

Mutations in both leptin and leptin receptor (*LEPR*) are associated with hypogonadotropic hypogonadism in addition to obesity and hyperphagia (Clement et al. 1998; Strobel et al.

1998). In 300 patients studied with severe early-onset obesity and hyperphagia, 3% had a mutation in the *LEPR*. These patients were characterised by altered immune systems and hypogonadotropic hypogonadism in addition to their obesity. Interestingly, they had relatively normal concentrations of leptin. Treatment with recombinant leptin in patients with leptin deficiency restores eugonadism. In one Brazilian kindred with leptin deficiency, before treatment, adults were hypogonadal; an adult male was prepubertal, he had no beard, bilateral gynaecomastia was present, pubic and axillary hair were scanty, the penis and testes were small, and the patient was azoospermic. Leptin replacement therapy with daily injection of recombinant methionyl human leptin given at night led to pubertal development and restoration of normal hypothalamo-pituitary-testicular function.

The *DAX1* gene

X-linked congenital adrenal hypoplasia (CAH) is associated with normosmic hypogonadotropic hypogonadism, and the *DAX-1* gene has been implicated in this relationship (Muscatelli et al. 1994). *DAX1* works during embryologic development to antagonise SRY and is therefore essential in sexual differentiation. It is also a transcriptional repressor of SF1 (Ito et al. 1997). *DAX1* encodes a nuclear receptor that is expressed in embryonic stem cells, steroidogenic tissues, the ventromedial hypothalamus and the pituitary gonadotrophs. The adrenal failure reflects a developmental abnormality in the transition of the fetal to adult zone, resulting in mineralocorticoid and glucocorticoid deficiency, whereas the aetiology of the hypogonadotropic hypogonadism involves a combined and variable deficiency of hypothalamic GnRH secretion and/or pituitary responsiveness to GnRH, resulting in low gonadotrophins and low testosterone. Treatment with exogenous gonadotrophins does not generally result in spermatogenesis. It is always the adrenal dysfunction that prompts investigation into the function of the hypothalamic-pituitary-gonadal axis as infants with CAH that are not recognised clinically are unlikely to survive until puberty.

GnRHR mutations

Whereas Kallmann syndrome genes are primarily involved in GnRH neuronal ontogeny, genes in which mutations lead to normosmic hypogonadotropic hypogonadism are involved in the regulation of the hypothalamic-pituitary-gonadal axis. *GnRHR* gene defects were the first identified cause of nonsyndromic CHH. Mutations in the *GnRHR* are responsible for roughly one-fifth of the sporadic cases and about half of autosomal recessive inherited cases of nIHH, whereas mutations in the gene for GnRH have proven rare, accounting for about 1% of cases (Bianco and Kaiser 2009). The most consistent characteristic of patients with *GnRHR* mutations is their pituitary resistance to pulsatile GnRH administration when the phenotype is severe and their spontaneous luteinizing hormone secretion is non-pulsatile. Mutations can affect GnRH binding, receptor activation or interaction with coupled effectors, but it has also been shown that GnRHR protein misfolding with misrouting may also be caused by mutations and lead to loss of human GnRHR function. High-dose GnRH may elicit a response in partial forms, with an increase in the luteinizing hormone pulse amplitude, and occasional pregnancies have been reported after pulsatile GnRH administration.

The *HS6ST1* gene

Insights from studies of cell-specific overexpression of *KAL-1* in a set of *Caenorhabditis elegans* interneurons that demonstrated a *KAL-1*-dependent axonal branching phenotype prompted a genetic modifier screen that uncovered mutations in the *C. elegans* HS 6-*o*-sulfotransferase gene (*HST-6*) as suppressors of a *KAL-1* gain-of-function phenotype. This finding supported earlier studies indicating that anosmin 1 required HS with specific 6-*o*-sulfate modifications for its in vivo action. Heparan 6-*o*-sulfation is also required for the function of FGFR1 and its ligand FGF8, with loss-of-function mutations in both genes being associated with human GnRH deficiency. The human *HST6ST1* homolog has been investigated as a candidate gene for GnRH deficiency, leading to the identification of mutations associated with reduced enzymatic activities in vivo and in vitro *HST6ST1* in 2% of patients with IHH (Tornberga et al. 2011).

The *WDR11* gene

By defining the chromosomal breakpoint of a balanced *t* (10;12) translocation from an individual with Kallmann syndrome and scanning genes in its vicinity in unrelated hypogonadal individuals, *WDR11* has been identified as an autosomal dominant gene involved in human puberty. Six patients with a total of five different heterozygous WDR11 missense mutations, including three alterations (A435T, R448Q and H690Q) in WD domains important for β propeller formation and protein–protein interaction, were identified (Kim et al. 2010). WDR11 has been shown to interact with EMX1, a homeodomain transcription factor involved in the development of olfactory neurons; moreover, missense alterations in WDR11 reduce or abolish this interaction. These findings suggested that impaired pubertal development in these patients resulted from a deficiency of productive WDR11 protein interaction.

FGF8 synexpression group

The hypothesis that mutations in genes encoding a broader range of modulators of the FGFR1 pathway might contribute to the genetics of CIHH as causal or modifier has been tested in a large group of IHH individuals and has revealed that mutations in members of the so-called FGF8 synexpression group, namely *FGF17, IL17RD, DUSP6, SPRY4* and *FLRT3*, harbour potential loss-of-function mutations in patients with CIHH (Miraoi et al. 2013). On the basis of their protein–protein interaction patterns with proteins known to be altered in CIHH, *FGF17* and *IL17RD* were predicted to be potentially important genes in IHH. Most of the *FGF17* and *IL17RD* mutations altered protein function in vitro. *IL17RD* mutations were found only in individuals with Kallmann syndrome and were strongly linked to hearing loss (six of eight individuals). Mutations in genes encoding components of the FGF pathway were found to be associated with complex modes of CIHH inheritance acting primarily as contributors to an oligogenic genetic architecture underlying CIHH.

The *SOX10* gene

The transcription factor *SOX10* plays an important role in the development of the neural crest and is involved in the maintenance of progenitor cell multipotency, lineage specification and cell differentiation. Mutations in *SOX10* have been implicated in Waardenburg syndrome, a rare disorder characterised by the association between pigmentation abnormalities and deafness. *SOX10* mutations cause a variable phenotype that spreads over the initial limits of the syndrome definition. On the basis of findings of olfactory bulb agenesis in individuals with Waardenburg syndrome, *SOX10* was hypothesised to be also involved in Kallmann syndrome. *SOX10* loss-of-function mutations were found in approximately one-third of individuals with Kallmann syndrome with deafness, indicating a substantial involvement in this clinical condition. Study of *SOX10*-null mutant mice revealed a developmental role of SOX10 in a sub-population of glial cells called olfactory ensheathing cells. These mice showed an almost complete absence of these cells along the olfactory nerve pathway, as well as defasciculation and misrouting of the nerve fibres, impaired migration of GnRH cells and disorganisation of the olfactory nerve layer of the olfactory bulbs (Pingault et al. 2013).

Neurokinin B and its receptor mutations

Neurokinin B (NKB/TAC3) and its receptor (NKBR/TAC3R) represent a further system whose malfunction is linked to normosmic (n)hypogonadotropic hypogonadism. NKB is highly expressed in the arcuate nucleus, a region of the brain that also expresses high levels of kisspeptin. In a study of four separate families with strong histories of normosmic hypogonadotrphic hypogonadism (nHH) without known mutations in other CIHH genes, affected individuals were found to have homozygous mutations in either the *TAC3* gene that encodes NKB or the *TAC3R* gene that encodes the NKBR (Guran et al. 2009; Topaloglu et al. 2009).

The anatomical and functional relationship between the GPR54/kisspeptin and NKB/NKBR has led to a greater understanding of the physiological regulation of GnRH release. Kisspeptin and NKB are directly involved in signalling between the arcuate nucleus and GnRH neurons and are found together with dynorphin 23 in these arcuate neurons. They may represent the GnRH pulse generator. Continuous kisspeptin infusion results in normal GnRH secretion in patients with loss-of-function mutations in TAC3 or TAC3R, suggesting that NKB is proximal to kisspeptin in the pathway for GnRH release possibly acting as a modulator of kisspeptin release.

NK3R is expressed on rodent GnRH-expressing neurons, and axons of neurons expressing neurokinin B are closely anatomically opposed to those of GnRH neurons within the median eminence where NKB-immunoreactive varicosities have been reported to be in direct contact with GnRH-immunoreactive axons. NKB expression is highest in the arcuate nucleus, where it colocalises with estrogen receptor-α and dynorphin 23, both of which are involved in progesterone feedback in response to GnRH secretion.

The *SEMA3A* gene

Cosegregation between the Kallmann syndrome phenotype and a heterozygous (i.e. autosomal dominant) SEMA3A deletion in a family with several affected members has been reported. If semaphorin 3A haploinsufficiency can be validated as causally linked to (irreversible) Kallmann syndrome, this relationship would contrast with the situation in model mice, in which only homozygous knockout leads to a similar phenotype. Interestingly, none of the family members with Kallmann syndrome reported had any other clinical neurological abnormalities, suggesting that the role of semaphorin 3A in neuronal migration is restricted in humans to olfactory system development and GnRH neuron migration, despite its expression in other neuronal and non-neuronal structures (Young et al. 2012).

The *SEMA3E* gene

SEMA3E encodes fibronectin leucine-rich transmembrane protein 3, a neurotrophic factor that delivers essential survival signals for GnRH neurons via PLXND1 and kinase insert domain receptor (KDR). It promotes survival of maturing GnRH neurons, and recently loss-of-function mutations have been associated with Kallmann syndrome (Cariboni et al. 2015).

Ataxia, dementia and hypogonadotropic hypogonadism

Whole-exome sequencing in a patient with ataxia and hypogonadotropic hypogonadism, followed by target sequencing of candidate genes in similarly affected patients, has revealed that the syndrome of ataxia, dementia and hypogonadotropic hypogonadism can be caused by inactivating mutations in RNF216, or by a combination of mutations in RNF216 and OTUD4, linking disordered ubiquitination to neurodegeneration and reproductive dysfunction (Margolin et al. 2013).

Reversible forms of congenital isolated hypogonadotropic hypogonadism

So-called reversible male forms of CIHH have been recognised for several decades (Quinton et al. 1999b; Raivio et al. 2007) and have been demonstrated with several CIHH genotypes, including *KAL1*, *FGFR1*, the GnRH receptor (*GnRHR*) gene and *PROKR2* (Pitteloud et al. 2005; Riberio et al. 2007; Sinisi et al. 2008). In these patients, very late activation of pulsatile gonadotropin secretion (due to late activation of the GnRH pulse generator, or gonadotroph responsiveness) occurs, such that gonadotropin secretion improves with time. This clinical variant, estimated to affect about 10% of cases, should be actively sought either by regular monitoring of testicular volumes or by periodic interruption of testosterone replacement therapy (TRT), and measurement of gonadotrophins with 09.00 testosterone. It is evident that when reversible forms occur before 20 years of age in an euosmic patient with no identifiable mutations, an alternative diagnosis is severe constitutional pubertal delay.

Oligogenic inheritance

Although normosmic CIHH and Kallmann syndrome have long been considered as monogenic disorders with a Mendelian inheritance pattern, several cases of possible digenic/oligogenic inheritance in Kallmann syndrome (Pitteloud et al. 2007) have been reported. Such digenic inheritance has been shown in both patients with Kallmann syndrome and patients with normosmic CIHH who bore mutations in both *PROKR2* and *PROK2*, in *FGFR1* and *NELF*, as well as in *PROKR2*, and *GnRH1*, *GnRHR* or *KISSR1* (Sykiotis et al. 2010). Defects in different genes could act synergistically to induce the CIHH or the Kallmann syndrome phenotype, or to modify the severity of the GnRH deficiency, partially explaining the phenotypic variability observed within and across families with CIHH and Kallmann syndrome.

When should clinical genetic testing be undertaken in Kallmann syndrome?

Given the large array of genetic defects that may be causally linked to both normosmic CIHH and Kallmann syndrome, what should the clinician's approach be to genetic testing in any one individual? The mode of inheritance is clearly of relevance and needs to be discussed with patients. In a study of eight Kallmann syndrome genes in six pathways (*KAL1, FGF8/FGFR1, PROK2/PROKR2, HS6ST1, NELF* and *CHD7*) conducted in 219 male and female patients with Kallmann syndrome (not nHH), it was hypothesised that mutations in these six pathways would exhibit specific phenotypes that could be used to direct genetic testing (Costa-Barbosa et al. 2013). Of 219 patients with Kallmann syndrome, 151 had rare sequence variants (RSVs) in at least one of these genes, and none was found in 68 patients.

Several phenotypes were examined: reproductive phenotype, presence of unilateral renal agenesis, bimanual synkinesis, hearing loss, presence of cleft palate, dental agenesis and skeletal anomalies. A severe reproductive phenotype was seen most commonly in *KAL1*, and renal agenesis in *KAL1* and also in the RSV-negative group. Synkinesia was seen in *KAL1* and *FGFR1* genotypes and also in other groups, including the RSV-negative groups, but not *HS6ST1*. Hearing loss was more common in the *CHD7* versus non-*CHD7* groups but was also seen in all other groups except *HS6ST1*. Cleft lip/palate was seen in all groups except *KAL1* and *PROK2/ PROKR2*. Dental agenesis was seen most commonly in the *FGFR1/FGF8* group but also identified in the *CHD7*/RSV-negative group. Syndactyly, polydactyly or camptodactyly were seen exclusively in the *FGFR1/ FGF8* group (Fig 19.3); scoliosis, kyphosis, excessive joint mobility, short fourth metacarpal bones, clinodactyly, foreshortened limb bones and flat feet were seen in all groups.

Treatment for congenital isolated hypogonadotropic hypogonadism

The treatment for both normosmic CIHH and Kallmann syndrome is that of the resulting hypogonadism. Treatment is first to initiate virilisation or breast development and second to develop fertility. Hormone replacement therapy, with testosterone for males and combined estrogen and progesterone for females, is required to stimulate the development of secondary sexual characteristics. When fertility is desired, either gonadotropins or pulsatile GnRH therapy is used to obtain testicular growth and sperm production in males or ovulation in females, although the therapy has been less successful in males who have a history of cryptorchidism. Both treatments restore fertility in the majority of affected individuals. It is still unknown whether transient hormone replacement therapy in affected male infants to simulate postnatal surge in gonadotropins could have later salutary impact on their sexual life and reproductive prognosis.

TREATMENT OF HYPOGONADOTROPIC HYPOGONADISM IN THE MALE PATIENT

Testosterone replacement therapy

TRT is available in a variety of formulations for clinical use, including oral, injectable esters, transdermal patch and gel preparations, each with its own unique pharmacokinetic profile. Treatment is commenced at a low dose initially and gradually increased at 6-month intervals to respect the normal cadence of puberty in the male. Tostran gel and Testim gel are particularly useful, allowing upward titration of the administered dose. Injectables (e.g. testosterone enanthate, 50mg every month) are given for 9 months, and the dose is gradually escalated to the adult dose of 200mg every 2 to 3 weeks over the course of 3 to 4 years.

Induction of spermatogenesis

In men desirous of fertility, options for spermatogenesis induction include exogenous gonadotrophins or pulsatile GnRH. GnRH substitution is more effective for hypothalamic than pituitary disorders, whereas administration of exogenous gonadotropins is suitable for patients with both pituitary and hypothalamic disorders. HCG, with its longer biological half-life, is used as a luteinizing hormone substitute, in conjunction with FSH in the form of either human menopausal gonadotrophins, highly purified urinary FSH preparations or recombinant FSH formulations (Gonal F, Puregon).

FSH is necessary for the maintenance of spermatogenesis, as evidenced by the findings in contraceptive trials using testosterone esters, where azoospermia was only attained in patients in whom serum FSH levels were fully suppressed (Behre et al. 1995). In a subset of patients with hypogonadotropic hypogonadism and larger testicular size, spermatogenesis can be stimulated with hCG alone (Burris et al. 1998), although it is likely that men with the fertile eunuch syndrome and sufficient endogenous FSH secretion to sustain normal spermatogenesis with hCG alone are well represented in this subgroup.

High intratesticular testosterone concentrations are essential for normal spermatogenesis. Thus, spermatogenesis can be induced by a combination of hCG and human menopausal gonadotropin (hMG), though not by a regimen of purified FSH and testosterone alone (Schaison et al. 1993).

Exogenous gonadotropin therapy

Traditionally, FSH has been administered using hMG derived from the urine of postmenopausal women. In this preparation, FSH activity predominates and luteinizing hormone activity is low, necessitating combined administration with hCG to achieve fertility (Buchter et al. 1998). Highly purified urinary FSH preparations give enhanced specific activity in comparison to hMG (10 000 vs. 150U/mg protein for hMG); however, these preparations have been superseded by recombinant human FSH (r-hFSH) formulations made in Chinese hamster ovary cells with a 48 ± 5h half-life and devoid of intrinsic luteinizing hormone activity (Puregon, Gonal F).

Recombinant gonadotrophins can be administered subcutaneously, a route that is as effective a mode of delivery as the intramuscular route, and is conducive to good compliance. hCG alone at a dose of 1 000U on alternate days, or 1 500U twice weekly (with dosage titration based on trough testosterone concentrations), is given initially. With larger initial testicular volume, spermatogenesis can be initiated with hCG alone, most likely due to residual FSH secretion (Finkel et al. 1985; Vicari et al. 1992).

Once there is a plateau in the response to hCG, and assuming no spermatozoa are seen in the ejaculate after 3–4 months of treatment, therapy with FSH (in one of the three forms described above) is added at a dose of 75U on alternate days initially, increasing to daily, if necessary (Mannaerts et al. 1996; European Metrodin HP Study Group 1998). Continuation of this combined regimen for 12–24 months induces testicular growth in almost all patients, with spermatogenesis in a large proportion and pregnancy rates in the range of 50%–80% (Mannaerts et al. 1996; European Metrodin HP Study Group 1998). Better outcome can be expected with larger baseline testicular size, and absence of previous cryptorchidism. Gynaecomastia is seen in up to 33% of patients on gonadotrophin therapy, the consequence of excessive secretion of oestrogen by Leydig cells in response to hCG, and is avoidable by using the lowest dose of hCG capable of maintaining serum testosterone concentrations towards the lower end of the normal range (Liu et al. 1988; Liu et al. 1999).

Gonadotrophin therapy to patients with hypogonadotropic hypogonadism rarely generates sperm concentration in the World Health Organisation (WHO) reference range. This result may be because initial 'priming' of testes did not occur during the minipuberty and also because of the high incidence of undescended testes. Failure to achieve normal sperm counts does not preclude fertility, however; and in one study the median sperm concentration achieved at conception was reported to be 5million/mL. The smaller the initial testicular volume, the longer the duration of treatment required, and it may take up to 24 months for spermatogenesis to be induced.

Given the aforementioned findings, it is sensible to start treatment 6–12 months before the time at which fertility is desired. Once pregnancy is achieved, therapy should be continued until at least the second trimester, and if a further conception is planned shortly thereafter, therapy with hCG alone should be continued. In contrast, if a longer interval is anticipated, testosterone therapy can be recommenced. The option of storing sperm for subsequent use in intrauterine insemination or intracytoplasmic sperm injection should also be discussed. In patients in whom the combination of hCG and FSH is required to induce spermatogenesis initially, treatment with hCG alone may be sufficient for subsequent pregnancies due to larger starting testicular size.

Pulsatile gonadotropin-releasing hormone therapy
The alternative to gonadotropin therapy is pulsatile administration of GnRH administered by a programmable, portable mini-infusion pump. Although intravenous administration produces the most physiological GnRH pulse contour and ensues luteinizing hormone response, the subcutaneous route is clearly more practical for the long-term treatment required to stimulate spermatogenesis. The frequency of GnRH administration recommended is every 2h at a dose of 25–600ng/kg/bolus, with the GnRH dose being titrated for each individual to ensure normalisation of testosterone, luteinizing hormone and FSH. Serum testosterone and gonadotropin concentrations should be monitored monthly, and once testicular volume reaches 8mL, regular semen analyses are obtained.

The majority of patients require treatment for at least 2 years to maximise testicular growth and achieve spermatogenesis, although, similar to the response to gonadotrophin therapy, the time taken to reach these endpoints tends to be shorter in patients with a larger initial gonadal size, and a poorer response is expected in patients with a history of bilateral cryptorchidism.

Effect of postnatal gonadotrophin therapy in males with hypogonadotropic hypogonadism

Because patients with hypogonadotropic hypogonadism may be diagnosed shortly after birth because of micropenis and cryptorchidism, combined with subnormal luteinizing hormone and FSH concentrations during the postnatal period, treating these patients with gonadotropins postnatally, to mimic physiological development, could improve testicular growth and fertility potential later in life. There has been one report of a hypogonadotropic hypogonadism male being treated by recombinant human luteinizing hormone and FSH in doses of 20 and 21.3 IU s.c. twice weekly, respectively, from 7.9 to 13.7 months of age. During treatment, concentrations of luteinizing hormone, FSH, inhibin B and oestradiol increased to values within normal limits, whereas serum testosterone remained undetectable. Penile length increased from 1.6cm to 2.4cm and testicular volume, assessed by ultrasound, increased by 170% (Main et al. 2002).

Management of hypogonadotropic hypogonadism in females

OESTROGEN REPLACEMENT THERAPY

Initial therapy is with ethinyloestradiol 5µg orally, for at least 6 months. A transdermal twice weekly oestradiol patch may be used as an alternative. Treatment is continued until breakthrough haemorrhage occurs, after which cyclical therapy with medroxyprogesterone acetate 5mg daily for 2 weeks is introduced. The dose of ethinyloestradiol is gradually increased over a 2- to 3-year period to a final dose of 20–30µg daily.

Gonadotropin therapy

Originally introduced more than 50 years ago, purified human urinary postmenopausal gonadotrophins (HMGs) containing luteinizing hormone to FSH bioactivity of 1:1 have been successfully used to induce ovulation in hypogonadotropic hypogonadal states. The availability of purified and highly purified urinary FSH, and recombinant human FSH (rFSH, >99% purity), has largely superseded HMG and can be given subcutaneously with none of the batch-to-batch variability observed with HMG. The aim of ovulation induction with gonadotrophins is the generation of a single dominant follicle.

Step-up and step-down protocols

A conventional step-up gonadotrophin protocol would involve a starting FSH dose of 37.5–75U/day designed to allow the FSH threshold to be reached gradually, minimising excessive stimulation and thereby reducing the risk of development of multiple follicles. The dose is increased only if, after 7 days, no response is documented on ultrasonography and serum oestradiol monitoring. The dose is incrementally increased at weekly intervals by 37.5–75U to a maximum of 225U/day, and the response is then monitored by ultrasonic cycle tracking with measurement of endometrial thickness and follicular diameter.

In the step-down protocol, therapy with 150U FSH/ day is started until a dominant follicle (>10mm) is seen on transvaginal ultrasonography, with the dose then being decreased to 112.5U/day, followed by a further decrease to 75U/day three days later, a dose that is continued until hCG is administered to induce ovulation.

Purified urinary FSH has some luteinizing hormone activity but rFSH does not. The experience with rFSH in hypogonadotropic hypogonadal women (WHO class 1) indicates that women who have very low serum luteinizing hormone concentrations (<0.5U/L) need exogenous hCG (or 75U/day s.c. recombinant luteinizing hormone) to maintain adequate oestradiol bio-synthesis and follicle development.

HCG at 5 000–10 000U i.m. is used to trigger ovulation when ovarian follicles >20mm are achieved and the endometrium is >10mm thick (Ludwig et al. 2003).

Cycle tracking

Transvaginal ultrasonography is used to measure follicular diameter and endometrial thickness, with an optimal scanning frequency of every two or three days in the late follicular phase. The criteria for follicle maturity are a follicle diameter of 18–20mm and/or a serum oestradiol >734pmol/L/dominant follicle.

HCG is given on the day that at least one follicle appears to be mature. If three or more follicles >15mm are present, stimulation is stopped, hCG is withheld, and a barrier contraceptive is advised to prevent multiple pregnancies and ovarian hyperstimulation. Pre-ovulatory concentrations of oestradiol above the normal range may predict ovarian hyperstimulation.

Pulsatile gonadotropin-releasing hormone therapy

Pulsatile administration of GnRH using an infusion pump stimulates the production of endogenous FSH and luteinizing hormone and can be used in patients whose hypogonadotropic hypogonadism is not caused by GnRHR loss-of-function mutations. The resulting serum FSH and luteinizing hormone concentrations remain within the normal range, so the chances of multifollicular development and ovarian hyperstimulation are low. The subcutaneous route can be used, and to mimic normal pulsatile GnRH release, the pulse interval is 60–90min and the dose is 2.5–10μg/pulse (Martin et al. 1990; Jansen 1993; Martin et al. 1993; Filicori et al. 1994). The lower dose should be used initially to minimise the likelihood of multiple pregnancies; the dose should then be increased to the minimum dose required to induce ovulation. Pulsatile GnRH administration may be discontinued after ovulation, and the corpus luteum supported by hCG.

Outcomes

Ovulation rates of 90% and pregnancy rates of 80% have been reported in women treated with pulsatile GnRH. Local complications such as phlebitis may occasionally occur.

Conclusion

To conclude, the last few years have seen major advances in our understanding of hypogonadotrophic hypogonadism and Kallmann syndrome; mutations in a number of genes have been identified in association with the condition. Digenic/oligogenic inheritance has been proposed in a number of cases, explaining some of the variability in phenotypic expression and penetrance. At the same time, novel therapeutic regimens are improving outcomes related to pubertal development, fertility and reproduction. However, a considerable amount of work is still required in the field in order to understand those cases of hypogonadotrophic hypogonadism and Kallmann syndrome that are still unexplained. Additionally, the prospects of fertility will continue to improve with the use of therapeutic regimens that will include novel approches.

REFERENCES

Andersson AM, Toppari J, Haavisto AM et al. (1998) Longitudinal reproductive hormonal profiles in infants: Peak of inhibin B levels in infant boys exceeds levels in adult men. *J Clin Endocrinol Metab* 83(2): 675–681.

Behre HM, Baus S, Kliesch S et al. (1995) Potential of testosterone buciclate for male contraception: Endocrine differences between responders and nonresponders. *J Clin Endocrinol Metab* 80: 2394–2403.

Bianco SD and Kaiser UB (2009) The genetic and molecular basis of idiopathic hypogonadotropic hypogonadism. *Nat Rev Endocrinol* 5: 569–576.

Bouligand J, Ghervan C, Tello JA et al. (2009) Isolated familial hypogonadotropic hypogonadism and a GNRH1 mutation. *N Engl J Med* 360: 2742–2748.

Buchter D, Behre HM, Kliesch S et al. (1998) Pulsatile GnRH or human chorionic gonadotropin/human menopausal gonadotropin as effective treatment for men with hypogonadotropic hypogonadism: A review of 42 cases. *Eur J Endocrinol* 139: 298–303.

Burris AS, Rodbard HW, Winters SJ et al. (1988) Gonadotropin therapy in men with isolated hypogonadotropic hypogonadism: The response to human chorionic gonadotropin is predicted by initial testicular size. *J Clin Endocrinol Metab* 66: 1144–1151.

Cariboni A, Andre V, Chauvet S et al. (2015) Dysfunctional SEMA3E signalling underlies GnRH neuron deficiency in Kallmann syndrome. *J Clin Invest* 125(6): 2413–2428.

Caronia LM, Martin C, Welt CK et al. (2011) A genetic basis for functional hypothalamic amenorrhea. *N Engl J Med* 364(3): 215–225.

Chan YM, de Guillebon A, Lang-Muritano M et al. (2009) GNRH1 mutations in patients with idiopathic hypogonadotropic hypogonadism. *Proc Natl Acad Sci USA* 106: 11703–11708.

Chung WC, Moyle SS and Tsai PS (2008) Fibroblast growth factor 8 signaling through Fgf receptor 1 is required for the emergence of gonadotropin-releasing hormone neurons. *Endocrinology* 149: 4997–5003.

Clement K, Vaisse C, Lahlou N et al. (1998) A mutation in the human leptin receptor gene causes obesity and pituitary dysfunction. *Nature* 392: 398–401.

Cole LW, Sidis Y, Zhang C et al. (2008) Mutations in prokineticin 2 (PROK2) and PROK2 receptor 2 (PROKR2) in human gonadotrophin-releasing hormone deficiency: Molecular genetics and clinical spectrum. *J Clin Endocrinol Metab* 93: 3551–3559.

Conrad B, Kriebel J and Hetzel WD (1978) Hereditary bimanual synkinesis combined with hypogonadotropic hypogonadism and anosmia in four brothers. *J Neurol* 218: 263–274.

Costa-Barbosa F, Balasubramanian R, Keefe KW et al. (2013) Prioritizing genetic testing in patients with Kallmann syndrome using clinical phenotype. *J Clin Endocrinol Metab* 98: E943–E953.

de Roux N, Genin E, Carel JC et al. (2003) Hypogonadotropic hypogonadism due to loss of function of the KiSS1- derived peptide receptor GPR54. *Proc Natl Acad Sci USA* 100: 10972–10976.

Dollfus H, Verloes A, Bonneau D et al. (2005) Update on Bardet–Biedl syndrome. *J Fr Ophtalmol* 28: 106–112.

European Metrodin HP Study Group (1998) Efficacy and safety of highly purified urinary follicle-stimulating hormone with human chorionic gonadotropin for treating men with isolated hypogonadotropic hypogonadism. *Fertil Steril* 70: 256–262.

Falardeau J, Chung WC, Beenken A et al. (2008) Decreased FGF8 signaling causes deficiency of gonadotropin- releasing hormone in humans and mice. *J Clin Invest* 118: 2822–2831.

Filicori M, Flamigni C, Dellai P et al. (1994) Treatment of an ovulation with pulsatile gonadotropin-releasing hormone: Prognostic factors and clinical results in 600 cycles. *J Clin Endocrinol Metab* 79: 1215–1220.

Finkel DM, Phillips JL and Snyder PJ (1985) Stimulation of spermatogenesis by gonadotropins in men with hypogonadotropic hypogonadism. *N Engl J Med* 313: 651–655.

Finkelstein JS, Klibanski A, Neer RM et al. (1987) Osteoporoais in men with idiopathic hypogonadotrophic hypogonadism. *Ann Intern Med* 106: 354–361.

Fromantin M, Gineste J, Didier A et al. (1973) Impuberism and hypogonadism at induction into military service. Statistical study. *Probl Actuels Endocrinol Nutr* 16: 179–199.

Goldstone AP, Holland AJ, Hauffa BP et al. (2008) Recommendations for the diagnosis and management of Prader–Willi syndrome. *J Clin Endocrinol Metab* 93: 4183–4197.

Gonzalez-Martinez D, Kim S, Hu Y et al. (2004) Anosmin-1 modulates fibroblast growth factor receptor 1 signaling in human gonadotropin-releasing hormone olfactory neuroblasts through a heparan sulfate-dependent mechanism. *JNeurosci* 24: 10384–10392.

Grumbach MM (2005) A window of opportunity: The diagnosis of gonadotropin deficiency in the male infant. *J Clin Endocrinol Metab* 90: 3122–3127.

Guran T, Tolhurst G, Bereket A et al. (2009) Hypogonadotropic hypogonadism due to a novel missense mutation in the first extracellular loop of the neurokinin B receptor. *J Clin Endocrinol Metab* 94: 3633–3639.

Hardelin J-P and Dodé C (2008) The complex genetics of Kallmann syndrome: KAL1, FGFR1, FGF8, PROKR2, PROK2 et al. *Sex Dev* 2: 181–193.

Hardelin J-P, Julliard AK, Moniot B et al. (1999) Anosmin-1 is a regionally restricted component of basement membranes and interstitial matrices during organogenesis: Implications for the developmental anomalies of X chromosome-linked Kallmann syndrome. *Dev Dyn* 215: 26–44.

Hébert JM, Partanen J, Rossant J et al. (2003) FGF signaling through FGFR1 is required for olfactory bulb morphogenesis. *Development* 130: 1101–1111.

Hu Y, Gonzalez-Martinez D, Kim S et al. (2004) Cross-talk of anosmin-1, the protein implicated in X-linked Kallmann's syndrome, with heparan sulphate and urokinase-type plasminogen activator. *Biochem J* 384: 495–505.

Ito M, Yu R and Jameson JL (1997) DAX-1 inhibits SF-1 mediated transactivation via a carboxy terminal domain that is deleted in adrenal hypoplasia congenital. *Mol Cell Biol* 17: 1476–1483.

Jansen RP (1993) Pulsatile intravenous gonadotrophin releasing hormone for ovulation induction: Determinants of follicular and luteal phase responses. *Hum Reprod* 8(Suppl 2): 193–196.

Kertzman C, Robinson DL, Sherins RJ et al. (1990) Abnormalities in visual spatial attention in men with mirror movements associated with isolated hypogonadotropic hypogonadism. *Neurology* 40: 1057–1063.

Kim H, Ahn JW, Kurth I et al. (2010) WDR11, a WD Protein that interacts with transcription factor EMX1, is mutated in idiopathic hypogonadotropic hypogonadism and Kallmann syndrome. *Am J Hum Genet* 87(4): 465–479.

Kim HG and Layman LC (2011) The role of CHD7 and the newly identified WDR11 gene in patients with idiopathic hypogonadotropic hypogonadism and Kallmann syndrome. *Mol Cell Endocrinol* 346: 74–83.

Kirk J, Grant D, Besser G et al. (1994) Unilateral renal aplasia in X-linked Kallmann's syndrome. *Clin Genet* 46: 260–262.

Klingmüller D, Duwes W, Krahe T et al. (1987) Magnetic resonance imaging of the brain in patients with anosmia and hypothalamic hypogonadism (Kallmann's syndrome). *J Clin Endocrinol Metab* 65: 581–584.

Krams M, Quinton R, Ashburner J et al. (1999) Kallmann's syndrome: Mirror movements associated with bilateral corticospinal tract hypertrophy. *Neurology* 52: 816–822.

Legouis R, Hardelin JP, Levilliers J et al. (1991) The candidate gene for the X-linked Kallmann syndrome encodes a protein related to adhesion molecules. *Cell* 67: 423–435.

Leroy C, Fouveaut C, Leclercq S et al. (2008) Biallelic mutations in the prokineticin-2 gene in two sporadic cases of Kallmann syndrome. *Eur J Hum Genet* 16: 865–868.

Lieblich JM, Rogol AD, White BJ et al. (1982) Syndrome of anosmia with hypogonadotropic hypogonadism (Kallmann syndrome). *Am J Med* 73: 506–519.

Lin L, Gu WX, Ozisik G et al. (2006) Analysis of DAX1 (NR0B1) and steroidogenic factor-1 (NR5A1) in children and adults with primary adrenal failure: Ten years' experience. *J Clin Endocrinol Metab* 91: 3048–3054.

Liu L, Banks SM, Barnes KM et al. (1988) Two-year comparison of testicular responses to pulsatile gonadotropin- releasing hormone and exogenous gonadotropins from the inception of therapy in men with isolated hypogonadotropic hypogonadism. *J Clin Endocrinol Metab* 67: 1140–1145.

Liu PY, Turner L, Rushford D et al. (1999) Efficacy and safety of recombinant human follicle stimulating hormone (Gonal-F) with urinary human chorionic gonadotrophin for induction of spermatogenesis and fertility in gonadotrophin-deficient men. *Hum Reprod* 14: 1540–1545.

Ludwig M, Doody KJ and Doody KM (2003) Use of recombinant human chorionic gonadotropin in ovulation induction. *Fertil Steril* 79: 1051.

Main KM, Schmidt IM, Toppari J et al. (2002) Early postnatal treatment of hypogonadotropic hypogonadism with recombinant human FSH and LH. *Eur J Endocrinol* 146(1): 75–79.

Mann DR, Smith MM, Gould KG et al. (1985) Effects of a gonadotropin-releasing hormone agonist on luteinizing hormone and testosterone secretion and testicular histology in male rhesus monkeys, Macaca fascicularis. *Fertil Steril* 43: 115–121.

Mannaerts B, Fauser B, Lahlou N et al. (1996) Serum hormone concentrations during treatment with multiple rising doses of recombinant follicle stimulating hormone (Puregon) in men with hypogonadotropic hypogonadism. *Fertil Steril* 65: 406–410.

Margolin DH, Kousi M, Chan Y-M et al. (2013) Ataxia, dementia and hypogonadotrophic hypogonadism caused by disordered ubiquitination. *N Engl J Med* 368: 1992–2003.

Martin KA, Hall JE, Adams JM and Crowley WF Jr (1993) Comparison of exogenous gonadotropins and pulsatile gonadotropin-releasing hormone for induction of ovulation in hypogonadotropic amenorrhea. *J Clin Endocrinol Metab* 77: 125.

Martin K, Santoro N, Hall J et al. (1990) Clinical review 15: Management of ovulatory disorders with pulsatile gonadotropin-releasing hormone. *J Clin Endocrinol Metab* 71: 1081A.

Massa G, de Zegher F and Vanderschueren-Lodeweyckx M (1992) Serum levels of immunoreactive inhibin, FSH, and LH in human infants at preterm and term birth. *Biol Neonate* 61(3): 150–155.

Matsumoto S, Yamazaki C, Masumoto KH et al. (2006) Abnormal development of the olfactory bulb and reproductive system in mice lacking prokineticin receptor PKR2. *Proc Natl Acad Sci USA* 103: 4140–4145.

Mayston MJ, Harrison LM, Quinton R et al. (1997) Mirror movements in X-linked Kallmann's syndrome. I. A neurophysiological study. *Brain* 120: 1199–1216.

Miraoi H, Dwyer AA, Sykiotis GP et al. (2013) Mutations in FGF17, IL17RD, DUSP6, SPRY4, and FLRT3 are identified in individuals with congenital hypogonadotropic hypogonadism. *Am J Hum Genet* 92(5): 725–743.

Molsted K, Kjaer I, Giwercman A et al. (1997) Craniofacial morphology in patients with Kallmann's syndrome with and without cleft lip and palate. *Cleft Palate-Craniofac J* 34: 417–424.

Monnier C, Dodé C, Fabre L et al. (2008) *ProKr2* missense mutations associated with Kallmann syndrome impair receptor signalling-activity. *Hum Mol Genet* 18(1): 75–81.

Muller F and O'Rahilly R (1989) The human brain at stage 17, including the appearance of the future olfactory bulb and the first amygdaloid nuclei. *Anat Embryol* 180: 353–369.

Murakami S, Seki T and Arai Y (2002) Structural and chemical guidance cues for the migration of GnRH neurons in the chick embryo. *Prog Brain Res* 141: 31–44.

Murray J and Schutte B (2004) Cleft palate: Players, pathways, and pursuits. *J Clin Invest* 113: 1676–1678.

Muscatelli F, Strom TM, Walker AP et al. (1994) Mutations in the DAX-1 gene give rise to both X-linked adrenal hypoplasia congenita and hypogonadotrophic hypogonadism. *Nature* 372: 672–676.

Muske L and Moore FL (1990) Ontogeny of gonadotropin-releasing hormone neuronal systems in amphibians. *Brain Res* 534: 177–187.

Netchine I, Sobrier ML, Krude H et al. (2000) Mutations in LHX3 result in a new syndrome revealed by combined pituitary hormone deficiency. *Nat Genet* 25: 182–186.

Ohtaki T, Shintani Y, Honda S et al. (2001) Metastasis suppressor gene KiSS-1 encodes peptide ligand of a G-protein- coupled receptor. *Nature* 411: 613–617.

Parhar IS (2002) Cell migration and evolutionary significance of GnRH subtypes. *Prog Brain Res* 141: 3–17.

Pingault V, Bodereau V, Baral V et al. (2013) Loss-of-function mutations in SOX10 cause Kallmann syndrome with deafness. *Am J Hum Genet* 92(5): 707–724.

Pinto G, Abadie V, Mesnage R et al. (2005) CHARGE syndrome includes hypogonadotropic hypogonadism and abnormal olfactory bulb development. *J Clin Endocrinol Metabol* 90: 5621–5626.

Pitteloud N, Acierno JS Jr, Meysing AU et al. (2005) Reversible Kallmann syndrome, delayed puberty, and isolated anosmia occurring in a single family with a mutation in the fibroblast growth factor receptor 1 gene. *J Clin Endocrinol Metab* 90: 1317–1322.

Pitteloud N, Meysing A, Quinton R et al. (2006) Mutations in fibroblast growth factor receptor 1 cause Kallmann syndrome with a wide spectrum of reproductive phenotypes. *Mol Cell Endocrinol* 254–255: 60–69.

Pitteloud N, Quinton R, Pearce S et al. (2007) Digenic mutations account for variable phenotypes in idiopathic hypogonadotropic hypogonadism. *J Clin Invest* 117: 457–463.

Pitteloud N, Zhang C, Pignatelli D et al. (2007) Loss-of- function mutation in the prokineticin 2 gene causes Kallmann syndrome and normosmic idiopathic hypogonadotropic hypogonadism. *Proc Natl Acad Sci USA* 104: 17447–17452.

Prevot V, Bellefontaine N, Baroncini M et al. (2010) Gonadotrophin-releasing hormone nerve terminals, tanycytes and neurohaemal junction remodelling in the adult median eminence: Functional consequences for reproduction and dynamic role of vascular endothelial cells. *J Neuroendocrinol* 22(7): 639–649.

Quinton R, Barnett P, Coskeran P et al. (1999a) Gordon Holmes spinocerebellar ataxia: A gonadotrophin deficiency syndrome resistant to treatment with pulsatile gonadotrophin-releasing hormone. *Clin Endocrinol* 51: 525–529.

Quinton R, Cheow HK, Tymms DJ et al. (1999b) Kallmann's syndrome: Is it always for life? *Clin Endocrinol* 50: 481–485.

Quinton R, Duke V, de Zoysa P et al. (1996) The neuroradiology of Kallmann's syndrome: A genotypic and phenotypic analysis. *J Clin Endocrinol Metab* 81: 3010–3017.

Quinton R, Duke VM, Robertson A et al. (2001) Idiopathic gonadotrophin deficiency: Genetic questions addressed through phenotypic characterization. *Clin Endocrinol* 55: 163–174.

Raivio T, Falardeau J, Dwyer A et al. (2007) Reversal of idiopathic hypogonadotrophic hypogonadism. *N Engl J Med* 357: 863–873.

Reynaud R, Barlier A, Vallette-Kasic S et al. (2005) An uncommon phenotype with familial central hypogonadism caused by a novel PROP1 gene mutant truncated in the transactivation domain. *J Clin Endocrinol Metab* 90: 4880–4887.

Ribeiro RS, Vieira TC and Abucham J (2007) Reversible Kallmann syndrome: Report of the first case with a Kal 1 mutation and literature review. *Eur J Endocrinol* 156: 285–290.

Roa J, Aguilar E, Dieguez C et al. (2008) New frontiers in kisspeptin/GPR54 physiology as fundamental gatekeepers of reproductive function. *Front Neuroendocrinol* 29: 48–69.

Salenave S, Chanson P, Bry H et al. (2008) Kallmann's syndrome: A comparison of the reproductive phenotypes in men carrying *Kal1* and *fGfr1/Kal2* mutations. *J Clin Endocrinol Metab* 93(3): 758–763.

Santen RJ and Paulsen CA (1972) Hypogonadotropic eunuchoidism. I. Clinical study of the mode of inheritance. *J Clin Endocrinol Metab* 36: 47–54.

Schaison G, Young J, Pholsena M et al. (1993) Failure of combined follicle-stimulating hormone-testosterone administration to initiate and/or maintain spermatogenesis in men with hypogonadotropic hypogonadism. *J Clin Endocrinol Metab* 77: 1545–1549.

Schwankhaus JD, Currie J, Jaffe MJ et al. (1989) Neurologic findings in men with isolated hypogonadotropic hypogonadism. *Neurology* 39: 223–226.

Schwanzel-Fukuda M (1999) Origin and migration of luteinizing hormone-releasing hormone neurons in mammals. *Microsc Res Tech* 44: 2–10.

Schwanzel-Fukuda M, Bick D and Pfaff DW (1989) Luteinizing hormone-releasing hormone (LHRH)-expressing cells do not migrate normally in an inherited hypogonadal (Kallmann) syndrome. *Mol Brain Res* 6(4): 311–326.

Schwanzel-Fukuda M and Pfaff DW (1989) Origin of luteinizing hormone-releasing hormone neurons. *Nature* 338: 161–164.

Seminara SB, Hayes FJ and Crowley WF Jr (1998) Gonadotropin-releasing hormone deficiency in the human (idiopathic hypogonadotropic hypogonadism and Kallmann's syndrome): Pathophysiological and genetic considerations. *Endocr Rev* 19: 521–539.

Seminara SB, Messager S, Chatzidaki EE et al. (2003) The GPR54 gene as a regulator of puberty. *N Engl J Med* 349: 1614–1627.

Sharpe RM, Fraser HM, Brougham MF et al. (2003) Role of the neonatal period of pituitary-testicular activity in germ cell proliferation and differentiation in the primate testes. *Hum Reprod* 18(10): 2110–2117.

Sinisi AA, Asci R, Bellastella G et al. (2008) Homozygous mutation in the prokineticin-receptor 2 gene (Val274Asp) presenting as reversible Kallmann syndrome and persistent oligozoospermia: Case report. *Hum Reprod* 23: 2380–2384.

Soussi-Yanicostas N, Hardelin J-P, Arroyo-Jimenez M et al. (1996) Initial characterization of anosmin-1, a putative extracellular matrix protein synthesized by definite neuronal cell populations in the central nervous system. *J Cell Sci* 109: 1749–1757.

Strobel A, Issad T, Camoin L et al. (1998) A leptin missense mutation associated with hypogonadism and morbid obesity. *Nat Genet* 18: 213–215.

Sykiotis GP, Plummer L, Hughes VA et al. (2010) Oligogenic basis of isolated gonadotropin-releasing hormone deficiency. *Proc Natl Acad Sci USA* 107: 15140–15144.

Topaloglu AK and Kotan LD (2010) Molecular causes of hypogonadotropic hypogonadism. *Curr Opin Obstet Gynecol* 22: 264–270.

Topaloglu AK, Reimann F, Guclu M et al. (2009) TAC3 and TACR3 mutations in familial hypogonadotropic hypogonadism reveal a key role for Neurokinin B in the central control of reproduction. *Nat Genet* 41: 354–358.

Topaloglu AK, Tello JA, Kotan LD et al. (2012) Inactivating KISS1 mutation and hypogonadotropic hypo-gonadism. *N Engl J Mede* 366: 629–635.

Tornberga J, Sykiotisb GP, Keefe K et al. (2011) Heparan sulfate 6-O-sulfotransferase 1, a gene involved in extracellular sugar modifications, is mutated in patients with idiopathic hypogonadotrophic hypogonad-ism. *Proc Natl Acad Sci USAmerica* 108(28): 11524–11529.

Trarbach EB, Costa EM, Versiani B et al. (2006) Novel fibroblast growth factor receptor 1 mutations in patients with congenital hypogonadotropic hypogonadism with and without anosmia. *J Clin Endocrinol Metab* 91: 4006–4012.

Uriarte MM, Baron J, Garcia HB et al. (1992) The effect of pubertal delay on adult height in men with isolated hypogonadotrophic hypogonadism. *J Clin Endocrinol Metab* 74: 436–440.

Vicari E, Mongioi A, Calogero AE et al. (1992) Therapy with human chorionic gonadotrophin alone induces spermatogenesis in men with isolated hypogonadotrophic hypogonadism—long-term follow-up. *Int J Androl* 15: 320–329.

Wegenke JD, Uehling DT, Wear JBJ et al. (1975) Familial Kallmann syndrome with unilateral renal aplasia. *Clin Genet* 7: 368–381.

Wray S (2001) Development of luteinizing hormone releasing hormone neurones. *J Neuroendocrinol* 13: 3–11.

Wray S, Grant P and Gainer H (1989) Evidence that cells expressing luteinizing hormone-releasing hormone mRNA in the mouse are derived from progenitor cells in the olfactory placode. *Proc Natl Acad Sci US A* 86: 8132–8136.

Young J, Metay C, Bouligand J et al. (2012) SEMA3A deletion in a family with Kallmann syndrome validates the role of semaphorin 3A in human puberty and olfactory system development. *Hum Reprod* 27(5): 1460–1465.

Young J, Rey R, Couzinet B et al. (1999) Antimüllerian hormone in patients with hypogonadotropic hypo-gonadism. *J Clin Endocrinol Metab* 84(8): 2696–2699.

Zhang X, Ibrahimi OA, Olsen SK et al. (2006) Receptor specificity of the fibroblast growth factor family. The complete mammalian FGF family. *J Biol Chem* 281: 15694–15700.

20
PRECOCIOUS PUBERTY

Jean-Claude Carel, Laetitia Martinerie, Dominique Simon, Delphine Zenaty,
Nicolas de Roux and Juliane Léger

Introduction

Premature sexual maturation is a frequent cause for referral in paediatric endocrinology. Although clinical evaluation will suffice to reassure the patient and family in a majority of cases, premature sexual maturation can reveal severe conditions and needs a thorough evaluation to identify its cause and potential for progression, in order to propose an appropriate treatment if needed. Most cases of precocious puberty result from the early activation of the gonadotropin-releasing hormone (GnRH) axis and the underlying mechanism is poorly understood. Peripheral or gonadotropin-independent forms of precocious puberty are rare, have been described in detail elsewhere (Carel and Leger 2008) and will not be described extensively in this chapter. Long-acting GnRH agonists are efficient and widely used in the treatment of central precocious puberty but questions remain regarding their optimal use (Carel et al. 2009). Among the several ongoing controversial issues in the area are the definition of normal pubertal development and the role of environmental disruptors.

Normal and premature sexual maturation

Normal pubertal development results from the increase of pulsatile release of GnRH in the hypothalamo-pituitary portal system and the activation of the hypothalamo-pituitary-gonadal axis. The onset of puberty is marked clinically by breast development in girls (Tanner 2 breast or B2; Fig 20.1) and testicular enlargement in boys (Tanner 2 genitalia or G2 or testicular volume greater than 4 ml or testicular length greater than 25 mm).

Defining the normal limits of pubertal development remains difficult, given the paucity of truly normative data and the number of components to consider including not only pubertal onset, but also progression of puberty and onset of menarche. Cross-sectional data obtained in the 1960s indicated a normal age range of pubertal onset (the age at which 95% of children reach Tanner stage 2) between 8 and 13 years in girls and 9.5 and 13.5 years in boys. Cross-sectional data obtained in the United States have shown that pubertal milestones were being reached earlier than previously thought by African American and to a lesser extent by Mexican American or non-Hispanic white girls (Herman-Giddens et al. 2004). A similar tendency has also been noted in Europe (Aksglaede et al. 2009) and in Asia (Ma et al. 2009). In girls examined in Copenhagen, the mean age at the B2 stage has decreased from 10.9 to 9.9 years between 1991 and 2006

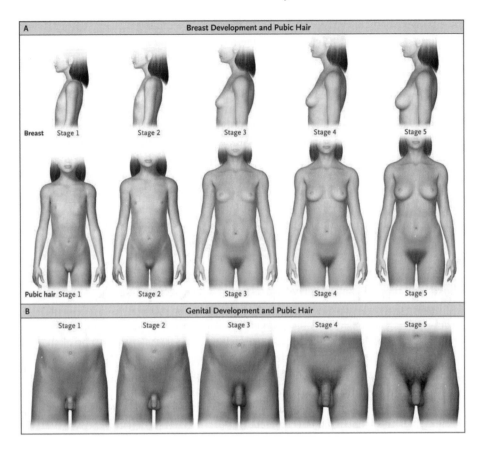

Figure 20.1. Classification of pubertal developmental stages according to Tanner. Reproduced with permission from Carel and Leger (2008).

(Aksglaede et al. 2009). Although the traditional limits of 8 years in girls and 9.5 years in boys are still used by most paediatric endocrinologists (Carel and Leger 2008, Carel et al. 2009), the cut-off limits should clearly be decreased (Kaplowitz and Oberfield 1999). Sexual hair development is a component of pubertal maturation that reflects the actions of androgen produced by the gonads or by the adrenals. Similarly, the traditional limits of pubic hair development have been set to 8 years in girls and 9.5 years in boys with wide ethnic variations.

In addition to the cross-sectional definitions and limits of the onset of puberty, there are several elements to consider to define normal and abnormal pubertal development. First, the activation of the gonadotropic axis is not an all or none phenomenon, but evolves over several years, starting 2 to 3 years before the clinical onset of puberty. Second, the mean duration of the transition from one stage to the next is generally close to 6 months on average, but varies among individuals. In slowly progressive puberty, pubertal development can remain at the B2 stage or revert to the B1 stage before resuming later. It is noteworthy that although the mean age at the B2 stage has decreased in the past decades, the age at menarche has been relatively stable, indicating a longer duration of puberty (Aksglaede et al. 2009). Third, the onset of puberty is affected by a number of factors in addition to ethnicity (Parent et al. 2003). Puberty occurs earlier in girls with early maternal menarche, low birthweight, excessive weight gain or obesity in infancy and early childhood, after international adoption (10 to 20 times increase in risk for unclear reasons; Teilmann et al. 2006) and possibly after exposure to estrogenic endocrine-disrupting chemicals or if no father is present in the household (Parent et al. 2003; Bogaert 2005; Carel and Leger 2008). These factors are generally not considered in definitions of normality in practice but should be kept in mind. It is important to recognise that a 'normal' timing of onset of pubertal development does not rule out a pathological condition (Midyett et al. 2003). The prevalence of precocious puberty is about 10 times higher in girls than in boys and has been estimated at 0.2% of girls and less than 0.05% of boys in Denmark (Teilmann et al. 2005).

Causes and mechanisms underlying premature sexual development
Premature sexual development (Fig 20.2) results from the action of sex steroids or compounds with sex steroid activity on target organs. The most common mechanism of premature sexual development is central precocious puberty due to the early activation of pulsatile GnRH secretion. Peripheral or gonadotropin-independent precocious puberty is due to the production of sex steroids by gonadal or adrenal tissue, independently of gonadotropins, which are generally suppressed. Exposure to exogenous sex steroids or to compounds with steroidal activity can also result in premature sexual development. It is also important to recognise variants of pubertal development that can mimic precocious puberty but do not lead to long-term consequences and are usually benign.

Central precocious puberty is due to the premature activation of GnRH secretion and results in a hormonal pattern that is similar to that of normal puberty, although early. Central precocious puberty can be due to hypothalamic tumours or lesions or may be idiopathic in the majority of cases, in particular in girls (Table 20.1; Fig 20.3). The mechanism by which hypothalamic lesions lead to accelerated activation of the GnRH axis is currently unknown. Hypothalamic hamartomas do not act as ectopic GnRH pulse generators but rather seem to interact with pubertal regulation by secreting factors such as transforming growth factor alpha (Parent et al. 2008). Paternally inherited loss of mutations in the makorin ring finger 3 (*MKRN3*) gene has been associated with central precocious puberty (Abreu et al. 2013) as have variants of the KISS1/KISS1R systems (Macedo et al. 2014). Understanding how *MKRN3* mutations lead to activation of puberty might also help understand how hypothalamic lesions lead to precocious puberty. Other genetic events have been associated with central precocious puberty occurring in complex developmental and neurological disorders.

Peripheral precocious puberty can result from gonadal, adrenal or human chorionic gonadotropin (hCG)-producing tumours, activating mutations in the gonadotropic pathway

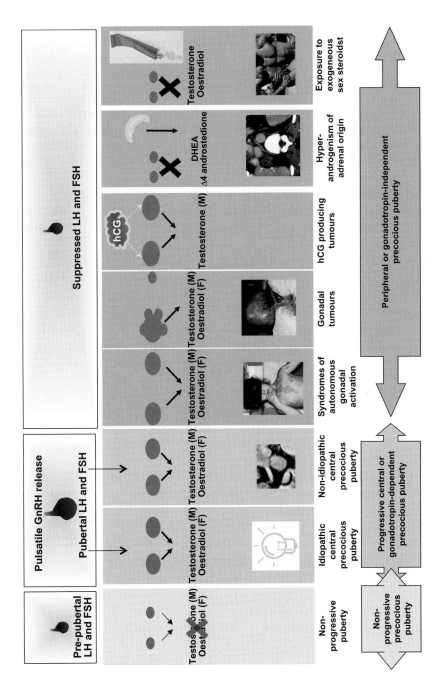

Figure 20.2. Principal mechanisms of premature sexual development.

331

TABLE 20.1
Clinical characteristics of the various forms of central precocious puberty

Cause	Symptoms and signs	Evaluation
Due to a CNS lesion		
Hypothalamic hamartoma	Possibly associated with gelastic (laughing attacks), focal or tonic-clonic seizures.	MRI: Mass in the floor of the third ventricle iso-intense to normal tissue without contrast enhancement
Other hypothalamic tumours: • Glioma involving the hypothalamus and/or the optic chiasm. • Astrocytoma, • Ependymoma, • Pinealoma, • Germ cell tumours.	Headache, visual changes, cognitive changes, symptoms/signs of anterior or posterior pituitary deficiency (eg decreased growth velocity, polyuria/polydipsia), fatigue, visual field defects. If CNS tumour (glioma) associated with neurofibromatosis, may have other features of neurofibromatosis (cutaneous neurofibromas, café au lait spots, Lisch nodules, axillary freckling)	MRI: contrast-enhanced mass that may involve the optic pathways (chiasm, nerve, tract), the hypothalamus (astrocytoma, glioma) or the pituitary stalk (germ cell tumour). May have evidence of intracranial hypertension. May have signs of anterior or posterior pituitary deficiency If germ cell tumour: ßhCG detectable in blood or CSF
Cerebral malformations involving the hypothalamus: • Suprasellar arachnoid cyst, • Hydrocephalus, • Septo optic dysplasia, • Myelomeningocele, • Ectopic neurohypophysis.	Neurodevelopmental deficits, macrocrania, visual impairment, nystagmus, obesity, polyuria/polydipsia, decreased growth velocity.	May have signs of anterior or posterior pituitary deficiency or hyperprolactinemia
Acquired injury: • Cranial irradiation, • Head trauma, • Infections, • Perinatal insults.	Relevant history. Symptoms and signs of anterior or posterior pituitary deficiency may be present.	MRI may reveal condition-specific sequelae or may be normal
Idiopathic - No CNS lesion	>95% of girls and ≈ 50% of boys. History of familial precocious puberty or adoption may be present. Paternally inherited loss of function mutations in the MKRN3 gene Other genetic factors have been implicated	No hypothalamic abnormality on the head MRI. The anterior pituitary may be enlarged.

(continued)

TABLE 20.1

(continued)

Cause	Symptoms and signs	Evaluation
Secondary to early exposure to sex steroids		Similar to other causes of central precocious puberty, but need to integrate the role of:
After cure of any cause of gonadotropin-independent precocious puberty.	Relevant history of one of the following group of conditions: Autonomous gonadal activation hCG or sex steroid producing tumours Adrenal disorders Environmental agents Severe untreated primary hypothyroidism	1. the variability of the control of the primary condition (as in congenital adrenal hyperplasia for instance) 2. the drugs used for the peripheral precocious puberty (such as aromatase inhibitors)

CNS, central nervous system; CSF, cerebrospinal fluid; hCG, human chorionic gonadotropin.

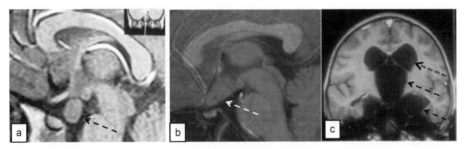

Figure 20.3. Hypothalamic lesions associated with precocious puberty: MRI findings in three cases. Typical examples of hamartoma of the tuber cinereum (a), optic chiasm glioma (b) and suprasellar archnoidal cysts (c), leading to dilatation of the ventricular system (double arrow).

and exposure to exogenous sex steroids. When peripheral precocious puberty is treated, it can rarely lead to secondary activation of pulsatile GnRH secretion and to central precocious puberty (Table 20.1).

It is essential to recognise that most cases of premature sexual maturation correspond to benign variants of normal development that can occur throughout childhood (Table 20.2). This is particularly true in girls below the age of 2 to 3 years, where the condition is known as premature thelarche. Similarly in older girls, at least 50% of cases of premature sexual maturation will regress or stop progressing and no treatment is necessary. Although the mechanism underlying these cases of non-progressive precocious puberty is unknown, the gonadotropic axis is not activated. Premature thelarche probably represents an exaggerated form of the physiological early gonadotropin surge that is delayed in girls relative to boys.

TABLE 20.2
Benign variants of premature sexual maturation

Condition	Characteristics	Management
Non-progressive precocious puberty	See table 20.4 for differential characteristics with progressive central precocious puberty	
Isolated precocious thelarche	Unilateral or bilateral breast development; particularly frequent before the age of 3 years.	No further evaluation needed in most cases
Isolated precocious pubarche	Pubic hair development can be associated with adult body odour, axillary hair or mild acne.	Normal cortisol precursors in serum, including normal concentrations of 17OH-progesterone after ACTH stimulation
Isolated precocious menarche	Isolated vaginal haemorrhage without breast development or pubic hair, and no genital trauma. It is important to evaluate clinically for a vaginal lesion (sex abuse, foreign body, tumour).	

Consequences of premature sexual maturation

Progressive premature sexual maturation can have consequences on growth and psychoso-cial development. Growth velocity is accelerated as compared to normal values for age and bone age is advanced in most cases. The acceleration of bone maturation can lead to pre-mature fusion of the growth plates and short stature. Several studies have assessed adult height in individuals with a history of precocious puberty. In earlier published series of untreated patients, mean heights ranged from 151 cm to 156 cm in boys and 150 cm to 154 cm in girls, corresponding to a loss of about 20 cm in boys and 12cm in girls relative to normal adult height (Carel et al. 2004). However, these numbers correspond to historical series of patients with early-onset precocious puberty, which are not representative of the majority of patients seen in the clinic today. Height loss due to precocious puberty is inversely cor-related with the age at pubertal onset, and currently treated patients tend to have later onset of puberty than those in historical series (Carel et al. 2004).

Parents often seek treatment in girls because they fear early menarche (Xhrouet-Heinrichs et al. 1997). However, there are few data to predict the age of menarche following early onset of puberty. In the general population, the time from breast development to menarche is longer for children with an earlier onset of puberty, ranging from a mean of 2.8 years when breast development begins at age 9 to 1.4 years when breast development begins at age 12 (Marti-Henneberg and Vizmanos 1997). Similarly, in the Danish study cited above showing a 1-year decrease in age at breast development, the corresponding decrease in age at first menses was only 3.5 months (Aksglaede et al. 2009).

Adverse psychosocial outcomes are also a concern, but the available data specific to patients with precocious puberty have serious limitations (Carel et al. 2009). In the general population, a higher proportion of early-maturing adolescents engage in exploratory behaviours (sexual intercourse and legal and illegal substance use) and at an earlier age than adolescents maturing within the normal age range or later (Michaud et al. 2006). In addition, the risk for sexual abuse seems to be higher in girls or women with early sexual maturation (Wise et al. 2009). However, the relevance of these findings to precocious puberty is unclear, and they should not be used to justify intervention. In addition, some data suggest an influence of psychosocial environment, in particular being raised in a stressful environment, with low income or separated from one's parents, on pubertal development (Belsky et al. 2007; Pesonen et al. 2008; Deardorff et al. 2011; Jean et al. 2011). Therefore, psychosocial outcomes of precocious puberty collected from epidemiological studies should not be unequivocally viewed as resulting from precocious puberty, since reverse causality could be involved.

Evaluation of the child with premature sexual development

The evaluation of patients with premature sexual development should address several questions: (1) Is sexual development really occurring outside the normal temporal range? (2) What is the underlying mechanism and is it associated with a risk of a serious condition, such as an intracranial lesion? (3) Is pubertal development likely to progress? and (4) Would this impair the child's normal physical and psychosocial development?

Clinical evaluation

A complete family history (age at onset of puberty in parents and siblings, with emphasis on the fact that paternal history is often difficult to collect) and personal history including the age at onset and progression of sexual development should be taken. Any evidence suggesting possible central nervous system disorder, such as headache, increased head circumference, visual impairment or seizures, should be collected. Growth should be evaluated by drawing a complete growth chart, because progressive precocious puberty is almost invariably associated with and sometimes preceded by an acceleration of growth velocity.

The stage of pubertal development should be classified according to Tanner (Fig 20.1). Careful assessment is needed in obese girls to avoid overestimating breast development. The development of pubic hair results from the effects of androgens, which may be produced by testes or ovaries in central precocious puberty. Acne, oily skin and hair may be present and result from the action of androgens. In girls, pubic hair in the absence of breast development is suggestive of adrenal disorders, premature pubarche or exposure to androgens. In boys, measurement of testicular volume may suggest the cause of puberty, as testicular volume increases in central precocious puberty as in normal puberty and in cases of peripheral precocious puberty due to testicular disorders (although generally less so), whereas it remains prepubertal in adrenal disorders, premature pubarche and other causes of peripheral precocious puberty. Physical examination should also assess for signs of specific causes of precocious puberty, such as hyperpigmented skin lesions suggesting neurofibromatosis or McCune-Albright syndrome. It is also important to recognise clinically the benign variants of precocious pubertal development with usually isolated and non-progressive secondary sexual characteristics (breast or pubic hair), normal or slightly increased growth velocity and no or slight bone age advancement, if performed (Table 20.2).

Premature sexual development can be associated with high levels of anxiety in girls and in parents and psychological evaluation of the child and of the familial environment may be useful.

LABORATORY EVALUATION AND IMAGING

Additional testing is generally recommended in all boys with precocious pubertal develop-ment, in girls who present with precocious Tanner 3 breast stage or higher or in girls with precocious B2 stage and additional criteria such as increased growth velocity, advanced bone age, symptoms or signs suggestive of central nervous system dysfunction or of periph-eral precocious puberty, implying that most girls with a precocious B2 stage without any additional manifestation should be carefully followed without additional testing.

Bone age

Bone age determined using the Greulich & Pyle or other methods evaluates the impact of sex steroids on epiphyseal maturation and is usually advanced in progressive precocious puberty. Caution should be taken in over-interpreting bone age, since there is a physiological scatter of approximately plus or minus 1 to 2 years of bone age versus chronological age in Caucasians and a systematic advance of bone age in children of Afro-Caribbean origin when using references obtained in Caucasians. Bone age can also be used to predict adult height, although with a low precision (95% confidence interval of about ± 6 cm) and a tendency to overestimate adult height in precocious puberty.

Hormonal measurements

Hormonal measurements that can be useful for the evaluation of premature sexual matura-tion are summarised in Table 20.3.

• Sex steroids should be determined in the morning, using assays with detection limits adapted to paediatric values. Most boys with precocious puberty have morning plasma testosterone concentrations in the pubertal range. In girls, serum oestradiol concentrations are highly variable and have a low sensitivity for the diagnosis of precocious puberty. Very high oestradiol concentrations are generally indicative of ovarian disease (cysts or tumours).

• Luteinizing hormone determinations are essential and should use ultrasensitive assays. Luteinizing hormone assays used should have a detection limit near 0.1 IU/L to discriminate prepubertal from pubertal luteinizing hormone concentrations. The measurement of gonad-otropins following GnRH (or GnRH agonist) stimulation is considered the criterion stan-dard. However, normative values are scarce and cut-off levels are not well validated. During normal puberty, the peak luteinizing hormone concentration increases progressively with a large overlap between successive pubertal stages resulting in an ability to fully discriminate only stage I and stage IV (Martinez-Aguayo et al. 2009). Peak luteinizing hormone concen-trations of 5–8 IU/l suggest progressive central precocious puberty (Resende et al. 2007).

TABLE 20.3
Hormonal evaluation for the evaluation of premature sexual maturation

	Technical requirements	Significance	Limitations	Use
Serum oestradiol (girls)	Use morning values due to circadian variation. Use assay with a lower limit of detection of ≈ 5 pg/ml (18 pmol/L) or lower.	Markedly elevated concentrations ≈ >100 pg/ml (367 pmol/L) suggest ovarian cyst or tumour.	Concentrations can be normal in authentic central precocious puberty. Difficulties in interpreting values measured with immuno-enzymatic methods (falsely high values close to the limit of detection of the assay).	First line test together with basal LH in girls. However, poor sensitivity to discriminate early pubertal from prepubertal concentrations.
Serum testosterone	Use morning values due to circadian variation. Use assay with a lower limit of detection of ≈ 0.1 ng/ml (0.35 nmol/L).	Boys: reliable marker of testicular activation. Girls: use if signs of hyperandrogenism; elevated testosterone concentrations suggest adrenal disorders.	Difficulties in interpreting values measured with immuno-enzymatic methods (falsely high values close to the limit of detection of the assay).	First line test with basal LH in boys. High sensitivity to confirm precocious puberty.
Serum LH	Use morning values due to circadian rhythm. Use ultrasensitive assays with a lower limit of detection of ≈ 0.1 UI/L or lower.	Basal LH measurement poorly discriminates between pre-pubertal and early pubertal children. Values >0.3 to 0.4 UI/L indicative of central precocious puberty with a high specificity and a low sensitivity in some series.	Wide interassay variations; assay characteristics must be taken into account.	First line screening test in association with oestradiol or testosterone measurement. If clearly elevated, obviates the need for a stimulation test.
Peak LH after stimulation with GnRH* or GnRH agonist	Can be performed at any time of the day; assay requirements similar to baseline measurements.	Peak LH concentration above the pubertal cutoff with elevated sex steroid concentrations indicate progressive central puberty. Suppressed peak LH concentration with elevated sex steroid concentrations indicate peripheral precocious puberty.	Wide interassay variations; assay characteristics must be taken into account. Paucity of normative values to define cut-offs; values of 5 to 8 UI/L are most often considered "high" in children aged from 4 to 8. Higher cutoffs to be used in younger children. Values vary with the stimulating agent (GnRH or GnRH agonist).	Criterion standard for the diagnosis of central precocious puberty.

(continued)

337

TABLE 20.3
(continued)

	Technical requirements	Significance	Limitations	Use
Peak FSH after stimulation with GnRH* or GnRH agonist		Peak LH/FSH ratio typically increases during puberty; high ratios are used as a secondary criterion for progressive central puberty.	Poorly validated, in particular with sandwich-antibody assays for gonadotropin measurements.	Can be useful as an additional criterion
Serum βhCG		Produced by germ cell tumours. Can be detected in serum (peripheral tumours) or in CSF (intra-cranial tumour).	Peripheral production of βhCG leads to pubertal development in boys and not in girls.	Measurement warranted in boys with peripheral precocious puberty to identify a germ cell tumour and in the CSF when a lesion compatible with a germ cell tumour is detected by MRI.
Serum dehydroepiandrosterone sulfate/Androstene-dione		Produced by the adrenals, marker of androgen-producing adrenal tumours or of adrenal enzymatic defect.	Also increased in precocious pubarche.	Measure if androgenic signs (pubic hair) predominate.
Serum 17OH-progesterone	Use morning (8 a.m.) values due to circadian rhythm or measure after ACTH stimulation.	Marker of adrenal enzymatic defects (congenital adrenal hyperpasia). Occasionally elevated with adrenal tumours.	Borderline elevations are frequent in unaffected carriers of non-classic congenital adrenal hyperplasia.	Measure if androgenic signs (pubic hair) predominate.

LH, luteinizing hormone; GnRH, gonadotropin-releasing hormone; FSH, follicle-stimulating hormone; hCG, human chorionic gonadotropin; CSF, cerebrospinal fluid; ACTH, adrenocorticotropic hormone.

- Random luteinizing hormone measurements have been proposed as an alternative but variable cut-off values have been proposed (Harrington et al. 2014). However, unless luteinizing hormone values are clearly elevated, we consider it preferable to confirm the diagnosis of progressive central precocious puberty by a stimulation test before initiating treatment. In girls below the age of 4 years, physiological gonadotropin levels are higher than in older prepubertal girls and caution should be taken when interpreting the values to avoid overdiagnosing precocious puberty (Bizzarri et al. 2014).
- Follicle-stimulating hormone (FSH) measurements provide less information than luteinizing hormone measurements since FSH concentrations vary little through pubertal development. However, the stimulated luteinizing hormone/FSH ratio may help differentiate progressive precocious puberty (which tends to have higher luteinizing hormone/FSH ratios) from nonprogressive variants that do not require GnRHa therapy.

Pelvic or testicular ultrasonography

In girls, pelvic ultrasonography can be used to detect ovarian cysts or tumours. Uterine changes due to oestrogen exposure can be used as an index of progressive puberty but the proposed cut-offs of a uterine volume greater than 2.0 ml or a uterine length of more than 34 mm are not universally validated (de Vries et al. 2006; Sathasivam et al. 2011). Testicular ultrasound scans should be performed if testicular volume is asymmetric or in peripheral precocious puberty, in order to detect Leydig cell tumours, which are generally not palpable.

Brain MRI

Brain MRI is important to detect hypothalamic lesions in progressive central precocious puberty (Stanhope 2003). The prevalence of such lesions is higher in boys (40 to 90% of cases) than in girls with precocious puberty, and is much lower when puberty starts after the age of 6 years in girls (2%–3%; Chalumeau et al. 2003; Pedicelli et al. 2014). It has been suggested that an algorithm based on age and oestradiol concentrations may obviate the need for MRI in one-third of girls, but this has not been extensively validated (Chalumeau et al. 2003; Stanhope 2003).

Genetic testing

The usefulness of screening for *MKRN3* mutations in familial cases with paternal transmission and in apparently sporadic cases remains to be evaluated (Simon et al. 2016).

INTEGRATING CLINICAL AND LABORATORY EVALUATION

Clinical evaluation, hormonal measurements and imaging usually allow identification of one of the following situations (Fig 20.2):

- *Peripheral (gonadotropin-independent) precocious puberty:* High serum testosterone in boys; generally high and, occasionally, very high serum oestradiol in girls; undetectable basal and low (suppressed) peak serum luteinizing hormone after GnRH stimulation; oestrogenised uterus on ultrasound examination; variable bone age.

- *Progressive central (gonadotropin-dependent) precocious puberty:* High serum testosterone in boys, variable serum oestradiol in girls, pubertal basal and peak serum luteinizing hormone after GnRH stimulation, advanced bone age and oestrogenised uterus on ultrasound examination.
- *Benign variants of precocious pubertal development:* Low serum sex-steroid concentrations, normal pelvic ultrasound examination and prepubertal basal and peak serum luteinizing hormone after GnRH stimulation (if done, not necessary in most cases).

Table 20.4 summarises the features that are useful in distinguishing between progressive central precocious puberty and non-progressive forms of precocious puberty. Although these criteria are not fully evidence-based, they can provide useful orientation. When discrepant results are obtained, it is recommended to wait a few months and reassess, to avoid unnecessary treatment (Leger et al. 2000).

Management of central precocious puberty

GnRH AGONISTS

GnRH agonists (Table 20.5) are generally indicated in progressive central precocious puberty. GnRH agonists continuously stimulate the pituitary gonadotrophs, leading to desensitisation and decreases in luteinizing hormone release and, to a lesser extent, FSH release (Lahlou et al. 2000). Several GnRH agonists are available in various depot forms and their approval for use in precocious puberty varies with countries. Despite nearly 30 years of use of GnRH agonists in precocious puberty, there are still ongoing questions on their optimal use, and an international consensus statement has summarised the available information and the areas of uncertainty as of 2007 (Carel et al. 2009).

GnRH agonist treatment should be followed by experienced clinicians and result in the regression or stabilisation of pubertal symptoms, decrease of growth velocity to normal prepubertal values and arrest of bone age advancement (Carel et al. 2009). Progression of breast or testicular development usually indicates poor compliance, treatment failure or incorrect diagnosis and requires further evaluation. Otherwise, routine biochemical monitoring using basal or stimulated luteinizing hormone measurements is not recommended (Carel et al. 2009; Lewis and Eugster 2013).

OUTCOMES AFTER GnRH AGONIST TREATMENT IN PRECOCIOUS PUBERTY

There are no randomised controlled trials assessing long-term outcomes of the treatment of central precocious puberty with GnRH agonists, and height outcomes have been mostly evaluated. Among approximately 400 girls treated until a mean age of 11 years, the mean adult height was about 160 cm and mean gains over predicted height varied from 3 cm to 10 cm (Carel et al. 2004). Individual height gains were very variable, but were calculated using predicted height, which is itself unreliable. Factors affecting height outcome include initial patient characteristics (lower height if bone age is markedly advanced and shorter predicted height at initiation of treatment) and, in some patients, duration of treatment (higher height gains in patients starting treatment at a younger age and with longer duration of treatment).

TABLE 20.4

Criteria to differentiate non-progressive forms and progressive central precocious puberty in girls

		Progressive central precocious puberty	*Non-progressive precocious puberty*
Clinical	Pubertal stages	Progression from one stage to the next in 3 to 6 months	Stabilization or regression of pubertal signs
	Growth velocity	Accelerated ($\approx$>6 cm/year)	Usually normal for age
	Bone age	Usually advanced by at least 1 year	Usually within 1 year of chronological age
	Predicted adult height	Below target height range or declining on serial determinations	Within target height range
Pelvic ultrasonography	Uterine development	Uterine volume >2.0 ml or length >34 mm Pear-like shaped uterus Endometrial thickening (endometrial echo)	Uterine volume $\leq$2.0 ml or length $\leq$34 mm Prepubertal, tubular shaped uterus
	Oestradiol	Usually measurable oestradiol concentration with advancing pubertal development	Oestradiol not detectable or close to the detection limit
Hormonal evaluation	Basal LH	Above threshold (to be validated depending on the assay used)	Below threshold (to be validated depending on the assay used)
	LH peak after GnRH or GnRH agonist	In the pubertal range	In the prepubertal range

LH, luteinizing hormone; GnRH, gonadotropin-releasing hormone.
Reproduced with permission from (Carel and Leger 2008)

TABLE 20.5
Long acting GnRH agonists used for the treatment of central precocious puberty

Depot GnRH agonists	Brand name	Usual Starting Dose**
Goserelin	Zoladex LA	3.6 mg every mo OR 10.8 mg every 3 mo
Buserelin	Suprefact depot	6.3 mg every 2 mo
Leuprolide	Enantone or Lupron-depot	3.75 mg every mo/ OR 11.25 mg every 3 mo
	Prostap SR	4–8 µg/kg/day
	Lupron-depot-PED	7.5, 11.25, or 15 mg every mo (0.2 to 0.3 mg/kg/mo) OR 11.25 mg OR 30 mg every 3 mo
Triptorelin	Decapeptyl, Gonapeptyl	3 or 3.75 mg every mo OR 11.25 mg every 3 mo
Histrelin	Supprelin LA	50 mg implant every year

**The availability and approval for use in precocious puberty of these medications vary throughout the world. Recommended dosages also vary around the world for the same drug. Reproduced with permission from Carel et al. (2009).

OTHER OUTCOMES

Other outcomes to consider include bone mineral density, risk of obesity and psychosocial outcomes. Bone mineral density may decrease during GnRH agonist therapy but subsequent bone mass accrual is preserved, and peak bone mass does not seem to be negatively affected by treatment (Carel et al. 2009). There have been concerns that the use of GnRH agonists may affect BMI but the available data indicate that long-term GnRH agonist treatment does not seem to cause or aggravate obesity, as judged from BMI (Carel et al. 2009). However, the risk of obesity is a concern in girls with precocious puberty and BMI should be closely monitored. Psychosocial evaluation data are scarce in patients with premature sexual maturation, and there is little evidence to show whether treatment with GnRH agonists is associated with improved psychological outcome (Carel et al. 2009).

Tolerance to GnRH agonist treatment
Tolerance is generally considered good; it may be associated with headaches and menopausal symptoms such as hot flushes. Local complications (3%–13%) such as sterile abscesses may result in a loss of efficacy and anaphylaxis has been exceptionally described (Carel et al. 2002; Johnson et al. 2012).

Interruption of treatment and resumption of gonadotropic axis activity
The *optimal time to stop treatment* has not been established and factors that could influence the decision to stop GnRH agonists include synchronising puberty with peers, ameliorating psychological distress or facilitating care of the developmentally delayed child. However, the only available data concern factors that affect adult height; chronological age, duration of therapy, bone age, height, target height and growth velocity have been proposed, alone or in combination, to decide as to when to stop treatment. However,

these variables are closely interrelated and cannot be considered independently, and retrospective analyses suggest that continuing treatment beyond the age of 11 years in girls is associated with no further gains (Carel et al. 1999). Therefore, it is reasonable to consider these parameters and informed parent and patient preferences, with the goal of menarche occurring near the population norms (Carel et al. 2009). Pubertal manifestations generally reappear within months of GnRH agonist treatment being stopped, with a mean time to menarche of 16 months for depot GnRH agonists, seemingly less for histrelin implants (Heger et al. 2006; Gillis et al. 2013). Long-term fertility has not been fully evaluated, but preliminary observations are reassuring (Heger et al. 2006; Lazar et al. 2014).

The addition of growth hormone (Pasquino et al. 1999) or oxandrolone (Vottero et al. 2006) when growth velocity decreases or if height prognosis appears to be unsatisfactory has been proposed, but data are limited on the efficacy and safety of these drugs in children with precocious puberty.

MANAGEMENT OF CAUSAL LESIONS

When precocious puberty is caused by a hypothalamic lesion (e.g. mass or malformation), management of the causal lesion has generally no effect on the course of pubertal development. Hypothalamic hamartomas should not be treated by surgery for the management of precocious puberty. Precocious puberty associated with the presence of a hypothalamic lesion may progress to gonadotropin deficiency.

Conclusion

The main concern when examining a patient with premature sexual development should be the existence of a malignant or potentially life-threatening lesion, either intra-cranial, in the gonads, the adrenals, or elsewhere. However, these lesions are exceedingly rare, in general, the main difficulty is with the differentiation of progressive and non-progressive forms of precocious puberty and with the decision to treat, particularly for girls with an onset of puberty between the ages of 6 and 8 years.

REFERENCES

Abreu AP, Dauber A, Macedo DB et al. (2013) Central precocious puberty caused by mutations in the imprinted gene MKRN3. *N Engl J Med* 368: 2467–2475.
Aksglaede L, Sorensen K, Petersen JH, Skakkebaek NE and Juul A (2009) Recent decline in age at breast development: The Copenhagen Puberty Study. *Pediatrics* 123: e932–e939.
Belsky J, Steinberg LD, Houts RM et al. (2007) Family rearing antecedents of pubertal timing. *Child Dev* 78: 1302–1321.
Bizzarri C, Spadoni GL, Bottaro G et al. (2014) The response to gonadotropin releasing hormone (GnRH) stimulation test does not predict the progression to true precocious puberty in girls with onset of premature thelarche in the first three years of life. *J Clin Endocrinol Metab* 99: 433–439.
Bogaert AF (2005) Age at puberty and father absence in a national probability sample. *J Adolesc* 28 541–546.
Carel JC, Eugster EA, Rogol A et al. (2009) Consensus statement on the use of gonadotropin-releasing hormone analogs in children. *Pediatrics* 123: e752–e762.
Carel JC, Lahlou N, Jaramillo O et al. (2002) Treatment of central precocious puberty by subcutaneous injections of leuprorelin 3-month depot (11.25mg). *J Clin Endocrinol Metab* 87: 4111–4116.

Carel JC, Lahlou N, Roger M and Chaussain JL (2004) Precocious puberty and statural growth. *Hum Reprod Update* 10: 135–147.

Carel JC and Leger J (2008) Clinical practice. Precocious puberty. *New England Journal of Medicine* 358: 2366–2377.

Carel JC, Roger M, Ispas S et al. (1999) Final height after long-term treatment with triptorelin slow-release for central precocious puberty: Importance of statural growth after interruption of treatment. *J Clin Endocrinol Metab* 84: 1973–1978.

Chalumeau M, Hadjiathanasiou CG, Ng SM et al. (2003) Selecting girls with precocious puberty for brain imaging: Validation of European evidence-based diagnosis rule. *J Pediatr* 143: 445–450.

de Vries L, Horev G, Schwartz M and Phillip M (2006) Ultrasonographic and clinical parameters for early differentiation between precocious puberty and premature thelarche. *Eur J Endocrinol* 154 891–898.

Deardorff J, Ekwaru JP, Kushi LH et al. (2011) Father absence, body mass index, and pubertal timing in girls: Differential effects by family income and ethnicity. *J Adolesc Health* 48: 441–447.

Gillis D, Karavani G, Hirsch HJ and Strich D (2013) Time to menarche and final height after histrelin implant treatment for central precocious puberty. *J Pediatr* 163: 532–536.

Harrington J, Palmert MR and Hamilton J (2014) Use of local data to enhance uptake of published recommendations: An example from the diagnostic evaluation of precocious puberty. *Arch Dis Child* 99: 15–20.

Heger S, Muller M, Ranke M et al. (2006) Long-term GnRH agonist treatment for female central precocious puberty does not impair reproductive function. *Mol Cell Endocrinol* 254–255: 217–220.

Herman-Giddens ME, Kaplowitz PB and Wasserman R (2004) Navigating the recent articles on girls' puberty in Pediatrics: What do we know and where do we go from here? *Pediatrics* 113: 911–917.

Jean RT, Wilkinson AV, Spitz MR, Prokhorov A, Bondy M and Forman MR (2011) Psychosocial risk and correlates of early menarche in Mexican-American girls. *Am J Epidemiol* 173: 1203–1210.

Johnson SR, Nolan RC, Grant MT et al. (2012) Sterile abscess formation associated with depot leuprorelin acetate therapy for central precocious puberty. *J Paediatr Child Health* 48: E136–E139.

Kaplowitz PB and Oberfield SE (1999) Reexamination of the age limit for defining when puberty is precocious in girls in the United States: Implications for evaluation and treatment. Drug and Therapeutics and Executive Committees of the Lawson Wilkins Pediatric Endocrine Society. *Pediatrics* 104: 936–941.

Lahlou N, Carel JC, Chaussain JL and Roger M (2000) Pharmacokinetics and pharmacodynamics of GnRH agonists: Clinical implications in pediatrics. *J Pediatr Endocrinol Metab* 13(Suppl 1): 723–737.

Lazar L, Meyerovitch J, de Vries L, Phillip M and Lebenthal Y (2014) Treated and untreated women with idiopathic precocious puberty: Long-term follow-up and reproductive outcome between the third and fifth decades. *Clin Endocrinol (Oxf)* 80: 570–576.

Leger J, Reynaud R and Czernichow P (2000) Do all girls with apparent idiopathic precocious puberty require gonadotropin-releasing hormone agonist treatment? *J Pediatr* 137: 819–825.

Lewis KA and Eugster EA (2013) Random luteinizing hormone often remains pubertal in children treated with the histrelin implant for central precocious puberty. *J Pediatr* 162: 562–565.

Ma HM, Du ML, Luo XP et al. (2009) Onset of breast and pubic hair development and menses in urban chinese girls. *Pediatrics* 124: e269–e277.

Macedo DB, Brito VN and Latronico AC (2014) New causes of central precocious puberty: The role of the genetic factors. *Neuroendocrinology* 100: 1–8.

Marti-Henneberg C and Vizmanos B (1997) The duration of puberty in girls is related to the timing of its onset. *Journal of Pediatrics* 131: 618–621.

Martinez-Aguayo A, Hernandez MI, Capurro T et al. (2009) Leuprolide acetate gonadotropin response patterns during female puberty. *Clin Endocrinol (Oxf)* 72: 489–95.

Michaud PA, Suris JC and Deppen A (2006) Gender-related psychological and behavioural correlates of pubertal timing in a national sample of Swiss adolescents. *Mol Cell Endocrinol* 254–255: 172–178.

Midyett LK, Moore WV and Jacobson JD (2003) Are pubertal changes in girls before age 8 benign? *Pediatrics* 111: 47–51.

Parent AS, Matagne V, Westphal M, Heger S, Ojeda S and Jung H (2008) Gene expression profiling of hypothalamic hamartomas: A search for genes associated with central precocious puberty. *Horm Res* 69: 114–123.

Parent AS, Teilmann G, Juul A, Skakkebaek NE, Toppari J and Bourguignon JP (2003) The timing of normal puberty and the age limits of sexual precocity: Variations around the world, secular trends, and changes after migration. *Endocr Rev* 24: 668–693.

Pasquino AM, Pucarelli I, Segni M, Matrunola M, Cerroni F and Cerrone F (1999) Adult height in girls with central precocious puberty treated with gonadotropin-releasing hormone analogues and growth hormone. *J Clin Endocrinol Metab* 84: 449–452.

Pedicelli S, Alessio P, Scire G, Cappa M and Cianfarani S (2014) Routine screening by brain magnetic resonance imaging is not indicated in every girl with onset of puberty between the ages of 6 and 8. *J Clin Endocrinol Metab* 99: 4455–61. doi: 10.1210/jc.2014-2702.

Pesonen AK, Raikkonen K, Heinonen K, Kajantie E, Forsen T and Eriksson JG (2008) Reproductive traits following a parent-child separation trauma during childhood: A natural experiment during World War II. *Am J Hum Biol* 20: 345–351.

Resende EA, Lara BH, Reis JD, Ferreira BP, Pereira GA and Borges MF (2007) Assessment of basal and gonadotropin-releasing hormone-stimulated gonadotropins by immunochemiluminometric and immunofluorometric assays in normal children. *J Clin Endocrinol Metab* 92: 1424–1429.

Sathasivam A, Rosenberg HK, Shapiro S, Wang H and Rapaport R (2011) Pelvic ultrasonography in the evaluation of central precocious puberty: Comparison with leuprolide stimulation test. *J Pediatr* 159: 490–495.

Simon D, Ba I, Mekhail N, Ecosse E, Paulsen A and Zenaty D (2016) Mutations in the maternally imprinted gene MKRN3 are common in familial central precocious puberty. *Eur J Endocrinol* 174: 1–8.

Stanhope R (2003) Gonadotrophin-dependent precocious puberty and occult intracranial tumors: Which girls should have neuro-imaging? *J Pediatr* 143: 426–427.

Teilmann G, Pedersen CB, Jensen TK, Skakkebaek NE and Juul A (2005) Prevalence and incidence of precocious pubertal development in Denmark: An epidemiologic study based on national registries. *Pediatrics* 116: 1323–1328.

Teilmann G, Pedersen CB, Skakkebaek NE and Jensen TK (2006) Increased risk of precocious puberty in internationally adopted children in Denmark. *Pediatrics* 118: e391–e399.

Vottero A, Pedori S, Verna M et al. (2006) Final height in girls with central idiopathic precocious puberty treated with gonadotropin-releasing hormone analog and oxandrolone. *J Clin Endocrinol Metab* 91: 1284–1287.

Wise LA, Palmer JR, Rothman EF and Rosenberg L (2009) Childhood abuse and early menarche: Findings from the black women's health study. *Am J Public Health* 99(Suppl 2): S460–S466.

Xhrouet-Heinrichs D, Lagrou K, Heinrichs C et al. (1997) Longitudinal study of behavioral and affective patterns in girls with central precocious puberty during long-acting triptorelin therapy. *Acta Paediatr* 86: 808–815.

21
PSYCHOLOGICAL AND BEHAVIOURAL CONSEQUENCES OF GONADAL HORMONE ABNORMALITY DURING EARLY DEVELOPMENT

Melissa Hines

Introduction

Gonadal steroids play a central role in physical sexual differentiation, as well as in sexual differentiation of behaviour and the brain. Experimental research in animals initially established the role of androgens and oestrogens in neurobehavioural development, and evidence from individuals with clinical conditions involving early hormone abnormalities has confirmed some similar influences in humans. These clinical conditions include classic congenital adrenal hyperplasia (CCAH), complete androgen insensitivity syndrome (CAIS), Turner syndrome, androgen biosynthetic deficiencies and other conditions causing abnormal penile development. This chapter will first summarise briefly the main points that have emerged from experiments where gonadal hormones have been manipulated in non-human species, and will then detail the evidence from studies of human clinical conditions that suggest similar effects in human beings. Finally, it will outline some implications for clinical care of individuals who experience gonadal steroid abnormalities early in life.

General principles from experimental research in non-human species

In most mammals the testes are active during very early development (prenatally and neonatally), are then quiescent during most of juvenile development and resume activity at puberty. The prenatal and neonatal periods of testicular activation produce higher concentrations of testosterone and its metabolites in developing males than females, and these hormones cause the external genitalia to develop as penis and scrotum (Wilson et al. 1981). In contrast to the testes, the ovaries do not produce substantial amounts of hormones before birth (Wilson et al. 1981), although there is an early postnatal surge of ovarian oestrogen (Bidlingmaier et al. 1974, 1987). The developmental importance of this surge is largely unknown, however, and oestrogen does not appear to be needed for the development of female physical phenotype (Wilson et al. 1981).

The same hormones that alter development of the external genitalia also influence behaviour (Hines 2004; Arnold 2009). For example, treating female rats or rhesus monkeys with testosterone during early development increases their male-typical behaviour and reduces their female-typical behaviour later in life. Similarly, removing testosterone from developing males has the opposite effects, reducing subsequent male-typical, and increasing subsequent female-typical, behaviour. The behaviours that are influenced include not only adult reproductive behaviours, but also other behaviours that show sex differences, including juvenile play and performance in spatial mazes (Hines 2004). Similar early hormone manipulations also influence brain structures that show sex differences in non-human mammals. The mechanisms involved in these neural effects include regulation of cell survival, anatomical connectivity and neurochemical specification (Alexander and Hines 1994; McCarthy et al. 2009). It is thought that the neural changes underlie the behavioural changes, although no specific neural change has yet been clearly implicated in producing a particular behavioural outcome.

The influences of ovarian hormones on sexual differentiation have not been studied as extensively as those of testicular hormones, perhaps because the removal of these hormones appears to have few physical, neural or behavioural effects (Goy and McEwen 1980; Hines 2004). There is some evidence, however, that ovarian hormones, particularly oestradiol, can have feminising influences on a small number of behavioural outcomes (Dunlap et al. 1978; Bakker and Baum 2008). In addition, because testosterone is converted to oestradiol within the brain, and interacts with oestrogen receptors to masculinise many aspects of neurobehavioural sexual differentiation, oestrogen also can promote male-typical neurobehavioural traits when administered to developing rodents (Goy and McEwen 1980; Bakker and Baum 2008). The role of oestrogen in male-typical neurobehavioural development of primates is debated, however (Hines 2004).

Several general principles have emerged from the thousands of experimental studies documenting gonadal steroid influences on neurobehavioural development in non-human species. First, gonadal steroids influence the development of behaviours that show sex differences, meaning that they differ on the average for males and females of the species. Second, the influences occur during critical periods of early development, corresponding to times when testosterone concentrations are higher in males than in females. Third, neurobehavioural sexual differentiation is multidimensional, there are different critical periods for hormonal influences on different behaviours and the specific mechanisms involved in hormonal influences on specific brain regions or behaviours can differ. For example, different behaviours can be influenced by different metabolites of testosterone, or exposure to gonadal steroids can prevent cell death in one brain region but promote it in another. These findings suggest that evidence of similar hormonal influences on one type of behaviour that shows a sex difference does not imply hormonal influences on all types of behaviours that show sex differences. These complexities also provide a mechanism whereby some sexually differentiated outcomes (e.g. juvenile play behaviour) can differ from other sexually differentiated outcomes (e.g. sex identity). Fourth, testosterone and its metabolites have been found to play some role in neurobehavioural sexual differentiation of many mammalian species, including mice, rats, hamsters, gerbils, guinea pigs, rabbits, dogs, sheep, marmoset monkeys and rhesus macaques. There are species differences, however, and, for a given behaviour, some species may show an influence of gonadal steroids, whereas others do not. Consequently, specific results of these studies of non-human mammals cannot be assumed to apply to human beings. Instead, the studies raise the possibility that similar effects might be seen in humans.

Evidence from clinical conditions involving gonadal hormone abnormality

Because gonadal hormones have been consistently found to influence neurobehavioural sexual differentiation in non-human mammals, human clinical conditions that cause abnormal production of, or sensitivity to, these hormones might have behavioural consequences. In particular, human behaviours that differ on the average for girls and boys, or men and women, might be hypothesised to be altered in these conditions. Evidence to date suggests that this is the case, at least for some behaviours.

CLASSIC CONGENITAL ADRENAL HYPERPLASIA

The most extensively studied condition involving early androgen abnormality is the autosomal recessive disorder, CCAH. CCAH is characterised by an enzymatic deficiency, typically of 21-hydroxylase (21-Ohase), causing impaired glucocorticoid production, and over-production of adrenal androgens, beginning prenatally (New 1998). The prenatal androgen elevation in females with CCAH produces genital virilisation (e.g. enlarged clitoris, partially fused labia) that is evident at birth, and usually leads to rapid diagnosis. Postnatally, hormone treatment is provided to regulate glucocorticoid and androgen concentrations, and girls with CCAH are typically assigned and reared as girls. Some girls with CCAH also have feminising genital surgery in infancy. Boys with CCAH are born with normal appearing male genitalia, and, in areas of the world without universal screening for CCAH, are usually diagnosed following salt wasting crises in infancy, or precocious puberty.

Childhood play

The most consistent finding regarding the psychological development of girls with CCAH is that they show increased male-typical, and reduced female-typical, childhood play behaviour, sometimes referred to as sex role behaviour (Hines 2010). For instance, studies observing toy choices in a playroom have found that girls with CCAH show increased interest in toys that are typically chosen by boys, such as vehicles and weapons, and reduced interest in toys that are typically chosen by girls, such as dolls and tea sets (Berenbaum and Hines 1992; Nordenstrom et al. 2002; Pasterski et al. 2005). Similarly, responses on questionnaires and in interviews suggest increased engagement in male-typical rough and tumble play, a type of behaviour that is characterised by overall body contact and playful aggression, as well as increased scores on broad measures of behavioural masculinity, that include toy, playmate and activity preferences (Ehrhardt and Baker 1977; Dittmann et al. 1990; Hines et al. 2004; Pasterski et al. 2011).

Sexual orientation

Later in life, females with CCAH appear to be less likely than other women to be exclusively or almost exclusively heterosexual (Money et al. 1984; Dittmann et al. 1992; Hines, Brook and Conway 2004; Meyer-Bahlburg et al. 2008; Frisén et al. 2009). Research to date suggests that about 70% of women with CCAH report being exclusively or almost exclusively heterosexual, in contrast to over 95% of other women. Thus, although sexual orientation is altered in women with CCAH as a group, most individual women with CCAH resemble women in general in regard to their sexual orientation. The mechanisms leading to altered sexual orientation in some women with CCAH have yet to be identified, although the more severe forms of the disorder (e.g. salt-wasting CCAH; null genotype) appear to be associated with a greater likelihood of not being exclusively or almost exclusively heterosexual, than are the less severe forms (e.g. simple virilising CCAH; I2splice or I172N genotypes) (Meyer-Bahlburg et al. 2008; Frisén et al. 2009). One possibility is that an early hormone-induced alteration in brain development somehow leads to altered sexual orientation. It also is possible, however, that other factors are involved. For instance, alterations in genital anatomy, caused by early androgen exposure or by genital surgery, could affect sexual behaviour or interest in some women with CCAH. These possibilities have not yet been systematically examined.

Sex identity

Women with CCAH are also more likely than other women to choose to live as men in adulthood, despite having been reared as girls (Meyer-Bahlburg et al. 1996; Zucker et al. 1996; Dessens et al. 2005). The likelihood of this outcome appears to be about 1%–2%, compared to far less than 0.01% for women in the general population. Thus, the likelihood of changing from living as a woman to living as a man is many hundreds of times as great if a woman has CCAH than if she does not. At the same time, however, the vast majority of females with CCAH evolve a female sex identity and choose to remain living as women in adulthood. There is conflicting evidence regarding variation in the strength of sex identity among girls and women with CCAH assessed dimensionally rather than in an either/or (living as male/female) manner. One study suggests that strength of female identity in girls with CCAH is similar to that in other girls (Meyer-Bahlburg et al. 2004), but results of another study of girls with CCAH suggest reduced female sex identity (Pasterski et al. 2015). In addition, a study of adults with CCAH found that women with CCAH who identify as female also show reduced strength of female sex identity compared to other women, and that the amount of this reduction relates to the amount of recalled male-typical behaviour in childhood (Hines, Brook and Conway 2004).

Girls with CCAH, as well as girls with other disorders that cause androgen elevation prenatally such as mixed gonadal dysgenesis, also are more likely than other girls to meet criteria for a diagnosis of sex identity disorder in childhood (Slijper et al. 1998). For both girls with CCAH and girls with other diagnoses causing androgen elevation, the incidence of sex identity disorder appears to be about 11%. Comparing these figures to those of women with CCAH who choose to live as men (described above), it appears that most sex dysphoric girls with CCAH evolve a female sex identity by adulthood, although the different outcome measures typically used in studies of women (choosing to live as a man) versus girls (meeting the criteria for a diagnosis of sex identity) could contribute to the apparent difference. Nevertheless, for most sex dysphoric children who do not have CCAH or any other evidence of atypical early exposure to gonadal steroids, sex dysphoria does not persist into adulthood. Thus, sex dysphoria in a young girl with CCAH does not necessarily predict adult sex change, or even adult sex dysphoria.

Interests and personality

There is also evidence suggesting that women with CCAH show increased interest in male-typical occupations, such as truck driver or car mechanic, and reduced interest in female-typical occupations, such as day care worker or teacher (Frisén et al. 2009; Beltz et al. 2011). Similarly, the interest of girls with CCAH in infants appears to be reduced compared to that of other females (Leveroni and Berenbaum 1998; Mathews et al. 2009). This reduced interest in female-typical occupations and in infants does not necessarily imply lack of interest in having a family. The amount of interest in these areas among females with CCAH, though significantly reduced in comparison to the average woman, is still similar to that of at least some other women without endocrine abnormality, and is no lower than that of boys and men, most of whom want and have families.

Regarding personality characteristics, females with CCAH have been reported to show enhanced interest and engagement in physically aggressive behaviour, as well as reduced empathy (Berenbaum and Resnick 1997; Mathews et al. 2009). Both outcomes represent increased male-typical behaviour, because physical aggression is higher, and empathy lower, in males than in females. Girls with CCAH have also been found to show increased scores on a questionnaire designed to tap characteristics associated with autistic spectrum disorders (ASD) (Knickmeyer et al. 2006). Boys typically score higher on the questionnaire than girls do, so the elevated scores in girls with CCAH again suggest more male-typical behaviour. None of the girls with CCAH had scores high enough to qualify for diagnosis of an ASD, however, and girls with CCAH are not viewed as being at increased risk of such a diagnosis.

Cognition

There may also be consequences of CCAH for cognitive abilities, although the results of some research in this area has been inconsistent and has included some misleading findings. Initially, for instance, individuals with CCAH were reported to have elevated general intelligence, because their intelligence quotient (IQ) scores were higher than standardised values (Masica et al. 1969). Subsequent research showed that this apparent advantage was artefactual, however. When individuals with CCAH were compared to their unaffected relatives, or to controls who had been carefully matched for demographic background, no IQ differences were seen (Hines 2004). More recently, general intelligence has been reported to be reduced in individuals with CCAH (Johannsen et al. 2006). This finding too is likely to be spurious, given the numerous other well-controlled studies finding no alterations in IQ or other measures of general intelligence in individuals with CCAH (Berenbaum et al. 2010).

Cognitive abilities that show sex differences might be more likely candidates than general intelligence for alteration in individuals with CCAH. Such abilities include mental rotations and mathematical problem solving, at which males excel on average, and verbal fluency and perceptual speed, at which females excel on average (Hines 2011). Here too, however, the evidence is inconsistent or sparse. Regarding mental rotations performance, some studies suggest enhancement in females with CCAH (Perlman 1973; Resnick et al. 1986; Berenbaum et al. 2012), but some others do not (Helleday et al. 1994; Hines et al. 2003b; Malouf et al. 2006). Looking at spatial abilities more broadly, including some that show smaller sex differences than shown with mental rotations, a meta-analysis concluded that CCAH gives girls an advantage (Puts et al. 2008), but this analysis did not include all of the relevant data from the studies, and the omissions increased the apparent CCAH-related advantage. Also, the effect of CCAH on spatial ability appears to be more dramatic in smaller studies than in larger studies, suggesting a spurious effect. In contrast to females with CCAH, males with CCAH show reduced mental rotations ability, and perhaps spatial ability more generally (Hampson et al. 1998; Hines et al. 2003b; Berenbaum et al. 2012). This reduction could relate to reduced androgen exposure during early infancy in boys with CCAH, caused by aggressive treatment with glucorticoids, by direct effects of glucocorti-coid treatment, or by hypoglycaemic episodes associated with salt-losing crises (Hines et al. 2003b). In regard to mathematical ability, there is no evidence of CCAH-related enhancement. On the contrary, both male and female individuals with CCAH have been found to show reduced arithmetic performance (Perlman 1973; Baker and Ehrhardt 1974; Sinforiani et al. 1994). Two studies have also reported reduced short-term memory, as assessed using digit span, in both males and females with CCAH (Brown et al. 2015; Collaer et al. 2015). One of these studies also linked the reduced short-term memory performance to reduced spatial/quantitative performance (Collaer et al. 2015).

There is less information on other syndromes involving gonadal steroid abnormality than on girls with CCAH, but there is some information on sex-related behaviour in individuals with Turner syndrome, individuals with CAIS, individuals with androgen bio-synthetic deficiencies and individuals with other conditions causing abnormal penile development.

TURNER SYNDROME

Turner syndrome occurs when the second X chromosome, or part of the chromosome, is missing (Bender et al. 1989; Ross and Zinn 1999). The syndrome involves a range of physi-cal problems, including short stature and primary gonadal failure in the vast majority of patients (Lippe 1991). Most individuals with Turner syndrome have impaired production of ovarian hormones, including androgens and oestrogens, beginning early in life (Singh and Carr 1966; Conte et al. 1975), although the degree of impairment varies somewhat across individuals (Rosenfield 1990; Saenger 1996).

Girls and women with Turner syndrome have normal verbal abilities, but show a well-documented reduction in spatial abilities (Money and Alexander 1966; Waber 1979; Rovet and Netley 1982; Downey et al. 1991; Kesler et al. 2004), perhaps representing decreased male-typical cognitive function, given that males tend to outperform females on many measures of spatial ability. There is also evidence of reduced social cognition in individuals with Turner syndrome (Downey et al. 1989; Skuse et al. 1997; Lawrence et al. 2003), an effect that represents decreased female-typical behaviour, given that girls and women perform better, on average, on measures of social cognition than do boys and men. One study suggests that girls with Turner syndrome show reduced performance on cognitive measures on which females typically excel (e.g. verbal fluency), as well as on those at which males excel (e.g. mental rotations), and that they show reduced male-typical as well as female-typical behaviour in other areas as well, including on measures of masculine and feminine personality traits and childhood activities (Collaer et al. 2002). These findings of reduced male-typical behaviour, as well as reduced female-typical behaviour, suggest that the gonadal steroids that are reduced in most individuals with Turner syndrome beginning early in development may be needed both for complete neurobehavioural masculinisation and for complete neurobehavioural feminisation. There is some evidence from experimental studies in other species that ovarian hormones are required for some aspects of feminisation, as well as masculinisation (Fitch and Denenberg 1998). However, this broad reduction in masculine as well as feminine behaviour is not as well established as the impaired spatial abilities in girls and women with Turner syndrome. It also has been suggested that the cognitive phenotype associated with Turner syndrome resembles nonverbal learning disability (Ross et al. 2006), and that this phenotype is linked to specific distal Xp chromosomal regions. It is possible that both genetic factors and early hormonal factors, as well as other consequences of Turner syndrome, contribute to the observed behavioural changes.

COMPLETE ANDROGEN INSENSITIVITY SYNDROME

CAIS is characterised by a cellular inability to respond to androgens, and consequent female-typical physical appearance in XY individuals. Because XY individuals with CAIS appear female at birth, they are usually assigned and reared as girls, with no awareness of the condition, sometimes until menstruation fails to occur. Some cases are diagnosed earlier with the presence of inguinal hernia or palpable gonads. Following diagnosis, treatment typically involves removal of the undescended testes and oestrogen replacement.

Individuals with CAIS almost always have female-typical sex identification and sexual orientation (Masica et al. 1971; Wisniewski et al. 2000; Hines et al. 2003a; Mazur 2005), despite their Y chromosome. This outcome is consistent with their insensitivity to androgen, and their assignment and rearing as girls. Individuals with CAIS also have been reported to recall female-typical toy preferences and sex role behaviour in childhood (Hines, Ahmed and Hughes 2003a), and there is some corroborative, contemporaneous evidence from children with CAIS of female-typical toy, activity and playmate preferences, as well (Jurgensen et al. 2007). One study reported reduced performance on spatial subtests of the Wechsler intelligence scales in adults with CAIS in comparison to both unaffected men and women (Imperato-McGinley et al. 1991), but there is, as yet, no reported replication of this finding. Finally, there is a case report of one individual with CAIS who, unlike the vast majority of individuals with this disorder, identifies as a man, and recalls male-typical behaviour in childhood (T'Sjoen et al. 2011). This unusual outcome remains to be explained.

DEFECTS OF ANDROGEN BIOSYNTHESIS

Androgen biosynthetic defects include 5α-reductase-2 deficiency and 17β-hydroxysteroid-dehydrogenase-3 deficiency (Miller 2002). Both of these rare disorders impair production of the full range of androgens, and lead to ambiguous or female-appearing genitalia at birth in 46,XY individuals. In many cases, sex assignment and rearing are therefore female, but physical virilisation occurs at puberty. Following physical virilisation, a substantial percentage of these individuals change to live as men. A review of the available reports suggests that 56%–63% of those with 5α-reductase-2 deficiency and 39%–64% of those with 17β-hydroxysteroid-dehydrogenase-3 deficiency, who were raised as girls, later chose to live as men (Cohen-Kettenis 2005). There appears to be no clear relationship between the degree of genital virilisation and an individual's choice to live as a man (Cohen-Kettenis 2005). It is possible that cultural factors, such as the higher social status of an infertile male than an infertile female in some societies, may be involved (Ghabrial and Girgis 1962; Wilson 1979; Rosler and Kohn 1983). Systematic surveys of sexual orientation in individuals with these disorders have yet to be conducted, and so it is not known if their sexual orientation accords with their social identity.

OTHER CONGENITAL GENITAL ABNORMALITIES

There are several rare conditions that cause a very small penis or its complete absence in 46,XY individuals. These conditions include aphallia, micropenis, cloacal exstrophy and penile ablation. In cases of aphallia, micropenis and cloacal exstrophy, the last of which often causes a small, bifid penis, some individuals have been assigned as girls and some as boys. In general, these individuals evolve a sex identity consistent with sex assignment, regardless of its direction (Meyer-Bahlburg 2005). One report suggested that many individuals with cloacal exstrophy, who had been assigned as females, subsequently indicated a desire to change to live as males (Reiner and Gearhart 2004). However, this is not the typical finding.

ACQUIRED GENITAL ABNORMALITIES

A final situation where sex assignment and identity are salient is in cases where a healthy male infant has penile ablation due to accident or injury. There are two cases where such infants have been reassigned as girls, and followed up in terms of adult sex identity, as well as sexual orientation. The first child was reassigned as female at the age of about 18 months, but in adulthood chose to live as a man, with a sexual orientation towards women (Diamond and Sigmundson 1997). The second child was reassigned by the age of 7 months, and, when assessed at 16 and 26 years of age, had a female sex identity and a bisexual sexual orientation (Bradley et al. 1998). Because these are only two cases, it is hard to know if the earlier age of the second child at reassignment accounts for the different outcomes. Regardless, for the second child, sex assignment and socialisation as female led to a female sex identity, despite a Y chromosome and exposure to both the prenatal and early postnatal surges of testosterone seen in typically developing boys, suggesting a remarkable ability of socialisation to shape human sex identity.

Conclusion

In summary, early exposure to testosterone clearly influences human neurobehavioural development. These influences are seen most clearly in children's sex role behaviour, including their toy interests. The evidence also consistently shows altered sexual orientation and sex identity in groups of girls and women with CCAH compared to groups of unaffected females, although the majority of women with CCAH have female-typical sexual orientation and almost all women with CCAH, assigned and reared as girls, have a female core sex identity. Individuals with androgen biosynthetic defects, raised as girls, are the most likely of any group with atypical early hormone exposures to decide to change sex as adults. This may be because physical virilisation makes it difficult to continue in the female role, or because living as a man in some cultures has large advantages. There is also some evidence of cognitive consequences for individuals with disorders involving early hormone abnormality. Both males and females with CCAH show reduced working memory and arithmetic ability and males with CCAH show reduced spatial abilities. Further research is needed to determine if these reductions relate to glucocorticoid treatment, to hypoglycaemic episodes or to other factors. Girls with Turner syndrome show impaired spatial ability and there is some evidence of reduced social cognition, as well as reduction in a range of female-typical as well as male-typical behaviours. These outcomes could relate to early hormone deficiency or to genetic information on the missing or incomplete X chromosome. In considering psychological development in children with these conditions it is useful to remember that sex development is multidimensional and proceeds over time. It is typical, for instance, for girls with CCAH to show male-typical toy interests and sex role behaviour in childhood, but this does not mean that they have a male sex identity, because these are different dimensions of psychological sex. In addition, a minority of girls with CCAH or other disorders involving early exposure to high concentrations of androgens may indicate a desire to be a boy, but this will not necessarily persist into adulthood, because sex development proceeds over time, and sex dysphoria of childhood often desists prior to adulthood.

REFERENCES

Alexander GM and Hines M (1994) Gender labels and play styles: Their relative contribution to children's selection of playmates. *Child Dev* in press.

Arnold AP (2009) The organizational-activational hypothesis as the foundation for a unified theory of sexual differentiation of all mammalian tissues. *Horm Behav* 55: 570–578.

Baker SW and Ehrhardt AA (1974) Prenatal androgen, intelligence and cognitive sex differences. In: Friedman RC, Richart RM and Vande Wiele RL (eds) *Sex Differences in Behavior*. New York: Wiley, 53–76.

Bakker J and Baum MJ (2008) Role for estrogen in female-typical brain and behavioral sexual differentiation. *Front Neuroendocrinol* 29: 1–16.

Beltz AM, Swanson JL and Berenbaum SA (2011) Gendered occupational interests: Prenatal androgen effects on psychological orientation to Things versus People. *Horm Behav* 60: 313–317.

Bender BG, Linden MG and Robinson A (1989) Verbal and spatial processing efficiency in 32 children with sex chromosome abnormalities. *Pediatr Res* 25: 577–579.

Berenbaum SA, Bryk K and Duck SC (2010) Normal intelligence in female and male patients with congenital adrenal hyperplasia. *Int J Pediatr Endocrinol* Article ID 853103, 6 pages

Berenbaum SA and Hines M (1992) Early androgens are related to childhood sex-typed toy preferences. *Psychol Sci* 3: 203–206.

Berenbaum SA, Korman Bryk KL and Beltz AM (2012) Early androgen effects on spatial and mechanical abilities: Evidence from congenital adrenal hyperplasia. *Behav Neurosci* 126: 86–96.

Berenbaum SA and Resnick SM (1997) Early androgen effects on aggression in children and adults with congenital adrenal hyperplasia. *Psychoneuroendocrinology* 22: 505–515.

Bidlingmaier F, Strom TM, Dörr G, Eisenmenger W and Knorr D (1987) Estrone and estradiol concentrations in human ovaries, testes, and adrenals during the first two years of life. *J Clin Endocrinol Metab* 65: 862–867.

Bidlingmaier F, Versmold H and Knorr D (1974) Plasma estrogens in newborns and infants. In: Forest M and Bertrand J (eds) *Sexual Endocrinology of the Perinatal Period*. Paris: Inserm, 299–314.

Bradley SJ, Oliver GD, Chernick AB and Zucker KJ (1998) Experiment of nurture: Ablatio penis at 2 months, sex reassignment at 7 months and a psychosexual follow-up in young adulthood. *Pediatrics* 102: 102–101.

Brown W, Hindmarsh PC, Pasterski V et al. (2015) Working memory performance is reduced in children with congenital adrenal hyperplasia. *Horm Behav* 67: 83–88.

Cohen-Kettenis PT (2005) Gender change in 46, XY persons with 5alpha-reductase-2 deficiency and 17beta-hydroxysteroid dehydrogenase-3 deficiency. *Arch Sex Behav* 34: 399–410.

Collaer ML, Geffner M, Kaufman FR, Buckingham B and Hines M (2002) Cognitive and behavioral characteristics of Turner Syndrome: Exploring a role for ovarian hormones in female sexual differentiation. *Horm Behav* 41: 139–155.

Collaer ML, Hindmarsh PC, Pasterski V, Fane BA and Hines M (2015) Reduced short term memory in congenital adrenal hyperplasia (CAH) and its relationship to spatial and quantitative performance. *Psychoneuroendocrinology* in press.

Conte FA, Grumbach MM and Kaplan SL (1975) A diphasic pattern of gonadotropin secretion in patients with the syndrome of gonadal dysgenesis. *J Clin Endocrinol Metab* 40: 670–674.

Dessens AB, Slijper FME and Drop SLS (2005) Gender dysphoria and gender change in chromosomal females with congenital adrenal hyperplasia. *Arch SexBehav* 34: 389–397.

Diamond M and Sigmundson HK (1997) Sex reassignment at birth: Long-term review and clinical implications. *Arch Pediatr Adolesc Med* 151: 298–304.

Dittmann RW, Kappes ME and Kappes MH (1992) Sexual behavior in adolescent and adult females with congenital adrenal hyperplasia. *Psychoneuroendocrinology* 17: 153–170.

Dittmann RW, Kappes MH, Kappes ME et al. (1990) Congenital Adrenal Hyperplasia I: Gender-related behavior and attitudes in female patients and sisters. *Psychoneuroendocrinology* 15: 401–420.

Downey J, Ehrhardt AA, Gruen R, Bell JJ and Morishima A (1989) Psychopathology and social functioning in women with Turner Syndrome. *J Nerv Ment Dis* 177: 191–201.

Downey J, Elkin EJ, Ehrhardt AA, Meyer-Bahlburg HFL, Bell JJ and Morishima A (1991) Cognitive ability and everyday functioning in women with Turner Syndrome. *J Learn Disabil* 24: 32–39.

Dunlap JL, Gerall AA and Carlton SF (1978) Evaluation of prenatal androgen and ovarian secretions on receptivity in female and male rats. *J Comp Physiol Psychol* 92(2): 280–288.

Ehrhardt AA and Baker SW (1977) Males and females with congenital adrenal hyperplasia: A family study of intelligence and gender-related behavior. In: Lee PA et al. (eds) *Congenital Adrenal Hyperplasia*. Baltimore MD: University Park Press, 447–461.

Fitch RH and Denenberg VH (1998) A role for ovarian hormones in sexual differentiation of the brain. *Behav Brain Sci* 21: 311–352.

Frisén J, Nordenstrom A, Falhammar H et al. (2009) Gender role behavior, sexuality, and psychosocial adaptation in women with congenital adrenal hyperplasia due to CYP21A2 deficiency. *J Clin Endocrinol Metab* 94: 3432–3439.

Ghabrial F and Girgis SM (1962) Reorientation of sex: Report of two cases. *Int J Fertil* 7: 249–258.

Goy RW and McEwen BS (1980) *Sexual Differentiation of the Brain*. Cambridge, MA: MIT Press.

Hampson E, Rovet J and Altmann D (1998) Spatial reasoning in children with congenital adrenal hyperplasia due to 21-hydroxylase deficiency. *Dev Neuropsychol* 14(2): 299–320.

Helleday J, Bartfai A, Ritzen EM and Forsman M (1994) General intelligence and cognitive profile in women with congenital adrenal hyperplasia (CAH). *Psychoneuroendocrinology* 19: 343–356.

Hines M (2004) *Brain Gender*. New York: Oxford University Press.

Hines M (2010) Sex-related variation in human behavior and the brain. *Trends in Cognitive Sciences* 14: 448–456.

Hines M (2011) Gender development and the human brain. *Annu Rev Neurosci* 34: 67–86.

Hines M, Ahmed SF and Hughes I (2003a) Psychological outcomes and gender-related development in complete androgen insensitivity syndrome. *Arch Sex Behav* 32: 93–101

Hines M, Brook C and Conway GS (2004) Androgen and psychosexual development: Core gender identity, sexual orientation and recalled childhood gender role behavior in women and men with congenital adrenal hyperplasia (CAH). *J Sex Res* 41: 75–81.

Hines M, Fane BA, Pasterski VL, Mathews GA, Conway GS and Brook C (2003b) Spatial abilities following prenatal androgen abnormality: Targeting and mental rotations performance in individuals with congenital adrenal hyperplasia (CAH). *Psychoneuroendocrinology* 28: 1010–1026.

Imperato-McGinley J, Pichardo M, Gautier T, Voyer D and Bryden MP (1991) Cognitive abilities in androgen-insensitive subjects: Comparison with control males and females from the same kindred. *Clin Endocrinol* 34: 341–347.

Johannsen TH, Ripa CPL, Reinisch JM, Schwartz M, Mortensen EL and Main KM (2006) Impaired cognitive function in women with congenital adrenal hyperplasia. *J Clin Endocrinol Metab* 91: 1376–1381.

Jurgensen M, Hiort O, Holterhus PM and Thyen U (2007) Gender role behavior in children with XY karyotype and disorders of sex development. *Horm Behav* 51: 443–453.

Kesler SR, Haberecht MF, Menon VWIS, Dyer-Friedman J, Neely EK and Reis AL (2004) Functional neuroanatomy of spatial orientation processing in Turner Syndrome. *Cereb Cortex* 14: 174–180.

Knickmeyer R, Baron-Cohen S, Fane B et al. (2006) Androgens and autistic traits: A study of individuals with congenital adrenal hyperplasia. *Horm Behav* 50: 148–153.

Lawrence K, Kuntsi J, Coleman M, Campbell R and Skuse D (2003) Face and emotion recognition deficits in Turner syndrome: A possible role for X-linked genes in amygdala development. *Neuropsychology* 17: 39–49.

Leveroni CL and Berenbaum SA (1998) Early androgen effects on interest in infants: Evidence from children with congenital adrenal hyperplasia. *Dev Neuropsychol* 14: 321–340.

Lippe B (1991) Turner syndrome. *Endocrinol Metab Clin North Am* 20: 121–152.

Malouf MA, Migeon CJ, Carson KA, Pertrucci L and Wisniewski AB (2006) Cognitive outcome in adult women affected by congenital adrenal hyperplasia due to 21-hydroxylase deficiency. *Horm Res* 65: 142–150.

Masica DN, Money J and Ehrhardt A (1971) Fetal feminization and female gender identity in the testicular feminizing syndrome of androgen insensitivity. *Arch Sex Behav* 1(2): 131–142.

Masica DN, Money J, Ehrhardt AA and Lewis VG (1969) IQ, fetal sex hormones and cognitive patterns: Studies in the testicular feminizing syndrome of androgen insensitivity. *Johns Hopkins Med J* 124: 34–43.

Mathews GA, Fane BA, Conway GS, Brook C and Hines M (2009) Personality and congenital adrenal hyperplasia: Possible effects of prenatal androgen exposure. *Horm Behav* 55: 285–291.

Mazur T (2005) Gender dysphoria and gender change in androgen insensitivity or micropenis. *Arch Sex Behav* 34: 411–421.

McCarthy MM, De Vries GJ and Forger NG (2009) Sexual differentiation of the brain: Mode, mechanisms, and meaning. In: Pfaff DW et al. (eds) *Hormones, Brain and Behavior*, 2nd edn, vol. 3. San Diego, CA: Academic Press, 1707–1744.

Meyer-Bahlburg HFL (2005) Gender identity outcome in female-raised 46, XY persons with penile agenesis, cloacal exstrophy of the bladder, or penile ablation. *Arch Sex Behav* 34: 423–438.

Meyer-Bahlburg HFL, Dolezal C, Baker SW and New MI (2008) Sexual orientation in women with classical or non-classical congenital adrenal hyperplasia as a function of degree of prenatal androgen excess. *Arch Sex Behav* 37: 85–99.

Meyer-Bahlburg HFL, Dollard J, Baker SW, Carlson AD, Obeid JS and New MI (2004) Prenatal androgenization affects gender-related behavior but not gender identity in 5–12-year-old girls with congenital adrenal hyperplasia. *Arch Sex Behav* 33: 97–104.

Meyer-Bahlburg HFL, Gruen RS, New MI et al. (1996) Gender change from female to male in classical congenital adrenal hyperplasia. *Horm Behav* 30: 319–332.

Miller WL (2002) Disorders of androgen biosynthesis. *Semin Reprod Med* 20: 205–216.

Money J and Alexander D (1966) Turner's syndrome: Further demonstration of the presence of specific cognitional deficiencies. *J Med Genet* 3: 47–48.

Money J, Schwartz M and Lewis V (1984) Adult erotosexual status and fetal hormonal masculinization and demasculinization: 46 XX congenital virilizing adrenal hyperplasia and 46 XY androgen-insensitivity syndrome compared. *Psychoneuroendocrinology* 9: 405–414.

New M (1998) Diagnosis and management of congenital adrenal hyperplasia. *Annu Rev Med* 49: 311–328.

Nordenstrom A, Servin A, Bohlin G, Larsson A and Wedell A (2002) Sex-typed toy play behavior correlates with the degree of prenatal androgen exposure assessed by CYP21 genotype in girls with congenital adrenal hyperplasia. *J Clin Endocrinol Metab* 87: 5119–5124.

Pasterski VL, Geffner ME, Brain C, Hindmarsh P, Brook C and Hines M (2005) Prenatal hormones and postnatal socialization by parents as determinants of male-typical toy play in girls with congenital adrenal hyperplasia. *Child Dev* 76: 264–278 (accessed 2005).

Pasterski VL, Geffner ME, Brain C, Hindmarsh PC, Brook C Hines M (2011) Prenatal hormones and childhood sex segregation: Playmate and play style preferences in girls with congenital adrenal hyperplasia. *Horm Behav* 59: 549–555.

Pasterski VL, Zucker KJ, Hindmarsh PC et al. (2015) Increased cross-gender identification independent of gender role behavior in girls with Congenital Adrenal Hyperplasia: Results from a standardized assessment of 4–11-year-old children. *Arch Sex Behav* 44: 1363–1375.

Perlman SM (1973) Cognitive abilities of children with hormone abnormalities: Screening by psychoeducational tests. *J Learn Disabil* 6: 21–29.

Puts DA, McDaniel MA, Jordan CL and Breedlove SM (2008) Spatial ability and prenatal androgens: Meta-analyses of congenital adrenal hyperplasia and digit ratio (2D:4D) studies. *Arch Sex Behav* 37: 100–111.

Reiner WG and Gearhart JP (2004) Discordant sexual identity in some genetic males with cloacal exstrophy assigned to female sex at birth. *N Engl J Med* 350(4): 333–341.

Resnick SM, Berenbaum SA, Gottesman II and Bouchard T (1986) Early hormonal influences on cognitive functioning in congenital adrenal hyperplasia. *Dev Psychol* 22: 191–198.

Rosenfield RL (1990) Spontaneous puberty and fertility in Turner syndrome. In: Rosenfeld RG and Grumbach MM (eds) *Turner Syndrome*. New York: Marcel Dekker, 131–148.

Rosler A and Kohn G (1983) Male pseudohermaphroditism due to 17 beta-hydroxysteroid dehydrogenase deficiency: Studies on the natural history of the defect and effect of androgens on gender role. *J Steroid Biochem* 19: 663–674.

Ross J, Roeltgen D and Zinn A (2006) Cognition and the sex chromosomes: Studies in Turner Syndrome. *Horm Res* 65: 47–56.

Ross JL and Zinn AR (1999) Turner syndrome: Potential hormonal and genetic influences on the neurocognitive profile. In: Tager-Flusberg H (ed) *Neurodevelopmental Disorders*. Cambridge, MA: MIT Press, 251–267.

Rovet J and Netley C (1982) Processing deficits in Turner's syndrome. *Dev Psychol* 18: 77–94.

Saenger P (1996) Turner's syndrome. *N Engl J Med* 335: 1749–1754.

Sinforiani E, Livieri C, Mauri M et al. (1994) Cognitive and neuroradiological findings in congenital adrenal hyperplasia. *Psychoneuroendocrinology* 19: 55–64.

Singh RP and Carr DH (1966) The anatomy and histology of XO human embryos and fetuses. *Anat Rec* 155: 369–384.

Skuse DH, James RS and Bishop DVM (1997) Evidence from Turner's syndrome of an imprinted X-linked locus affecting cognitive function. *Nature* 387: 705–708.

Slijper FME, Drop SLS, Molenaar JC and de Muinck Keizer-Schrama SMPF (1998) Long-term psychological evaluation of intersex children. *Arch Sex Behav* 27: 125–144.

T'Sjoen G, De Cuypere G, Monstrey S et al. (2011) Male gender identity in complete androgen insensitivity syndrome. *Arch Sex Behav* 40: 635–638.

Waber DP (1979) Neuropsychological aspects of Turner's syndrome. *Dev Neurol* 21: 58–70.

Wilson JD (1979) Sex hormones and sexual behavior. *N Engl J Med* 300: 1269–1270.

Wilson JD, George FW and Griffin JE (1981) The hormonal control of sexual development. *Science* 211: 1278–1284.

Wisniewski AB, Migeon CJ, Meyer-Bahlburg HFL et al. (2000) Complete androgen insensitivity syndrome. Long-term medical, surgical, and psychosexual outcome. *J Clin Endocrinol Metab* 85: 2664–2669.

Zucker KJ, Bradley SJ, Oliver G, Blake J, Fleming S and Hood J (1996) Psychosexual development of women with congenital adrenal hyperplasia. *Horm Behav* 30: 300–318.

22
DIABETES AND THE DEVELOPING BRAIN

Fergus J Cameron, Elisabeth A Northam and Terrie E Inder

Introduction

Glucose is the primary metabolic fuel for the central nervous system (CNS). Diabetes, particularly type 1 diabetes, is a chronic disease that primarily disrupts the stability of plasma glucose concentrations. Developing brains are more susceptible to metabolic insults than the mature CNS. Thus it is not surprising that type 1 diabetes during childhood and adolescence impacts upon neural and brain development. As the emphasis of diabetes care during childhood broadens from the avoidance of acute metabolic disturbance and micro-vascular complications such as renal and retinal disease, there is an increasing interest in the impact of diabetes upon the pre-eminent developmental task of childhood – that of CNS ontogeny.

Aspects of brain metabolism relevant to type 1 diabetes

Type 1 diabetes remains the most common form of diabetes during childhood and adolescence (Sabin et al. 2009). It is characterised by an auto-immune process that results in pancreatic β-cell damage and loss of insulin production. Prior to diagnosis, patients experience increasing hyperglycaemia, osmotic diuresis, catabolism of muscle, fat and stored glycogen and subsequent ketogenesis. If untreated, the ultimate consequence of this catabolic state is the life-threatening complication of diabetic ketoacidosis (DKA). The mainstay of diabetes therapy is the exogenous replacement of insulin via a variety of subcutaneous delivery strategies which can be intermittent or continuous, using either recombinant human insulin or structurally manipulated analogue insulins. Routinely used capillary or subcutaneous glucose-sensing techniques are also remote from the physiologic entero-pancreatic-hepatic milieu of glucose regulation. Consequently, contemporary techniques of insulin delivery and glucose sensing are far from ideal, with unavoidable delays in glucose sensing and insulin delivery, causing non-physiologic perturbations of plasma glucose that can occur on an hourly basis (Fig 22.1).

Brain energy consumption (accounting for 25% of total body glucose utilisation in adults) is predominantly to maintain ion gradients and facilitate ion transport and subsequent neural activity. Glucose is the primary energy substrate for the brain and is used to generate pyruvate and lactate to fuel the tricarboxylic acid cycle as well as being incorporated into lipids, proteins and acting as the precursor to neurotransmitters

(a)

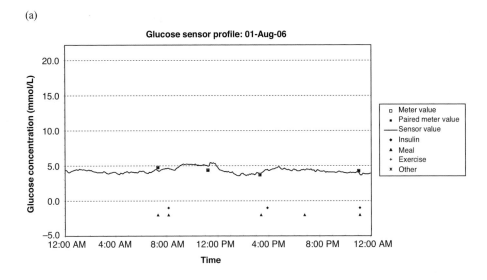

(b)

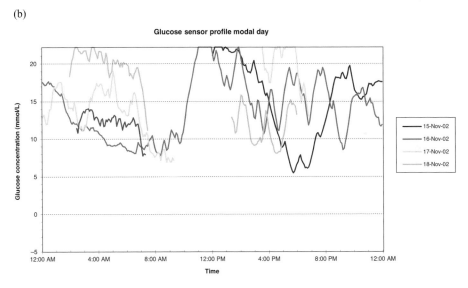

Figure 22.1. Continuous glucose sensing traces from (a) a person without diabetes and (b) a child with type 1 diabetes. (A colour version of this figure can be seen in the plate section at the end of the book.)

gamma-aminobutyric acid (GABA), glutamate and acetylcholine. Other secondary energy sources include ketone bodies (acetoacetate, β-hydroxybutyrate), free fatty acids, pyruvate and lactate (Qutub and Hunt 2005). The uptake of glucose and other hexoses into most mammalian cells is mediated by the SLC2 (solute carrier) family of 13 glucose transporter proteins, GLUTs 1–12 and HMIT (H-myo-inositol transporter). Unlike peripheral, metabolically active, tissues such as liver, fat and skeletal muscle that rely on insulin-mediated GLUT2 and GLUT4 glucose uptake, glucose uptake in astrocytes and neurons occurs via an insulin-independent mechanism (Simpson et al. 2007). Most GLUTs are expressed within the brain; however, GLUT1 and GLUT3 appear to be the dominant CNS glucose transporters and are up-regulated in an insulin-independent fashion in response to hypoglycaemic or hypoxic stimuli. GLUT1 and GLUT 3 are facilitative bi-directional transporters that mediate glucose equilibration, not accumulation, by glial and neural cells, respectively. The intracellular conversion of glucose to glucose-6-phosphate catalysed by hexokinase is the first of the 10-step glycolysis process that ultimately yields pyruvate and adenosine triphosphate. Under physiologic conditions, it is considered that the rate-limiting step of brain glycolysis is related to hexokinase activity and not to glucose transport (Qutub and Hunt 2005). Decreased frontal cortex levels of GLUT1 and GLUT3 and abnormalities in glycolysis in frontal, temporal, parietal and cingulate cortices have been associated with Alzheimer disease (Hunt et al. 2007; Liu et al. 2008). Monocarboxylic acids (lactate and pyruvate) and ketone bodies (acetoacetate and β-hydroxybutyrate) are transported via monocarboxylate transporters (MCT's) 1, 2 and 4 (Simpson et al. 2007). Both GLUTs and MCTs are thought to be up-regulated as a neuroprotective response in patients who experience recurrent hypoglycaemia with intensively controlled diabetes (Herzog et al. 2011).

BRAIN ENERGY SUBSTRATES

Glucose

Glucose is presented to the brain via the cerebral microvasculature and blood–brain barrier (BBB) – characterised by extremely tight endothelial junctions (50–100 times tighter than in peripheral capillaries) opposed to peri-vascular astrocytic processes (Abbott 2002). Astrocytes, whose processes cover 99% of the BBB endothelia (Qutub and Hunt 2005), are responsible for the active uptake of glucose using transmembrane GLUT1. Heterozygous mutations in the gene that codes for GLUT1 (the *SLC2A1* gene) result in impaired transport of glucose across the BBB and a debilitating neurologic phenotype, De Vivo disease (De Vivo et al. 1991; Seidner et al. 1998). Areas of the brain that are histologically distant from microvasculature (luminal membranes) receive energy substrates supplied via astrocytic gap junctions (abluminal membranes) that are permeable to glucose, and its derivative metabolites glucose-6-phosphate, lactate and glutamate and glutamine (Tabernero et al. 2006).

Microdialysis studies in humans have shown that the brain extracellular fluid (ECF) concentrations of glucose are approximately 30% those of the plasma concentrations of glucose and that in induced hyper- and hypoglycaemia there is a 20- to 30-minute equilibration lag time between brain ECF and plasma glucose concentrations (Abi-Saab et al. 2002). Glucose transport into the neuron itself is facilitated by GLUT3 which is expressed predominantly on axons and dendrites. Neurologic phenotypes of heterozygous *SLC2A3* gene mutations in humans have yet to be described; however, homozygous mutation in animal models results in embryonic lethality. The carbohydrate reserve of the brain is glycogen which is several-fold higher in concentration than that of cerebral glucose under physiologic conditions (Oz et al. 2007). Cerebral glycogen granules are mostly stored in astrocytes and appear to have varying euglycaemic and hypoglycaemic functions not the least of which is to act as a neuronal energy reserve (Oz et al. 2009; DiNuzzo et al. 2011).

A number of in vitro and in vivo studies have shown that stable glucose concentrations in a narrow 'euglycaemic' range are critical for neuronal function. Whilst it has been known for some time that exposure of cultured neural cells to low- or high-ambient glucose concentrations reduces cell survival and mitochondrial activity (Sima 2010; Tomlinson and Gardiner 2008), recent studies have indicated that exposing such cells to non-physiologic *fluctuations* in glucose appears to be the most toxic environment for neural activity (Russo et al. 2012). Such glycaemic fluctuations are of course the day-to-day reality for most patients with type 1 diabetes (Fig 22.1). In animal models antecedent hypoglycaemia has been shown to increase glucose transport across the BBB into neurons via up-regulation of GLUT1 and 3, although in humans the significance of this adaptive response remains controversial (McNay and Cotero 2010).

Ketone bodies

Ketone bodies are formed after periods of prolonged energy restriction by metabolism of acetyl Co-A in the liver. Ketone bodies (primarily β-hydroxybutyrate during periods of insulinopaenia associated with ketosis or ketoacidosis) are the principal alternative to glucose as an energy substrate for the brain. Under non-diabetic fasting conditions in adults, ketone bodies can provide up to 60% of the brain's energy requirement (Owen et al. 1967). Ketone bodies originate predominantly from the liver but are also produced by astrocytes themselves (Guzmán and Blázquez 2004).

The rate of ketone body metabolism by the brain depends primarily upon circulating concentrations of ketones, levels of MCT1 to facilitate ketone passage across the BBB and less well-characterised levels of relevant metabolic enzymes within the brain (Morris 2005). Interestingly, in human ketosis associated with fasting, intracerebral β-hydroxybutyrate levels increase to a greater extent than when exogenous β-hydroxybutyrate is administered intravenously in the non-fasted state (Pan et al. 2000). Rat studies have indicated that this occurs via increased MCT1 expression at the BBB (Leino et al. 2001). In the human brain, astrocytes express MCT1 whereas neurons express both MCT1 and MCT2 (Simpson et al. 2007). Mouse studies have shown that both acetoacetate and β-hydroxybutyrate have effects upon the BBB by increasing endothelial production of the vasoconstrictor endothelin-1 and vascular permeability factor, respectively (Isales et al. 1999). Metabolism of β-hydroxybutyrate and acetoacetate within mitochondria to acetyl-CoA fuels the tricarboxylic acid cycle in a pyruvate-independent fashion. Ketone bodies may exert neuroprotective effects as is evidenced by the beneficial effects of ketogenic diets in some seizure disorders, and rat studies of administered β-hydroxybutyrate decreasing infarction and oedema in hypoxic mediated injury (Guzmán and Blázquez 2004).

However, in two recent studies, ketosis in DKA was associated with cerebral injury. In a diabetic rat model, ketosis was found to independently cause reductions in high-energy phosphate metabolites and cerebral blood flow (Glaser et al. 2012). In another recent prospective study of brain morphology over the medium term, children presenting with ketoacidosis were found to have significant white and grey matter cortical volume changes in the first week after diagnosis. Lower pH was associated with greater volume change independent of haemodynamic status and other electrolyte imbalances implying ketone bodies may have both protective and injurious effects upon the brain (Cameron et al. 2014).

Free fatty acids and amino acids

Free fatty acids (FFAs) are one of the body's most important forms of stored energy. FFAs are released through either the metabolism of stored or ingested triglycerides. Stored tri-glycerides are mobilised from adipose tissue during hypoglycaemia due to interactions between glucagon, adrenaline and noradrenaline with hormone sensitive lipase. When glucose concentrations are high, hormone sensitive lipase activity is inhibited by insulin. FFAs are metabolised within mitochondria to acetyl Co-A, a substrate for the tricarboxylic acid cycle. FFAs are actively transported across the BBB via fatty acid transport proteins (FATPs) – predominantly FATP-1 and FATP-4 (Mitchell et al. 2011). FFAs are a very effective alternative fuel source for the brain. In one insulin clamp study of induced hypoglycaemia in adults with diabetes, simultaneous administration of FFAs reversed all aspects of hypoglycaemia-induced memory impairment (Page et al. 2009).

Amino acids are the most important substrate for hepatic and renal gluconeogenesis, accounting for greater than 90% of overall gluconeogenesis (Gerich 1993). Amino acids are also neurotransmitters or neurotransmitter precursors in their own right. There are several amino acid transport systems across the BBB which facilitate the movement of amino acids both into and out of the brain (Hawkins et al. 2006). In a hypoglycaemic insulin clamp study of individuals with and without diabetes, the concomitant oral administration of a mix of 19 amino acids significantly improved performance on 10 out of 12 cognitive tasks (Rossetti et al. 2008).

Lactate and pyruvate

Lactate and pyruvate, substrates of the tricarboxylic acid cycle, are secondary energy sources for the brain. However, unlike glucose, under physiologic conditions brain ECF lactate concentrations are three-fold higher than plasma (Abi-Saab et al. 2002). Lactate and pyruvate passage across the BBB during hypoglycaemia is increased by the up-regulation of MCTs. Patients with well-controlled diabetes have a two-fold increase in monocarboxylic acid uptake across the BBB (Mason et al. 2006). Dynamic radio-labelled lactate studies have shown that under physiologic conditions the human brain (particularly neurons) is able to support up to 10% of its energy need by lactate consumption and at times of stress (such as hypoglycaemia) this can increase to 60% (Boumezbeur et al. 2010). Lactate and pyruvate that are generated within the CNS through glycolysis can also act as significant energy substrates.

Interest, in particular, has focused on the potential link between astrocyte glycolysis and neuronal energy uptake. The astrocyte-neuron lactate shuttle (ANLS) hypothesis suggests that glycolysis from glycogen within astrocytes and a lactate shuttle to neurons is the dominant glutamatergic energy pathway to neurons under activated conditions (Pellerin et al. 2007). The role ANLS plays under physiologic conditions is controversial given that neurons also have the ability to take up glucose directly via GLUT3 and can undertake glycolysis directly. It is also apparent that under physiologic conditions there may in fact be a reverse net neuron to astrocyte shuttle of lactate (Mangia et al. 2009). Thus whether the primary source of neuronal energy during neurotransmission is lactate derived from astrocyte glycolysis is an area of ongoing debate. There may be a therapeutic role for exogenous lactate and pyruvate to mitigate neuronal injury caused by hypoglycaemia. In humans, intravenous administration of lactate (within the physiologic range) improved brain function and lowered the threshold for disturbed cognition in insulin-induced hypoglycaemia (Maran et al. 1994). In a rat model of insulin-induced severe hypoglycaemia, intraperitoneal administration of pyruvate reduced neuronal death by 70%–90% with a concomitant sustained improvement in cognitive performance (Suh et al. 2005).

NEUROTRANSMITTERS

Glutamate

Glutamate is the most abundant free amino acid in the brain and acts as an excitatory neurotransmitter in the mammalian nervous system (Meldrum 2000). Glutamate plays a key role in synaptic plasticity and thus is important in cognitive functioning, particularly in the areas of learning and memory (McEntee and Crook 1993). Glucose metabolism by astrocytes fuels glutamate uptake and glutamine biosynthesis (Vannucci et al. 1997). The BBB is not very permeable to glutamate and CNS uptake depends upon glutamate channels expressed upon both astrocyte and neuronal membranes (Hawkins 2009). Glutamate is taken up by astrocytes, converted to glutamine via glutaminase and then released and taken up by presynaptic neuronal terminals and converted back to glutamate via glutamate decarboxylase (GAD) – the so-called glutamate–glutamine cycle. GAD also catalyses the conversion of glutamate to the dominant inhibitory neurotransmitter GABA. GAD expression has been found to be reduced in patients with bipolar disorder and schizophrenia (Kalkman and Loetscher 2003). Antibodies to GAD are seen both in type 1 diabetes and in some neurologic conditions such as stiff person syndrome and schizophrenia (Yarlagadda et al. 2007; Vincent 2008). The degree to which GAD antibodies cross the BBB and that to which they are immuno-pathogenic or merely markers of tissue damage remain unclear.

Under physiologic conditions the glutamate–glutamine cycle prevents excitotoxicity – a process of neuronal cell death due to excessive uptake of glutamate seen in some pathologic conditions. Glutamate itself is also produced as a by-product of glucose metabolism. After glycolysis the tricarboxylic acid cycle generates α-ketoglutarate. Transamination of α-ketoglutarate produces glutamate. A logical postulate is that the combination of higher ambient cerebral glucose levels and GAD antibodies would lead to higher cerebral glutamate levels. Interestingly a study of young adult type 1 diabetes patients did indeed find higher prefrontal glutamate levels in diabetes than in controls as well as correlations between these levels and mild depression and lower global cognitive performance (Lyoo et al. 2009). Hypoglycaemia in human controls has been found to reduce intracerebral glutamate concentrations. Loss of this response has been documented in patients with type 1 diabetes and implicated as a potential mechanism of 'hypoglycaemia unawareness' (Bischof et al. 2006).

HORMONES

Insulin

Insulin is actively transported across the BBB (Schwartz et al. 1991) and insulin receptors are widely distributed throughout the brain (Havrankova et al. 1978). Whilst not required for glucose transport, insulin plays a direct role in energy homeostasis and cognitive function within the CNS (Hallschmid and Schultes 2009). Alterations in neuronal insulin and insulin-like growth factor 1 (IGF-1) signalling have been implicated as a causative mechanism for the increased incidence of Alzheimer disease seen in type 2 diabetes (Zemva and Schubert 2011). Impaired insulin signalling within the brain has also been implicated in Huntington disease, Parkinson disease and amyotrophic lateral sclerosis (Cardoso et al. 2009). Both intravenous (crosses the blood BBB) and intranasal (bypasses the BBB) administration of insulin under peripheral euglycaemic conditions improves declarative memory in adults (Benedict et al. 2011). Functional MRI studies have indicated that possible mechanisms for this include insulin potentiating hippocampal activity (important in the development and maintenance of memory) via specific impacts upon long-term depression and potentiation of synaptic transmission. In addition animal models have shown insulin increases synapse density and dendritic plasticity in visual pathways as well as glucose utilisation of neuronal networks (Ott et al. 2012). The peripheral delivery of exogenous insulin means that most children with type 1 diabetes experience chronic hyperinsulinaemia. The extent to which this might mitigate against glycaemically mediated neuronal injury is an open question.

C-peptide

Insulin is produced from pro-insulin by the removal of the C-peptide fragment in the endoplasmic reticulum of the β cell. C-peptide has been known for some time to cross the BBB and enter brain cells (Dorn et al. 1983). In a series of experiments using the streptozocin diabetic rat model, exogenously administered C-peptide was found to prevent neurobehavioural deficits that were otherwise seen (Sima 2010). There is in vivo evidence that both insulin and C-peptide deficiencies impact upon neural survival through withdrawal of trophic factors (such as IGF-1 and nerve growth factor) leading to grey matter atrophy, and increased oxidative stress leading to neural apoptosis and white matter atrophy (Sima 2010). Intriguingly C-peptide may prove to be a mediating factor between the age of diagnosis and cognitive outcome. Cognitive outcomes have been found to be worse in those patients diagnosed in early life (particularly under 2 years of age; McCrimmon et al. 2012). This has hitherto been assumed to relate to the increased sensitivity of the immature brain to glycaemic perturbation. However, this same age group is also more likely to have lower C-peptide levels at presentation and have a greater incidence of DKA (Mortensen et al. 2010). Deficient C-peptide levels may prove to be an exacerbating factor in CNS injury in this very young group of patients.

Counter-regulatory hormones

Acute responsiveness of the counter-regulatory hormones (glucagon, adrenaline, noradrenaline, cortisol and growth hormone) to hypoglycaemia is often impaired in type 1 diabetes.

Whilst hypoglycaemia-associated autonomic failure in this disease is primarily mediated by peripheral failure of the counter-regulatory hormone response, central impairment of neurogenic symptom response is also contributory (Cryer 2010). Counter-regulatory hormones can also either directly or indirectly affect cognitive processes within the brain (McGaugh et al. 1975). Emotional arousal with its associated counter-regulatory hormonal changes is strongly linked to long-term memory consolidation (McIntyre et al. 2012). The teleological purpose of this is to ensure that significant experiences are not forgotten. Drugs that enhance the adrenal release of adrenaline and cortisol have been shown to improve learning in humans (McIntyre et al. 2012). Adrenaline crosses the BBB poorly and its effect appears to be mediated via ascending vagal fibres that terminate in the nucleus of the solitary tract within the brainstem. Fibres from the nucleus of the solitary tract (with some influence from the locus coeruleus) then regulate noradrenaline release from the amygdala. Noradrenaline in turn promotes plasticity in cortical and hippocampal synapses. The relationship between adrenaline and noradrenaline levels and brain function in type 1 diabetes is yet to be investigated.

Glucocorticoids (cortisol) and corticotropin-releasing hormone interact directly with the brain, the cytokine system and other hormone systems such as the growth hormone/IGF-1 and CNS noradrenergic systems (O'Connor et al. 2000). Glucocorticoids bind to both glucocorticoid and mineralocorticoid receptors; cortisol binding to the mineralocoticoid receptor occurs with 10 times the affinity of the glucocorticoid receptor. Cortisol freely crosses the BBB and both of its receptors are found throughout the brain (Gomez-Sanchez 2010). Despite often exhibiting a blunted cortisol response to recurrent hypoglycaemia (Brock Jacobsen et al. 2011), patients with type 1 diabetes have decreased 5α-reductase activity, resulting in reduced metabolism of cortisol and net hypercortisolaemia (Remer et al. 2006). In mouse and rat models of streptozocin-induced diabetes, chronic hypercortisolism was associated with impaired cognitive function and hippocampal morphological changes. Blockade of the glucocorticoid receptor with mifepristone reversed these changes (Revsin et al. 2009; Zuo et al. 2011).

In rat models of cerebral hypoxia, glucagon increases metabolism of ketones by neural cells (Kirsch and Alecy 1984); however, glucagon itself appears to have little direct effect on cognitive processes. On the other hand, the alternative cleavage product of pro-glucagon, glucagon-like peptide-1 (GLP-1), does have direct effects in terms of inducing satiety by binding to GLP-1 receptors in the arcuate nucleus of the hypothalamus. Rats that over-express GLP-1 receptors have shown enhanced memory and learning (During et al. 2003). Reduced GLP-1 activity on the other hand has been implicated as a causal link between type 2 diabetes and neurodegeneration (Mossello et al. 2011).

Growth hormone and its intermediary hormone IGF-I are both synthesised within the CNS along with their respective receptors and binding proteins (Lobie et al. 2000). Growth hormone is also able to cross the BBB to a varying extent. In the developing brain, growth hormone and IGF-1 affect brain size and morphology, as well as influencing differentiated cell function and cognitive development (Lobie et al. 2000). In the adult brain, growth hormone and IGF-1 have been found to increase progenitor cell proliferation and new neurons, oligodendrocytes and blood vessels in the dentate gyrus of the hippocampus

(Isgaard et al. 2007). As mentioned above, IGF-1 has some molecular overlap with insulin signalling. Impaired IGF-1 signalling impacting upon neuroprotection, regeneration and plasticity has been mechanistically implicated in several neurodegenerative conditions. In type 1 diabetes, circulating insulin-like growth factor 1 (IGF-1) and insulin-like binding protein 3 (IGFBP-3) are reduced whereas growth hormone and IGFBP-1 are increased (Dunger et al. 2005). These changes are most marked during puberty and are associated with a reduction in insulin sensitivity. The contributory CNS roles of endocrine versus paracrine IGF-1 remain unknown; however, one study using the streptozocin-diabetic adult rat showed that peripherally administered IGF-1 could fully ameliorate diabetes impaired cognition (Lupien et al. 2003).

OTHER BIOCHEMICAL VARIABLES

In the context of DKA, serum urea, plasma osmolality and sodium (often expressed as 'corrected serum sodium') are thought to have significant associations with the rare complication of fulminant cerebral oedema (Glaser et al. 2001; Hoorn et al. 2007). Mechanisms remain unclear and these biochemical variables may prove to be proxies for other metabolic processes that affect fluid movement across the BBB. The Na-K-Cl co-transporter on the luminal membrane of the BBB is responsible for up to 30% of brain interstitial fluid generation. Inhibition of this transporter with bumetanide in a rat model of DKA was found to improve levels of high-energy phosphate metabolites in the brain after insulin and saline rescue (Glaser et al. 2010). Whilst such data are yet to be replicated in the human context, the implication is that in DKA, potential peripheral biochemical changes that predispose to brain injury may be ameliorated by manipulation of the porosity of the BBB.

Neuroimaging insights in type 1 diabetes

MAGNETIC RESONANCE IMAGING TECHNIQUES

Magnetic resonance imaging (MRI) provides valuable insight into neuroanatomical, biochemical and functional alterations in the acute, subacute and chronic phases of diabetes to understand the cerebral impact during childhood of diabetes, hyperglycaemia, hypoglycaemia and ketoacidosis. There are multiple imaging techniques that can be applied using MRI. We shall summarise those of greatest relevance that have been applied in studies related to the neurological impact in diabetic children with type 1 diabetes.

Conventional anatomic imaging

Conventional MRI methods provide high-resolution anatomical images based on the detection of the ^{1}H nuclei of ordinary water (^{1}H$_2$O). In concrete terms, if a nuclear spin system (e.g. a brain containing H$_2$O) is placed in a magnetic field, it is possible to excite the nuclei (hydrogen or ^{1}H atoms in the water) using a radiofrequency pulse. This excitation causes the ^{1}H atomic nuclei to make the transition between ground and excited spin states and vice versa as predicted by quantum mechanics. The energies of these transitions are very small, many orders of magnitude smaller than the typical energy of a chemical bond. Using these methods, it is possible to obtain magnetic resonance images so that there is image contrast between tissues (e.g. water in white matter versus grey matter). This is because white and grey matter provide different microenvironments for water molecules and this affects some of their magnetic resonance properties. Two such properties are the T1 and T2 relaxation time constants when applied producing T1-weighted and T2-weighted images, respectively.

Conventional magnetic resonance images provide a neuro-anatomical framework and define the presence and severity of cerebral injury which may result acutely from cerebral oedema related to DKA. Importantly, high-resolution conventional imaging forms the substrate for volumetric and surface-based analyses.

Diffusion MRI

The image contrast for diffusion-weighted imaging (DWI) is due to water displacements. With this method, water displacements on the order of tens of micron are typically detected. Since these displacements are strongly affected by local cell architecture (i.e. hindered by cell membranes), this method can be used to probe tissue microstructure. Among the parameters available from DWI is the overall water displacement value for each image voxel, known as the apparent diffusion coefficient (ADC). In addition to providing ADC, diffusion imaging also provides information that can be used to characterise the microstructural organisation of cerebral tissue. For example, when diffusion is evaluated in myelinated white matter, ADC values are greater when measured parallel to the direction of the axons (axial diffusivity) as compared to the perpendicular direction (radial diffusivity). This is likely because water motion perpendicular to axons is relatively hindered by the necessity of crossing the membrane layers of myelin, whereas water motion parallel to axons can take place within myelin layers without the necessity of crossing membranes. This spatial variation of ADC values is known as diffusion anisotropy. Being sensitive to underlying brain microstructure, diffusion tensor imaging (DTI) measurements have been used to quantify the nature of cerebral oedema in the setting of DKA. Investigators have utilised DTI to attempt to distinguish vasogenic oedema, resulting from disturbances in the BBB or ion transporters, from cytotoxic oedema with cerebral cellular swelling, particularly in astrocytes.

Magnetic resonance spectroscopy

In ^{1}H magnetic resonance spectroscopy (MRS), magnetic resonance signal is obtained from non-water protons enabling the detection of a number of metabolites including choline, creatine, N-acetyl-aspartate (NAA) and lactate. Choline is associated with high turnover of lipid membranes, and tends to be relatively elevated in tumors and during brain development. Creatine levels are relatively constant, and the choline resonance is often used as a reference for normalisation of other resonances. NAA is a neuronal marker, and a decrease in NAA is an indicator of neuronal loss. Lactate is a product of anaerobic metabolism.

Functional MRI

Sensitivity to local magnetic field distortions provides the basis of functional magnetic resonance imaging (fMRI). When a brain region is activated during a task, cerebral blood flow (oxygen delivery) increases out of proportion to the change in oxygen consumption. As a result, local deoxyhemoglobin levels decrease. This leads to less distortion of the local magnetic field, which is manifest as an increase in the T2* relaxation time constant of local water (^{1}H$_2$O). This change in T2* can be used to identify areas of neural activation.

Volumetric MRI/surface-based analysis

Conventional magnetic resonance images can be used to measure cerebral volumes. Images of different contrasts, such as T1, T2, and proton-density weighted, can be analysed to classify tissue as CSF, grey matter or white matter. The number of image elements, or voxels, corresponding to each class can be summed to compute volumes in units of millilitres. There is not yet a consensus as to the optimal means for assessing and comparing these volumes, particularly with respect to how to apportion various brain areas for statistical analysis. A potentially more sophisticated approach, sometimes called voxel-based morphometry, consists of applying statistical methods to compare the volume of the brain of interest to that of a 'standard' brain on a voxel-by-voxel basis. This method provides parametric maps of the regions for which volumes are statistically different, similar to the maps generated for fMRI studies.

CURRENT INSIGHTS IN DIABETES IN CHILDHOOD

Acute diabetic ketoacidosis

On conventional MRI, investigators have documented findings consistent with cerebral swelling, effacement of sulci and decreased grey–white contrast. If progressive, then infarction in the deep nuclear grey matter, periaqueductal grey matter and pons can occur (Muir et al. 2004). More subtle alterations in FLAIR imaging within the medial frontal lobes have also been reported by our group in new onset DKA without clinical symptoms suggestive of DKA (Cameron et al. 2005).

MRI has been applied to define the basis for the DKA-related cerebral oedema. Some data from MRI studies in children indicate that the oedema developing during DKA treatment may be vasogenic, with elevated ADC values and increased cerebral blood flow (Glaser et al. 2004). The elevated ADC results from the increased extravascular water content. If cytotoxic cell swelling was the dominant mechanism, then one would expect a restriction in the ADC values.

Finally, a third mechanism of alterations in MRI during acute DKA may be involved – hypoxic-ischaemic cerebral injury. This is supported by animal studies that suggest that the characteristics of cerebral perfusion, metabolism and oedema during DKA are similar to those observed during cerebral ischaemia and reperfusion. For example, untreated DKA is characterised by low ADC values (suggesting cytotoxic oedema) and low cerebral blood flow (Yuen et al. 2008; Glaser et al. 2012). Brain lactate levels are elevated and levels of high-energy phosphates are decreased (Glaser et al. 2010). In contrast, during DKA treatment, cerebral blood flow is elevated and vasogenic oedema develops. Brain levels of high-energy phosphates and ratios of *N*-acetylaspartate to creatine (an indicator of neuronal health) decline during initial treatment with insulin and saline (Glaser et al. 2010) in a similar fashion to that which occurs during the phases of cerebral injury from hypoxia-ischemia.

In a further MRI study aimed at differentiating vasogenic from cytotoxic oedema (Figueroa et al. 2005) DTI and T2 relaxometry (T2R) were obtained in paediatric patients presenting with severe DKA 6–12h after initial DKA treatment and stabilisation and 96h after correction of DKA. T2R changes in an age-related manner across the lifespan. During early development, T2R time shortens, mainly reflecting the progression of myelination in white matter. In this paediatric DKA, cohort T2R was significantly increased during treatment in both white and grey matter, in comparison to the absolute T2R values 96h after correction of DKA. Classic intracellular cytotoxic oedema could not be detected, based on the lack of a statistically significant decrease in ADC values. ADC values were instead elevated, implying a large component of cell membrane water diffusion, correlating with the elevated white and grey matter T2R. This study further supported the presence of vasogenic oedema during the early treatment phase of DKA.

Importantly, a recent study in children 8–18 years presenting with DKA with type 1 diabetes were randomised to receive two different forms of fluid hydration during their acute rehydration and insulin therapy. MRI were undertaken at 3–6h after therapy, 9–12h after therapy and >72h after therapy. The authors found an increased ADC, consistent with their previous findings, with no difference in relation to the speed of rehydration (Glaser et al. 2013).

MRS has established acute disturbances during DKA and its medical therapy including increased ketones and lactate (Wootton-Gorges et al. 2005) which have been associated with alterations in mental function. In addition, this same group has established both an acute reduction in NAA, a measure of neuronal integrity, during DKA therapy (Wootton-Gorges et al. 2007) and a progressive decline in an adolescent who had recurrent DKA without any clinical cerebral oedema (Wootton-Gorges et al. 2010) suggestive of neuronal loss. Finally, our own group demonstrated increased taurine and myoinositol levels in new onset DKA (Cameron et al. 2005). Taurine has been postulated in both in vivo and in vitro studies to be a mediator of cellular oedema in diabetes (Koves et al. 2012). Thus, MRS provides valuable complementary information on the acute and chronic impact of hypo- and hyperglycaemia on brain metabolism and development.

Hypoglycaemia

Profound hypoglycaemia is a recognised aetiology for severe cerebral injury within the cortex, particularly the temporal and hippocampal regions, basal ganglia and substantia nigra (Jung et al. 2005; Rankins et al. 2005). In addition to neuronal injury, there also appears to be axonal injury with white matter T2-weighted and diffusion hyperintensities, with particular involvement of major white matter tracts such as the corpus callosum and internal capsule (Lo et al. 2006). These diffusion restrictions have been observed to be reversible in some instances (Maekawa et al. 2006).

The role of hypoglycaemia in mediating cerebral injury in children with diabetes remains under investigation. Although case series, as described above, demonstrate a severe end of the spectrum, there is an increasing awareness of the contribution of recurrent hypoglycaemia to brain growth and development (Aye et al. 2011). Early-onset diabetes with severe hypoglycaemia has been shown to be a high risk for mesial temporal lobe sclerosis and reduction in hippocampal grey matter volume (Ho et al. 2008). In addition, studies suggest that recurrent hypoglycaemia in adults with diabetes and the development of hypoglycaemic unawareness may be associated with alterations in cerebral blood flow with blunted changes in the setting of hypoglycaemia (Mangia et al. 2012).

Chronic diabetes throughout childhood and brain morphometry

Brain volumetry has been most commonly applied in defining the impact of long-standing diabetes on cerebral development. In a young cohort of children with diabetes aged 3–10 years, Aye et al. (2011) documented that the normative linear increase in white matter volume with age did not occur in children with type 1 diabetes. A similar trend was detected for hippocampal volume. Children with type 1 diabetes who had experienced hypoglycaemic seizures showed significantly reduced grey matter and white matter volumes relative to children with type 1 diabetes who had not experienced seizures.

In an older cohort of children with diabetes aged 7–17 years, Perantie et al. (2007) used voxel-based morphometry to determine the relationships of prior hypo- and hyperglycaemia to regional grey and white matter volumes across the whole brain. No significant differences were found between healthy controls and those with diabetes in total grey or white matter volumes. However, in those with diabetes, a history of severe hypoglycaemia was associated with smaller grey matter volume in the left superior temporal region. Greater exposure to hyperglycaemia was associated with smaller grey matter volume in the right cuneus and precuneus, smaller white matter volume in a right posterior parietal region and larger grey matter volume in a right prefrontal region. In a similar study of late adolescent/early adult aged young people with type 1 diabetes with longer duration of disease (Northam et al. 2009; Pell et al. 2012), the group with diabetes showed significantly lower NAA in frontal lobes and basal ganglia and higher myoinositol and choline in frontal and temporal lobes and basal ganglia the control group. The group with diabetes also had decreased grey matter in bilateral thalami and right parahippocampal gyrus and insular cortex. White matter was decreased in bilateral parahippocampi, left temporal lobe and middle frontal area. T2 in individuals with type 1 diabetes was increased in left superior temporal gyrus and decreased in bilateral lentiform nuclei, caudate nuclei and thalami, and right insular area. Significant age-related reductions were noted in grey matter volume of the lentiform and thalamic nuclei and insular and cingulate cortices, and decreasing T2 relaxation times in the cortical and subcortical brain regions, including frontal and temporal cortices (Fig 22.2; Northam et al. 2009; Pell et al. 2012).

Finally in an adult cohort of patients with type 1 diabetes aged 25–40 years, lower densities of grey matter in several brain regions including the left posterior cingulate, right parahippocampal gyrus, left hippocampus and left superior temporal gyrus were noted. In this cohort there were associations between grey matter loss and a history of chronic hyperglycaemia and severe hypoglycaemia (Musen et al. 2006). There were no changes noted in white matter (Weinger et al. 2008). Combined, these varying studies of magnetic resonance outcomes in differing age groups of patients with type 1 diabetes demonstrate varying associations between disease characteristics and brain volume outcomes – perhaps the most consistent findings being an association between episodes of severe hypoglycaemia and grey matter regional volume changes (Table 22.1).

Brain function in type 1 diabetes

Given the pathophysiological changes to brain that result from disturbed glucose/insulin homeostasis, it is not surprising that neurocognitive deficits have been described in type 1 diabetes. Meta-analytic studies have documented subtle decrements in overall IQ in both

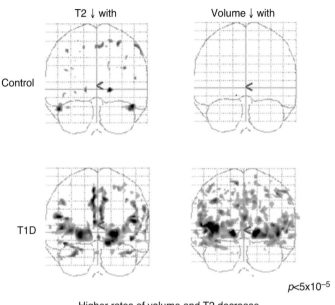

T2 ↓ with   Volume ↓ with

Control

T1D

$p<5x10^{-5}$

Higher rates of volume and T2 decrease
observed in widespread regions across the
brain

Figure 22.2. 'Accelerated' age-related decrease of brain volume and T2 signal in type 1 diabetes during childhood and adolescence. The black specked areas on the image are areas of the brain where the age regression slope is significant. The figures on the left demonstrate a significant relationship between older age and decreased volume in participants with diabetes in widespread areas across the brain but only minimal effects in the controls. A degree of age-related change is expected with normal ageing. However, the effect is far more pronounced in participants with diabetes, who show a faster and more widespread T2 signal decrease with age, relative to controls. The figures presented here demonstrate a significant relationship between increasing age and decreased volume and T2 signal in both groups in areas fairly widespread across the brain. As the control T2 image shows, a certain degree of age-related change is expected with normal ageing. However, the effect is far more pronounced in individuals with diabetes, who show a faster and more widespread volume and T2 decrease with age relative to controls.

adults (Brands et al. 2005) and children (Gaudieri et al. 2008; Naguib et al. 2009) with the disease, as well as mild deficits in specific cognitive skills including attention, executive functions, psychomotor efficiency and information-processing speed. Somewhat surprisingly, memory and learning deficits are either not evident (Brands et al. 2005) or limited to those with early-onset disease and/or a history of severe hypoglycaemia (Naguib et al. 2009). The magnitude of cognitive dysfunction in adults is moderate, with effect sizes ranging from 0.3 to 0.8 SD units, raising the possibility of some cumulative impact of the disease on cognition with increasing age and longer duration of the illness. Indeed, Biessels et al. have suggested that the chronic disturbance of glucose and insulin homeostasis inherent in type 1 diabetes elicits a form of 'accelerated brain ageing' (Biessels et al. 2006), particularly during critical periods of brain change such as neurodevelopment and neurodegeneration (Biessels et al. 2008).

TABLE 22.1
Summary of brain MRI studies in type 1 diabetes

	Age studied	Duration of diabetes	Differences between controls and diabetes patients in grey/white matter regional volume changes	Associations between severe hypoglycaemia and grey/white matter regional volume changes	Associations between chronic hyperglycaemia and grey/white matter regional volume changes
Aye et al. 2011	4–9yrs	3.6yrs	–/+	+/+	–/–
Perantie et al. 2007	7–17yrs	5.7yrs	–/–	+/–	+/+
Perantie et al. 2011	7–17yrs	5–7yrs	–/–	–/+	+/–
Northam et al. 2009; Pell et al. 2011	13–28yrs	13yrs	+/+	+/–	–/–
Musen et al. 2006; Weinger et al. 2008	25–40yrs	20yrs	+/–	+/–	+/–

Even subtle decrements in cognitive capacity can impact on children engaged in ongoing learning and skill development. An early-onset sample of Finnish children were at increased risk for academic difficulties independent of metabolic control history (Hannonen et al. 2012), similar findings to those reported in a population-based study of children in Sweden (Dahlquist and Källén 2007). Adolescents with diabetes had lower rates of school completion and work/study participation than healthy controls in a longitudinal cohort study (Northam et al. 2010), despite having similar IQ at diabetes onset 12 years previously. Subtle cognitive dysfunction may impair daily living skills and impact on independent decision making in self-management of diabetes. For example, a recent study (McNally et al. 2010) reported an association between deficits in executive skills such as goal setting, planning, organisation, working memory and mental flexibility, reduced treatment adherence and poor metabolic control although they were unable to discern the direction of effects in a cross-sectional design.

The functional implications of the pathophysiological brain changes described above are not limited to cognition and academic achievement. McIntyre et al. (2010) point out that the brain regions subserving affective and cognitive functions, such as the hippocampus, prefrontal cortex and limbic structure, overlap; hence diabetes-related biochemical disturbances in brain are also likely to affect mental health. Meta-analytic reviews confirm that depression and other affective disorders occur more commonly in both children (Reynolds and Helgeson 2011) and adults (Lustman et al. 2000; Anderson et al. 2001) with type 1 diabetes than in healthy controls and are associated with poor metabolic control. Traditionally, findings such as these have been interpreted as an indirect effect of a stressful illness impacting on emotional well-being but recent findings raise the possibility that an increased vulnerability to affective disorders may also result directly from altered brain biochemistry. For example, Lyoo et al. (2009) reported elevations in prefrontal glutamate-glutamine-y-aminobutyric acid levels and in mild depression in young adults with type 1 diabetes, with both biochemical changes and affective symptoms showing a linear relationship with lifetime hyperglycaemia exposure. In another report, children spent increased time in normoglycaemia and exhibited improved behaviour and mood after commencing on insulin pump therapy, consistent with the possibility that a reduction in diabetes-related biochemical abnormalities is associated with improvements in mental health (Knight et al. 2009).

Attempts to identify specific diabetes-related risk factors for cognitive deficits in type 1 diabetes populations have produced mixed findings. An association between early disease onset and cognitive impairment is the most robust finding (Ferguson et al. 2005; Lin et al. 2010; Kaufmann et al. 2012), with the magnitude of effects sizes increasing from small to moderate in children with onset prior to 5–6 years compared to age-matched controls (Gaudieri et al. 2008). Associations between cognitive impairment and glycaemic perturbations are less consistent. Given the obvious alterations in conscious state that accompany falling blood glucose concentrations, it is not surprising that the focus has traditionally been on hypoglycaemia as the explanation for cognitive deficits in type 1 diabetes. In fact, the 'early-onset' effect just described is often interpreted as a proxy for recurrent severe hypoglycaemia which is common, and often unrecognised, in small children. Positive associations between early hypoglycaemic seizure history and cognitive deficit have been documented in paediatric samples (Asvold et al. 2010; Aye et al. 2011; Ly et al. 2011), particularly compromising verbal intelligence (Rovet and Ehrlich 1999; Northam et al. 2010) and memory (Hershey et al. 2005; Perantie et al. 2008). However, the Diabetes Control and Complications Trial (Jacobson et al. 2007) failed to find any evidence for hypoglycaemia-related cognitive decline in young adults followed prospectively over an 18-year period, suggesting that even if an association between hypoglycaemia and cognitive deficit exists in the young child, the adult brain exhibits some form of cerebral adaptation to hypoglycaemia.

In adults, long-term exposure to hyperglycaemia increases the risk of hypertension and microvascular disease, including nephropathy, retinopathy and neuropathy, which, in turn, are associated with cognitive deficits (Ferguson et al. 2003; Jacobson et al. 2007). There is now an increasing awareness that chronically elevated blood glucose concentrations may be a risk factor for cognitive difficulties from much earlier in the course of the illness. For example, Aye et al. (2011) found a significant negative association in a paediatric sample between a time-weighted average HbA1c level and verbal IQ, a similar association to that found by Perantie et al. (2008). Overall cognitive abilities were poorer in those with a history of chronic hyperglycaemia in the study of pre-school-aged children by Patino-Fernandez et al. (2010), suggesting that poor control in the very young child may have a pervasive impact on cognitive development in general.

In seeking to understand the relationship between diabetes-related brain changes and cognitive deficit in type 1 diabetes, there is a clear need to broaden our focus beyond the glycaemic extremes of hypo- and hyperglycaemia to incorporate other aspects of dysglycaemia into our explanatory models. Constantly fluctuating glucose concentrations, as well as disturbances in insulin homeostasis, C peptide, IGF-1 and neurotransmitter functions, as well as altered counter-regulatory hormone responses, may all be important in explaining cognitive changes. In fact, Sima (2010) argues based on animal models that cognitive deficits in type 1 diabetes result from insulin and C-peptide deficiencies and their impaired signalling rather than hyperglycaemia per se. The methodological challenges of this research are many. Reliable ascertainment of metabolic control history is problematic particularly when gathered retrospectively and in vivo measurement of many of the variables listed above is difficult, or indeed impossible, given current technologies. Furthermore, putative neural insults may be cumulative and/or synergistic and their impact on the CNS is likely to be influenced by stage of neurodevelopment at the time they occur, thus confounding attempts to identify causal mechanisms. However there is a clear clinical imperative to pursue such research as treatments targeting aberrant neurochemistry hold promise for neuroprotective therapies which over time may reduce morbidity in both cognition and affective state.

Conclusion

A constant supply of glucose to the brain is critical for normal cerebral metabolism, with both hypoglycaemia and hyperglycaemia affecting activity, survival and function of neural cells (Tomlinson and Gardiner 2008). Uni-dimensional in vivo and in vitro models of diabetic dysglycaemia consistently demonstrate adverse consequences in neural cell survival and function. The multidimensional clinical model involving multiple variables such as age, duration of disease and dysglycaemia in the context of other metabolic and endocrine disturbance has been less consistent in terms of outcome. Such inconsistency is probably reflective of the difficulties inherent in non-invasive studies of the human brain, varying measurement techniques and poorly understood interactive mechanisms between metabolites and hormones at the neural cellular level.

REFERENCES

Abbott NJ (2002) Astrocyte–endothelial interactions and blood–brain barrier permeability. *J Anat* 200: 629–638.

Abi-Saab WM, Maggs DG, Jones T et al. (2002) Striking differences in glucose and lactate levels between brain extracellular fluid and plasma in conscious human subjects: Effects of hyperglycemia and hypoglycemia. *J Cereb Blood Flow Metab* 22: 271–279.

Anderson RJ, Freedland KE, Clouse RE and Lustman P (2001) The prevalence of comorbid depression in adults with diabetes. *Diabetes Care* 24: 1069–1078.

Asvold B, Sand T, Hestad K and Bjorgaas M (2010) Cognitive function in type 1 diabetic adults with early exposure to severe hypoglycaemia. *Diabetes Care* 33: 1945–1947.

Aye T, Reiss A, Kesler S et al. (2011) The feasibility of detecting neuropsychologic and neuroanatomic effects of type 1 diabetes in young children. *Diabetes Care* 34: 1458–1462.

Benedict C, Frey WH II, Schiöth HB, Schultes B, Born J and Hallschmid M (2011) Intranasal insulin as a therapeutic option in the treatment of cognitive impairments. *Exp Gerontol* 46(2–3): 112–115.

Biessels GJ, Deary IJ and Ryan CM (2008) Cognition and diabetes: A lifespan perspective. *Lancet Neurology* 7:184–190.

Biessels GJ, Staekenborg S, Brunner E, Brayne C and Scheltens P (2006) Risk of dementia in diabetes mellitus: A systematic review. *Lancet Neurol* 5: 64–74.

Bischof MG, Brehm A, Bernroider E et al. (2006) Cerebral glutamate metabolism during hypoglycaemia in healthy and type 1 diabetic humans. *Eur J Clin Invest* 36: 164–169.

Boumezbeur F, Petersen KF, Cline GW et al. (2010) The contribution of blood lactate to brain energy metabolism in humans measured by dynamic 13C nuclear magnetic resonance spectroscopy. *J Neurosci* 30: 13983–13991.

Brands AM, Biessels GJ, de Haan EH, Kappelle LJ and Kessels RP (2005) The effects of type 1 diabetes on cognitive performance: A meta-analysis. *Diabetes Care* 28: 726–735.

Brock Jacobsen I, Vind BF, Korsholm L et al. (2011) Counter-regulatory hormone responses to spontaneous hypoglycaemia during treatment with insulin Aspart or human soluble insulin: A double-blinded randomized cross-over study. *Acta Physiol (Oxf)* 202: 337–347.

Cameron FJ, Kean MJ, Wellard RM, Werther GA, Neil JJ and Inder TE (2005) Insights into the acute cerebral metabolic changes associated with childhood diabetes. *Diabet Med* 22: 648–653.

Cameron FJ, Scratch S, Nadebaum C et al. (2014) Neurological consequences of diabetic ketoacidosis at initial presentation of type 1 diabetes in a prospective cohort of children. *Diabetes Care* 37: 1554–1662.

Cardoso S, Correia S, Santos RX et al. (2009) Insulin is a two-edged knife on the brain. *J Alzheimers Dis* 18: 483–507.

Cryer PE (2010) Hypoglycemia in type 1 diabetes mellitus. *Endocrinol Metab Clin North Am* 39: 641–654.

Dahlquist G and Källén B (2007) School performance in children with type 1 diabetes-a population-based register study. *Diabetologia* 50: 957–964.

De Vivo DC, Trifiletti RR, Jacobson RI, Ronen GM, Behmand RA and Harik SI (1991) Defective glucose transport across the blood-brain barrier as a cause of persistent hypoglycorrhachia, seizures, and developmental delay. *N Engl J Med* 325: 703–709.

DiNuzzo M, Maraviglia B and Giove F (2011) Why does the brain (not) have glycogen? *Bioessays* 33: 319–326.

Dorn A, Rinne A, Bernstein HG, Hahn HJ and Ziegler M (1983) Insulin and C-peptide in human brain neurons. *J Hirnforsch* 24: 495–499.

Dunger DB, Regan FM and Acerini CL (2005) Childhood and adolescent diabetes. *Endocr Dev* 9: 107–120.

During MJ, Cao L, Zuzga DS et al. (2003) Glucagon-like peptide-1 receptor is involved in learning and neuroprotection. *Nat Med* 9: 1173–1179.

Ferguson SC, Blane A, Perros P et al. (2003) Cognitive ability and brain structure in type 1 diabetes: Relation to microangiopathy and preceding severe hypoglycaemia. *Diabetes* 52: 149–156.

Ferguson SC, Blane A, Wardlaw J, Perros P, McCrimmon RJ and Deary I (2005) Influence of an early-onset age of type 1 diabetes on cerebral structure and cognitive function. *Diabetes Care* 28: 1431–1437.

Figueroa RE, Hoffman WH, Momin Z, Pancholy A, Passmore GG and Allison J (2005) Study of subclinical cerebral edema in diabetic ketoacidosis by magnetic resonance imaging T2 relaxometry and apparent diffusion coefficient maps. *Endocr Res* 31: 345–355.

Gaudieri PA, Greer TF, Chen R and Holmes CS (2008) Cognitive function in children with type 1 diabetes: A meta-analysis. *Diabetes Care* 31: 1892–1897.

Gerich JE (1993) Control of glycaemia. *Baillieres Clin Endocrinol Metab* 7: 551–586.

Glaser N, Barnett P, McCaslin I et al. (2001) Risk factors for cerebral edema in children with diabetic ketoacidosis. The Pediatric Emergency Medicine Collaborative and Research Committee of the American Academy of Pediatrics. *N Engl J Med* 344: 264–269.

Glaser N, Ngo C, Anderson S, Yuen N, Trifu A and O'Donnell M (2012) Effects of hyperglycemia and effects of ketosis on cerebral perfusion, cerebral water distribution, and cerebral metabolism. *Diabetes* 61: 1831–1837.

Glaser NS, Wootton-Gorges SL, Buonocore MH et al. (2013) Subclinical cerebral edema in children with diabetic ketoacidosis randomized to 2 different rehydration protocols. *Pediatrics* 131: e73–e80.

Glaser NS, Wootton-Gorges SL, Marcin JP et al. (2004) Mechanism of cerebral edema in children with diabetic ketoacidosis. *J Pediatr* 145: 164–171.

Glaser N, Yuen N, Anderson SE, Tancredi DJ and O'Donnell ME (2010) Cerebral metabolic alterations in rats with diabetic ketoacidosis: Effects of treatment with insulin and intravenous fluids and effects of bumetanide. *Diabetes* 59: 702–709.

Gomez-Sanchez EP (2010) The mammalian mineralocorticoid receptor: Tying down a promiscuous receptor. *Exp Physiol* 95: 13–18.

Guzmán M and Blázquez C (2004) Ketone body synthesis in the brain: Possible neuroprotective effects. *Prostaglandins Leukot Essent Fatty Acids* 70: 287–292.

Hallschmid M and Schultes B (2009) Central nervous insulin resistance: A promising target in the treatment of metabolic and cognitive disorders? *Diabetologia* 52: 2264–2269.

Hannonen R, Komulainen J, Rikonen R et al. (2012) Academic skills in children with early-onset type 1 diabetes: The effects of diabetes-related risk factors. *Dev Med Child Neurol* 54: 457–463.

Havrankova J, Roth J and Brownstein M (1978) Insulin receptors are widely distributed in the central nervous system of the rat. *Nature* 272: 827–829.

Hawkins RA (2009) The blood-brain barrier and glutamate. *Am J Clin Nutr* 90: 867S–874S.

Hawkins RA, O'Kane RL, Simpson IA and Viña JR (2006) Structure of the blood-brain barrier and its role in the transport of amino acids. *J Nutr* 136: 218S–226S.

Hershey T, Perantie DC, Warren SL, Zimmerman EC, Sadler M and White NH (2005) Frequency and timing of severe hypoglycaemia affects spatial memory in children with type 1 diabetes. *Diabetes Care* 28: 2372–2377.

Herzog RI, Sherwin RS and Rothman DL (2011) Insulin-induced hypoglycemia and its effect on the brain: Unraveling metabolism by in vivo nuclear magnetic resonance. *Diabetes* 60: 1856–1858.

Ho MS, Weller NJ, Ives FJ et al. (2008) Prevalence of structural central nervous system abnormalities in early-onset type 1 diabetes mellitus. *J Pediatr* 153: 385–390.

Hoorn EJ, Carlotti AP, Costa LA et al. (2007) Preventing a drop in effective plasma osmolality to minimize the likelihood of cerebral edema during treatment of children with diabetic ketoacidosis. *J Pediatr* 150: 467–473.

Hunt A, Schönknecht P, Henze M, Seidl U, Haberkorn U and Schröder J (2007) Reduced cerebral glucose metabolism in patients at risk for Alzheimer's disease. *Psychiatry Res* 155: 147–154.

Isales CM, Min L and Hoffman WH (1999) Acetoacetate and beta-hydroxybutyrate differentially regulate endothelin-1 and vascular endothelial growth factor in mouse brain microvascular endothelial cells. *J Diabetes Complications* 13: 91–97.

Isgaard J, Aberg D and Nilsson M (2007) Protective and regenerative effects of the GH/IGF-I axis on the brain. *Minerva Endocrinol* 32: 103–113.

Jacobson AM, Musen G, Ryan CM et al. (2007) Long-term effect of diabetes and its treatment on cognitive function. *N Engl J Med* 356: 1842–1852.

Jung SL, Kim BS, Lee KS, Yoon KH and Byun JY (2005) Magnetic resonance imaging and diffusion-weighted imaging changes after hypoglycemic coma. *J Neuroimaging* 15: 193–196.

Kalkman HO and Loetscher E (2003) GAD(67): The link between the GABA-deficit hypothesis and the dopaminergic- and glutamatergic theories of psychosis. *J Neural Transm* 110: 803–112.

Kaufmann L, Pixner S, Starke M et al. (2012) Neurocognition and brain structure in pediatric patients with type 1 diabetes. *J Pediatr Neuroradiol* 1: 25–35.

Kirsch JR and D'Alecy LG (1984) Glucagon stimulates ketone utilization by rat brain slices. *Stroke* 15: 324–328.

Knight S, Northam E, Donath S et al. (2009) Improvements in cognition, mood and behaviour following commencement of continuous subcutaneous insulin infusion therapy in children with type 1 diabetes mellitus: A pilot study. *Diabetologia* 52: 193–198.

Koves I, Russo VC, Higgins S, Pitt J, Cameron FJ and Werther GA (2012) An in vitro paradigm for diabetic cerebral oedema and its therapy – A critical role for taurine and water channels. *Neurochem Res* 37:182–192.

Leino RL, Gerhart DZ, Duelli R, Enerson BE and Drewes LR (2001) Diet-induced ketosis increases mono-carboxylate transporter (MCT1) levels in rat brain. *Neurochem Int* 38: 519–127.

Lin A, Northam EA, Rankins D, Werther GA and Cameron FJ (2010) Neuropsychological profiles of young people with type 1 diabetes 12 yr after disease onset. *Pediatric Diabetes* 11: 235–243.

Liu Y, Liu F, Iqbal K, Grundke-Iqbal I and Gong CX (2008) Decreased glucose transporters correlate to abnormal hyperphosphorylation of tau in Alzheimer disease. *FEBS Lett* 582: 359–364.

Lo L, Tan AC, Umapathi T and Lim CC (2006) Diffusion-weighted MR imaging in early diagnosis and prognosis of hypoglycemia. *AJNR Am J Neuroradiol* 27: 1222–1224.

Lobie PE, Zhu T, Graichen R and Goh EL (2000) Growth hormone, insulin-like growth factor I and the CNS: Localization, function and mechanism of action. *Growth Horm IGF Res* 10: S51–S56.

Lupien SB, Bluhm EJ and Ishii DN (2003) Systemic insulin-like growth factor-I administration prevents cognitive impairment in diabetic rats, and brain IGF regulates learning/memory in normal adult rats. *J Neurosci Res* 74: 512–523.

Lustman PJ, Anderson RJ, Freedland KE, de Groot M, Carney RM and Clouse RE (2000) Depression and poor glycemic control: A meta-analytic review of the literature. *Diabetes Care* 23: 934–942.

Ly T, Anderson M, McNamara K, Davis E and Jones T (2011) Neurocognitive outcomes in young adults with early-onset type 1 diabetes. *Diabetes Care* 34: 2192–2197.

Lyoo IK, Yoon SJ, Musen G et al. (2009) Altered prefrontal glutamate-glutamine-gamma-aminobutyric acid levels and relation to low cognitive performance and depressive symptoms in type 1 diabetes mellitus. *Arch Gen Psychiatry* 66: 878–887.

Maekawa S, Aibiki M, Kikuchi K, Kikuchi S and Umakoshi K (2006) Time related changes in reversible MRI findings after prolonged hypoglycemia. *Clin Neurol Neurosurg* 108: 511–513.

Mangia S, Simpson IA, Vannucci SJ and Carruthers A (2009) The in vivo neuron-to-astrocyte lactate shuttle in human brain: Evidence from modeling of measured lactate levels during visual stimulation. *J Neurochem* 109(Suppl 1): 55–62.

Mangia S, Tesfaye N, De Martino F et al. (2012) Hypoglycemia-induced increases in thalamic cerebral blood flow are blunted in subjects with type 1 diabetes and hypoglycemia unawareness. *J Cereb Blood Flow Metab* 32: 2084–2090.

Maran A, Cranston I, Lomas J, Macdonald I and Amiel SA (1994) Protection by lactate of cerebral function during hypoglycaemia. *Lancet* 343: 16–20.

Mason GF, Petersen KF, Lebon V, Rothman DL and Shulman GI (2006) Increased brain monocarboxylic acid transport and utilization in type 1 diabetes. *Diabetes* 55: 929–934.

McCrimmon RJ, Ryan CM and Frier BM (2012) Diabetes and cognitive dysfunction. *Lancet* 379: 2291–2299.

McEntee WJ and Crook TH (1993) Glutamate: Its role in learning, memory, and the aging brain. *Psychopharmacology (Berl)* 111: 391–401.

McGaugh JL, Gold PE, Van Buskirk R and Haycock J (1975) Modulating influences of hormones and catecholamines on memory storage processes. *Prog Brain Res* 42: 151–162.

McIntyre CK, McGaugh JL and Williams CL (2012) Interacting brain systems modulate memory consolidation. *Neurosci Biobehav Rev* 36: 1750–1762.

McIntyre RS, Kenna HA, Nguyen HT et al. (2010) Brain volume abnormalities and neurocognitive deficits in diabetes mellitus: Points of pathophysiological commonality with mood disorders?. *Adv Ther* 27: 63–80.

McNally K, Rohan J, Pendley J, Delamater A and Drotar D (2010) Executive functioning, treatment adherence, and glycemic control in children with type 1 diabetes. *Diabetes Care* 33: 1159–1162.

McNay EC and Cotero VE (2010) Mini-review: Impact of recurrent hypoglycemia on cognitive and brain function. *Physiol Behav* 100: 234–238.

Meldrum BS (2000) Glutamate as a neurotransmitter in the brain: Review of physiology and pathology. *J Nutr* 130: 1007S–10015S.

Mitchell RW, On NH, Del Bigio MR, Miller DW and Hatch GM (2011) Fatty acid transport protein expression in human brain and potential role in fatty acid transport across human brain microvessel endothelial cells. *J Neurochem* 17: 735–746.

Morris AA (2005) Cerebral ketone body metabolism. *J Inherit Metab Dis* 28: 109–121.

Mortensen HB, Swift PG, Holl RW et al. (2010) Hvidoere Study Group on Childhood Diabetes. Multinational study in children and adolescents with newly diagnosed type 1 diabetes: Association of age, ketoacidosis, HLA status, and autoantibodies on residual beta-cell function and glycemic control 12 months after diagnosis. *Pediatr Diabetes* 11: 218–226.

Mossello E, Ballini E, Boncinelli M et al. (2011) Glucagon-like peptide-1, diabetes, and cognitive decline: Possible pathophysiological links and therapeutic opportunities. *Exp Diabetes Res* 2011. doi: 10.1155/2011/281674.

Muir AB, Quisling RG, Yang MC and Rosenbloom AL (2004) Cerebral edema in childhood diabetic keto-acidosis: Natural history, radiographic findings, and early identification. *Diabetes Care* 27: 1541–1546.

Musen G, Lyoo IK, Sparks CR et al. (2006) Effects of type 1 diabetes on gray matter density as measured by voxel-based morphometry. *Diabetes* 55: 326–333.

Naguib JM, Kulinskaya E, Lomax Cl and Garralda ME (2009) Neuro-cognitive performance in children with type 1 diabetes – A meta-analysis. *J Pediatr Psychol* 34: 271–282.

Northam EA, Lin A, Finch S, Werther GA and Cameron FJ (2010) Psychosocial well-being and functional outcomes in youth with type 1 diabetes 12 years after disease onset. *Diabetes Care* 33: 1430–1437.

Northam EA, Rankins D, Lin A et al. (2009) Central nervous system function in youth with type 1 diabetes 12 years after disease onset. *Diabetes Care* 32: 445–450.

O'Connor TM, O'Halloran DJ and Shanahan F (2000) The stress response and the hypothalamic-pituitary-adrenal axis: From molecule to melancholia. *QJM* 93: 323–333.

Ott V, Benedict C, Schultes B, Born J and Hallschmid M (2012) Intranasal administration of insulin to the brain impacts cognitive function and peripheral metabolism. *Diabetes Obes Metab* 14: 214–221.

Owen OE, Morgan AP, Kemp HG, Sullivan JM, Herrera MG and Cahill GF Jr (1967) Brain metabolism during fasting. *J Clin Invest* 46: 1589–1595.

Oz G, Kumar A, Rao JP et al. (2009) Human brain glycogen metabolism during and after hypoglycemia. *Diabetes* 58: 1978–1985.

Oz G, Seaquist ER, Kumar A et al. (2007) Human brain glycogen content and metabolism: Implications on its role in brain energy metabolism. *J Physiol Endocrinol Metab* 292: E946–E951.

Page KA, Williamson A, Yu N et al. (2009) Medium-chain fatty acids improve cognitive function in intensively treated type 1 diabetic patients and support in vitro synaptic transmission during acute hypoglycemia. *Diabetes* 58: 1237–1244.

Pan JW, Rothman TL, Behar KL, Stein DT and Hetherington HP (2000) Human brain beta-hydroxybutyrate and lactate increase in fasting-induced ketosis. *J Cereb Blood Flow Metab* 20: 1502–1507.

Patino-Fernandez AM, Delamater AM, Applegate EB et al. (2010) Neurocognitive functioning on preschool-age children with type 1 diabetes. *Pediatr Diabetes* 11: 424–430.

Pell GS, Lin A, Wellard RM et al. (2012) Age-related loss of brain volume and T2 relaxation time in youth with type 1 diabetes. *Diabetes Care* 35: 513–519.

Pellerin L, Bouzier-Sore AK, Aubert A et al. (2007) Activity-dependent regulation of energy metabolism by astrocytes: An update. *Glia* 55: 1251–1262.

Perantie DC, Lim A, Wu J et al. (2008) Effects of prior hypoglycaemia and hyperglycaemia on cognition in children with type 1 diabetes mellitus. *Pediatr Diabetes* 9: 87–95.

Perantie DC, Wu J, Koller JM et al. (2007) Regional brain volume differences associated with hyperglycemia and severe hypoglycemia in youth with type 1 diabetes. *Diabetes Care* 30: 2331–2337.

Qutub AA and Hunt CA (2005) Glucose transport to the brain: A systems model. *Brain Res Rev* 49: 595–617.

Rankins D, Wellard RM, Cameron F, McDonnell C and Northam E (2005) The impact of acute hypoglycemia on neuropsychological and neurometabolite profiles in children with type 1 diabetes. *Diabetes Care* 28: 2771–2773.

Remer T, Maser-Gluth C, Boye KR, Hartmann MF, Heinze E and Wudy SA (2006) Exaggerated adrenarche and altered cortisol metabolism in type 1 diabetic children. *Steroids* 71: 591–598.

Revsin Y, Rekers NV, Louwe MC et al. (2009) Glucocorticoid receptor blockade normalizes hippocampal alterations and cognitive impairment in streptozotocin-induced type 1 diabetes mice. *Neuropsychopharmacology* 34: 747–758.

Reynolds KA and Helgeson V (2011) Children with diabetes compared to peers: Depressed? Distressed? *Ann Behav Med* 42: 29–41.

Rossetti P, Porcellati F, Busciantella Ricci N et al. (2008) Effect of oral amino acids on counterregulatory responses and cognitive function during insulin-induced hypoglycemia in nondiabetic and type 1 diabetic people. *Diabetes* 57: 1905–1917.

Rovet JF and Ehrlich RM (1999) The effect of hypoglycaemic seizures on cognitive function in children with diabetes: A 7-year prospective study. *J Pediatr* 134: 503–506.

Russo V, Higgins S, Werther GA and Cameron FJ (2012) Effects of fluctuating glucose levels on neuronal cells in vitro. *Neurochem Res* 37: 1768–1782.

Sabin MA, Cameron FJ and Werther GA (2009) Type 1 diabetes–still the commonest form of diabetes in children. *Aust Fam Physician* 38: 695–697.

Seidner G, Alvarez MG, Yeh J-I et al. (1998) GLUT-1 deficiency syndrome caused by haploinsufficiency of the blood-brain barrier hexose carrier. *Nature Genetics* 18: 188–191.

Sima AA (2010) Encephalopathies: The emerging diabetic complications. *Acta Diabetol* 47: 279–293.

Simpson IA, Carruthers A and Vannucci SJ (2007) Supply and demand in cerebral energy metabolism: The role of nutrient transporters. *J Cereb Blood Flow Metab* 27: 1766–1791.

Schwartz MW, Bergman RN, Kahn SE et al. (1991) Evidence for entry of plasma insulin into cerebrospinal fluid through an intermediate compartment in dogs. Quantitative aspects and implications for transport. *J Clin Invest* 88: 1272–1281.

Suh SW, Aoyama K, Matsumori Y, Liu J and Swanson RA (2005) Pyruvate administered after severe hypoglycemia reduces neuronal death and cognitive impairment. *Diabetes* 54: 1452–1458.

Tabernero A, Medina JM and Giaume C (2006) Glucose metabolism and proliferation in glia: Role of astrocytic gap junctions. *J Neurochem* 99: 1049–1061.

Tomlinson DR and Gardiner NJ (2008) Glucose neurotoxicity. *Nat Rev Neurosci* 9: 36–45.

Vannucci SJ, Maher F and Simpson IA (1997) Glucose transporter proteins in brain: Delivery of glucose to neurons and glia. *Glia* 21: 2–21.

Vincent A (2008) Stiff, twitchy or wobbly: Are GAD antibodies pathogenic? *Brain* 131: 2536–2537.

Weinger K, Jacobson AM, Musen G et al. (2008) The effects of type 1 diabetes on cerebral white matter. *Diabetologia* 51: 417–425.

Wootton-Gorges SL, Buonocore MH, Caltagirone RA, Kuppermann N and Glaser NS (2010) Progressive decrease in N-acetylaspartate/Creatine ratio in a teenager with type 1 diabetes and repeated episodes of ketoacidosis without clinically apparent cerebral edema: Evidence for permanent brain injury. *AJNR Am J Neuroradiol* 31: 780–781.

Wootton-Gorges SL, Buonocore MH, Kuppermann N et al. (2005) Detection of cerebral {beta}-hydroxy butyrate, acetoacetate, and lactate on proton MR spectroscopy in children with diabetic ketoacidosis. *AJNR Am J Neuroradiol* 26: 1286–1291.

Wootton-Gorges SL, Buonocore MH, Kuppermann N et al. (2007) Cerebral proton magnetic resonance spectroscopy in children with diabetic ketoacidosis. *AJNR Am J Neuroradiol* 28: 895–899.

Yarlagadda A, Helvink B, Chou C and Clayton AH (2007) Blood brain barrier: The role of GAD antibodies in psychiatry. *Psychiatry (Edgmont)* 4: 57–59.

Yuen N, Anderson SE, Glaser N, Tancredi DJ and O'Donnell ME (2008) Cerebral blood flow and cerebral edema in rats with diabetic ketoacidosis. *Diabetes* 57: 2588–2594.

Zemva J and Schubert M (2011) Central insulin and insulin-like growth factor-1 signaling: Implications for diabetes associated dementia. *Curr Diabetes Rev* 7: 356–366.

Zuo ZF, Wang W, Niu L et al. (2011) RU486 (mifepristone) ameliorates cognitive dysfunction and reverses the down-regulation of astrocytic N-myc downstream-regulated gene 2 in streptozotocin-induced type-1 diabetic rats. *Neuroscience* 190: 156–165.

23
CENTRAL ACTIONS OF INSULIN

Benjamin G Challis and Robert K Semple

Introduction

Insulin is the quintessential hormone of plenty, its release tightly coupled to the ingestion and absorption of nutrients, and its actions serving to orchestrate the body's response to availability of anabolic substrates. Specifically, insulin activates intracellular signalling pathways required for uptake, utilisation and storage of glucose, amino acids and fatty acids, while simultaneously inhibiting the catabolic processes involved in the breakdown of glycogen, fat and protein. Decades of research have focused on uncovering the intricate insulin signalling network in the liver, skeletal muscle and adipose tissue, which have long been regarded as the canonical insulin-responsive tissues essential for the systemic actions of insulin.

Insulin has pleiotropic biological effects in multiple tissues beyond this traditional trio of 'insulin-responsive' tissues, however, and at least some of these are likely to subserve important physiological effects. The tight entrainment of blood insulin concentrations to acute nutritional state, and its tendency to rise in the face of long-term caloric excess and increased adipose tissue accumulation, means that it has properties well suited to a role in the central nervous system (CNS) sensing of nutritional state in both the short and the longer term. Indeed a potential role of insulin in the CNS has been the focus of study since the 1960s, almost exclusively in animal model systems, and core aspects of these studies have been reviewed (Plum et al. 2005; Porte et al. 2005). In this chapter the key findings from animal studies will be summarised, and an attempt will be made to gauge the extent to which available evidence supports an important physiological role for insulin in the human CNS.

Does insulin have access to the brain?

Like other peptide hormones, insulin can access CNS tissue directly from the perivascular space at sites of permeability of the blood–brain barrier such as the area postrema and periventricular organs (Plum et al. 2005; Porte et al. 2005). However, insulin was originally thought to be unable to cross the blood–brain barrier at other sites. This notion was challenged in the early years after development of the insulin radioimmunoassay by the demonstration that increasing concentrations of immunoreactive insulin could be detected in the cerebrospinal fluid (CSF) of anaesthetised dogs following peripheral insulin infusion (Margolis and Altszuler 1967). It has subsequently become clear that the efficiency of insulin transit into the CSF varies markedly among different species, but many studies have confirmed that the concentration of CSF insulin does mirror basal plasma insulin concentrations. Nevertheless CSF concentrations of insulin are markedly attenuated compared to those in plasma, with, for example, intravenous pulses of insulin resulting in an increase in CSF insulin levels of less than 1% in dogs (Woods and Porte 1977).

Insulin crosses the blood–brain barrier via a saturable, receptor-mediated transport process (Woods and Porte 1977), although the precise mechanism underlying this remains unclear. The relative delay in the rise in CSF insulin concentration following its peripheral infusion suggests that insulin must diffuse through interstitial fluid following transit across the blood–brain barrier before eventually reaching the CSF.

It has more recently been suggested that insulin may act as a bona fide neuropeptide through its *de novo* synthesis in the CNS. There are two insulin-encoding genes in rats and mice, and many reports have described expression of both preproinsulin I and II mRNAs, encoded by *Ins1* and *Ins2*, in the fetal rat brain. A more recent study has suggested, however, that *Ins2*, but not *Ins1*, is expressed in the mouse brain (Mehran et al. 2012). In humans, too, expression of the sole insulin-encoding mRNA has been found throughout the adult brain including the cortex, hippocampus and hypothalamus (Mehran et al. 2012); secretion of insulin peptide into the human CNS has yet to be proven, and so the significance of central insulin production and its relative contribution to central insulin signalling remain the subject of speculation only.

Insulin signalling in the central nervous system
Once in the brain, the actions of insulin, as in peripheral tissues, are initiated by its binding to the insulin receptor (InsR), a member of the tyrosine kinase receptor family. Abundant InsR expression has been described in the olfactory bulb, cerebral cortex, cerebellum, hippocampus, striatum and key hypothalamic nuclei implicated in metabolic homeostasis including the arcuate nucleus (Mehran et al. 2012).

Following insulin binding to the extracellular α-subunits of its dimeric receptor, allosteric conformational change activates the tyrosine kinase activity of the intracellular β-subunits, resulting in their autophosphorylation, and subsequently in the phosphorylation of downstream effector molecules including insulin receptor substrate (IRS) proteins and Src homology and collagen-like (Shc). Tyrosine-phosphorylated IRS-1 or IRS-2 act as docking sites for Src-homology 2 (SH2) domain containing proteins, including the p85 regulatory subunit of phosphatidylinositol 3-kinase (PI3K) and the growth factor receptor binding protein 2 (Grb2). Binding of these proteins to tyrosine phosphorylated IRS results in their activation and subsequent stimulation of downstream signalling cascades including the Ras-Raf-MAPK and PI3K-AKT-FoxO1 pathways, which mediate the diverse cellular actions of insulin. The insulin signalling pathway is schematised in Figure 23.1.

Evidence for central insulin action in the regulation of energy homeostasis
From the preceding discussion it is clear not only that insulin can gain access to the CNS, albeit at low levels, but also that the cellular machinery exists there to respond to it. This circumstantial evidence does not, however, prove that central insulin action is physiologically significant. More direct evidence for this comes from experiments in rodents.

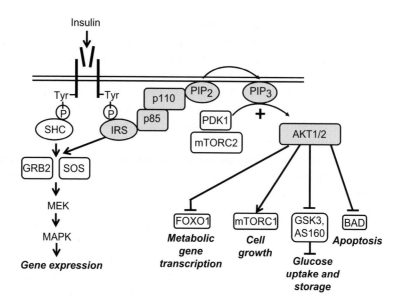

Figure 23.1. Simplified schematic of insulin signal transduction pathway. Core components of the phosphaitidylinositol-3-kinase/(PI3K)AKT pathway are shaded in grey. P85 is the regulatory subunit of PI3K and p110 the catalytic subunit. PIP2 and PIP3 are the lipid substrate and product of PI3K, respectively. SHC, Src homology and collagen-like; GRB2, growth factor receptor-bound protein 2; SOS, Son of Sevenless; MEK, mitogen-activated protein kinase kinase; MAPK, mitogen-activated protein kinase; IRS, insulin receptor substrate; PDK1, phosphoinositide-dependent protein kinase 1; mTORC, mammalian target of rapamycin complex 1; GSK, glycogen synthase kinase; AS160, Akt substrate of 160 kDa; BAD, Bcl-2-associated death.

Pharmacological studies provided the first evidence for such a central role of insulin signalling with the observation that chronic intracerebroventricular (ICV) or intrahypothalamic delivery of insulin to baboons or rodents reduced food intake and body weight. In contrast, central administration of either high affinity anti-insulin antibodies or InsR anti-sense oligonucleotides stimulated food intake and promoted weight gain in rodents (reviewed in [Porte et al. 2005]). Furthermore complete neuron-specific inactivation of the *InsR* gene in mice (producing so-called NIRKO mice) resulted in hyperphagic obesity and reproductive defects (Bruning et al. 2000), while, more indirectly, selective ablation of neurons with an active insulin promoter produced thin, hypophagic mice (Rother et al. 2012). These observations provide strong evidence that central insulin action exerts important neuroendocrine effects, at least in mice.

More recently intensive efforts to elucidate the neurocircuitry mediating these anorexigenic effects of insulin have been made. A key focus of investigation has been the melanocortin pathway, which has been well established to play a critical role in both energy and glucose homeostasis. The melanocortin system consists of two distinct neuronal populations within the hypothalamic arcuate nucleus that sense peripheral humoral signals, including insulin, and convey this information to higher CNS centres: one population expresses proopiomelanocortin (POMC) from which the potent anorectic peptide α-MSH is derived, and the second co-expresses the orexigenic peptides, neuropeptide Y (NPY) and agouti-related peptide (AGRP). Activation of NPY/AGRP neurons increases food intake and decreases energy expenditure, whereas depolarisation of POMC neurons suppresses feeding and increases energy expenditure. InsR expression is enriched within the mouse arcuate nucleus, and, more specifically, on POMC and NPY/AGRP neurons, where insulin appears to regulate them in a reciprocal manner: intracerebroventricular delivery of insulin into the third ventricle increases *POMC* expression while decreasing *NPY* expression (Schwartz et al. 1992; Benoit et al. 2002), whereas central administration of an α-MSH antagonist abrogates insulin-mediated anorexia, thereby supporting an important role for the melano-cortin pathway in central insulin signalling (Benoit et al. 2002).

Since the demonstration that these neuronal populations are insulin responsive, many laboratories have begun to address the question of which components of the insulin signalling cascade are required to mediate insulin's neuronal effects. Irs1 and Irs2 are widely expressed in the brain. Irs1 is expressed throughout the CNS but is not found within the ventral hypothalamus, and mice lacking *Irs1* are growth retarded and insulin resistant but not obese. Irs2, in contrast, is concentrated within the arcuate nucleus and is co-expressed with the InsR in POMC and NPY/AGRP neurons (Pardini et al. 2006). *Irs2*$^{-/-}$ mice develop diabetes due to impaired β-cell function and female *Irs2*$^{-/-}$ mice are obese and infertile. Furthermore, brain-specific deletion of *Irs2* results in obesity, insulin resistance and glucose intolerance (Taguchi et al. 2007). Surprisingly, however, mice with selective inactivation of *Irs2* in POMC neurons are not obese (Choudhury et al. 2005). This has been taken to suggest either redundancy within intracellular insulin signalling cascades, or alternatively that additional, distinct neuronal populations exist that are insulin-responsive and that contribute to the maintenance of energy homeostasis.

A caveat to studies involving germline deletion of insulin signalling molecules is suggested by the observation that male *Irs2*-deficient mice also exhibit a global reduction in brain size. This is attributed to defective neuronal proliferation during development, and is consistent with the well-recognised role of peripheral insulin/insulin-like growth factor-1 signalling in the regulation of somatic growth. It is plausible that some physiological differences in energy homeostasis in animals with lifelong genetic perturbations may reflect subtle developmental defects instead of, or in addition to, acute disturbance of function of anatomically normal neuronal networks.

More distal components of the cellular insulin signalling apparatus have also been examined in the brain. Phosphatidylinositol 3 kinase (PI3K) activity is co-located with *Irs2* expression within arcuate POMC neurons. It is activated by centrally administered insulin and insulin-induced anorexia is blocked by third ventricle delivery of PI3K inhibitors (Niswender et al. 2003). Many of the metabolically important transcriptional responses to insulin in peripheral tissues, such as the suppression of hepatic expression of gluconeogenic genes, are mediated by its ability to reduce activity of the transcription factor FoxO1. In the hypothalamus, insulin decreases FoxO1 activity to suppress feeding, whereas fasting activates FoxO1 to promote food intake, in part, through transcriptional activation of *NPY* and *AGRP* (Kim et al. 2006) (Fig 23.2).

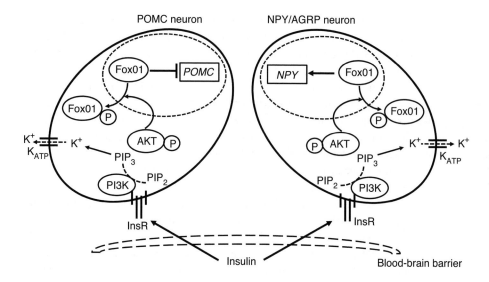

Figure 23.2. Schematic of reciprocal insulin action on key hypothalamic neurons controlling appetite. Insulin acts *via* its receptor (InsR) to stimulate phosphatidylinositol-3-kinase and generate PIP3. This may exert direct actions on ion channels to alter membrane potential, and also increases transcription of anorexigenic proopiomelanocortin, while repressing expression of orexigenic NPY.

PI3K activation may also alter neuronal behaviour through changes in the electrophysiological properties of neurons, mediated, for example, by modulation of function of adenosine triphosphate (ATP)-dependent potassium (K_{ATP}) channels. Akin to the channels in pancreatic β-cells, these hyperpolarising K_{ATP} channels are inactivated by increasing concentrations of intracellular ATP, leading to membrane depolarisation and neuronal firing. This effectively couples cellular energy change to neuronal activity. Conversely, insulin stimulates accumulation of phosphatidylinositol-3,4,5-trisphosphate (PIP3), the membrane phospholipid product of PI3K, to promote K_{ATP} channel opening, membrane hyperpolarisation and thereby neuronal silencing. Pre-treatment with PI3K inhibitors such as wortmannin or LY249002 blocks this effect (Spanswick et al. 2000) (Fig 23.2).

Although discussion of studies involving PI3K manipulation are often couched in terms of insulin signalling, it is important to remember that PI3K is a highly promiscuous signal transducer, co-opted to receptors for many hormones and neuropeptides including leptin. There is moreover considerable potential for crosstalk among the signalling pathways activated in response to such stimuli. Thus the extent to which targeted perturbation of PI3K and its downstream pathways can be said to indicate true physiological actions of insulin alone is doubtful.

Evidence for central insulin action in the regulation of glucose homeostasis

Insulin-mediated alterations in central mechanisms subserving energy homeostasis would be expected ultimately to alter adiposity, and thereby to exert indirect effects on glucose homeostasis through changes in insulin sensitivity. However studies performed over the past 10 years suggest that central insulin action may also have acute effects on peripheral glucose metabolism, in particular through effects on hepatic glucose production (HGP) that are distinct from the well-established direct action of insulin on hepatocytes.

The case for central insulin signalling in the regulation of HGP was first made by the demonstration that ICV delivery of insulin or a small molecule insulin mimetic diminished HGP in rats, and that the effect could be abolished through blockade of hypothalamic K_{ATP} channels (Obici et al. 2002b). In contrast to the rapid suppression of HGP by peripherally administered insulin, the effect of central insulin to suppress HGP required several hours of continuously administered ICV insulin, and was only discernible after use of somatostatin and insulin co-infusion to 'clamp' peripheral insulin production.

Genetically modified mouse models have also lent support to a role for central insulin signalling in glucose metabolism. For example, HGP is attenuated in mice lacking InsR expression in the brain (Koch et al. 2008) and hypothalamus (Obici et al. 2002a), while genetic or pharmacological disruption of insulin signalling in POMC and AGRP neurons induces insulin resistance. This suggests that, in addition to having key roles in energy balance, these neurons are required for normal insulin sensitivity. More recently, insulin-mediated activation of extracellular signal-regulated kinase 1/2 (Erk1/2) within the dorsal vagal complex has been shown to suppress peripheral glucose production in mice and rats, suggesting that extrahypothalamic sites may also be important in glucose metabolism (Filippi et al. 2012).

The best-characterised efferent mechanism coupling central insulin signalling in rodents to HGP involves autonomic neural input to the liver. Thus, the reduced hepatic expression of gluconeogenic enzymes including glucose-6-phosphatase and phosphoenolpyruvate kinase expression seen after central insulin exposure is abolished following vagal nerve transaction (Pocai et al. 2005). However, the tools available to dissect different components of autonomic nervous system function are at present relatively blunt, and so a refined understanding of exactly how insulin-induced modulation of autonomic function influences peripheral metabolism remains elusive. Interestingly, the relationship between insulin action and the autonomic nervous system is also two-way, with insulin having a well-established ability to stimulate sympathetic outflow from the brain (Scherrer and Sartori 1997).

For all the residual uncertainty about detailed mechanism, these rodent data collectively provide strong evidence that central insulin can, in some circumstances, alter peripheral glucose metabolism and energy homeostasis. However, it has recently been argued cogently that some aspects of these studies over-emphasise the physiological importance of this central effect of insulin (Ramnanan et al. 2012). While a detailed explanation of these is beyond the scope of this chapter, concerns may broadly be grouped into those that pertain to the normal metabolic homeostasis of rodents, and those that relate to the specific design of the key studies. Mice are known to have higher basal levels of glucose production and to deplete hepatic glycogen stores more rapidly than larger animals on fasting. Hence they are more reliant on gluconeogenic pathways, which are thus under tighter control by multiple regulatory mechanisms. It has also been argued that artefactual alteration of peripheral:portal insulin ratios and the suppression of glucagon with somatostatin infusion may create highly non-physiological artificial conditions which unduly overemphasise the importance of changes in HGP. Finally the intra-CSF route of insulin administration may not faithfully recapitulate the distribution of insulin to the CNS that is observed when it is delivered by the vascular system (Ramnanan et al. 2012).

The dog has been used as a larger animal model to address some of these concerns. Canine studies have demonstrated that modest hyperinsulinemia at non-hepatic tissues, including the brain, does suppress hepatic glucose output, but that the mechanism predominantly depends on acute inhibition of adipose tissue triglyceride lipolysis (Sindelar et al. 1997). Moreover acute CNS hyperinsulinemia, achieved by bilateral carotid and vertebral artery insulin infusion during a pancreatic clamp to maintain basal hepatic insulin and glucagon concentrations, fails to acutely influence HGP despite activating hypothalamic AKT and suppressing gluconeogenic gene expression in the liver (Ramnanan et al. 2011). Eventually, but only after several hours of insulin delivery, hepatic glucose flux is reduced, and this is associated with increased glycogen synthase activity. ICV treatment with a PI3K inhibitor completely blocks these effects (Ramnanan et al. 2011).

These studies have been interpreted as demonstrating on one hand that, as in the rodent, the CNS in the dog is capable of sensing acute changes in plasma insulin and conveying this signal to the liver to drive changes in transcription of gluconeogenic genes, but on the other that this makes a negligible contribution to acute physiological regulation of canine HGP.

Relevance of central insulin action to human physiology and disease

Thus, although the notion of a human brain–liver axis that can both sense energy availability and also initiate a rapid neural response to maintain blood glucose, the preferred fuel of the brain, has considerable appeal, the inconsistencies reported in model animal studies mean that its existence in humans remains, at best, unproven. Even if insulin action in the brain is not important as an acute modulator of HGP, it is possible that insulin serves a role in the brain as a higher order modulator of basal expression of gluconeogenic genes in the liver. However, the observation that in humans with type 2 diabetes hyperinsulinemia is not associated with changes in gluconeogenic gene expression challenges even this view (Samuel et al. 2009).

It is very difficult to conceive of ethical human studies to test the metabolic actions of central insulin directly. Although humans with genetic defects in insulin action are known, the signalling dysfunction affects all insulin-responsive tissues, confounding attempts to assess central defects. Some aspects of the prevailing model of central insulin's actions on liver metabolism via the autonomic nervous system can be tested, however, by comparison of glucose metabolism between patients after orthotopic liver transplantation, which involves stable denervation of the donor liver, and patients with other solid organ transplants and similar immunosuppressive regimens. Several studies have exploited this to demonstrate no major changes in fasting glucose and insulin, nor in HGP suppression during hyperinsulinaemic euglycaemic clamp (reviewed in [Ramnanan et al. 2012]). Nevertheless these studies neglect the possibility of a more nuanced or 'asymmetric' influence of central insulin on parasympathetic and sympathetic supply to the liver. Most studies to date, in mice and humans, have also failed to address the possibility that the central effect of insulin on glucagon secretion from the pancreas may play a role in central effects of insulin on metabolism.

Conclusion

Insulin has strong credentials *a priori* as a neuromodulatory peptide, sending continuous signals to the hypothalamus and other centres about acute and, to a lesser extent, chronic, nutritional state. However, although a large and fairly coherent body of evidence has accumulated in rodent studies over the past 20 years that insulin acting in the CNS can alter both energy homeostasis and acute hepatic glucose metabolism, studies in dogs have cast doubt on the physiological importance of insulin's central effects on glucose metabolism. Studies in humans are extremely challenging, but opportunistic observations have failed to provide strong supportive evidence to date for a major role of hepatic autonomic innervation in glucose control. Nevertheless the case for a key role of centrally acting insulin in the control of human energy and glucose homeostasis is best regarded as 'not proven' at present. Further studies are warranted.

REFERENCES

Benoit SC, Air EL, Coolen LM et al. (2002) The catabolic action of insulin in the brain is mediated by melanocortins *J Neurosci* 22: 9048–9052.

Bruning JC, Gautam D, Burks DJ et al. (2000) Role of brain insulin receptor in control of body weight and reproduction. *Science* 289: 2122–2125.

Choudhury AI, Heffron H, Smith MA et al. (2005) The role of insulin receptor substrate 2 in hypothalamic and beta cell function. *J Clin Invest* 115: 940–950.

Filippi BM, Yang CS, Tang C and Lam TK (2012) Insulin activates Erk1/2 signaling in the dorsal vagal complex to inhibit glucose production. *Cell Metab* 16: 500–510.

Kim MS, Pak YK, Jang PG et al. (2006) Role of hypothalamic Foxo1 in the regulation of food intake and energy homeostasis *Nat Neurosci* 9: 901–906.

Koch L, Wunderlich FT, Seibler J et al. (2008) Central insulin action regulates peripheral glucose and fat metabolism in mice. *J Clin Invest* 118: 2132–2147.

Margolis RU and Altszuler N (1967) Insulin in the cerebrospinal fluid *Nature* 215: 1375–1376.

Mehran AE, Templeman NM, Brigidi GS et al. (2012) Hyperinsulinemia drives diet-induced obesity independently of brain insulin production. *Cell Metab* 16: 723–737.

Niswender KD, Morrison CD, Clegg DJ et al. (2003) Insulin activation of phosphatidylinositol 3-kinase in the hypothalamic arcuate nucleus: A key mediator of insulin-induced anorexia *Diabetes* 52: 227–231.

Obici S, Feng Z, Karkanias G, Baskin DG and Rossetti L (2002a) Decreasing hypothalamic insulin receptors causes hyperphagia and insulin resistance in rats. *Nat Neurosci* 5: 566–572.

Obici S, Zhang BB, Karkanias G and Rossetti L (2002b) Hypothalamic insulin signaling is required for inhibition of glucose production. *Nat Med* 8: 1376–1382.

Pardini AW, Nguyen HT, Figlewicz DP et al. (2006) Distribution of insulin receptor substrate-2 in brain areas involved in energy homeostasis. *Brain Res* 1112: 169–178.

Plum L, Schubert M and Bruning JC (2005) The role of insulin receptor signaling in the brain. *Trends Endocrinol Metab* 16: 59–65.

Pocai A, Obici S, Schwartz GJ and Rossetti L (2005) A brain-liver circuit regulates glucose homeostasis. *Cell Metab* 1: 53–61.

Porte D Jr, Baskin DG and Schwartz MW (2005) Insulin signaling in the central nervous system: A critical role in metabolic homeostasis and disease from C. elegans to humans. *Diabetes* 54: 1264–1276.

Ramnanan CJ, Edgerton DS and Cherrington AD (2012) Evidence against a physiologic role for acute changes in CNS insulin action in the rapid regulation of hepatic glucose production. *Cell Metab* 15: 656–664.

Ramnanan CJ, Saraswathi V, Smith MS et al. (2011) Brain insulin action augments hepatic glycogen synthesis without suppressing glucose production or gluconeogenesis in dogs. *J Clin Invest* 121: 3713–3723.

Rother E, Belgardt BF, Tsaousidou E et al. (2012) Acute selective ablation of rat insulin promoter-expressing (RIPHER) neurons defines their orexigenic nature. *Proc Nat Acad Sci USA* 109: 18132–18137.

Samuel VT, Beddow SA, Iwasaki T et al. (2009) Fasting hyperglycemia is not associated with increased expression of PEPCK or G6Pc in patients with Type 2 Diabetes. *Proc Natl Acad Sci USA* 106: 12121–12126.

Scherrer U and Sartori C (1997) Insulin as a vascular and sympathoexcitatory hormone: Implications for blood pressure regulation, insulin sensitivity, and cardiovascular morbidity. *Circulation* 96: 4104–4113.

Schwartz MW, Sipols AJ, Marks JL et al. (1992) Inhibition of hypothalamic neuropeptide Y gene expression by insulin. *Endocrinology* 130: 3608–3616.

Sindelar DK, Chu CA, Rohlie M, Neal DW, Swift LL and Cherrington AD (1997) The role of fatty acids in mediating the effects of peripheral insulin on hepatic glucose production in the conscious dog. *Diabetes* 46: 187–196.

Spanswick D, Smith MA, Mirshamsi S, Routh VH and Ashford ML (2000) Insulin activates ATP-sensitive K+ channels in hypothalamic neurons of lean, but not obese rats. *Nat Neurosci* 3: 757–758.

Taguchi A, Wartschow LM and White MF (2007) Brain IRS2 signaling coordinates life span and nutrient homeostasis. *Science* 317: 369–372.

Woods SC and Porte D Jr (1977) Relationship between plasma and cerebrospinal fluid insulin levels of dogs. *Am J Physiol* 233: E331–E334.

INDEX

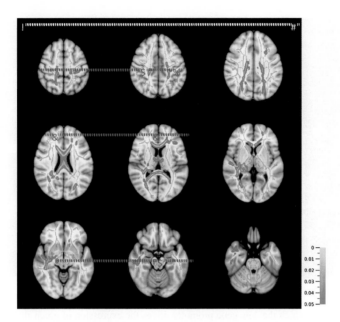

Figure 4.1. (p 49) Functional MRI and tract-based spatial statistics analysis comparing fractional anisotropy in children with isolated growth hormone deficiency (GHD) and children with short stature. Areas of the mean fractional anisotropy skeleton in green represent regions where there were no significant differences in fractional anisotropy values; areas in red/yellow are regions where the fractional anisotropy was significantly lower in the isolated GHD group, as observed in the corpus callosum (a), right and left corticospinal tract (b and c). Colour map indicates the degree of significance for red and yellow regions. Adapted from Webb et al., *Brain* 2012; 135:216–227, Oxford University Press, with permission.

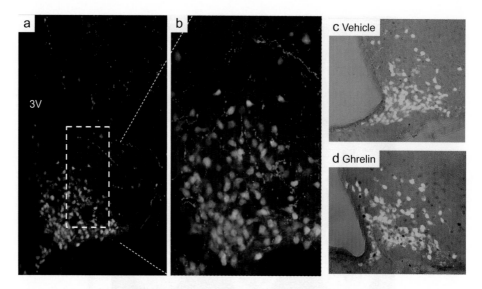

Figure 9.4. (p 124) (a) Fluorescently labelled NPY neurones in the arcuate nucleus of a transgenic *Npy*-GFP mouse in which the *Npy* gene promoter drives the expression of green fluorescent protein and (b) increased magnification of the same photomicrograph. The section has been dual labelled to demonstrate orexin-containing neuronal fibres intermingling with the NPY neurones and (c) section from a similar mouse given a systemic, control injection of isotonic saline. The section has been dual labelled for the cellular activity marker, c-Fos, and (d) a mouse given a systemic injection of the gut-derived hormone, ghrelin. NPY neurones have been activated, as demonstrated by the induction of c-Fos (black cell nuclei). 3V, third cerebral ventricle.

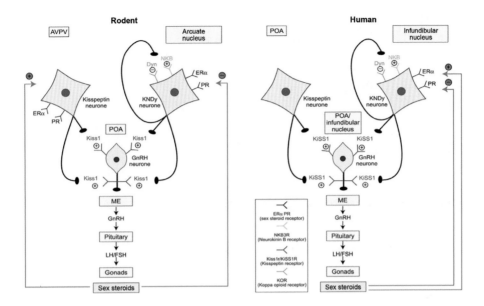

Figure 18.4. (p 273) Organization of the kisspeptin–GnRH pathway and KNDy/GnRH neurons in rodents and humans. Kisspeptin signals directly to kisspeptin receptor-expressing GnRH neurons. The location of kisspeptin neuron populations within the hypothalamus is species-specific, residing within the anteroventral periventricular nucleus (AVPV) and the arcuate nucleus in rodents, and within the preoptic area (POA) and the infundibular nucleus in humans. Kisspeptin neurons in the infundibular (humans)/arcuate (rodents) nucleus co-express neurokinin B and dynorphin (KNDy neurons), which via neurokinin B receptor and kappa opioid peptide receptor autosynaptically regulate pulsatile kisspeptin secretion, with neurokinin B being stimulatory and dynorphin inhibitory. Negative (red) and positive (green) sex steroid feedback is mediated via distinct kisspeptin populations in rodents, via the AVPV and the arcuate nucleus, respectively. In humans, KNDy neurons in the infundibular nucleus relay both negative (red) and positive (green) feedback. The role of the POA kisspeptin population in mediating sex steroid feedback in humans is incompletely explored. ME, median eminence; +, stimulatory; −, inhibitory; ERα, estrogen receptor alpha; PR, progesterone receptor; KISS1/KiSS1, kisspeptin; NKB, neurokinin B; Dyn, dynorphin.

(a)

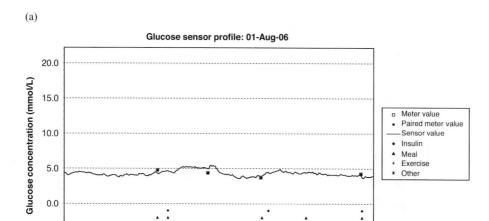

(b)

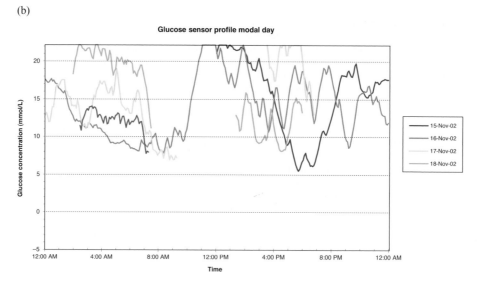

Figure 22.1. (p 359) Continuous glucose sensing traces from (a) a person without diabetes and (b) a child with type 1 diabetes.

Recent titles from Mac Keith Press www.mackeith.co.uk

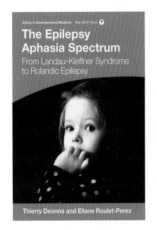

The Epilepsy Aphasia Spectrum: From Landau-Kleffner Syndrome to Rolandic Epilepsy
Thierry Deonna and Elaine Roulet-Perez

Clinics in Developmental Medicine
Winter 2016 ▪ 200pp ▪ hardback ▪ 978-1-909962-76-7
£50.00 / €62.94 / $75.00

Landau-Kleffner syndrome (LKS) is a rare childhood epilepsy, now considered to be at the severe end of the 'epilepsy-aphasia spectrum'. This book is aimed at the large range of professionals involved in the diagnosis, therapy and rehabilitation of children on the spectrum. The authors discuss work-up and management strategies and the reader will find chapters on topics such as the link between LKS and developmental language and communication disorders.

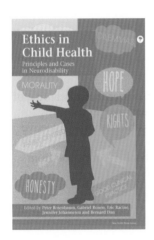

Ethics in Child Health: Principles and Cases in Neurodisability
Peter L. Rosenbaum, Gabriel M. Ronen, Eric Racine, Jennifer Johannesen and Bernard Dan (Editors)

2016 ▪ 396pp ▪ softback ▪ 978-1-909962-63-7
£39.95 / €50.00 / $60.00

This book explores the ethical dimensions of issues that have either been ignored or not recognised. Each chapter is built around an illustrative scenario and discusses how ethical principles can be utilised to inform decision-making. 'Themes for Discussion' at the end of each chapter will help professionals and policy makers put practical ethical thinking at the heart of care.

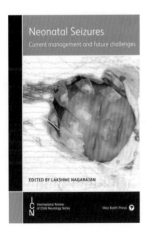

Neonatal Seizures: Current Management and Future Challenges
Lakshmi Nagarajan (Editor)

International Review of Child Neurology Series
2016 ▪ 214pp ▪ hardback ▪ 978-1-909962-67-5
£44.99 / €58.40 / $65.00

This book distils what is known about the many advances in the management of neonatal seizures into one scholarly yet practical text. Chapters cover the neonatal neuron, the use of video EEG in diagnosis, advances in neurophysiology, genetics and neuroprotective strategies, as well as outcomes. This volume will be of use to neonatologists, paediatricians, neurologists and all health professionals involved in the care of neonates experiencing seizures.

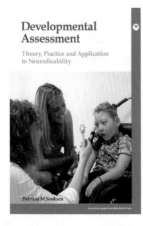

Developmental Assessment: Theory, Practice and Application to Neurodisability
Patricia M. Sonksen

A practical guide from Mac Keith Press
2016 ▪ 384pp ▪ softback ▪ 978-1-909962-56-9
£39.95 / €56.50 / $65.00

This handbook presents a new approach to assessing development in preschool children that can be applied across the developmental spectrum. The reader is taught how to confirm whether development is typical, and if it is not, is signposted to the likely nature and severity of the impairments with a plan of action. The author uses numerous case vignettes from her 40 years' experience to bring to life her approach with clear summary key points and helpful illustrations.

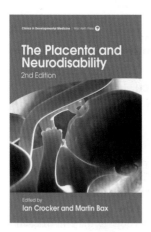

The Placenta and Neurodisability, 2nd Edition
Ian Crocker and Martin Bax (Editors)

Clinics in Developmental Medicine
2015 ▪ 176pp ▪ hardback ▪ 978-1-909962-53-8
£50.00 / €67.50 / $80.00

This comprehensive and authoritative book discusses the critical role of the utero-placenta in neurodisability, both at term and preterm. It examines aspects of fetal compromise and possible cerebro-protective interventions, recent evidence on fetal growth and mental illness, as well as cerebro-therapeutics. Throughout the book, information from the basic sciences is placed within the clinical context.

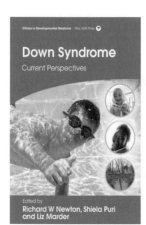

Down Syndrome: Current Perspectives
Richard W. Newton, Shiela Puri and Liz Marder (Editors)

Clinics in Developmental Medicine
2015 ▪ 320pp ▪ hardback ▪ 978-1-909962-47-7
£95.00 / €128.30 / $150.00

Down syndrome remains the most common recognisable form of intellectual disability. The challenge for doctors today is how to capture the rapidly expanding body of scientific knowledge and devise models of care to meet the needs of individuals and their families. *Down Syndrome: Current Perspectives* provides doctors and other health professionals with the information they need to address the challenges that can present in the management of this syndrome.